NUTRITION IN INFANCY AND CHILDHOOD

NUTRITION IN INFANCY AND CHILDHOOD

EDITED BY

CRISTINE M. TRAHMS, M.S., R.D., C.D., F.A.D.A.

Lecturer, Division of Pediatric Genetics,
Department of Pediatrics, School of Medicine; and Head, Nutrition,
Center on Human Development and Disabilities
University of Washington, Seattle

PEGGY L. PIPES, R.D., M.P.H.

Emeritus, Parent and Child Nursing, School of Nursing
University of Washington, Seattle

SIXTH EDITION
illustrated

WCB/McGraw-Hill

A Division of The McGraw-Hill Companies

WCB/McGraw-Hill

A Division of The **McGraw·Hill** *Companies*

TRAHMS, PIPES: NUTRITION IN INFANCY AND CHILDHOOD

3 4 5 6 7 8 9 10   FGRFGR   9 9

ISBN 0–8151–8455–7

Publisher: *Ed Bartell*
Executive editor: *Vicki Malinee*
Developmental editor: *Jean Babrick*
Senior marketing manager: *Pamela S. Cooper*
Project manager: *Donna Nemmers*
Design freelance coordinator: *Mary Christianson*
Cover designer: *Ben Neff*
Cover illustrator: *Jason Dowd*
Compositor: *Shepherd, Inc.*
Typeface: *10/11 Galliard*

Library of Congress Catalog Card Number 97–70088

http://www.mhcollege.com

Contributors

BETTY LUCAS, M.P.H.

Lecturer, Parent and Child Nursing, School of Nursing;
Nutritionist, Center on Human Development and Disabilities,
University of Washington, Seattle, Washington

MARY J. O'LEARY, PH.D., R.D.

Nutrition Consultant, Private Practice,
Albuquerque, New Mexico

SALLY M. O'NEIL, PH.D.

Behavioral Psychologist, Private Practice,
Seattle, Washington

ROBIN PRITKIN GLASS, M.S., O.T.R.

Occupational Therapist,
Children's Hospital and Medical Center, Seattle, Washington

JANE MITCHELL REES, M.S., R.D.

Lecturer, Division of Adolescent Medicine,
Department of Pediatrics, School of Medicine;
Director, Nutrition and Education Services, Adolescent Health Program,
University of Washington, Seattle, Washington

JOAN ZERZAN, M.S., R.D.

Neonatal Nutritionist,
University of Washington Medical Center, Seattle, Washington

In memory of
Miriam Lowenberg, Ph.D.
A friend and supportive colleague,
whose professional contributions
to the nourishment of children endure.

Preface

From its first edition the goal of *Nutrition in Infancy and Childhood* has been to offer nutrition information related to both growth and development and also normal and abnormal conditions in infancy and childhood. The primary intended audience consists of students and providers of clinical services in the nutrition-related medical environment. However, we recognize that the general public has an increased interest in nutrition. Accordingly, we have tried to develop materials in such a way that the book is not only geared to professionals but also to the interested general reader. In doing so, we have not compromised the scientific content of the material.

Most parents are aware that nutrition plays a major role not only in the growth and development of their child but also in the prevention of disease. However, despite, or perhaps because of, the many nutrition-related articles that can be found in the popular press, many parents have questions about how best to feed their children. Some parents have questions about which foods provide needed nutrients or appropriate diet modifications for their children. Others have questions about how to create an environment in which children will consume the needed foods. Answers to these questions are provided in these chapters. The sixth edition of *Nutrition in Infancy and Childhood* is updated and expanded to best meet the twin goals of providing useful information to both professionals and the general reader.

CONTENT FEATURES

The organization of this sixth edition strives to maintain a chronological approach and to combine a consistent progression from the general or usual to the specific or unusual circumstances of nourishment, growth and development. The first chapters of *Nutrition in Infancy and Childhood* present background materials and tools that will be used in later chapters: growth and development, nutrient needs of infants and children, and the clinical approach to assessing and collecting food intake information. The next chapters focus on nourishment of well infants and the special needs of preterm and low-birth-weight infants. The following chapters deal with behavior; how food patterns are developed, shaped, and changed. The chapter originally prepared by Miriam Lowenberg, Ph.D., one of the major pioneers in nutrition and feeding of children, remains in its original format. This chapter can now be considered a classic nutrition work. The next chapter focuses on more current issues related to the development of food patterns for young children. The discussion then moves to parent and child interactions as they influence food patterns and the use of behavior modification techniques to achieve the acceptance of foods and teach feeding skills to young children. Discussions of the application of nutrition in special circumstances follow. These include the child who is vegetarian and the prevention of chronic diseases by dietary intervention.

The chronological grouping of chapters continues with emphasis on children of various ages: preschool, school-age, and adolescent children. After a discussion of adolescent growth and nutritional needs, special circumstances in adolescence that require emphasis on nourishment are presented. These include discussions of pregnancy management for adolescent females, nutritional concerns in athletic competition, and situations of disordered eating: anorexia nervosa, bulimia nervosa, and obesity. The final chapter deals with children who have special health care and nutritional needs.

To aid the student in application, review questions are a part of every chapter. Developmental and behavioral parameters are integrated into the chapter discussions. Case studies are added to each chapter to enhance application of the principles presented. The suggested learning activities and case studies provide strategies for clinical approaches that utilize the information presented in the chapters.

The implementation of nutrition plans for children, especially those with special needs, and when medical or psychosocial factors play a role in the etiology of the nutrition concern, requires an interdisciplinary assessment and management model. Therefore the interdisciplinary approach has been emphasized. In fact, an interdisciplinary group of professionals including an occupational therapist and a nurse with expertise in behavioral management techniques, as well as nutritionists known for their skills in nutrition intervention for specific age groups and conditions, contributed to the book. A variety of general readers, students, and health care professionals—especially those interested in nutrition/dietetics, maternal and child nursing, occupational therapy, and physical therapy—will find the book useful.

ACKNOWLEDGMENTS

In the preparation of any manuscript, many individuals make significant contributions. Parents of clients and clients themselves at the Center on Human Development and Disabilities, University of Washington, willingly discussed their nutrition concerns. They provided detailed information on what their children ate and factors that influenced their acceptance of foods and food plans. Parents of clients, and clients themselves, asked many thoughtful questions and helped shape the approach to nutrition services we present in this book. The nutrition trainees and students asked many probing and important questions and shaped our viewpoint on nutrition assessment and services. The contributors developed their chapters to meet an additional deadline in their already busy schedules. The encouragement from our friends and supporters in the federal Maternal and Child Health Bureau is much appreciated.

We found Jean Babrick, our editor at McGraw-Hill, to be especially helpful in providing guidance and patience as the sixth edition became a reality.

We are also grateful to the reviewers who gave of their time and expertise to help us develop a useful text. We are especially grateful to Judy Powell, MS, RD, CDE, Pediatric Nutrition Specialist; Gail Kieckhefer, Ph.D., Parent and Child Nursing, University of Washington; and Mary Story, Ph.D., Division of Epidemiology, University of Minnesota.

We appreciate the technical skills of Greg Owen whose expertise in graphics is shown in the growth charts, and Ann LeVasseur and Dorothea Trahms-Allen, whose photographs enhance the text. Finally, we thank our family members and friends who supported us as we struggled to bring the sixth edition to fruition.

Cristine M. Trahms
Peggy L. Pipes

Contents

6   FOOD PATTERN DEVELOPMENT IN YOUNG CHILDREN

Miriam E. Lowenberg

13   NUTRITION FOR ADOLESCENTS

Jane Mitchell Rees
Peggy L. Pipes

14   ADOLESCENT NUTRITION IN SPECIAL SITUATIONS

Jane Mitchell Rees
Cristine M. Trahms

15 NUTRITION AND SPECIAL HEALTH CARE NEEDS

Peggy L. Pipes
Robin Pritkin Glass

1

Growth, Development, and Nutrition

Cristine M. Trahms
Peggy L. Pipes

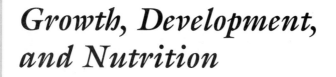

+++

Objectives

After studying this chapter, the student should:

✔ *Understand the effect of nutrition on physical growth and development.*

✔ *Understand characteristics of cell growth and the concept of critical stages of growth and development.*

✔ *Recognize appropriate equipment necessary to secure accurate measurements of height, weight, and skinfolds.*

✔ *Recognize if anthropometric parameters are secured in a manner that provides accurate data.*

✔ *Be able to interpret growth data on individual children in relation to guidelines.*

A healthy child grows at a genetically predetermined rate that can be compromised or accelerated by undernutrition, imbalanced nutrient intake, or overnutrition. Progress in physical growth is one criterion used to assess the nutritional status of populations and of individual children. It is therefore important that persons concerned with nutrition and feeding of infants and children be familiar with the process and parameters of growth, as well as the charts used to assess it.

Although every aspect and component of growth is thought to be influenced by nutrition, this discussion focuses on those parameters dealt with by persons concerned with children's food intake: increases in linear growth and weight, changes in body composition, how to secure accurate measurements of growth, and how to

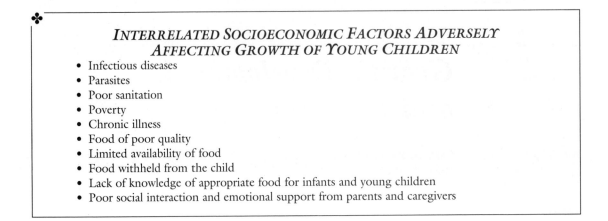

❖
INTERRELATED SOCIOECONOMIC FACTORS ADVERSELY AFFECTING GROWTH OF YOUNG CHILDREN

- Infectious diseases
- Parasites
- Poor sanitation
- Poverty
- Chronic illness
- Food of poor quality
- Limited availability of food
- Food withheld from the child
- Lack of knowledge of appropriate food for infants and young children
- Poor social interaction and emotional support from parents and caregivers

interpret physical growth patterns of normal children. Patterns of catch-up growth after an episode of wasting (when there is a greater deficit in weight than length) and stunting (when deficits of both height and weight are present) are discussed.

NUTRITION AND PHYSICAL GROWTH

The relationship between nutrition and physical growth of infants and young children is complex. There are many broad social, economic, biologic, and psychological factors that affect the growth of the infant and young child. Many efforts have been dedicated to understanding these relationships and mechanisms. As shown in the box above, the nutrition component of depressed physical growth may be related to limited availability of foods or the poor quality of food consumed. These factors may lead to an insufficiency of energy and/or protein or an insufficient intake of one or more other nutrients. Chronic illness, parasites, or poor sanitation are also significant factors. Nutrition to support typical growth requires a minimum intake of energy, protein, and nutrients appropriate for age and body size. For the rapidly growing infant, nutrient needs closely parallel growth.

Children who are undernourished are shorter and weigh less than their well-nourished peers.

The rate of gain in weight is affected more than is the rate of gain in height, but if the nutritional deficit is severe enough and continues long enough, linear growth will be deficient or may cease and pubertal maturation and **epiphyseal closure** may be delayed. Linear growth is delayed when energy intake is adequate but protein intake is deficient. Weight gain is depressed when energy intake is deficient, and linear growth will eventually be deficient (table 1-1).

Physical growth is a sign of positive interaction between nutrition, genetics, and time. Nutrition functions within the boundaries of an individual's genetic background and current environment to maximize growth potential. Growth is one measure of nutritional effectiveness in early life and is controlled by complex interrelated external and internal factors. General categories of factors affecting growth are (1) genes, (2) hormones, and (3) environmental influences that include (a) nutrition, (b) secular trends among groups of people, (c) immigration, (d) socioeconomic status, and (e) health and emotions.

SECULAR AND GENETIC INFLUENCES ON GROWTH

Growth patterns of children of racial groups whose members have been believed to be genetically small increase under conditions of improved

TABLE 1-1 *Guidelines for Assessment of Growth*

	Length/Height	Weight	Head Circumference
Typical growth	In channel*	In channel	In channel
Energy deprivation	In channel	Depressed	In channel
Protein-energy malnutrition	Depressed	Depressed	In channel
Severe malnutrition	Depressed	Depressed	Depressed
Various disease states	Depressed	Depressed	Often depressed
Recovery or catch-up growth	Accelerated	Accelerated	Accelerated

In channel is defined as the usual growth pattern of the child between the 10th and 90th percentiles.

nutrition. Especially striking was the change in the growth pattern of Japanese children born in the post–World War II period compared with those institutionalized during the prewar period. In 1962, boys at 14 years of age were found to be 7.6 cm taller and girls at 11 years of age 6.6 cm taller than prewar children of the same ages. The change in growth patterns was credited to an increase in the intake of animal protein.[1] A 1960 survey of children in Japanese orphanages whose food budgets were limited found heights to be significantly less than those of the national averages for children of the same age and sex. Adolescents, as a group, were shorter than their age-group average than were younger children.[2] During the subsequent 10 years the provision of 180 gm of milk and one egg per day, as well as increases in food budgets resulted in improvements in the quality and quantity of protein, as well as in the total amount of nutrients consumed. Increases in average stature were greater than expected.[2]

The long-term effects of malnutrition on physical growth during infancy and early childhood have been studied in children. Asian children tend to be smaller than black children or white children. However, growth status of refugee East Asian children increased between 1978 and 1989 and is now similar to or approaching that of other ethnic groups in the United States. The researchers at the Centers for Disease Control suggest that these studies may indicate that children of different ethnic origins have similar growth potentials.[3]

Differences have been noted in rates of growth of population groups in the United States. These differences are largely attributable to socioeconomic status. American black infants are smaller than American white infants at birth. American black infants grow more rapidly during the first 2 years, and from that age through adolescence are taller than American white boys and girls of the same age groups. The Hispanic Health and Nutrition Examination Survey, 1982 to 1984, found only minor differences in height of Mexican-American children before adolescence compared with white children in the second National Health and Nutrition Examination Survey. However, differences increased during adolescence. Mexican-American teenagers were shorter than white teenagers.[4] Mexican-American children over 6 years of age had a relatively high prevalence of overweight and relatively low prevalence of thinness compared with the U.S. population of children as a whole. The mean body mass index (BMI) of American Indian schoolchildren was higher than that of children in the overall U.S. population. This suggests the prevalence of overweight is likely to be higher for these children than for other children in the United States.[5]

CHARACTERISTICS OF GROWTH

Growth may be defined as an increase in the physical size of the body as a whole or as an increase in any of its parts associated with an increase in cell number or cell size. Development is defined as the acquisition of function associated with **cell differentiation** and maturation of individual organ systems or as a change from a lower to a more advanced stage of complexity for greater facility in functioning. Growth and development are affected by genetic, hormonal, environmental, and behavioral factors that interact to determine an individual's growth pattern.

Individual children have their own genetically predetermined growth patterns. Growth and development, however, proceed in an orderly and predictable sequence. Each organ and organ system has its own period of rapid growth marked by rapid cell differentiation, changes in form, and susceptibility to physical and environmental influences. Growth is the composite of many tissues that are growing at different rates. Skeletal muscle growth approximates whole body growth. The brain, lymphoid, adrenal, and reproductive tissue follow different patterns as shown in figure 1-1. The head reaches 90% of its adult size by 6 years of age, whereas growth of the reproductive system proceeds slowly until puberty when sexual maturation occurs. The lymph tissue grows rapidly until puberty and then reduces in size.

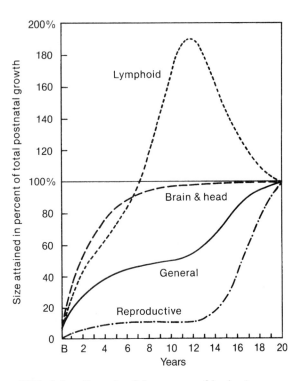

FIG. 1-1   Growth of four types of body tissue as percent of adult size.

(From Scammon RE: Measurement of the body in childhood. In *The measurement of man*, Minneapolis, 1930, University of Minnesota Press.)

PERIODS OF GROWTH

Increases in physical size are achieved by increases in both the number and the size of cells. Cell growth in any organ proceeds in three stages: **hyperplasia,** in which an increase occurs in cell number; **hypertrophy** and hyperplasia, in which increases occur in both the size and the number of cells; and hypertrophy, in which only the size of the cells increases. Growth in both the number and the size of cells can be assessed by calculation of the rates of weight to deoxyribonucleic acid (DNA) or the rates of protein to DNA.

There is a time when cell division stops before the organ attains its full size, and there is a phase when cell size, not cell number, increases. Some tissues, like the brain, reach a full adult complement of DNA sometime in the second year, whereas other tissues, such as muscle, continue to increase in DNA throughout adolescence.[6]

Rats malnourished by restriction of total food intake during the period of increase in cell number but given normal diets during later growth had a reduction in the number of brain cells. Those malnourished later in life and rehabilitated had normal numbers and sizes of cells.[7] Studies of muscle and liver cells of rats found that restriction of energy resulted in fewer cells, whereas restriction of protein and energy resulted in a decrease in both cell size and number.[8]

GROWTH IN HEIGHT AND WEIGHT

The birth weight is determined by the length of gestation, the mother's prepregnancy weight, and weight gain during pregnancy. The average weight of the typical full-term newborn is approximately 3500 gm. However, about 7% of infants born in the United States are of low birth weight (LBW), weighing less than 2500 gm, or are of very low birth weight (VLBW), weighing less than 1500 gm.[9] Infants may be of LBW because of a premature delivery or because of a deficient rate of growth in utero. An infant small for gestational age whose intrauterine weight gain was poor, but whose linear and head growth is appropriate for gestational age, has experienced **asymmetric** intrauterine growth retardation. A small for gestational age infant whose length and head circumference are also below the National Center for Health Statistics (NCHS) 10th percentile is said to be symmetrically growth deficient. The symmetrical type of growth deficiency reflecting early and prolonged intrauterine nutritional deficit is more detrimental to later growth and development.

After birth a genetic period of catch-up or lag-down growth may occur.[10] The majority of infants who are genetically determined to be longer shift channels (percentile ratings) of growth during the first 3 to 6 months. However, many infants born at or below the 10th NCHS percentile who are determined to be of average length may not achieve a new channel until 1 year of age. Larger infants whose genotypes are for smaller sizes grow at their fetal rates for several months before the lag-down in growth becomes evident. Figure 1-2 illustrates this natural phenomenon. Appropriate lag-down and catch-up growth are shown for two typical breast-fed infants the same age. Often a new channel of physical growth is not apparent until the child is 13 months of age.[10]

Immediately after birth there is a weight loss resulting from a loss of fluid and some catabolism of tissue. The loss averages 6% of body weight but occasionally exceeds 10%. Thereafter, weight gain in infancy proceeds at a rapid but decelerating rate. Table 1-2 shows expected weight gain for a healthy full-term infant.

Males double their birth weight earlier than do females, and smaller newborns double their birth weights sooner than do heavier infants. The weight increment during the second year is slightly less than the birth weight. Table 1-3 shows the expected weights of a typical infant.

TABLE 1-2 *Average Expected Weight Gains for Infants*

Age (mo.)	Average Weight Gain (gm/day)	Expectation
0–4	20–25 gm/day	Double birth weight by 4–5 months
5–12	15 gm/day	Triple birth weight by 12 months

TABLE 1-3 *Expected Weights of a Typical Infant*

Age	Weight (kg)
Birth	3.5
4–6 months	7
12 months	10.5
2 years	13

Thereafter, the yearly increments in weight proceed at a slower but constant rate averaging 2.3 kg/year until the ninth or tenth year, when the rate of gain shows a steady increase. This rate continues until adolescence, when a rapid increase in rate of gain occurs.

Height, like weight, increases at a rapid but decelerating rate until adolescence when the adolescent growth spurt occurs (fig. 1-3). Infants usually increase their lengths by 50% by 1 year of age, double them by 4 years of age, and triple them by 13 years of age. The average increase in length from infancy to preadolescence is shown in table 1-4. Between 6 years of age and puberty sex differences can be noted. At age 6 years boys are taller and heavier than girls. By 9 years of age the height of the average girl is the same as the 9-year-old boy but her weight is greater.

The range of chronological ages at which children of either sex enter adolescence and at

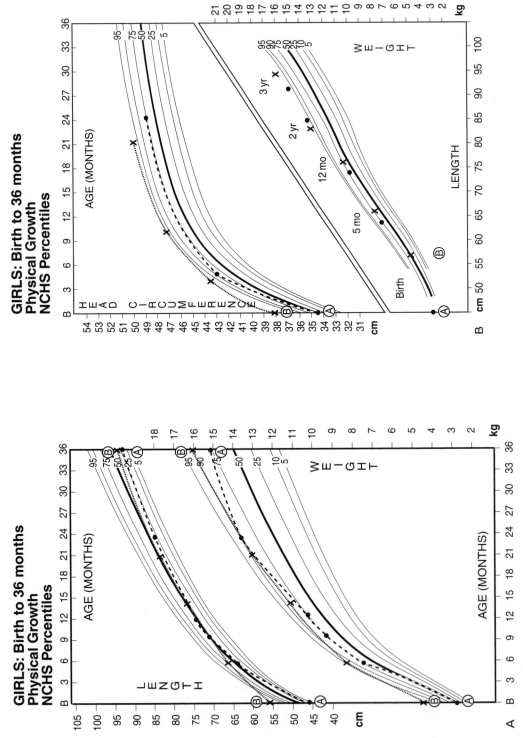

FIG. 1-2 Example of appropriate changing of growth channels by breast-fed infants. **A.** Infant A weighed 3120 gm (50th percentile) at birth; birth length was at the 5th percentile. Infant B weighed 4770 gm (>95th percentile) at birth; birth length was >95th percentile. By 4 to 6 months of age Infant A had changed channels in weight upward and Infant B had changed channels downward. **B.** Despite the difference in body size and growth velocity, the weight for length for both infants was nearly the same proportion for the first three years.

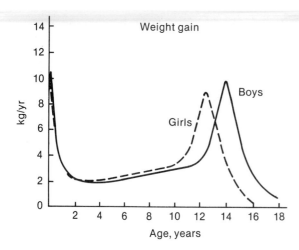

FIG. 1-3 Mean weight gain for age of males and females between infancy and 18 years of age.

(From Hamill PVV, Johnston FE, Lemeshow S: *Heights and weights of youths 12-17 years,* United States, 1966-1970. Vital and Health Statistics, Series II, No 124. DHEW Pub No [HSM] 73-1606, Washington, DC, 1973, Government Printing Office.)

TABLE 1-4 *Expected Increase in Length/ Stature from Infancy to Preadolescence*

Age	Length/Stature (cm)
Birth	50
1 year	74–76
4 years	100–105
Preadolescent	150–155

which specific events occur is wide. Females enter prepubescence at a younger age than do males. Males have a more intense growth spurt that lasts longer. Typically girls become taller than boys shortly after the age of 11 years because of their growth spurt. However, by 14.5 years of age boys experience their growth spurt and are taller than the average girl. At approximately 9 years of age, girls become heavier than boys and remain so until approximately 14.5 years of age when boys surpass them in weight (fig. 1-3).

Growth during adolescence is under the control of androgens and growth hormones. Testosterone, other androgens, and estrogen exert an effect on linear growth and accelerate skeletal maturation. Growth hormone, thyroid hormone, and sex hormones are all necessary for growth.

CHANGES IN BODY PROPORTIONS

Increases in height and weight are accompanied by changes in body proportions. The head at birth accounts for approximately one-fourth of the total body length; however, the head is one-eighth of the body length by the time growth has ceased. Brain growth is 75% complete by the end of the second year, and the brain is 100% of adult size by age 6 to 10 years. Leg length increases from approximately three-eighths to one-half of total body length between birth and adulthood (fig. 1-4).

BODY COMPOSITION

Changes occur not only in height and weight during growth but also in the components of the tissues. Increases in height and weight and skeletal maturation are accompanied by changes in body composition—in adiposity, lean body mass, and hydration. Estimates of the changes in body composition have been made from chemical analysis of human bodies and of individual tissues, from indirect measurements of water and electrolyte levels, from excretions of **creatinine** and **hydroxyproline,** and from estimates of fatness. Indirect measurements of body fat have been attempted by several methods, including measurement of the density of the whole body, measurements of total body weight minus lean body mass, use of fat-soluble gases, measurement of the thickness of fat by **roentgenographic studies,** and measurements of subcutaneous fat layers. Although there is more to be learned about body composition, there is data that can be related to physical growth and nutrient needs.

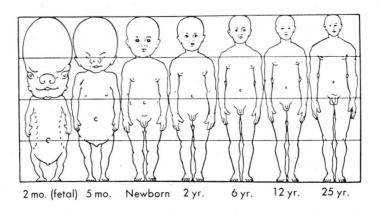

2 mo. (fetal)   5 mo.   Newborn   2 yr.   6 yr.   12 yr.   25 yr.

FIG. 1-4   Changes in body proportions from second fetal month to adulthood.
(From Robbins WJ and others: *Growth*, New Haven, Conn, 1928, Yale University Press.)

TABLE 1-5   *Percentage of Water in Fat-Free Mass of Reference Infants*

Age	Male Reference Infant Percentage of Water in Fat-Free Mass	Female Reference Infant Percentage of Water in Fat-Free Mass
4 months	78	80
12 months	79	79
3 years	78	78
10 years	75	77

Adapted from Fomon, *Nutrition in Infancy,* Mosby–Year Book, 1993.

Determinations of total body water alone or in combination with other measurements such as density or potassium have been used as a basis for estimations of lean body mass. Total body water as a percentage of body weight decreases throughout infancy from approximately 70% at birth to 60% at 1 year of age. Reduction of body water is almost entirely extracellular. Extracellular water decreases from 42% of body weight at birth to 32% of body weight at 1 year of age. This change results from decreases in the water content of adipose tissue, increases in adipose tissue, and relative increases in lean body mass.[11] The percentage of weight of water in lean body mass at any age is relatively stable. In other words, there is a direct relationship between total body water and lean body mass. Water is estimated to be responsible for 80% of the weight of fat-free mass at birth and 72% to 73% of the weight of fat-free mass of an adult. Reference infants were used to estimate the percentage of water in fat-free mass of the body (table 1-5). Adipose tissue contains about 15% water.

The potassium concentration (grams per kilogram of body weight) increases from the first year of life, reaches a maximum at 8 or 9 years of age, and then declines sharply. After this, sex differences become apparent. The decline continues in females, but an increase is noted in males between 14 and 16 years of age, followed by another decline.[12]

Using data on total body water and total body potassium, knowledge of the concentration of potassium in extracellular and cellular water, and

TABLE 1-6 *Estimates of Body Composition of Children*

Age (mo.)	Weight (kg)	Fat (gm)	Body Weight as Protein (%)	Body Weight as Osseous Minerals (%)	Body Weight as Carbohydrate (%)
Males					
Birth	3.6	485	12.9	2.6	0.5
6	8.0	2035	12.0	2.3	0.4
12	10.2	2290	12.9	2.3	0.5
18	11.5	2380	13.5	2.5	0.5
Females					
Birth	3.3	495	12.8	2.6	0.5
6	7.3	1915	12.0	2.2	0.4
12	9.2	2175	12.9	2.3	0.5
18	10.8	2345	13.5	2.4	0.5

Adapted from Fomon, *Nutrition in Infancy,* Mosby–Year Book, 1993.

the mineral content of the body, Fomon and others[11] have estimated the body composition of children between birth and 10 years of age. Male and female infants grow at slightly different rates from early infancy. Although female infants weigh less than males, the absolute amount of body fat and percentage of body fat is slightly higher at all ages. The proportion of the body that is protein, osseous mineral, and carbohydrate is similar for males and females during infancy (table 1-6).

Forbes,[13] in studies of persons 7.5 to 10.5 years of age, with a K^{40} counter (a chamber used to measure body composition), found a linear relationship between height and lean body mass at any age and an exponential relationship between lean body mass, height, and age groups. Sex differences in lean body mass and height ratios were noted in the earlier years, although they were not great enough to be significant. Males had greater amounts of lean body mass per centimeter of height than did females. After 12.5 years of age the lean body mass/height ratio increased rapidly in the male, whereas the increase was more gradual in the female. The female's lean body mass/height ratio maximum, which was about two-thirds

that of the male maximum value, appeared to be attained at 16 years of age, 3 years earlier than in the male. At 20 years of age males had one and a half times more lean body mass per centimeter of height than did females.

Fat is found in adipose tissue, in sites in the bone marrow, in phospholipids in the brain and the nervous system, and as a part of cells. It is the component of the body in which the greatest differences between children, age groups, and sexes are seen. The fat content of the body increases slowly during early fetal development, then increases rapidly in the last trimester. Total body fat of the newborn infant has a mean value of 16%.[14] Fat accumulates rapidly during infancy until approximately 9 months of age.

Between 2 and 6 months of age the increase in adipose tissue is more than twice as great as the increase in the volume of muscle. Sex-related differences appear in infancy, with the female depositing a greater percentage of weight as fat than the male.

During childhood the yearly increments for fat show a steady decrease. In many children a prepubertal fat spurt occurs before the true growth spurt. When growth proceeds most rapidly in height, adipose tissue increases least rapidly in the female. In the male there is an actual decrease and loss of fat during high velocity periods of growth.

EXAMPLES OF GROWTH IN SPECIAL SYSTEMS

Brain and adipose cellular development have been intensively studied in relation to nutritional status and nutrient intake. Although the long-term physiological and behavioral effects have yet to be clarified, many investigators think that events during early growth of these two systems are important to an individual's growth and development.

Brain Growth

The most rapid and critical period of brain growth in humans begins 9 months before birth and during the first months of postnatal life. During this time there is rapid cell multiplication and increasing differentiation. Thereafter, there is an increase only in cell size with a resulting increase in mass.

Severe malnutrition early in development typically results in spontaneous abortion. Moderate malnutrition throughout pregnancy or severe malnutrition in later pregnancy generally allows continuous fetal development but results in changes in the growth of the placenta and fetus. Animal studies indicate that inadequate maternal energy and protein intakes are associated with LBW infants who have decreased brain weight and decreased numbers of neurons and glial cells. There is also insufficient myelination and impairment of the dendritic development. These changes cannot be reversed by later nutritional rehabilitation.

Postnatal malnutrition is associated with a permanent reduction in the number of glial cells but not with a reduction in the number of neurons. Synaptogenesis and myelination of axons may be inhibited. Some degree of recovery will occur if adequate nutrition is provided.[15]

There have been few studies of cellular growth of the brain in humans. A study comparing brain growth of marasmic (severely malnourished) and typical infants who died in the first year of life demonstrated significant reductions in wet weight, dry weight, total protein content, and total DNA in the cerebrum, cerebellum, and brain stems of marasmic infants compared with typical infants. The brain stem was less affected.[16] Brains of children thought to be adequately fed in the first year of life but malnourished at an older age have been found to have a normal complement of DNA but reduced brain weight. This indicates a normal cell number but reduced cell size, further defining the critical period of increase in cell number of the brain.[17]

Most neuronal cell division, at least in the cerebrum, occurs prenatally during the second trimester. Glial cell division is a postnatal event that peaks at 3 months of age. Growth in DNA in the total brain and its two major regions continues into the second year of postnatal life, probably reaching a plateau at approximately 18 months of age.[18]

The rapid increase in brain mass is accompanied by rapid increases in head circumference. Head circumference achieves two-thirds of its postnatal growth by 24 months of age. Head circumferences of malnourished children have been found to be smaller than those of their well-nourished peers.

Studies of the long-term effects of malnutrition on behavior in humans are difficult to interpret because malnutrition rarely can be isolated as the sole cause of functional deficits. Malnourished children usually live in deprived environments and poverty. Often these families are unable to provide adequate housing, nurturing, or medical care. Also, malnutrition is associated with symptoms of behavior that may functionally isolate children from their environment and delay behavioral development. Children with protein energy malnutrition are typically irritable, apathetic, and withdrawn.

Early studies found that children malnourished in early infancy, even when they had been nutritionally rehabilitated, performed less well on a variety of tests of cognitive development than did control subjects. However, subsequent studies recognizing that environments that produce malnourished infants and children are depressed and nonnurturing have suggested social and environmental factors as more important variables. Children subjected to malnutrition prenatally because of war-induced famine or during infancy because of disease or anomalies, and who have been discharged to families that provided sufficient food and nurturing, have been able to make up any nutritionally induced deficit.[19] Malnourished children adopted by nurturing families have been able to catch up in mental development.[20]

Postnatal growth and cognition. Data from populations in which malnutrition is endemic indicate a relationship between growth deficiency of infants and young children and low performance on tests of mental development. Of special interest is the follow-up study of all children in Barbados who were given a diagnosis of marasmus or kwashiorkor in early life as compared to a matched group of adequately nourished children. Those children who were malnourished in infancy and tested at 5 to 11 years of age performed less well academically than did well-nourished control subjects, an effect mediated by deficits in classroom behavior (e.g., lack of attention, poor memory, poor motivation, and easy distractibility).[21] Testing of the same children at 11 to 18 years of age found that the generalized deficits in cognitive functioning persisted into adolescence. The IQ scores of children malnourished in early childhood remained lower than those of children who had not suffered a nutritional insult.[22,23]

Marginal malnutrition is more common in all parts of the world than severe states of malnutrition. Severe malnutrition such as starvation and protein energy malnutrition frequently occur in conditions of famine and other disasters. Mild malnutrition of young children occurs in poor countries of the world. After years of research the question still remaining is: Does mild malnutrition affect the functional and intellectual capacity of individuals? A large-scale study, the Nutrition Collaborative Research Support Program (Nutrition CRSP)[24] observed groups of children in Kalama, Egypt, Embu, Kenya, and the Solis Valley of Mexico. Growth faltering or slowing for these children started at about 3 months of age. Most growth faltering had occurred by 22 months of age. Both length and weight were affected. Children with diarrhea between 3 and 6 months of age were most affected. Growth was relatively normal after this

age.[24] The findings support the results of previous studies on the relationship of poor nutrition and its impact on growth and cognition. Growth-stunted children of all ages tended to perform less well on cognitive tests than their better grown peers.

Adipose Cell Size and Number

Adipose tissue is distributed throughout the body. However, cell size varies within a site and the range of cell size varies from one site to another. Estimates of fat, number, or size of cells based on a single biopsy may not be representative of body fat.

The number of adipose cells in children who became obese in the first year of life was higher than the number of adipose cells in children who became obese in later childhood.[25,26] Children who were low weight for their age and who suffered an insult to growth in infancy had a profound deficit in adipose cell number. In older nonobese children, little change in cell size was found during childhood and it was hypothesized that the increase in body fat during childhood must be a result of a gradual increase in number of adipose cells and that variations in body fatness must be caused by differences in cell size.[25] The adipose organ grows by increases in both cell size and number during childhood and increases in cell number do not occur after puberty.

Whether an increased adipose cell number at any age predisposes a child to later obesity or has an influence on the prognosis for weight reduction and maintenance of normal weight remains unknown. There is, however, evidence that obesity in school-age years is likely to continue into adolescence and adulthood and that early-onset obesity is much more resistant to therapy than onset of obesity in later life.[27] The accumulation of excessive numbers of adipose cells or larger cells is to be discouraged at any age.

METHODS OF ASSESSMENT

It is important that persons concerned with a child's nutrient intake be aware of how growth progresses. Assessments are made by periodic

---

❖

ASSESSMENT OF TYPICAL GROWTH OF YOUNG CHILDREN

- Weight and length or stature measurements between the 25th and 75th percentiles
- Measurements between the 10th to 25th and 75th to 90th percentiles may or may not be appropriate
  - Should assess:
    - pattern of previous measures
    - genetic factors
    - environmental factors
- Measurements <10th or >90th percentile should be rechecked and carefully evaluated
- Crossing channels is not unusual depending on age and health status

---

determinations of height, weight, and head circumference. The measurements must be determined accurately, and they must be interpreted in relation to the child's current stage of growth. Individual children whose growth does not appear to be proceeding typically may require additional methods of assessment, such as bone-age and skinfold measurements.

Growth Charts

Growth charts for height, weight, and head circumference make it possible to visualize how a child's growth is proceeding. Comparative data for bone age permit an estimate of physiological maturity. Skinfold and arm circumference charts provide a basis for determining whether a child is lean, typical, overweight with greater than average muscle and average fat, or obese.

Height, weight, and head circumference. Charts for expected growth have been devised from studies in which large numbers of healthy children of the same race and socioeconomic group were carefully measured at various ages and the data ranked in percentiles. The number in the percentile indicates the position that a measurement would hold in a series of 100.[28] Data from these studies are in tables, charts, and graphs. Growth curves and charts have been designed to measure how far the child has grown (distance curves) or how fast the child has grown (velocity curves). These growth charts are used in health evaluation to give some indication of how a child is growing and are often used in the assessment of nutritional status. Guidelines for evaluation of typical growth are

shown in the box titled Assessment of Typical Growth of Young Children.

The charts are prepared so that age values lie along the axis and height or weight values or changes in height or weight values are plotted along the abscissa. Height and weight values plotted for one age give information as to how a child ranks in size in relation to other children of the same sex and age, and information pertaining to the relationship of weight and height as compared with other children. Several measurements of height and weight at different ages plotted on the charts enable the practitioner to visualize if the child's growth is progressing as might be expected. Most children stay in approximately the same percentile during infancy and childhood. Growth, however, does not proceed in a smooth curve as the charts might indicate. Children grow in spurts, and changes may not adhere to the typical curve. A child may have no gain in weight or stature one month but considerable gain the next. During adolescence the growth patterns of many individuals change in percentile, with the early maturer moving to a higher percentile and the later maturer moving to a lower percentile. Both patterns usually return to the original percentiles by the time growth is complete. It is for this reason that the maturational stages become important in adolescence.

The most commonly used growth charts in the United States are those prepared by an expert committee for the National Center for Health Statistics (NCHS).[28] Data from the Fels Research Institute were used to determine the

TABLE 1-7 *Comparison of Populations Used for Reference Growth Curves*

Age	Fels 0–3 Years	NCHS 2–18 Years
Study design	Longitudinal	Cross-sectional
Population	White, middle class	Representative of U.S. children
Stature measure	Recumbent (length)	Standing (stature)

Fels: Fels Research Institute
NCHS: National Center for Health Statistics

percentiles for children from birth to 36 months of age. These data included only bottle-fed infants. The committee used data from the Health Examination Surveys and the Health Nutrition Examination Survey to prepare charts for children from 2 to 18 years of age.

See the appendix for NCHS curves for male and female infants birth to 3 years of age for length, weight, head circumference, and weight for length, and curves for males and females aged 3 to 18 years for weight, stature, and weight for stature. The NCHS charts are derived from two populations of children as shown in table 1-7. It is important for the clinician to know the basis of the reference data used to assess the growth of children.

Velocity charts provide an indication of how fast a child is growing.[29] Children tend not to stay nearly as close to a given velocity percentile as they do to a distance percentile. However, change in percentile rating does signal an important acceleration or deceleration. These charts are particularly useful in adolescence when children and parents often become concerned about height and weight in relation to peers and about final stature.

Tanner prepared both distance and velocity growth charts from the same data for children from 2 to 19 years of age.[29] The distance velocity growth charts for males and females are shown in the appendix. The changing velocity of normal growth for a male is shown in figure 1-5.

If the clinician is concerned about the physical growth of a child whose parents are very short or very tall, a correction using midparent

height can be made using data collected at the Fels Institute.[30] These tables are shown in the appendix.

In addition to graphs that reflect gains in weight and height, the committee constructed body weight for length or stature graphs that are appropriate for plotting values for infants, young children, and prepubescent boys and girls.

Appropriate use of growth charts requires that measurements be made in the same manner in which the reference data were secured. Weight values for the child less than 36 months of age should be obtained while the child is unclothed, using calibrated beam balance scales (fig. 1-6). Length values should be of recumbent length (fig. 1-7) and stature values should be of upright height (fig. 1-8). Children older than 36 months of age are weighed standing on a beam balance scale as shown in figure 1-9. The charts for children 2 to 18 years of age use measurements of children in stocking feet and light indoor clothing.

If infants and children are weighed and measured accurately and plotted carefully, longitudinal growth charts can be used to assess inadequate intake of energy and consequent faltering growth. The effect of adequate nourishment on improved growth can also be documented. The effect of undernutrition on a female infant subjected to inadequate energy intake because of a dilute formula is shown in figure 1-10. Figure 1-11 shows the effect of a restriction in food intake on the growth of a preschool boy.

Measurements of head circumference are made in health examinations by passing a cloth

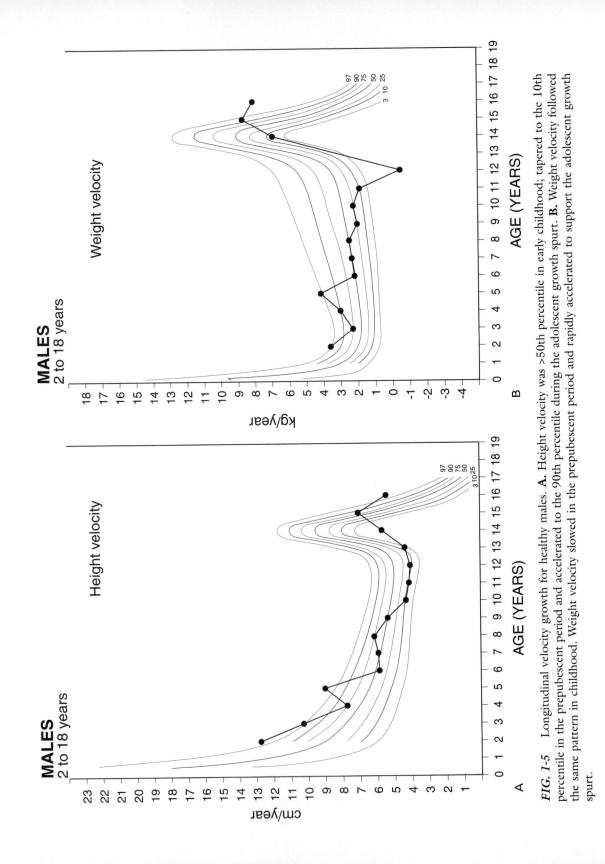

FIG. 1-5 Longitudinal velocity growth for healthy males. **A.** Height velocity was >50th percentile in early childhood; tapered to the 10th percentile in the prepubescent period and accelerated to the 90th percentile during the adolescent growth spurt. **B.** Weight velocity followed the same pattern in childhood. Weight velocity slowed in the prepubescent period and rapidly accelerated to support the adolescent growth spurt.

FIG. 1-6   Infant is weighed unclothed on calibrated beam balance scale. Procedure: • Use calibrated beam scale or electronic scale • Remove infant's clothing and diapers • Center the infant in the scale tray • Weigh infant to the nearest 0.01 kg • Write the weight on the infant's growth chart • Repeat the process and compare weights • Weight should agree within 0.02 kg • If infant is too active, postpone the measure until later • If a weight is required, and the infant is not cooperative, note this on the chart, e.g., "infant moving, about 5.0 kg" • Plot weight measurement on growth chart appropriate for age and gender • Report weight to parents; convert weight from kg to lb. at parents' request.

FIG. 1-7   Recumbent length is measured with suitable measuring board. Procedure: • Use a calibrated length board with a fixed headboard and movable footboard perpendicular to the surface of the table • Measure recumbent length for children less than 24 months of age or children 24–36 months who cannot stand unassisted • Measure infant without his/her shoes and wearing light underclothing or diaper • One person holds the infant's head so the infant is looking vertically upward and the crown of the head is against the headboard • A second person aligns the infant's trunk and legs, extends both legs, and brings the footboard firmly against the feet • Measure infant to the nearest 0.1 cm • Record measure to the nearest 0.1 cm • Write length measurement on chart • Reposition and remeasure infant • Measurements should agree to the nearest 0.2 cm • Plot length measurement on the birth to 36-month growth chart appropriate for age and gender • Report length to parents; convert cm to in. at parents' request.

FIG. 1-8 The child is measured with heels, buttocks, shoulders, and head touching wall. Procedure: • Measure stature for children over age 3 • Use a calibrated vertical stadiometer with a right-angle headboard • Child should stand against the stadiometer without shoes, with heels together, legs straight, arms at sides, shoulders relaxed. Heels, buttocks, shoulders, and head should touch the stadiometer • Child looks straight ahead • Bring the perpendicular headboard to touch the crown of the head • Measurer's eyes should be parallel with the headboard • Read the measurement to the nearest 0.1 cm and record it on the chart • Reposition and remeasure the child • Measures should agree within 0.2 cm • Plot the measurement on a growth chart appropriate for age and gender • Report measure to parents; convert from cm to ft. and in. at parents' request.

FIG. 1-9 A child older than 36 months is weighed standing on a beam balance scale. Procedure: • Use calibrated beam balance or electronic scale • Child can stand without assistance • Child is wearing lightweight undergarments, gown, or lightweight outer clothing • Child stands on center of platform • Record weight to the nearest 0.1 kg • Reposition and repeat weight measurement • Write weight on child's growth chart • Compare measures; they should agree within 0.2 kg • Plot weight measurement on growth chart appropriate for age and gender • Report measure to parents; convert from kg to lb. at parents' request.

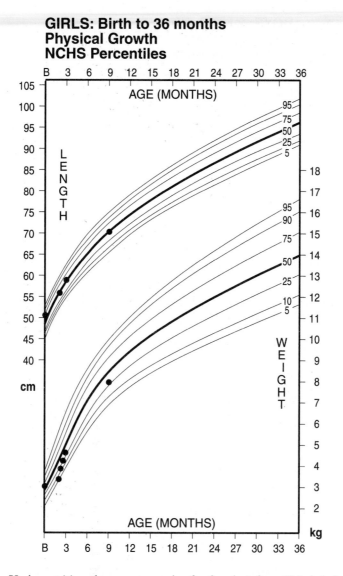

GIRLS: Birth to 36 months
Physical Growth
NCHS Percentiles

FIG. 1-10 Undernutrition depresses growth of a female infant. This baby's mother was worried because the baby was spitting up. A neighbor suggested adding more water to the formula. When the baby continued to spit up, the mother diluted the formula even more. At 10 weeks of age, a nutritional evaluation showed that the baby had gained only 460 gm since birth. Her rate of weight increase had dropped from the 50th to the 5th percentile on the NCHS chart. She was consuming a large volume of formula but only 190 to 225 kcal/day, approximately 50 kcal/kg. Changing to a concentrated formula (24 kcal/oz) resulted in a gain of 500 gm the first week and 240 gm the second week. The rapid rate of gain continued until she reached and remained at the 25th percentile.

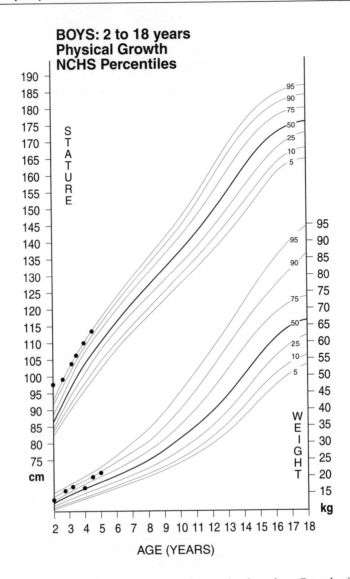

BOYS: 2 to 18 years
Physical Growth
NCHS Percentiles

FIG. 1-11 Undernutrition depresses growth of a preschool-age boy. Growth of a preschool-age boy was depressed because a sudden change in family income meant that the parents were unable to buy as much food as they had previously. Catch-up growth occurred when the family applied for and received food stamps, and the child was given his normal ration of food.

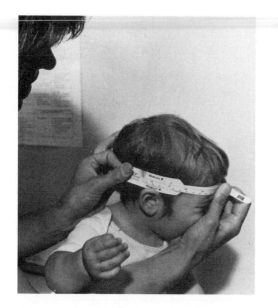

FIG. 1-12 Head circumference is measured over most prominent part of occiput and just above supra-orbital ridges. Procedure: • Use a flexible nonstretchable measuring tape • Position tape just above the eyebrows, above the ears, and around the biggest part of the head • Pull tape snugly to compress the hair • Read the measurement to the nearest 0.1 cm • Write the measurement on the chart • Reposition the tape and remeasure the head circumference • Measures should agree within 0.2 cm • Plot the measurement on a chart appropriate for age and gender • Report measure to parents; convert from cm to in. at parents' request.

or paper tape measure over the most prominent part of the occiput and just above the supraorbital ridges (fig. 1-12).

The NCHS growth charts include data on changes in head circumference from birth to 36 months of age in percentiles. Nellhaus prepared a graph of head circumference measurements from birth to 18 years of age.[31] This graph reflects weighted averages of variance and standard deviations from published reports.

The NCHS head circumference chart is used for children less than 36 months of age and the Nellhaus chart for children over 3 years of age. Sequential measurements plotted on these charts can be used to identify children whose cranial growth is deviating from typical. A rapid increase in the rate of growth may indicate hydrocephalus. A slowdown in the rate of growth may indicate a condition that can cause developmental delays. Such slowdowns have been noted in children who were subjected to severe undernutrition.

INCREMENTAL GROWTH

Assessment of growth increments is a valuable adjunct to evaluation of growth, especially for children in whom adequate growth attainment has been a problem and intervention strategies have been implemented. The change in growth velocity is more evident when increments of growth are plotted. The growth increments reflect the impact of malnutrition and rehabilitation more readily than the longitudinal charts, which reflect linear growth.

Incremental changes in length or height and weight are ideally plotted at 6-month intervals on the age- and gender-specific charts[32,33] (see appendix) and should be used in conjunction with the NCHS longitudinal charts. For infants the interval is 1 month.[34] Children who remain at the upper or lower percentiles for incremental growth for long periods are of most concern. Increments in the higher percentiles on charts are expected when a child is being rehabilitated and increments in the lower percentiles during periods of restriction of energy intake. Figure 1-13 shows typical growth increments for a child.

Midparent Height

Length and stature tend to be similar within families. A child's length can be adjusted for the stature of parents if both parents are tall or short. These adjustments remove the influence of parent stature from the child's measurement and make it easier to recognize potential growth problems. Tables for parent specific adjustment for stature are shown in the appendix.

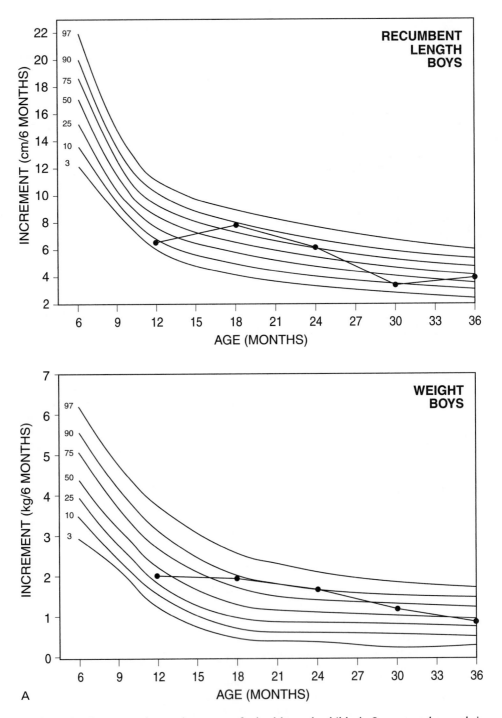

FIG. 1-13 Incremental growth pattern of a healthy male child. **A.** Incremental growth in recumbent length and weight are relatively stable during infancy. Note the predictable tapering of growth after infancy.

FIG. 1-13, Cont'd. Incremental growth pattern of a healthy male child. **B.** Incremental stature and weight gains for the child are appropriate and comparable to velocity growth pattern shown in figure 1-5.

Gestational Age

Because rate of growth and maturity are closely related, maturity status is particularly important for the interpretation of the growth of infants. Gestational age should be taken into account when interpreting the growth status of infants who are premature. First, the actual age and measurements are plotted on the growth chart. For interpretation of growth, the degree of prematurity is recorded on the growth chart and subtracted from actual age before plotting adjusted growth. The adjustment for prematurity is based on a gestational age of 40 weeks. For example, the adjusted growth data for an infant born at 30 weeks (10 weeks premature) would be plotted after subtracting 2.5 months from the actual age the infant was measured. Adjustments for prematurity are applied until age 18 months for head circumference, 21 months for weight, and 36 months for length.[35]

Skeletal Maturation

Fusion of the epiphyses and the appearance of ossification centers occur in a predictable bone order. As a result, skeletal maturation can be assessed by observation of the various centers of ossification and the fusion of the epiphyses on roentgenographic studies. Standards of bone age have been devised from longitudinal roentgenographic studies of hands and wrists of children. The most commonly used standards are those of Greulich and Pyle, which were based on 100 hand films of children who were examined periodically from birth to 18 years of age.[36]

Bone age is often used to assess the physiological maturity of a child whose linear growth appears to be proceeding at a very slow or very rapid rate. It is an especially useful tool in adolescence when parents or children or both become concerned about late and early maturation. Bone age correlates with secondary sex characteristics and with mature height.

Undernutrition delays skeletal ossification. Insufficient energy intake slows bone growth and delays calcification of the ossification centers. Also, the bone appears normal but often is thinner. Protein malnutrition, caused by an insufficient intake of protein, an intake of poor quality protein, or both, results not only in a reduction in bone growth but also in delays in the appearance of ossification centers and possible alterations in the sequence of ossification.[36] Obese children have been found to have advanced skeletal ages.

Skinfold Thickness

Since approximately half of the total body fat is deposited in subcutaneous adipose tissue, the fatness of an individual can be estimated by measuring the thickness of the skinfold at selected sites with special calipers that have been calibrated to provide a constant tension. It is important that proper calipers be used. Plastic calipers are generally not adequate.[37,38] In general, one truncal (subscapular) measurement and one limb (triceps) measurement are advised. If only one measurement is to be used, measurement of the triceps is preferred. The triceps is the easiest site to measure and is representative of body fatness (fig. 1-14).

The triceps measurement is taken midway between the acromion and olecranon processes. The client stands with the back to the measurer, right arm relaxed with palm facing the lateral thigh. The tips of the acromial and olecranon processes are palpated, and a point halfway between is marked on the skin. The skinfold is picked up over the posterior surface on the triceps muscle 1 cm above the mark on the vertical line, and the jaws of the caliper are applied to the marked level. The jaws of the caliper are permitted to exert full pressure as the trigger level of the caliper is released. The dial is read to the nearest 0.5 mm. Measurement error can be minimized by averaging three measurements.

Percentiles for triceps skinfold measurement are shown in the appendix. Triceps skinfold measurements were compiled from a cross-sectional study of white subjects from 1 to 75 years of age and are included in the Health and Nutrition Examination Survey I (1971–1974) (table 1-8).[39] Such measurements are useful as a complement to growth charts in the evaluation of children's growth and in the decision as to the necessity to modify energy or nutrient intake. Athletic, muscular children may appear overweight or obese if only height and weight are used as criteria for judgment. On the other hand, children with

FIG. 1-14 Triceps skinfold measurements are taken midway between the acromion and olecranon processes. Procedure: • Use a flexible, nonstretchable tape measure to identify the midpoint between the shoulder and the elbow on the back of the left arm. • Child's elbow is flexed at 90° • Mark the midpoint between the shoulder and the elbow • Grasp a vertical fold of skin about 1 cm above the midpoint • Gently pull the skinfold away from the muscle and hold it while applying the caliper • Record the measurement to the nearest 0.1 cm • Record the measurement on the chart • Reposition the child and remeasure the skinfold • Compare measures; they should agree within 0.2 cm • Plot the measurement on the chart appropriate for age and gender.

TABLE 1-8   *Percentiles for Triceps Skinfold (mm²) for Whites of the United States: Health and Nutrition Examination Survey I of 1971 to 1974*

| | Males | | | | | | | | Females | | | | | | | |
Age Group (Years)	n	5	10	25	50	75	90	95	n	5	10	25	50	75	90	95
1–1.9	228	6	7	8	10	12	14	16	204	6	7	8	10	12	14	16
2–2.9	223	6	7	8	10	12	14	15	208	6	8	9	10	12	15	16
3–3.9	220	6	7	8	10	11	14	15	208	7	8	9	11	12	14	15
4–4.9	230	6	6	8	9	11	12	14	208	7	8	8	10	12	14	16
5–5.9	214	6	6	8	9	11	14	15	219	6	7	8	10	12	15	18
6–6.9	117	5	6	7	8	10	13	16	118	6	6	8	10	12	14	16
7–7.9	122	5	6	7	9	12	15	17	126	6	7	9	11	13	16	18
8–8.9	117	5	6	7	8	10	13	16	118	6	8	9	12	15	18	24
9–9.9	121	6	6	7	10	13	17	18	125	8	8	10	13	16	20	22
10–10.9	146	6	6	8	10	14	18	21	152	7	8	10	12	17	23	27
11–11.9	122	6	6	8	11	16	20	24	117	7	8	10	13	18	24	28
12–12.9	153	6	6	8	11	14	22	28	129	8	9	11	14	18	23	27
13–13.9	134	5	5	7	10	14	22	26	151	8	8	12	15	21	26	30
14–14.9	131	4	5	7	9	14	21	24	141	9	10	13	16	21	26	28
15–15.9	128	4	5	6	8	11	18	24	117	8	10	12	17	21	25	32
16–16.9	131	4	5	6	8	12	16	22	142	10	12	15	18	22	26	31
17–17.9	133	5	5	6	8	12	16	19	114	10	12	13	19	24	30	37
18–18.9	91	4	5	6	9	13	20	24	109	10	12	15	18	22	26	30
19–24.9	531	4	5	7	10	15	20	22	1060	10	11	14	18	24	30	34

From Frisancho AR: *Am J Clin Nutr* 34:2540, 1981.

poor muscle tone often plot in a lower percentile for weight than height even though they have an adequate amount of adipose tissue.

It must be noted that data in these reference curves are derived from white children. Population differences have been noted in measured fat thickness. Puerto Rican children demonstrated greater fat measurements than U.S. white and black children. Black children have a greater deposition of adipose tissue from infancy through 4 years of age than do their white peers. After 4 years of age the differences are reversed.[39] Group and genetic differences must be considered in interpreting skinfold measurements.

Mid–Upper Arm Circumference

Measurement of mid–upper arm circumference combined with triceps skinfold is one method used to estimate muscle and fat. The mid–upper arm circumference measurement, like the triceps skinfold, is made at the midpoint of the upper part of the left arm. A flexible, nonstretchable tape is used (fig. 1-15). The subject is positioned with the right arm completely relaxed and extended by the side. A mark is drawn on the lateral side of the arm midway between the acromion and the olecranon. The tape is passed around the arm so that it is touching the skin but not compressing the tissue. It is important to ensure that the tape is on a plane perpendicular to the long axis of the arm.[38] Arm circumference is measured to the nearest 0.1 cm. Arm muscle diameter may be estimated by the following formula:

$$\text{Arm muscle diameter (mm)} = \frac{\text{Arm circumference (mm)} - \text{Triceps skinfold (mm)}}{\pi}$$

Data for arm muscle diameter and arm circumference have been derived from the Health and Nutrition Examination Survey.

Clinicians must be carefully trained to perform accurate, valid, and reliable skinfold and circumference measurements. These measurements, though deceptively simple, are difficult to perform in a reliable and accurate manner. Small differences in positioning of the child or technique of the measurer can render these

FIG. 1-15 Mid–upper arm circumference is measured with paper insertion tape that touches skin but does not compress tissue. Procedure: • Use a flexible, nonstretchable tape measure to identify the midpoint between the shoulder and the elbow on the back of the left arm • Have the child's elbow flexed at 90° • Measure down the back of the arm from the shoulder to the elbow • Mark the midpoint between the shoulder and the elbow • Measure the circumference of the arm over the midpoint mark without compressing the tissue of the arm • Measure the circumference to the nearest 0.1 cm • Write the measurement on the chart • Reposition and remeasure the arm circumference • Compare measures; they should agree within 0.2 cm.

measurements invalid. Measurement error is likely to be higher in infants and young children because it is difficult for them to maintain a standard position while the measurement is being performed. If measurements are carefully and reliably performed, it is reasonable to proceed with calculations of arm muscle diameter and interpolation of body composition.

Weight-height indexes of relative body weight have been developed. Several that are reliable for adults are not applicable for children. Durant and Linder[40] found that the weight-length index calculated by the following formula was the most appropriate for children:

$$WLI = \frac{A}{B} \times 100$$

where

$$A = \frac{Actual\ weight\ (kg)}{Actual\ height\ (cm)}$$

$$B = \frac{50th\ percentile\ expected\ weight\ (kg)\ for\ age}{50th\ percentile\ expected\ height\ (cm)\ for\ age}$$

The normal range for children is between 90 and 109. Those who score below 89 can be considered lean; those over 110, overweight; and those over 120, obese. The method does classify muscular children as overweight. However, skinfold measures can validate or negate the assumption.[40,41]

Body Mass Index

Body mass index (BMI) has been used as a noninvasive clinically convenient manner of assessing chronic energy deficiency and overweight in children over 1 year of age. BMI is expressed as a ratio of weight in kg to height in m².[42]

$$BMI = \frac{Weight\ (kg)}{Height\ (m^2)} \times 100$$

The resulting percentage can be used to grade the degree of impact of inadequate or excessive nourishment. If accurate length or height measures are obtained regularly in the clinical setting, the calculation of BMI adds a useful dimension in the assessment of body composition. This index of weight relative to length or stature can be used to monitor relative changes in BMI over time as well as a comparison to the recently developed percentile curves for BMI and the NCHS gender- and age-specific growth charts (fig. 1-16, fig. 1-17). A higher percentile BMI in childhood is a useful predictor for overweight in adulthood.[43] Regardless of effect on cognition, low BMI is related to starvation, deficiencies of the immune system, illness, morbidity, and mortality.

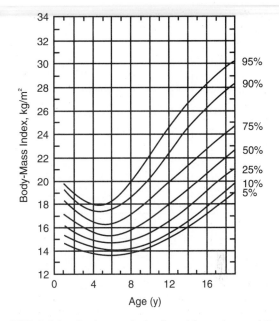

FIG. 1-16 Body mass index for white males aged 1 to 19 years. Percentiles were computed using data from the First National Health and Nutrition Examination Survey, 1971 to 1974.

Hammer, LD and others: *Am J Dis Child* 145, 1991.

Bioelectric impedance. Much research effort has been expended to determine more precise measurements and determination of body composition. This effort has focused on measurements of the components of body compartments electronically. It appears that measurement of resistance of the trunk is a predictor of the percentage of body fat in 6- to 18-year-old boys and adults.[44,45]

Although bioelectric impedance measures are a relatively accurate measure of the percentage of body fat, especially when used in conjunction with stature, weight, and skinfold thickness, they are difficult to perform because of the technology and difficult to interpret because of the lack of reference data for infants and children.

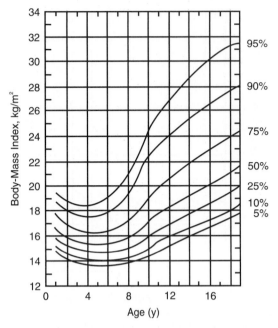

FIG. 1-17 Body mass index for white females aged 1 to 19 years. Percentiles were computed using data from the First National Health and Nutrition Examination Survey, 1971 to 1974.

Hammer, LD and others: *Am J Dis Child* 145, 1991.

COMPROMISED GROWTH

In the United States, depressed physical growth has been called failure to thrive, growth faltering, failure to grow, or failure to gain weight. The label used has depended on the situation and the severity of the depression of growth. The term *failure to thrive* is generally used to describe infants and young children whose growth is substantially less than that of their peers. Depressed physical growth is a symptom of health problems, not a disorder in itself. The usual description of failure to thrive is a decreased rate of weight gain or weight loss. Generally, two types of failure to thrive are described: (1) Organic failure to thrive describes children with a specific diagnosis that affects growth. In a relative state of health ordinary illnesses like upper respiratory infections (URI) are not severe or prolonged enough to significantly affect growth. However, chronic, repeated, or severe illness can cause depression or slowing of growth. It has been estimated that 20% to 40% of children called failure to thrive are in this category. (2) Nonorganic failure to thrive describes children with no obvious cause for poor growth and thus implies that the cause of failure to thrive is external to the infant. The majority of children called failure to thrive are in this category.[46]

The first step in the evaluation of children with failure to grow is to evaluate the adequacy of nutrients and energy provided by the food offered and of the food consumed. The children may be offered inadequate food because of poverty and lack of food, poor feeding techniques, or neglect. Impaired parent-child interactions may lead to a child who refuses to eat sufficient food or a parent who does not offer appropriate foods. This often results from inadequate bonding or psychosocial deprivation.

Observations of a feeding time during the evaluation can give important information when appropriate foods are offered but not consumed (see chapter 3). If the cause of poor growth is suspected to result from neurological problems, observations of oral motor skills to assess the child's ability to suck, chew with rotary movements, and self-feed will give information needed to plan intervention (see chapters 3 and 15).

If a disturbance of parent-child interaction is suspected, the parent's feelings about her child and her expectations about appropriate feeding patterns for the child need to be explored. Such children are often viewed as having had feeding problems in infancy and difficulty in accepting semisolid foods. They frequently consume more food when it is offered by another caregiver. When placed in an environment that provides adequate nurturing and stimulation, they consume large quantities of food; they catch up. Intervention for poor growth must be directed to correction of the psychosocial difficulties that caused the disturbed parent-child relationship.

Before using the term failure to thrive to describe the growth of an infant or young child one must understand and acknowledge normal variations in growth velocity. An example of changed growth velocity is the growth pattern of exclusively breast-fed infants whose growth is slowed compared with formula-fed infants from 2 months of age until age 1 year. Is this pattern delayed growth or typical growth for healthy exclusively breast-fed infants?

Questions have been raised about the apparent differences in growth between typical exclusively breast-fed and bottle-fed infants. Functional outcomes (activity level, behavioral development, and risk of morbidity) have been evaluated. Breast-fed infants grew more rapidly in the first 2 months of life and less rapidly from 3 to 12 months when compared with current NCHS growth charts. In the second year of life these infants gained weight more rapidly than suggested by the reference data.[47] The introduction of complementary foods at 4 to 6 months of age did not have an impact on the growth of exclusively breast-fed infants in two groups of low-income families in Honduras.[48]

A World Health Organization (WHO) Working Group evaluated the data available on the growth of infants. Breast-fed infants were at a weight for age less than the NCHS curves from 2 to 12 months. The decline in length was not as great. Mean weight for length was less than the NCHS charts at 12 months. There was a return toward the current NCHS curves at 12 to 24 months. There is a need also to evaluate the effects of nutritional quality of complementary foods on growth and other outcomes from 4 months onward. There are no data to suggest that slower weight gain is associated with deleterious functional consequences.[49] Based on the criteria used, breast-fed infants have lower rates of illness than formula-fed infants.[47] Further, the WHO Working Group concluded that a single reference would be preferable to separate charts for breast-fed and formula-fed infants.

The WHO Working Group that looked at the question of appropriate growth and appropriate evaluation of growth differentiated between "reference data," which is a tool that provides a common basis for comparison, and a "standard," which is a concept of normative growth or a target to be achieved.[49] In general, growth curves are comprised of reference data and are a guide for screening and monitoring. They are not a diagnostic tool to be used to define malnutrition or pathology. In practice, growth curves are often (inappropriately) used as standards. WHO suggests that interpretation of maintenance of adequate growth can vary depending on which reference curve is used.

CATCH-UP GROWTH

During recovery from malnutrition or illness that has halted or depressed growth, the child grows at a rate above that expected for his or her age. As the more rapid growth proceeds, the child catches up with his or her growth curve. Gain in weight proceeds rapidly until the child reaches the correct weight for height, then proceeds at a slower rate as height and weight increase together. During the second phase, growth proceeds at a height-expected rather than age-expected rate (fig. 1-18).

The range and magnitude of growth deficits vary with the condition and severity of the disorder that caused the growth deficiency. Catch-up growth is, however, possible in all situations, even when growth depression has been severe and prolonged, provided the epiphyses have not closed and the condition that caused the deficit has been remedied.

It is not unusual for children recovering from malnutrition, who were both wasted and stunted, to gain weight at rates 20 times faster than healthy age group peers until their weight is appropriate for their height; then, the rate of gain approximates that of children who were only wasted. The average catch-up rate of weight gain for children who are only stunted is approximately three times faster than would be expected for chronological age.[50]

Children who have experienced growth deficiency because of malnutrition and continue to live with marginal or insufficient food may have little opportunity for catch-up growth. For these

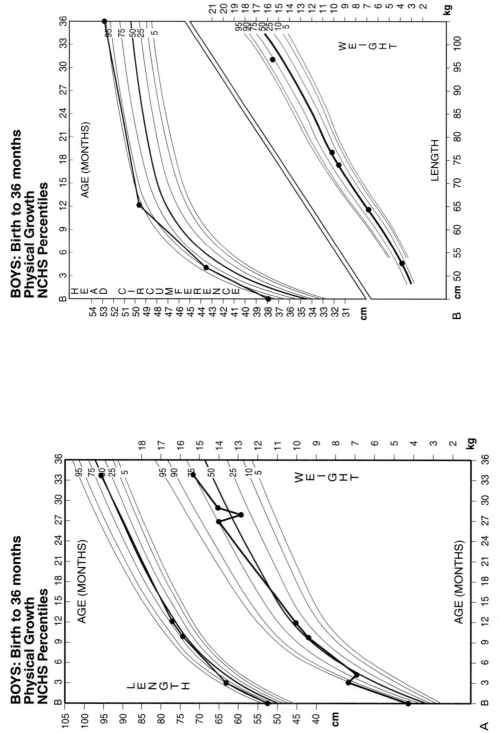

FIG. 1-18 This infant was at the 95th percentile for weight and the 90th percentile for length at birth and was exclusively breast-fed for 6 months. The infant changed channels for weight attainment and velocity at 3 to 5 months of age and established a new and consistent growth pattern at about the 50th percentile for weight and length. At age 27 months this toddler became critically ill. This illness was reflected in a precipitous weight loss. Two months later at resolution of the illness, the toddler demonstrated catch-up growth with an intake of about 150 kcals/kg until growth was resumed at the previous channel. Appetite decreased when the previous channel was attained. Length was not affected by this illness.

children, pubertal development is delayed. In some cases catch-up growth occurs because of prolongation of the growth period. In other instances children severely malnourished in early childhood who continue to live with a marginal food intake do not catch up in growth even though pubertal development may be delayed 2 years.[50]

Anthropometry is often used to assess nutritional status. Low weight for height, often called wasting or thinness, reflects failure to gain weight or loss of weight. Low height for age—often called stunting, short stature, or linear growth deficiency—is often associated with poor overall economic conditions or repeated exposure to adverse conditions. Long-term energy deficiency in childhood does cause stunting and reduction in the final attained stature. Weight for age is a composite index of both weight for height and height for age, yet it fails to distinguish tall, thin children from short children of adequate weight. Weight for age is not a good predictor of wasted children in the United States. Children who have suffered wasting are best identified by weight for height; children who have suffered stunting are best identified by height for age.[51] Children of all ages who have low weight for height or who have experienced growth faltering (in terms of weight for height) are likely to respond to intervention or treatment of the cause. Appropriate treatment of children less than 2 years old generally results in increased stature; but this is not true for older children.

Summary

Children grow at their individual predictable rates; the range of growth rates at any age is large. When plotted on growth charts, measurements of growth provide information as to whether children are expressing their genetic potential for growth. Skinfold measurements taken with calibrated instruments provide important information when children are suspected to be undernourished or overnourished. If children are not growing as expected, the ade-quacy of their energy and nutrient intake should be investigated.

As physical growth proceeds, changes in body composition occur. During adolescence, the deposition of lean body mass per inch of height is greater in the male than in the female. At maturity, males have one and a half times the lean body mass of females.

There are critical stages of development during cell growth when the number of cells in an organism is increasing and an organ is most vulnerable to deprivation. Even so, catch-up growth appears possible if rehabilitation occurs and if sufficient foods and nurturing are provided.

REVIEW QUESTIONS

1. Describe the long-term effects of malnutrition in infancy and early childhood on physical growth and mental development.
2. Why do health care professionals plot heights, weights, and head circumferences on growth charts?
3. When is it appropriate to use an incremental growth chart?
4. Which measurements of body composition are clinically useful?
5. What is catch-up growth?
6. How does one interpret growth data plotted on the NCHS growth chart for non-Caucasians?

SUGGESTED LEARNING ACTIVITIES

1. Obtain heights and weights of a child over several years from a school health record or medical chart, plot them on a growth chart, and interpret the curves on the chart.
2. Describe how you would interpret, to a school-age boy and his parents, the physical growth of a child growing at the 10th percentile whose neighbor of the same age and sex is growing at the 95th percentile.
3. Describe measuring devices and scales that provide valid information.
4. Demonstrate how to correctly measure mid–upper arm circumference and triceps skinfold thickness.

❖ ❖ ❖

Growth of a Healthy Male Child

Longitudinal measures of weight, length/stature, and head circumference for a normally grown boy are shown in figures 1-19 and 1-20. Figure 1-19A shows the pattern of growth for weight and length from early infancy until age 3. Although this boy crossed channels for both length and weight, his growth was appropriately consistent. Figure 1-19B shows head circumference measures for the same child; these measures too were appropriately consistent at the 50th percentile. Plotting of weight for length measures shows that as an infant he was "long" and "lean" with weight for length at the 5th percentile; as he aged, his weight for length increased to the 50th percentile. Figure 1-20A shows a gradual regression toward the mean for stature; and for weight. Figure 1-20B

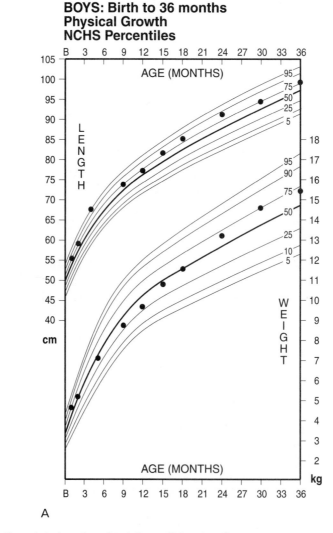

A

FIG. 1-19   **A.** Growth in length and weight until 3 years of age.

❖ ❖ ❖

CASE STUDY

Growth of a Healthy Male Child—cont'd

shows that weight for length proportions were at the 50th percentile for most of childhood.

Figure 1-13A (p. 21) shows the incremental increases in length and weight for the same male child. Figure 1-13B shows incremental increases in weight and length throughout childhood and into adolescence. Note the changes in channels when viewed longitudi-

nally. This demonstrates periods of rapid growth and periods of slower growth during childhood and then a rapid acceleration during adolescence. Figure 1-5 (p. 14) demonstrates the same data on a velocity growth chart for height and weight. Again, periods of rapid and of slower growth are clearly shown.

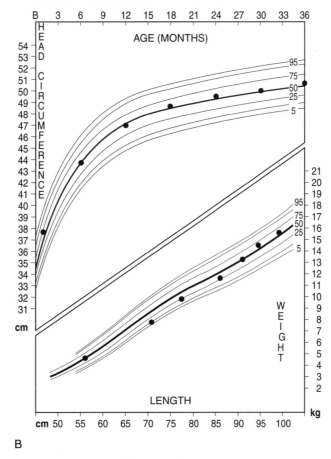

FIG. 1-19, Cont'd. **B.** Growth in head circumference and weight/length until age 3 years.

Continued.

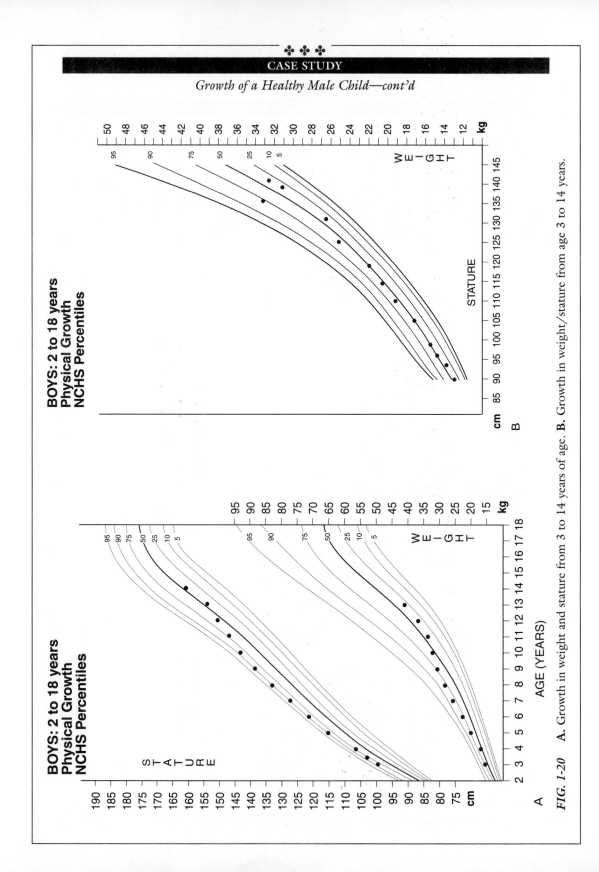

FIG. 1-20 **A.** Growth in weight and stature from 3 to 14 years of age. **B.** Growth in weight/stature from age 3 to 14 years.

REFERENCES

1. Mitchell HS: Nutrition in relation to stature, *J Am Diet Assoc* 40:521, 1962.
2. Mitchell HS, Santo S: Nutritional improvement in Nokkaido orphanage children—1960–1970, *J Am Diet Assoc* 72:506, 1978.
3. Yip R, Scanion K, Trowbridge F: Improving growth status of Asian refugee children in the United States, *JAMA* 127:937, 1992.
4. Martorell R and others: Genetic and environmental determinants of growth in Mexican-Americans, *Pediatrics* 84:864, 1989.
5. Community Nutrition Institute: *Nutrition Week,* 26:4, March 15, 1996.
6. Winick M, Noble A: Quantitative changes in DNA, RNA, and protein during prenatal and postnatal growth in the rat, *Dev Biol* 12:451, 1965.
7. Winick M, Noble A: Cellular growth in rats during malnutrition at various ages, *J Nutr* 89:300, 1966.
8. Elliott DA, Cheek DB: Muscle and liver cell growth in rats with hypoxia and reduced nutrition. In Cheek DB, editor: *Human growth, body composition, cell growth, energy, and intelligence,* Philadelphia, 1968, Lea & Febiger.
9. Johnson K, Rosenbaum S, Simons J: *The data book: the nation, states and cities,* Washington, DC, 1985, Children's Defense Fund.
10. Smith D and others: Shifting linear growth during infancy: illustration of genetic factors in growth from fetal life through infancy, *J Pediatr* 89:225, 1976.
11. Fomon SF and others: Body composition of reference children from birth to 10 years, *Am J Clin Nutr* 35:1169, 1982.
12. Anderson EC, Langham WH: Average potassium concentration of the human body as a function of age, *Science* 130:713, 1959.
13. Forbes GB: Relation of lean body mass to height in children and adolescents, *Pediatr Res* 6:32, 1972.
14. Widdowson EM, Spray CM: Chemical development in utero, *Arch Dis Child* 26:205, 1951.
15. Kanarek RB, Marks-Kaufman RM: *Nutrition and behavior,* New York, 1991, Van Nostrand Reinhold.
16. Winick M, Rosso P, Waterlow J: Cellular growth of cerebrum, cerebellum, and brain stem in normal and marasmic children, *Exp Neurol* 26:393, 1970.
17. Winick M: Nutrition and nerve cell growth, *Fed Proc* 29:1510, 1970.
18. Brasel JA, Gruen RK: Cellular growth of brain, liver, muscle, and lung. In Falkner F, Tanner JM, editors: *Human growth,* vol 2, New York, 1978, Plenum Publishing.
19. Beardslee WR and others: The effect of infantile malnutrition on behavioral development, a follow-up study, *Am J Clin Nutr* 35:1437, 1982.
20. Graham GG, Adrianzen TB: Late "catch-up" growth after severe infantile malnutrition, *Johns Hopkins Med J* 131:204, 1972.
21. Galler JR, Ramsey F, Solimano G: The influence of early malnutrition on subsequent development. III. Learning disabilities as a sequel to malnutrition, *Pediatr Res* 18:309, 1984.
22. Galler JR and others: Long-term effects of early kwashiorkor compared with marasmus. II. Intellectual performance, *J Pediatr Gastroenterol Nutr* 6:847, 1987.
23. Galler JR and others: Long-term effect of early kwashiorkor compared with marasmus. III. Fine motor skills, *J Pediatr* 6:855, 1987.
24. Allen, LH: The Nutrition CRSP: What is marginal malnutrition, and does it affect human function? *Nutr Rev* 51:255, 1993.
25. Brook CGD: Cellular growth: adipose tissue. In Falkner F, Tanner JM, editors: *Human growth,* vol 2, New York, 1978, Plenum Publishing.
26. Brook CGD: Cell growth in man, *Am Heart J* 86:571, 1973.
27. Committee on Nutrition, American Academy of Pediatrics: Nutritional aspects of obesity in infancy and childhood, *Pediatrics* 68:880, 1981.
28. National Center for Health Statistics: NCHS growth charts, 1976, *Monthly Vital Statistics Report,* vol. 25, no 3, Suppl (HRA) 76-1120, Rockville, Md, 1976, Health Resources Administration.
29. Tanner JM, Davies PSW: Clinical longitudinal standards for height and weight velocity for North American children, *Pediatrics* 107:317, 1985.
30. Himes JH and others: Parent-specific adjustments for evaluation of recumbent length and stature of children, *Pediatrics* 75:304, 1985.
31. Nellhaus G: Head circumference from birth to 18 years, *Pediatrics* 41:106, 1968.
32. Roche AF, Himes JH: Incremental growth charts, *Am J Clin Nutr* 33:2041, 1980.
33. Incremental growth charts—boys and incremental growth charts—girls. Ross Growth and Development Program, Columbus, Ohio, 1981, Ross Laboratories.

34. Guo S and others: Reference data on gains in weight and length during the first two years of life. *J Pediatr* 119:355, 1991.

35. Moore WM, Roche AF: *Pediatric anthropometry,* 2nd ed. Ross Growth and Development Program, Ross Laboratories, Columbus, OH, 1983.

36. Greulich WW, Pyle PI: *Radiographic atlas of skeletal development of the hand and wrist,* Stanford, Calif, 1959, Stanford University Press.

37. Gray GE, Gray LK: Anthropometric measurements and their interpretation: principles, practices, and problems, *J Am Diet Assoc* 77:534, 1980.

38. Lohman TG, Roche AF, Martorell R, editors: *Anthropometric standardization reference manual,* Champaign, Ill, 1988, Human Kinetics Books.

39. Frisancho AR: New norms of upper limb fat and muscle areas for assessment of nutritional status, *Am J Clin Nutr* 34:2540, 1981.

40. Durant RN, Linder CW: An evaluation of five indexes of relative body weight for use with children, *J Am Diet Assoc* 78:35, 1981.

41. Cronk CE, Roche AF: Race- and sex-specific reference data for triceps and subscapular skinfolds and weight stature, *Am J Clin Nutr* 35:347, 1982.

42. Hammer LD, Kraemer HC, Wilson DM, Ritter PL, Dornbusch SM: Standardized percentile curves of body-mass index for children and adolescents. *Am J Dis Child* 145:259, 1991.

43. Guo SS, Roche AF, Chumlea WC, Gardner JD, Siervogel RM: The predictive value of childhood body mass index for overweight at age 35 y. *Am J Clin Nutr* 59:810, 1994.

44. Baumgartner RN, Chumlea WC, Roche AF: Bioelectric impedance phase angle and body composition, *Am J Clin Nutr* 48:16, 1988.

45. Chumlea WC, Baumgartner RN, Roche AF: Specific gravity used to estimate fat-free mass from segmental body measures of bioelectric impedance, *Am J Clin Nutr* 48:7, 1988.

46. Magioni A, Lifshitz, F: Nutritional management of failure to thrive, *Ped Clin N Amer* 42:791, 1995.

47. Dewey KG, Peerson JM, Brown KH and others: Growth of breast-fed infants deviates from current reference data: a pooled analysis of US, Canadian, and European data, *Pediatrics* 96:495, 1995.

48. Cohen RJ, Brown KH et al: Determinants of growth from birth to 12 months among breast-fed Honduran infants in relation to age of introduction of complementary foods, *Pediatrics* 96:504, 1995.

49. WHO Working Group on Infant Growth: An evaluation of infant growth: the use and interpretation of anthropometry in infants, *Bull World Health Org* 73:165, 1995.

50. Ashworth A, Millward DJ: Catch-up growth in children, *Nutr Rev* 44:157, 1986.

51. Gorstein J, Sullivan K, Yip R and others: Issues in the assessment of nutritional status using anthropometry, Bull World Health Org 72:272, 1994.

2

Nutrient Needs of Infants and Children

Cristine M. Trahms
Peggy L. Pipes

++

Objectives

After studying this chapter, the student should:

✔ *Understand the rationale for recommended intakes of nutrients and energy in infancy and childhood.*

✔ *Recognize appropriate foods as sources of nutrients and energy for infants and children.*

✔ *Be aware of the reasons for the wide range of acceptable energy intakes in infancy and childhood.*

✔ *Be able to make appropriate recommendations for the use of nutrient supplements in infancy and childhood.*

✔ *Understand factors that affect the bioavailability of nutrients.*

Children must consume sufficient high-quality proteins, vitamins, minerals, and energy if acceptable growth is to occur. Energy generated from the metabolism of fats, carbohydrates, and proteins provides the fuel that supports the maintenance of body functions and provides for activity and growth. Protein supplies amino acids for the synthesis of new tissues and nitrogen for the maturation of existing tissues in early childhood.

Vitamins function in a variety of metabolic processes that make protein synthesis and energy metabolism possible. Their requirements are therefore determined by intakes of energy, protein, and other nutrients. Minerals are essential components of body tissue. Their requirements are influenced by rates of growth and the interrelationships they share with other nutrients.

TABLE 2-1 *Comparison of Recommended Daily Intakes for Infants (0–6 Months of Age)*

	RDA	FAO/WHO	RNI	U.S. RDA
Protein (gm)	13	2.04 gm/kg to 1.73 gm/kg or 9–12 gm/day	11–14	18–25
Energy (kcal)	115–105 kcal/kg or 650–950 kcal/day	108 kcal/kg	120–95 kcal/kg or 500–700 kcal/day	
Calcium (mg)	400		350	600
Iron (mg)	6		5	15
Vitamin D (μg)	7.5		10	400 IU

RDA: Recommended Dietary Allowances, 10th ed., United States, 1989.[1]
FAO/WHO: Food and Agricultural Organization/World Health Organization, 1985.[3]
RNI: Recommended Nutrient Intakes for Canadians, Health and Welfare Canada, 1983.[4]
U.S. RDA: Required on food labels in the United States.

A wide range of opinions exists as to optimal intakes of nutrients for individuals at all ages. The most recent edition of the Recommended Dietary Allowances (RDA), 1989,[1] was controversial at its introduction. In its recommendations the Food and Nutrition Board, National Academy of Sciences attempts to include the most recent data from nutrient balance studies, biochemical measurements of tissue saturation, nutrient intake data, epidemiological observations, and when appropriate, extrapolation from animal studies.

It is important to remember that the RDAs are recommendations for planning food supplies to meet the needs of populations and for designing public nutrition intervention and education programs. The RDAs are a statistical concept. They are determined for a particular group of individuals with specific characteristics who consume a specified diet and refer to the average need for nutrients over a reasonable period of time. The RDAs are levels of intake of nutrients considered to be adequate to meet known nutrient needs of practically all healthy people. The RDAs do not address possible interactions of nutrients and other dietary components. The RDAs assume the individual's needs for energy are met. When the RDAs are used as guidelines in assessing food intake patterns of children,

they should not be confused with the U.S. RDA designation on food labels. They are not designed to define individual requirements or to assess the adequacy of an individual's intake.

The RDAs should not be used to diagnose nutritional deficits for individuals.[2] Since the energy and nutrient needs of individual children vary, assessment of appropriate nutrient intake should be based on clinical outcome and professional clinical judgment and not directly related to arbitrary RDA units. If, however, one is knowledgeable about the data used to establish the guidelines and the safety factors added, one can use this knowledge to identify infants and children at risk and to plan diets for infants and children. Combined with growth data and a knowledge of foods as sources of nutrients, such information can be used to identify a need for change in the dietary intake of an individual infant or child.

Commonly used reference guidelines for nutrient intakes are shown in table 2-1. The recommendations are intended to be sufficient for the maintenance of health in nearly all people of the designated population group. The values differ because of the judgment factors applied to each set of guidelines, which are based on food availability and average intake of the group of people for whom the guidelines are intended.

TABLE 2-2   *Recommended Energy Intake*

| Category | Age (Years) | Weight | | Height | | REE* (kcal/day) | Average Energy Allowance (kcal)† | | |
		kg	lb	cm	in		Multiples of REE	Per kg	Per day[1]
Infants	0.0–0.5	6	13	60	24	320		108	650
	0.5–1.0	9	20	71	28	500		98	850
Children	1–3	13	29	90	35	740		102	1300
	4–6	20	44	112	44	950		90	1800
	7–10	28	62	132	52	1130		70	2000
Males	11–14	45	99	157	62	1440	1.70	55	2500
	15–18	66	145	176	69	1760	1.67	45	3000
Females	11–14	46	101	157	62	1310	1.67	47	2200
	15–18	55	120	163	64	1370	1.60	40	2200

Modified from *Recommended dietary allowances,* ed 10, National Research Council, Washington, DC, 1989, National Academy Press.

*Calculation based on WHO equations, then rounded.[3] *REE,* Resting energy expenditure.

†In the range of light to moderate activity, the coefficient of variation is ±20%.

The U.S. RDA values are those that appear on food labels in the United States.

The chronic misuse of the RDAs, plus newer scientific information, has led to a discussion of major revisions in the proposed 11th edition of the RDAs by the Food and Nutrition Board. It has been suggested that four levels of intake be described: (1) *deficient* (level of nutrient intake below which healthy people can be expected to experience deficiency symptoms), (2) *average requirement* (mean level of nutrient intake that appears sufficient to maintain biochemical/ physiological function in a population), (3) *recommended dietary allowance* (intake of nutrient considered to meet the nutritional needs of practically all healthy persons), and (4) *upper safe* (level of intake beyond which there appears to be risk of toxicity over time).[5]

NUTRIENT NEEDS

Many factors determine an individual's needs for nutrients, including age, gender, body size, rate of growth, physical activity, basal energy expenditure, and reserves acquired in utero by the fetus or from dietary intake by the infant and older child.

Energy

Total energy requirements reflect that expended for basal metabolism, specific dynamic action, activity, and growth. Because of wide variations in all of the parameters at any age, ranges of recommended intake have been suggested. The recommended energy intakes are shown in table 2-2.

The energy requirement is very high per unit of body size in a child's first few months of life but declines as the rate of growth decreases. A higher basal metabolic demand in infancy is thought to be caused by a larger loss of heat because of a relatively greater body surface and by a larger proportion of metabolic tissue. Males expend greater amounts of basal energy than do females. The differences are small during the preadolescent years but become pronounced during adolescence.

Maintenance requirements approximate 1.5 times the basal metabolic expenditure, since some movement occurs even during sleep, and the specific dynamic action is estimated to be 7% to 8% of ingested energy for infants and about 5% for older children. Table 2-2 shows estimated resting energy expenditure (REE). Energy costs of growth have been estimated to approximate 4.4 to 5.7 kcal/gm of tissue gained or 15 to 25 kcal/kg/day.[3] Decreasing rates of growth result in decreasing requirements for energy per unit of size (kcal/kg). In other words, as children grow older, they need greater numbers of kcalories because of larger body sizes but their need for energy per unit of size decreases.

The contribution of physical activity to total energy expenditure is variable among children and in individual children from day to day. At all ages, activity patterns among children show wide ranges in both the time spent in the various activities and the intensity of the activities. Some infants, for example, may be quiet, cuddly, and satisfied to explore their environment with their eyes, but others may expend more energy in crying, kicking, and physical movement to see the world around them. Some older children engage in such sedentary activities as looking at books or watching television, whereas their peers may be engaged in physical activities that demand running, jumping, and general body movements.

Established methods of predicting energy expenditure are felt to be outdated. New predictive equations for energy requirements from measures of body composition and estimates of energy expenditure in activity are being developed.[6] The newest estimates of the energy requirements of infants combine the requirements of energy for growth with a measure of total energy expenditure. These estimates are completed using the doubly labeled water technique and are shown in table 2-3. Total energy expenditure as determined by this method was 25% less than the current RDA for young children.[7] It has also been suggested that for infants and children, age and fatness are predictors of sedentary energy expenditure and basal metabolic rate.[8]

Energy requirements, which are greatest per unit of size in infancy, decline until adolescent growth is complete. During adolescence the energy requirement is a reflection of the adolescent growth spurt. Since adolescents enter the growth spurt at different ages, recommendations established for a given age must be applied with caution.

TABLE 2-3   *Calculated Energy Needs of Infants Using Doubly Labeled Water Technique*

Age (mo.)	Energy (kcal/kg/day)
1	110
3	95
6	85
9	83
12	83
24	84
36	85

Adapted from Davies, 1989,[9] Lucas, 1987,[10] Prentice et al. 1988.[11]

During a period of catch-up growth after illness or malnutrition, the requirement for energy and nutrients is greatly increased. Total intakes of 150 to 250 kcal/kg of body weight have been recommended for children of preschool age with 50 to 80 kcal/kg supporting the increased growth. An intake of 200 kcal/kg/day should produce a weight gain of 20 gm/kg/day.[12]

The energy needs of individual children of the same size, age, and gender vary. Reasons for these differences remain unexplained. Differences in physical activity, in the metabolic cost of minimal and excessive protein intakes at equivalent levels of energy intake, and in the efficiency with which individuals utilize energy have all been hypothesized to exert an influence.

In 1930 an expert committee, after reviewing energy intake data in relation to physical parameters, stated that height appeared to be the most appropriate criterion on which to base studies of energy needs.[13] The observation was never used. In estimating energy needs of children, body surface area or weight has continued to be used as a reference for suggested energy intakes of children. Energy per centimeter of height has proved clinically, however, to be a useful reference in estimating energy needs and designing diets for individual children. It is an especially useful reference for children who are genetically short.

TABLE 2-4 *Selected Foods as Sources of Energy for Infants*

Food	Energy kcal/oz	Energy kcal/T
Milk		
Human milk	22	11
Commercially available infant formula	20	10
Whole cow's milk	19	9
Commercially available infant foods (average value)		
Dry infant cereals	129	14
Strained and junior fruits	16	8
Strained and junior vegetables	12	5
Strained and junior meats	34	14
Strained egg yolks	65	28
Strained and junior dinners		
Vegetables with meat	22	9
Lean meat dinners	22	9
Strained and junior desserts	25	11

TABLE 2-5 *Selected Foods as Sources of Energy for Children*

Food	Portion Size	Average Energy (kcal)
2% milk with nonfat milk solids	½ c	69
Meat, poultry, or fish	1 oz	72
Egg	1 medium	75
Peanut butter	1 T	94
Cheese	½ oz	57
Legumes, cooked	¼ c	58
Enriched bread	½ slice	33
Ready-to-eat cereals (not sugar-coated)	¾ c	67
Cooked cereal	½ c	73
Saltine crackers	1	12
Rice, macaroni, spaghetti, cooked	¼ c	66
Potato (boiled)	½ medium	58
Potato chips	5	52
Green beans	¼ c	9
Carrots		
Cooked	¼ c	17
Raw	2 medium sticks	14
Apple	1 small	81
Banana	1 medium	105
Orange	1 small	62
Orange juice	½ c	56
Sugar	1 t	15
Jam or jelly	1 t	17
Butter, margarine, oil, mayonnaise	1 t	33
Cookies, assorted	1	50–60
Ice cream	¼ c	67

The best evaluation of the adequacy of infants' and childrens' energy intake is the adequacy of their growth rates in length and weight. If upward or downward changes in weight percentiles occur without changes in length percentiles, undernutrition or overnutrition should be suspected.

The recommended energy allowances from the 1989 RDAs represent the average needs of individuals at various ages and weights. The weights are median weights from NCHS data[14] and not arbitrary ideal weights. From birth to 6 months the recommendation is 108 kcal/kg/day and from 6 months to 1 year it is 98 kcal/kg/day. As shown in table 2-2 these recommended energy allowances are those reported by the World Health Organization (WHO).[3]

Food sources. Energy values of foods commonly consumed in infancy and childhood are given in tables 2-4 and 2-5. It can be seen that the energy density (energy content per portion of food) varies widely. Choices of foods offered to the infant and young child can greatly affect the total energy intake and consequently the rate of growth and weight gain. Table 2-6 indicates the increase in variety, texture, and quantity of foods to support and appropriate energy intake for young children.

TABLE 2-6   *Food Patterns That Provide Appropriate Energy Intakes for Young Children of Various Ages*

Age	2 Months	6 Months	10 Months	4 Years
Weight (kg)	6	7.5	9	20
Recommended Energy Needs (kcal)	650	750	850	1800
Foods that provide appropriate energy intake	28–32 oz human milk or infant formula	28 oz human milk or infant formula 4 T dry infant cereal 4 oz fruit juice 5 T strained fruit	24 oz infant formula 8 T dry infant cereal 14 T junior fruit 8 T junior vegetable 4 T junior meat ½ slice toast 1 oz chopped chicken 1 T mashed green beans 1 sm. banana 2 T ice cream 1 graham cracker	24 oz milk 6–8 oz fruit juice 3 slices bread ½ to ¾ c dry cereal 2 T peanut butter 1 t jelly 2 oz lean hamburger patty ¼ c macaroni and cheese ¼ c green beans ⅛ c ice cream 1 graham cracker 1 med. apple 1 sm. banana

Protein and Amino Acid Requirements

Protein provides energy but also serves a more important and complex function. Protein is the basic component of the protoplasm in cells; therefore an adequate intake of protein is essential if normal growth is to occur. Increases in body protein average 3.5 gm/day for the first 4 months and 3.1 gm/day for the next 8 months, with the body protein increasing from 11% to 14.6% in the first year.[15]

Amino acid requirements of infants have been estimated from studies in which pure amino acids were supplied in proportions of amino acids of human milk.[16] The requirement of an amino acid was defined as the least amount required to maintain satisfactory nitrogen retention and weight gain when nitrogen levels and other amino acids were held constant. Fomon and others,[17] as well as Fomon and Filer,[18] have estimated amino acid requirements from intakes of infants between 8 and 112 days of age who

were fed whole protein in cow's milk formulas and soy formulas. Satisfactory linear growth and weight gain, nitrogen balance, and serum concentrations of albumin equivalent to those of normal breast-fed infants were used as criteria of adequacy.

The current estimates of amino acid requirements for infants and children are based on composite data from several studies. The criteria of growth and nitrogen accumulation were used for infants and the amount of intake needed to maintain positive nitrogen balance was used as the criterion for children (table 2-7).

Investigators have found amino acid requirements for 10- to 12-year-old children to be two to three times greater than those for adults. Requirements of males in all cases exceeded those of females.[21] Histidine is essential in infancy but not in the older child.

Protein needs for growth (expressed as percentages of requirement) decrease as rates of growth decline. Of the protein requirement,

TABLE 2-7 *Estimates of Amino Acid Requirements*

Amino Acid	Requirements, mg/kg/day, by Age Group		
	Infants, Age 3–4 mo*	Children, Age ~2 yr†	Children, Age 10–12 yr‡
Histidine	28	?	?
Isoleucine	70	31	28
Leucine	161	73	42
Lysine	103	64	44
Methionine plus cystine	58	27	22
Phenylalanine plus tyrosine	125	69	22
Threonine	87	37	28
Tryptophan	17	12.5	3.3
Valine	93	38	25
Total without histidine	714	352	214

Modified from *Recommended dietary allowances,* ed 10, National Research Council, Washington, DC, 1989, National Academy Press.

*Based on amounts of amino acids in human milk or cow's milk formulas fed at levels that supported good growth. Data from Fomon and Filer (1967).[18]

†Based on achievement of nitrogen balance sufficient to support adequate lean tissue gain (16 mg N/kg/day). Data from Pineda and others (1981).[19]

‡Based on upper range of requirement for positive nitrogen balance. Recalculated by Williams and others (1974)[20] from data of Nakagawa and others (1964).[21]

50% is used for growth in the first 2 months of life. This declines to 11% at 2 to 3 years of age and is gradually reduced to zero after an increase during the adolescent growth spurt. Amino acids required for growth differ from those required for maintenance.

Recommended intakes. The recommendations for daily protein intakes for infants and children have assumed an adequate intake of energy. These recommendations are based on ingestion of milk protein in infancy and a mixed diet that provides protein that has an efficiency of utilization of 75% in older children.[1] Table 2-8 shows the recommended protein intakes by age.

Fomon and others[17] have suggested that during infancy, amino acid and protein requirements expressed per unit of energy consumed (reflecting both size and rate of growth) are more meaningful than expressions of requirements on the basis of body weight alone. They estimate the protein requirement to be 1.6 gm/100 kcal for children 1 to 4 months of age

and 1.4 gm/100 kcal for children 8 to 12 months of age.

Fomon[22] has proposed a factorial method of estimating the protein requirement for infants. The requirement for growth plus the requirement of replacement of losses in urine, feces, and skin is shown in table 2-9. This requirement decreased by 5 months of age and then remained stable to about 12 months of age. The Recommended Dietary Intake (RDI) proposed by Fomon at 1 month is 2.6 gm/kg/day and by 5 months it is 1.4 gm/kg/day; this recommendation is stable for the remainder of the first year of life. The 1989 Recommended Dietary Allowances suggest an average protein intake of 1.68 gm/kg/day between birth and 3 months with the reference protein as human milk.[1]

Based on nitrogen balance studies, it was concluded that an appropriate protein allowance for 7- to 10-year-old children would be 45 gm or more per day.[23] Reported protein intakes of children in the United States have shown actual

TABLE 2-8   *Recommended Allowances of Reference Protein and U.S. Dietary Protein*

Category	Age (Years)	Weight (kg)	Derived Allowance of Reference Protein (gm/kg)	Recommended Dietary Allowance gm/kg*	Recommended Dietary Allowance gm/day
Both sexes	0–0.5	6	2.20†	2.2	13
	0.5–1	9	1.56	1.6	14
	1–3	13	1.14	1.2	16
	4–6	20	1.03	1.1	24
	7–10	28	1.00	1.0	28
Males	11–14	45	0.98	1.0	45
	15–18	66	0.86	0.9	59
Females	11–14	46	0.94	1.0	46
	15–18	55	0.81	0.8	44

Modified from *Recommended dietary allowances,* ed 10, National Research Council, Washington, DC, 1989, National Academy Press.

*Amino acid score of typical U.S. diet is 100 for all age groups, except young infants.

Digestibility is equal to reference proteins. Values have been rounded upward to 0.1 gm/kg.

†For infants 0 to 3 months of age, breastfeeding that meets energy needs also meets protein needs. Formula substitutes should have the same amount and amino acid composition as human milk, corrected for digestibility if appropriate.

TABLE 2-9   *Estimate of Protein Requirement and Recommended Protein Intakes for Infants*

	Calculated Requirement for Growth/Replacement*		Recommended Dietary Intake (RDI)		1989 Recommended Dietary Allowances (RDA)
Age	gm/kg	gm/100 kcal	gm/kg	gm/100 kcal	gm/kg
0–1 month	1.98	1.65	2.6	2.2	2.2
5–12 months	1.18	1.31	1.4	1.6	1.6

*Requirement based on requirements for growth and replacement of losses from urine, feces, and skin.

Adapted from Fomon, *Nutrition of normal infants,* Mosby–Year Book, 1993.[15]

protein intakes to be 10% to 15% of energy consumed. During periods of catch-up growth, protein requirements increase. Milk protein intakes of 3.2 gm/kg when energy intakes are adequate have been suggested to support catch-up growth for infants.[12]

The Committee on Nutrition of the American Academy of Pediatrics[24] has set minimum protein standards for infant formula of 1.8 gm/100 kcal or 7.2% of kcal with a protein efficiency ratio to that of **casein.**

The protein requirement for any child depends on the rate of growth and the quality of protein in the diet. This implies that evaluation of a child's protein intake must be approached on the basis of the adequacy of the rate of growth, the quality of protein in the foods ingested, the combinations of foods that provide amino acids consumed together, and the adequacy of those nutrients (minerals and vitamins) and energy that are necessary for protein synthesis.

TABLE 2-10 *Approximate Protein Contents of Various Milks and Foods Fed to Infants*

Food	Protein (gm/oz)
Human milk	0.3
Commercial infant formulas	0.5
Commercial soy infant formula	0.5
Homogenized milk	1.0
Evaporated milk, prepared	1.1
Infant cereals, high protein, dry (12 T)	11
Infant cereals, rice (12 T)	2.8
Strained chicken noodle dinners	0.6
Strained vegetable and meat dinners	0.6–0.8
Strained beef and vegetable dinners	2.0
Strained turkey and vegetable dinners	1.9
Strained egg yolk	2.8
Strained beef	3.9
Strained veal	3.8

TABLE 2-11 *Selected Foods as Sources of Protein for Preschool Children*

Food	Portion Size	Protein (gm)
Yogurt, made from whole milk	½ c	3.9
Cottage cheese, creamed	2 T	3.5
Cheddar cheese	1 oz	7.1
Hamburger patty, lean	2 oz	14.0
Chicken drumstick	1	13.2
Peanut butter	1 T	4.5
Egg	1 large	6.2
Tuna	¼ c	11.5
Nonfat milk solids, dry	1 T	1.5
Milk	½ c	4.9
Ready-to-eat cereals	½ c	0.5–3.0

Food sources. Protein of high quality is available to most infants in developed countries as human milk and modified cow's milk formula. Infants who have allergic reactions to cow's milk are often fed formulas prepared from water-soluble soy isolates. These commercial formulas support appropriate growth and intake of nutrients.

As discussed in chapter 4, commercially prepared formulas are manufactured so that all nutrients are provided in the appropriate amounts if consumed in recommended quantities. Home preparation of soy formulas is discouraged because parents may not be careful to heat the soy milk sufficiently to achieve inactivation of the trypsin inhibitor and may discard the residue of soy material from which the milk was made. In so doing, much of the protein and many of the other essential nutrients are discarded.

Table 2-10 lists foods commonly consumed in infancy that contribute protein. Protein intakes of infants can be greatly increased depending on the choice and quantity of foods offered to the infant.

As children grow older and accept table food, they receive additional foods that provide high-quality protein. Examples of foods acceptable to preschoolers that provide high-quality protein are given in table 2-11. The protein density of these foods is generally greater than that of infant foods. Judicious food choices can be used to easily meet the protein needs of the young child.

Examples of combinations of foods that meet the recommended intakes for protein for 2-month-old, 6-month-old, 10-month-old, and 4-year-old children are given in table 2-12. The examples given include much less protein than most children consume. In fact, it would be difficult to provide sufficient energy in the diet if protein intakes were restricted to the recommended amounts. For example, 4-year-old children who consume the food listed receive approximately 500 kcal/day from these sources, leaving 1300 kcal that needs to be met from vegetables, fruits, fat, and sweets without additional protein from meats, breads, nuts, other cereal grains, or cheese (table 2-12).

The protein intakes of some children are a matter of concern. **Protein energy malnutrition** (PEM) has been reported in infants whose parents purposely withheld milk after episodes of vomiting or diarrhea and who were treated with clear liquids and in children from families who live in extreme poverty where there was

TABLE 2-12   *Foods That Provide Appropriate Protein Intakes for Young Children*

Age	2 Months	6 Months	10 Months	4 Years
Weight (kg)	6	7.5	9	20
Recommended protein intake (gm)	13	13	14	24
Foods to meet daily protein needs	38 oz human milk or 26 oz infant formula	38 oz human milk or 26 oz infant formula	24 oz iron fortified infant formula and 2 oz yogurt	16 oz milk, 1 T peanut butter, and 3 oz low-fat yogurt

marked restriction of protein intake. Children with multiple allergies often learn to control their feeding environment by refusing all protein-rich foods. Often they demonstrate catch-up growth when encouraged through reinforcement techniques to accept meats and other protein-rich foods to which they had no allergic reactions. Children who are hypersensitive in the oral area frequently refuse meat, eggs, milk, and dairy products if unlimited amounts of carbohydrates such as starches and sugars are available to them. Limited financial resources restrict the amounts of high-quality protein parents can purchase for their children. Without careful planning, the quality of a child's protein intake may be compromised. However, peanut butter and whole wheat bread sandwiches, beans and rice, eggs, and powdered milk are inexpensive high-quality protein sources.

Fat

Fat, the most energy concentrated nutrient, supplies between 40% and 50% of the energy consumed in infancy and approximately 40% of the energy consumed after infancy by individuals in developed countries. Because it is *energy* concentrated, it may be very important in the diet of children who are lean, physically active, and have a small appetite or in the diet of children with oral motor problems who can consume a limited volume of food. However, heavy, inactive children should limit the quantity of fat they consume to mediate their total energy intake and prevent a too rapid weight gain.

Essential fatty acids. Polyunsaturated **linoleic acid** has been conclusively proven to be an essential nutrient for both children and adults. Although arachidonic acid performs some of the same functions, it is considered to be an essential fatty acid only when linoleic acid intake is deficient.

Some investigators consider linolenic acid to be essential, although no specific deficiency of linolenic acid has been reported in humans.

One of the earliest manifestations of fatty acid deficiency recognized in animals was an increased basal metabolic rate. Infants who are fed formulas low in the essential fatty acid consume greater numbers of kcalories of energy than do those who consume adequate quantities of linoleic acid to maintain normal growth. Energy utilization has been reported to vary with intakes of linoleate up to 4% to 5% of total energy. It has been suggested that the ratio of triene/tetraene fatty acids in the blood serum can be used in assessing nutritional status of linoleic acid. A triene/tetraene ratio of 0.4 or less is considered indicative of normal fatty acid status, and a ratio greater than 0.4 is indicative of an insufficient intake of essential fatty acid.[25] Such biochemical evidence of deficiency appears when linoleic acid is less than 1% of the total energy. On this basis the minimal requirements for linoleic acid are considered to be approximately 1% of the kcalories consumed, and an optimal intake is thought to be 4% to 5% of the energy consumed.[26]

Recommended intakes. If less than 30% of energy intakes are derived from fat, a dry and unpalatable diet may result.

TABLE 2-13   *Foods as Sources of Fat for Infants*

Food	Fat (gm/oz)
Infant cereal, dry (12 T/oz)	1.2–2.4
Vegetable and meat dinners	.3–.6
Meat and vegetable dinners	.8–1.2
Strained and junior meats	1.5–2.9
Strained egg yolks	5.2
Commercial infant formula	1.1
Commercial infant soy formula	1.1

TABLE 2-14   *Foods as Sources of Fat for Preschool Children*

Food	Portion Size	Fat (gm)
Margarine	1 T	12
Mayonnaise	1 T	4.9
Butter	1 t	3.8
Cheddar cheese	1 oz	10
Peanut butter	1 T	8.1
Frankfurter, 5″ by ³/₄″	1	17
Broiled hamburger patty	2 oz	10.4
Chicken drumstick, skin	1	15.4
Egg	1 medium	4.9
Tuna, drained	¼ c	3.3
Ice cream	¼ c	3.5
Potato chips	10	7.0
Chicken breast, no skin	¼	1.6
Whole milk (3.3% fat)	½ c	4.1
2% milk	½ c	2.3
Yogurt, lowfat	½ c	1.8
Yogurt, whole milk	½ c	3.7

Recommended intakes of fat are controversial, especially in view of the recent work on blood lipid levels and future disease. However, the Healthy People 2000: Nutrition Objectives[27] list a reduction of dietary fat to an average of 30% of energy or less and an average saturated fat intake to less than 10% of energy intake for people 2 years and older. This recommendation is controversial. It has been calculated that food patterns containing 30% to 40% of energy as fat are more appropriate and more likely to support normal energy intakes and growth.[28] It has been suggested that diets that provide less than 30% of total energy or greater than 50% of total energy should be avoided for infants and young children.[15,29]

Food sources. Human milk, cow's milk, and commercially available infant formulas provide approximately 50% of energy as fat. Approximately 4% of the total energy in human milk and 1% of the energy in cow's milk are provided by linoleic acid. Commercially available infant formulas contain blends of vegetable oils and contribute greater amounts of linoleic acid.

The Committee on Nutrition of the American Academy of Pediatrics[24] has recommended that infant formulas contain a minimum of 300 mg of 18:2 fatty acids/100 kcal (2.7% of the energy content).

Prepared infant foods are relatively low in fat as compared with foods consumed by older children. Tables 2-13 and 2-14 list the amounts of fat provided by foods commonly consumed by infants and preschool children.[8]

Table 2-15 shows a sample of foods that provide the recommended 30% to 40% of energy as fat intake for a young child and provide adequate energy intake. Other nutrients, such as calcium and iron, may be limited on this restricted menu pattern.

Carbohydrates

Carbohydrates are the principal sources of dietary energy and supply between 40% and 50% of the energy consumed by most infants and children in the United States. Sugars and complex carbohydrates are the most important dietary carbohydrate sources.

Recommended intakes. Since glucose can be synthesized from amino acids and the glycerol moiety of fat, no specific recommendations for intake have been made. The Food and Nutrition Board of the National Research Council suggests that more than half the energy requirement

TABLE 2-15   *Sample Menu for a Young Child to Meet Guidelines for Fat Intake*

Age	Recommended Energy Intake (kcals)	Foods to Provide 30–40% of Energy Intake as Fat			
		Food	Amount	Energy	Fat (gm)
2 years	1300	Milk, 2%	20 oz	310	12
		Toast	2 sl	130	2
		Margarine	2 t	65	8
		Jelly	2 t	35	0
		Applesauce	½ c	100	trace
		Vegetable soup	½ c	30	1
		Saltines	4	60	1
		Rice	¼ c	65	trace
		Green beans	¼ c	10	0
		Margarine	2 t	65	8
		Chopped chicken	¼ c	100	4
		Graham crackers	2	70	3
		Cheddar cheese	1 oz	95	7
		Apple juice	6 oz	90	trace
		Ice cream	½ c	145	8
		TOTAL		1380	54
		% total energy intake as fat			35

beyond infancy be provided by carbohydrates with an emphasis on complex carbohydrates rather than sugars. They recommend minimum intakes of 50 to 100 gm/day.

Dietary fiber plays a role in prevention of many diseases. The Committee on Nutrition of the American Academy of Pediatrics[30] stated that more work must be done on the effect of a high-fiber diet on mineral status before firm recommendations can be made. However, the committee recommends a substantial intake of fiber to ensure normal laxation. As much fiber as 170 to 300 mg/kg may be desirable.[31] The inclusion of whole grain cereals, breads, fruits, and vegetables in the diet of preschool, school-age, and adolescent children is important.

Food sources. The predominant carbohydrate in the young infant's diet is lactose, found in human milk and cow's milk. It has become a common practice for parents to add starch (in the form of prepared cereals and ingredients of commercially prepared infant foods) and sucrose (which is added to fruits and some vegetables) to the infant's diet at 4 to 6 months of age (table 2-16). Many foods that provide complex carbohydrates for energy for the young child are relatively limited in fat content and provide a variety of other important nutrients.

Some foods contain carbohydrates and few other nutrients, whereas others contribute carbohydrates and other essential nutrients. Candy, cookies, and potato chips, for example, provide primarily energy, whereas cereal grains are important sources of the B vitamins; legumes offer amino acids, iron, and B vitamins as well as carbohydrates. Therefore, careful attention to the nutrients carried by the carbohydrate-containing foods is important in planning diets for children.

Most children prefer sweet foods. In fact, infants at birth appear to distinguish sugar water from plain water. They accept larger quantities

TABLE 2-16   Carbohydrates in Foods for Infants

Food	Carbohydrate (gm/oz)
Human milk	2.1
Prepared infant formulas	2.1
Homogenized milk	1.5
Infant cereals, dry	14.8–26.2
Strained and junior desserts	5.3–6.7
Strained and junior vegetable and meat dinners	2.5–3.2
Strained and junior meat and vegetable dinners	2.2–2.5
Strained and junior fruits	3.7–5.9
Strained and junior vegetables	1.9–4.7

of sugar-sweetened solutions than unsweetened mixtures.[32] Indiscriminate consumption of candy, cookies, carbonated beverages, and other sweetened drinks dulls the appetite for nutrient-rich foods, contributes to overweight, dental caries, and general poor nourishment and should be discouraged. The impact of these sucrose-containing foods on the incidence of dental caries is discussed in chapter 12.

Water

Even more important to the body than food is water. It functions as an essential component of body structure and as a solvent for minerals and other physiologically important compounds. It transports nutrients to and waste products from the cells and helps to regulate body temperature.

The percentage of body weight provided by water decreases from approximately 75% at birth to 60% at 1 year of age (see chapter 1). After 1 year of age intracellular water accounts for approximately 60% and extracellular water for 40% of total body water. The usual daily turnover of water for infants is about 15% of total body weight.

Recommended intakes. Water is lost by evaporation through the skin and respiratory tract (**insensible water loss**), through perspiration when the environmental temperature is elevated, and by elimination in the feces and the urine. During growth a positive water balance is necessary since additional water is obligated as a constituent of tissue and for increases in the volume of body fluids. The amount of water required for growth, however, is very small at all ages.

Water lost by evaporation in infancy and early childhood accounts for more than 60% of that needed to maintain homeostasis, as compared with 40% to 50% in the adult. At all ages approximately 24% of the basal heat loss is by evaporation of water through the skin and respiratory tract.[33] This amounts to 45 ml of insensible water loss per 100 kcal expended. Fomon[15] estimates evaporative water loss at 1 month of age to average 210 ml/day and at 1 year of age, 500 ml/day. Evaporative losses increase with fever and higher environmental temperature. Increases in humidity decrease respiratory loss. Loss of water in the feces averages 10 ml/kg/day in infancy.[34]

The volume of urine, in general, reflects fluid intake. It includes both water required to concentrate the solutes presented to the kidney for excretion and water in excess of the individual's need. The renal water requirement is determined by the diet and by the concentrating power of the kidney.

Ziegler and Fomon[34] developed a method for estimating the renal solute load by calculating the amount of dietary sodium, chloride, potassium, and urea (estimated to be 4 mOsm/gm of protein). The urinary water requirement can then be estimated from the sum of these values and is estimated at 1.5 ml/kcal of energy expenditure for infants. Balance studies of 5-year-old children showed intakes of 1100 ml/day; metabolic water contributed an additional 200 ml/day. Water intakes averaged 0.7 ml/kcal/day.[35] Ranges of average water requirements of infants and children are given in table 2-17.

Food sources. Fluid in liquids and food consumed are the primary source of water. In addition, metabolic water is created from the metabolism of protein, fat, and carbohydrate: 1 gm protein produces 4.1 ml water, 1 gm carbohydrate produces 5.5 ml water, and 1 gm fat produces 1.07 ml water. Table 2-18 gives the water content of representative foods consumed in infancy and early childhood. When milk is boiled the liquid evaporates and protein and electrolytes are concentrated. Boiled milk is an inappropriate food for infants.

Infants are vulnerable to water imbalance because of their relatively greater demand for insensible water and a renal concentrating capacity that may be less than that of adults.

Under normal environmental conditions infants do not need additional water.

Difficulties arise when formulas are improperly prepared (see chapter 4), when infants ingest limited volumes of milk during illness, and when renal losses are greater than usual, such as during episodes of vomiting and diarrhea.[15] To ensure adequate water intakes, infant formula should not be concentrated to more than 100 kcal/100 ml (30 kcal/oz).

As children grow older, the concentrating power of the kidney increases. Children learn to communicate and ask for water when they become thirsty. For older children difficulties in achieving water balance are unlikely in the absence of vomiting or diarrhea.

Minerals

Although minerals contribute only 3% to 4% of body weight, they play important roles in the regulation of body fluids, acid-base balance, and metabolic processes. Table 2-19 indicates the RDA recommended intake for minerals.

Calcium and phosphorus. Calcium and phosphorus occur in three systems in the body. In general, the calcium content of the body is about 2% of body weight and bone contains 99% of body calcium; the remaining 1% is found in body fluids and striated muscle. Bone contains 80% of body phosphorus; the remaining

TABLE 2-17   *Water Requirements of Infants and Children*

Age	Water Requirement (ml/kg/day)
3 days	80–100
10 days	125–150
3 months	140–160
6 months	130–155
1 year	120–135
2 years	115–125
6 years	90–100
10 years	70–85
14 years	50–60

From Barness LA: *Nutrition and nutritional disorders.* In Berman RE, Kliegman, RM: *Nelson textbook of pediatrics,* ed 14, Philadelphia, 1992, WB Saunders.

TABLE 2-18   *Percentage of Water in Selected Foods*

Food	Water (%)	Food	Water (%)
Human milk	85.2	Strained carrots	92.3
Cow's milk	87.4	Hamburger patty	68.3
Infant cereals, high protein	6.1	Chicken, cooked, dark meat	64.4
Infant cereals, rice	6.7	Egg, hard boiled	73.7
Strained macaroni and cheese	87.1	Oatmeal, cooked	83.6
Strained chicken with vegetables	90.0	Bread, white, enriched	35.6
Strained beef with vegetables	85.4	Carrots, cooked	91.2
Strained applesauce	88.6	Peas, canned	81.5
Strained peaches	80.1	Banana	75.7
Strained beef	80.6	Pears, canned	91.1
Strained peas	87.5		

From Gebhardt SE, Cutrufelli R, Matthews RH: *Composition of foods, baby foods, raw processed, prepared,* Agriculture Handbook No 8-3, Washington, DC, 1978, US Department of Agriculture.

TABLE 2-19   *Food and Nutrition Board, National Academy of Sciences—National Research Council Recommended Dietary Allowances, 1989, Designed for the Maintenance of Good Nutrition of Practically All Healthy People*

Category	Age (Years)	Calcium (mg)	Phosphorus (mg)	Magnesium (mg)	Iron (mg)	Zinc (mg)	Iodine (µg)
				Minerals			
Infants	0.0–0.5	400	300	40	6	5	40
	0.5–1.0	600	500	60	10	5	50
Children	1–3	800	800	80	10	10	70
	4–6	800	800	120	10	10	90
	7–10	800	800	170	10	10	120
Males	11–14	1200	1200	270	12	15	150
	15–18	1200	1200	400	12	15	150
Females	11–14	1200	1200	280	15	12	150
	15–18	1200	1200	300	15	12	150

Modified from *Recommended dietary allowances,* ed 10, National Research Council, Washington, DC, 1989, National Academy Press.

20% is found in striated muscle and blood serum. Calcium has a role in directing cell function and nerve impulses. Phosphorus is primarily involved in energy metabolism.

Plasma calcium and phosphorus levels are higher in children than in adults. Serum concentrations of the minerals are highest during early childhood, then decrease, paralleling decreases in the parathyroid hormone. The levels stabilize between 6 and 12 years of age and decline to adult values during adolescence.[36]

Calcium requirements vary throughout the lifetime of an individual. Calcium needs are greater during periods of rapid growth in childhood and adolescence. For children the optimal calcium intake refers to the levels of calcium consumption necessary for that individual to maximize peak adult bone mass. The calcium content of the body reflects both gender and stature. The amount of calcium accumulated during growth depends on the rate of growth and final stature attained. It has been estimated that the fetus acquires an average calcium intake of 97 mg/day.[37] The body of the full-term newborn infant has been estimated to contain approximately 27 gm of calcium.

TABLE 2-20   *Threshold Intake for Maximum Retention of Calcium*

Age Group	Threshold Intake (mg/day)	Retention (mg)
Infants	1090	503
Children	1390	246
Adolescents	1480	396
Young adults	957	114

Adapted from Matkovic AJCN 245S-60S, 1991.[38]

Skeletal requirements for calcium and phosphorus depend on body size and rates of growth. Requirements are greatest for taller, more rapidly growing children at any age. It has been demonstrated that body retention of calcium increases with increasing calcium intake to a threshold, beyond which calcium intake causes no further increase in calcium retention. These levels differ with age and are shown in table 2-20. Threshold at which balance no longer increased with intake were higher than the current RDA.[38]

TABLE 2-21   Calcium Intake and Absorption from Breast Milk and Formula for Infants

Age (mo.)	Feeding Method	Calcium Intake (mg)	Absorption (%)	Retention (mg)	RDA (mg/day)
0–6	Exclusively breast-fed	250–330	55–60	150–200	400
0–6	Formula, cow milk base	500–660	40	150–200	400
0–6	Formula, soy base	500–660	40	150–200	400

Adapted from NIH Consensus Statement, 1994.[40]

Recommended intakes. Attempts to establish recommended intakes of calcium have caused considerable controversy. Populations that have adapted to intakes of 200 to 400 mg/day without adverse effects have been identified, yet calcium accretion may be at that level during the pubertal growth spurt.[39] The recommended intake of 400 mg/day for the first 6 months of life has been planned to meet the needs of formula-fed infants who retain 25% to 30% of the calcium consumed in cow's milk. Although breast-fed infants ingest less calcium, estimated at 240 mg calcium from 750 ml of human milk, they retain approximately two-thirds of intake. The differences in calcium intake, absorption, and retention in breast milk– and cow milk–based formula for infants are shown in table 2-21.

Children may need two to four times as much calcium as adults since they are growing; thus 600 mg/day is recommended for the last half of the first year and 800 mg/day for 1 to 10 years of age. The adolescent growth spurt presents an added imperative for adequate calcium intake. Table 2-22 shows the remarkable increase in skeletal accumulation of calcium during early puberty. It is suggested that an intake of 1200 to 1500 mg calcium/day for growing adolescents might result in a higher peak adult bone mass. The National Institutes of Health proposed a calcium intake greater than the RDA in childhood and adolescence to support the development of adult peak bone mass (table 2-23).

Food sources. Milk and dairy products are the richest sources of calcium in the North American diet. Table 2-24 shows the calcium contribution

TABLE 2-22   Calcium Accumulation for Preadolescent and Pubertal Individuals

Age	Intake (mg/day)	Accumulation (mg/day)
Preadolescent	500–1000	140–165
Pubertal	500–1000	400–500

Adapted from NIH Consensus Statement, 1994.[40]

TABLE 2-23   Comparison of Current Recommendations for Calcium Intake

Age (years)	NIH Recommendation (mg/day) (a)	RDA Recommendation (mg/day) (b)
Infants, 0.0–0.5	400	400
Infants, 0.5–1.0	600	600
1–5	800	800
6–10	800–1200	800
11–24	1200–1500	1200

NIH: NIH Consensus Statement, 1994[40]
RDA: Recommended Dietary Allowances, 1989[1]
(a) assumed absorption rate of 30%
(b) assumed absorption rate of 40%

of selected milk and dairy products. Most dark green leafy vegetables also contribute appreciable amounts of calcium. Absorption of calcium fluctuates from 30% to 60% of intake and may be

TABLE 2-24   *Calcium in Milk and Dairy Products*

Food	Household Measure	Calcium (mg)
Human milk	4 oz	40
Cow's milk	4 oz	176
Powdered milk, nonfat, instant dry	⅓ c	276
Cheddar cheese	1 oz	204
Yogurt	½ c	207
Custard, baked	½ c	149
Chocolate pudding, cooked with milk	½ c	133
Chocolate pudding, instant	½ c	187
Ice cream	½ c	88

as high as 75% during rapid growth. Lactase increases absorption. Phytic and oxalic acid reduce absorption while vitamin D promotes calcium absorption. Protein and phosphorus intake may affect the metabolism of calcium but generally have little effect on calcium balance if calcium is ingested at recommended levels. Calcium absorption from carbonate, acetate, gluconate, citrate salts of calcium, and whole milk are similar.[41]

Phosphorus is found in combination with calcium in dairy products but also occurs in foods that contain little calcium. It occurs in most protein-rich foods such as meats, eggs, nuts, and legumes and is found in grains. Phosphate-containing additives are ingredients of many carbonated beverages, processed meats, cheese, and refrigerated bakery goods.

In a recent survey, calcium intakes of children whose food patterns included cow's milk were an average of 790 mg/day, calcium intakes of children who received milk substitutes were an average of 415 mg/day and calcium intakes of children receiving neither were an average of 200 mg/day.[42]

Plasma concentrations of calcium and phosphorus are greater in cord blood than in maternal blood. During the first two to three days of life the levels of calcium fall significantly. In healthy, full-term infants the decline is greatest in those who are formula-fed and least in those who receive human milk. The fall in plasma calcium levels is accompanied by a rise in plasma inorganic phosphorus levels.

After the initial decline, plasma calcium levels stabilize and tend to rise by the tenth day of life, the level being dependent on the calcium/phosphorus ratio of milk. Serum calcium concentrations in breast-fed infants are greater than those in formula-fed infants. Serum concentrations of phosphorus reflect the phosphorus content of the milk consumed.

One of the striking differences between human milk and cow's milk is the content of calcium and phosphorus. Cow's milk contains more than three times as much calcium and six times as much phosphorus as does human milk.

Manufacturers of infant formulas reduced the quantity of phosphorus in cow's milk formulas. The current recommendation for infant formulas is a 1.5:1.0 calcium to phosphorus ratio in early infancy and a 1.0:1.0 ratio after 1 year of age. Monitoring the amount of phosphorus consumed by infants in the early neonatal period continues to be important.[43]

Magnesium. Approximately 50% of the body's magnesium is deposited with calcium and phosphorus in bone, 25% is in muscle, and the remainder is found in soft tissue. Magnesium is the fourth most abundant mineral in the body and the second most abundant intercellular cation.

Recommended intakes. Although the data on magnesium requirements are sparse, Harris and Wilkinson[44] state that the newborn infant needs to retain 10.2 mg/day of magnesium to satisfy the requirement for growth. Fomon[15] estimates the requirement to be 16.5 mg/day during the first 4 months and suggests an intake of 25 mg/day. The average intake in early infancy is 30 mg/day, and the allowance is set at 40 mg/day for young infants and 60 mg/day for older infants. An intake of 6 mg/kg is recommended for ages 1 to 15 years.

Food sources. Magnesium is found in many foods. Nuts, soybeans, whole grains, and legumes are excellent sources. Magnesium also exists in all green plants as a component of chlorophyll. The magnesium content of human milk and cow's milk is approximately 4 mg/100 ml and 12 mg/100 ml, respectively.

Iron. Iron is the most abundant trace mineral in the body, accounting for approximately 75 mg/kg of the newborn infant.

The concentration of **hemoglobin** at birth averages 17 to 19 gm/100 ml of blood. During the first 6 to 8 weeks of life it decreases to approximately 10 to 11 gm/100 ml because of a shortened life span of the fetal cell and decreased **erythropoiesis.** After this age there is a gradual increase in hemoglobin concentration to 13 gm/100 ml at 2 years of age. During adolescence a sharp increase occurs in males at the time of the growth spurt. Infants, children, and adolescents need iron not only to maintain hemoglobin but also to increase the iron mass related to growth increases in body size.

Iron deficiency is the most common nutritional deficiency in North America. It occurs most frequently in 12- to 36-month-old children, in adolescent males, and in females during their childbearing years.[45] It may result from inadequate iron intakes, impaired absorption, or blood loss.

Iron deficiency. Iron deficiency results when body iron is diminished. There are three stages of depletion. The first is a decrease in iron status represented by a drop in plasma **ferritin.** The second is normocytic-iron deficient erythropoiesis, in which red blood cell protoporphyrin is elevated and transferrin saturation is reduced. The third stage is iron deficiency anemia, when red blood cells are **microcytic** and hypochromic and hemoglobin levels are reduced. Iron deficiency anemia is diagnosed when **transferrin** saturation falls below 16%; anemia is diagnosed when hemoglobin concentrations fall below 11 gm/100 ml and **hematocrit** values fall below 33%. Iron status is regulated by both absorption and bioavailability of iron from foods. Absorption of iron depends on the size of the iron stores. Absorption increases with iron depletion and decreases when stores are increased. Absorption is also increased when a greater supply of iron is needed for erythropoiesis (e.g., iron deficiency anemia).

Recommended intakes. Iron requirements of individual children vary with rates of growth, increasing blood volumes, iron stores, variations in menstrual losses of iron of adolescent females, and the timing of growth spurts of adolescents. Larger, more rapidly growing children have the greatest requirement for iron at any age.

Because of stored iron the healthy newborn can maintain satisfactory hemoglobin levels solely from human milk for 3 months, but beginning at age 3 months and continuing to age 3 years, a daily intake of 1 mg/kg to a maximum of 15 mg/day is usually considered appropriate. The RDA for 6 months to 3 years is set at 10 mg/day and considered adequate for most healthy children as shown in table 2-19. Iron loss during menstruation varies widely among females but is consistent from month to month in individuals. Average losses of blood of 15-year-old girls in a Swedish study were 33.8 ml per period, equivalent to an iron loss of approximately 0.5 mg/day.[46] To attain stores of 300 mg for both sexes by age 20 to 25 years, an intake of 10 mg/day is recommended for children. An additional 2 mg/day intake is recommended for males during the pubertal growth spurt and 5 mg/day for females starting with the pubertal growth spurt and menstruation and continuing through the menstrual years.[47]

Food sources. Diets in the United States have been estimated to provide iron amounts of 6 mg/1000 kcal. Muscle meats provide the richest and most usable sources. Other food sources include nuts, green vegetables, whole wheat flour, bread, and fortified cereal products.

Of the iron in pork, liver, and fish, 30% to 40% is in the form of heme iron, and of the iron in beef, lamb, and chicken, 50% to 60% is in the form of heme iron. These foods are sources of nonheme iron also, as are greens, vegetables, grains, legumes, and eggs. The iron content of human milk and cow's milk is 0.5 to 1.0 mg/L. During infancy, iron-fortified formulas and cereals fortified with reduced iron are primary food

TABLE 2-25   Selected Food Sources of Iron

Food	Household Measure	Iron (mg)
Iron-fortified formula	8 oz	2.9
Infant cereals, high protein	1 T	1.7
Infant cereals, rice	1 T	1.7
Strained vegetables with ham	2 T	0.1
Strained chicken with vegetables	2 T	0.1
Strained beef with vegetables	2 T	0.1
Strained beef	2 T	0.5
Hamburger, cooked	2 oz	1.2
Chicken, dark meat	1 oz	1.2
Frankfurter, 5″ by ¾″	1	0.7
Egg	1 medium	0.7
Pork and beans	¼ c	1.1
Peanut butter	1 T	0.3
Bread, enriched white	1 slice	0.7
Macaroni, enriched, cooked	¼ c	0.5
Carrots, cooked	¼ c	0.2
Orange	1 medium	0.1
Canned pears	¼ c	0.1
Cheerios	½ c	1.2
Rice Chex	½ c	1.0

sources. Table 2-25 lists representative sources of iron for infants and children.

Iron absorption from food. The percentage of iron absorbed from food depends on the presence of heme iron or nonheme iron, the combinations of food consumed together, and the iron reserves of the individual. Individuals with inadequate iron stores absorb approximately 35%; those with adequate iron stores absorb 25% of heme iron consumed. Individuals with deficient iron reserves may absorb as much as 20% of nonheme iron, whereas iron-replete individuals may absorb as little as 2%.[48] The presence of meat, which offers heme iron and the addition of ascorbic acid, increases the absorption of nonheme iron. Absorption is decreased by the inclusion of phytate and bran in the foods consumed at the same time. Absorption of nonheme iron varies widely depending on the composition of the meal. Overall, about 50% of the iron in human milk, 10% of the iron in cow's milk, and 4% of the iron in iron-fortified formula is absorbed. The addition of strained vegetables to the infant's diet significantly reduces the availability of iron from human milk.[49]

Many foods are fortified with iron salts. Of particular importance to persons concerned with the iron intakes of infants and children are those iron salts used to fortify the commercially prepared infant formulas, cereal grains, and cereals consumed so abundantly by children. Iron-fortified formulas contain 12 mg of iron per liter as ferrous sulfate. Cereals and baked products may be fortified with reduced iron, sodium iron pyrophosphate, or ferric orthophosphate.

Ferrous sulfate is the most bioavailable of the iron salts, but it is seldom used to fortify food because of difficulties in manufacturing. The percentage of absorption of reduced iron depends on the particle size, surface area, and porosity of the salts, which in turn determine the extent to which the particles dissolve in the acid of the stomach. Human studies indicated absorption is about 5% of that of ferrous sulfate. Fomon[45] feels this iron salt is not a reliable source of iron for infants.

Some pediatricians believe it may be advantageous for infants over 6 months of age to receive one feeding that includes not milk but iron-fortified cereal, vegetables, and fruit or fruit juice containing vitamin C.

A desirable iron status can be compromised by a low-energy diet, poor selection of foods, or any dietary extremes. Assuming that a well-chosen diet contains iron intakes of approximately 6 mg/1000 kcal, adolescents dieting to lose weight will be receiving minimal iron intakes. In addition to this, the common practice of choosing foods such as yogurt and cottage cheese as primary protein foods in a reducing diet results in an even lower dietary iron intake plus reducing absorption.

Ideally, regular monitoring of iron status should be provided for infants and adolescents, especially those with limited high-iron foods or those practicing various dietary extremes or restrictions.

The addition of iron to infant formulas has been controversial because of a belief that additional iron causes gastrointestinal distress. Because of the lack of evidence for gastrointestinal change caused by iron fortification of infant formulas and the positive effect fortification has had on the decrease of iron deficiency anemia in young children, the American Academy of Pediatrics has recommended that iron-fortified infant formulas be used for all formula-fed infants.[50] This view is supported by the general improvement of iron status as a result of increased iron intake from fortified formulas by those infants and young children enrolled in the Special Supplemental Food Program for Women, Infants, and Children (WIC).[51] Long-term follow-up of iron- and non–iron-supplemented children indicates a developmental advantage for those children who did not suffer from anemia.[52]

Zinc. Zinc is distributed throughout all cells and tissues. The fetus contains approximately 20 mg/kg. During infancy, serum zinc levels are determined primarily by the zinc content of the milk consumed.[53]

Poor growth reflected as poor weight gain and linear growth and depressed immune function have been reported from many countries.[54,55]

It appears that many preschool and school-age children from low-income and middle-income families may be ingesting inadequate amounts of zinc. Studies in Denver of Head Start children 3.5 to 6 years of age whose heights were less than the 5th percentile revealed that 69% had low plasma and hair zinc concentrations. Improvement was noted by increasing daily zinc intake from 0.4 to 0.8 mg/kg/day.[56]

Recommended intakes. Recommendations for intake have been made from studies of zinc intakes of apparently well-nourished individuals and from studies of zinc balance. Growth velocity is the main determinant of the zinc requirement in childhood. The infant is born without zinc stores and rapidly becomes dependent on an adequate supply of biologically available zinc.

Variations in plasma zinc concentrations during growth reflect the continual utilization and depletion of body stores of zinc. Declines occur during periods of rapid growth. Requirement for zinc at 4 to 6 months of age is 50% less than at 1 month.[53] Breast-fed infants receive an average of 2 mg/day during the first month and show no signs of depletion because of the high bioavailability of zinc in breast milk.[57] The recommendation for infants is 5 mg/day during the first year of life and 10 mg/day during childhood. Intakes of children 1 to 3 years of age are estimated to average 5 mg/day; those of children 3 to 5 years of age, 5 to 7 mg/day; and those of adolescents, 13 mg/day.[58]

Food sources. Seafoods and meats are rich sources of bioavailable zinc. Cereals and legumes also contain significant amounts, but refining processes destroy much zinc. Frequently zinc is added back to foods, especially breakfast cereals. Fiber and phytate in plants tend to bind zinc and decrease absorption. The bioavailability ranges from 20% to 30%. Estimates of zinc in human milk and cow's milk range from 3 to 5 mg/L. Picciano and Guthrie[59] found ranges of 0.14 to 3.95 mg/L in milk of 50 lactating women. Colostrum contains 20 mg/L, three to five times as much as later milk. Levels of zinc in human milk decline after two months of lactation and may fall below 1 mg/L. Infant formulas are supplemented with zinc and contain 3 to 4 mg/L. Table 2-26 gives the zinc content of representative foods consumed by infants and children.

Iodine. Of the iodine in the human adult, 70% to 80% is concentrated in the thyroid gland, which synthesizes its only functional compounds, thyroxine and triiodothyronine. The remaining iodine in the body is distributed in the blood, skin, and other tissues.

Recommended intakes. The breast-fed infant has an iodine intake of 10 to 20 μg/100 kcal from an adequately fed lactating mother. The current recommendations are 40 and 50 μg for younger and older infants. This recommendation increases from 70 to 150 μg/day throughout childhood. It has been suggested that requirements for 8- to 16-year-old children may not be much greater than 56 μg/day.[15] Average

TABLE 2-26   Selected Food Sources of Zinc

Food	Household Measure	Zinc (mg)
Cow's milk	4 oz	0.5
Ground beef, cooked	2 oz	3.0
Chicken drumstick	1	1.4
Egg	1 large	0.5
Oatmeal, cooked	½ c	0.6
Bread, white	1 slice	0.2
Bread, whole wheat	1 slice	0.5
Green beans, canned	¼ c	0.2
Spinach	½ c	0.7
Banana	½ medium	0.1
Orange	1 medium	0.1

intakes of iodine in the United States are five to ten times the recommended amounts. However, wide variations in iodine intakes may be experienced by individuals, depending on sources of food and geographical locations.

Food sources. Iodized salt, bread made with iodate as a dough conditioner, milk, and seafood are excellent sources of dietary iodine. The fact that the iodine content of food is determined by the soil in which it is grown is no longer significant in the etiology of iodine deficiency. Food consumed in one area is often transported from another. The iodine content of milk and dairy products depends on whether the cattle have been given iodine-supplemented feed or iodized salt blocks. Milk iodine levels may be as high as 450 µg/L.

The amounts of iodine absorbed from environments polluted by the combustion of fossil fuels and organic matter can be significant.

Selenium. It is difficult to assess both selenium intake and status because humans apparently have the capability to adjust homeostasis over a wide range of intakes, thus invalidating balance studies. Little is known about the selenium requirements of children, so the recommendations have been extrapolated from adult values plus a generous factor for growth. The recommendations are for 10 to 15 µg/day selenium for the first year of life and 20 to 30 µg/day during childhood.

Food sources. Seafood, kidney, and liver are primary food sources of selenium. Other meats and grains are lesser sources of this nutrient.

Remaining Trace Elements

The fact that only safe and adequate intakes have been recommended for the remaining trace minerals—copper, manganese, fluoride, chromium, and molybdenum—indicates the lack of information necessary to define specific needs during the life cycle. These estimated safe values are shown in table 2-27.

Less than adequate intake during infancy and childhood may occur in cases of generalized malnutrition or in infants maintained on nutrient-deficient formulas. Infants and children who consume a variety of foods are likely to consume appropriate quantities of these nutrients.

Fluoride. Fluoride in the body is concentrated in the bones and teeth. The concentration in bones increases linearly with increased intakes.

The role of fluoride as an essential trace mineral lies in its ability to reduce the incidence of dental caries. It has not been proved essential to survival. Epidemiological studies have repeatedly proved that there is a close relationship between tooth decay and the amount of fluoride ingested during tooth development.[60] When the fluoride content of community drinking water has been adjusted to a level of 1 ppm (1 mg/L), the incidence of dental caries has been reduced 40% to 60%. Although the effect is especially important during tooth development, fluoride has also been shown to be beneficial to adults.

Recommended intakes. The Committee on Nutrition of the American Academy of Pediatrics[61] recommends that supplemental fluoride dosages be adjusted to the fluoride content of the water supply (table 2-28). In communities with a fluoride content less than 0.7 mg/L in the water supply, fluoride supplements of 0.25 mg/day are recommended from 2 weeks to 2 years of age, 0.5 mg/day between 2 and 3 years of age, and 1 mg/day after 3 years of age. It is suggested that children whose drinking water

TABLE 2-27   *Estimated Safe and Adequate Daily Dietary Intakes of Selected Vitamins and Minerals*

		Vitamins	
Category	Age (Years)	Biotin (µg)	Pantothenic Acid (mg)
Infants	0–0.5	10	2
	0.5–1	15	3
Children and adolescents	1–3	20	3
	4–6	25	3–4
	7–10	30	4–5
	11+	30–100	4–7

		Trace Elements†				
Category	Age (Years)	Copper (mg)	Manganese (mg)	Fluoride (mg)	Chromium (µg)	Molybdenum (µg)
Infants	0–0.5	0.4–0.6	0.3–0.6	0.1–0.5	10–40	15–30
	0.5–1	0.6–0.7	0.6–1.0	0.2–1.0	20–60	20–40
Children and adolescents	1–3	0.7–1.0	1.0–1.5	0.5–1.5	20–80	25–50
	4–6	1.0–1.5	1.5–2.0	1.0–2.5	30–120	30–75
	7–10	1.0–2.0	2.0–3.0	1.5–2.5	50–200	50–150
	11+	1.5–2.5	2.0–5.0	1.5–2.5	50–200	75–250

From *Recommended dietary allowances,* ed 10, National Research Council, Washington, DC, 1989, National Academy Press.
†Since the toxic levels for many trace elements may be only several times usual intakes, the upper levels for the trace elements given in this table should not be habitually exceeded.

TABLE 2-28   *Supplemental Fluoride Dosage Schedule (mg/day)* *

	Concentration of Fluoride in Drinking Water (ppm)		
Age	<0.3	0.3–0.7	>0.7
2 weeks to 2 years	0.25	0	0
2 to 3 years	0.50	0.25	0
3 to 16 years	1.00	0.50	0

From Committee on Nutrition: *Pediatrics* 63:150, 1979.
*2.2 mg of sodium fluoride contains 1 mg of fluoride.

contains between 0.3 and 0.7 mg of fluoride ppm receive 0.25 mg between 2 and 3 years of age and 0.5 mg between 3 and 16 years of age.

Food sources. All foods and water contain very small amounts of fluoride. Seafood contains greater amounts. Food produced and prepared in areas in which the water is fluoridated reflect the fluoride content of the water. Cow's milk has a fluoride content of about 20 µg/L[62] and human milk contains 5 to 25 µg/L and reflects maternal intake.[63] Average intakes of 15- to 19-year-old males are estimated to be 1.85 mg/day in areas with fluoridated water supplies and 0.86 mg/day in those with nonfluoridated water. Beverages and water contributed approximately 75% of intake.[64]

The recommendation of a safe intake of fluoride for younger children is set at a maximum of 2.5 mg to avoid tooth mottling. Suggested safe ranges of intake are 0.5 to 1.0 mg for the first year and 0.5 to 1.5 mg until 3 years of age.

Infants who ingest low levels of fluoride, that is, those who receive human milk or formulas prepared with nonfluoridated water, should receive fluoride supplements of 0.25 mg/day until 2 years of age.

There is an increasing concentration of fluoride in the food chain. Processing food with fluoridated water significantly increases its fluoride content. The fluoride content of ready-to-drink fruit juices increases five to twenty times when fluoridated water is used in processing. The fluoride content of infant cereals is influenced by the fluoride content of the water in which they were produced. Mechanically deboning meat increases the fluoride content of the end products because bone chips are incorporated during processing. Infant formula is no longer manufactured with fluoridated water. Infants who drink ready-to-feed formula do not receive fluoride; those whose formula is prepared with water often do receive some fluoride, depending on the quantity in the water supply.

Mottling and fluorosis of tooth enamel. When the fluoride concentrations of drinking water increase above 2 ppm, mottling (a brown stain on the teeth) during tooth development occurs. The incidence and severity of the manifestation increase as the fluoride content of the water increases. At levels of 8 ppm almost all individuals who consumed the water during tooth development have extensively mottled teeth.[65] In areas with a high natural concentration of fluoride, it has become a practice to dilute fluoride in water supply to no more than 1.2 ppm.

Fluorosis, usually manifested as opaque spots or streaks on the enamel of permanent teeth and not discernible by the layperson, has been noted in 63% of children by the time they were 7 to 12 years of age in a community without fluoridated water when the use of fluoride supplements was common.[65] Leverett suggests that the definition of the optimum concentration of fluoride in community water supplies needs to be reassessed.

Copper. Although copper deficiency is rare in humans, it has been demonstrated in severely malnourished children. About half of the copper that accumulates during gestation is in the fetal liver and offers some protection against early deficiency. Again efficient homeostatic mechanisms rule out determination of requirements by the use of balance studies.

Breast-fed infants have thrived on a copper intake of about 40 to 60 µg/kg/day;[66] thus the estimation for an intake of 0.4 to 0.6 mg/day. Infant formulas are supplemented with copper to the level of 60 µg/100 kcal of energy. The relatively stable need for copper of 40 µg/kg/day is demonstrated in the estimation of 1 to 2 mg/day in childhood.[26]

Manganese. Manganese status is difficult to assess. Little is known about the manganese requirement of infants, and manganese deficiency has not been demonstrated in infants. The estimated safe intake for infants and children is derived and set at 0.3 to 1.0 mg in the first year and 1 to 3 mg/day in childhood.

Chromium. The difficulty in assessing chromium status and requirement has led to extrapolation of safe intakes based on expected food intake. This is made more difficult by the limited data on chromium content of foods. These factors have led to the wide range of estimated safe intakes of 10 to 60 µg/day in infancy and 20 to 200 µg/day in childhood.

Molybdenum. Human milk contains small amounts of molybdenum. Little is known about bioavailability. Because deficiency has not been easily demonstrated, it is assumed that the requirement is small and that it can be met with usual intakes of food.

Vitamins

Because of vitamins' functions in metabolic processes, the amounts required are determined by intakes of energy, protein, and fats. Exact needs are difficult to define.

Most vitamins cross the placenta and accumulate in the fetus at greater concentrations than in the mother. Maternal hypovitaminemia will be reflected in the fetus.

Vitamins A and E and beta-carotene concentrations are lower in the newborn infant's blood than in the mother's. The concentration of water-soluble vitamins in the blood of the neonate is higher than in that of the mother.[67]

Fat-soluble vitamins in excess of need are not excreted but are stored. Reserves can be

TABLE 2-29   *Food and Nutrition Board, National Academy of Sciences—*
National Research Designed for the Maintenance
of Good Nutrition of Practically All Healthy People

Category	Age (Years)	Fat-Soluble Vitamins			
		Vitamin A (μg RE)[a]	Vitamin D (μg)[b]	Vitamin E (mg α-TE)[c]	Vitamin K (μg)
Infants	0.0–0.5	375	7.5	3	5
	0.5–1.0	375	10.0	4	10
Children	1–3	400	10.0	6	15
	4–6	500	10.0	7	20
	7–10	700	10.0	7	30
Males	11–14	1000	10.0	10	45
	15–18	1000	10.0	10	65
Females	11–14	800	10.0	8	45
	15–18	800	10.0	8	55

Modified from *Recommended dietary allowances,* ed 10, National Research Council, Washington, DC, 1989, National Academy Press.
[a]Retinol equivalents. 1 retinol equivalent = 1 μg retinol or 6 μg β-carotene.
[b]As cholecalciferol. 10 μg cholecalciferol = 400 IU of vitamin D.
[c]α-Tocopherol equivalents. 1 mg d-α tocopherol = 1 α-TE.

accumulated. The **toxicity** of excessive intakes of vitamins A and D is well documented.

In contrast to vitamins A, D, E, and K, the water-soluble vitamins are stored in small amounts and deficiencies can be expected to occur in a relatively short period if the nutrient is absent from dietary intake.

Fat-soluble Vitamins

Vitamin A. The term "vitamin A" is used for a group of compounds needed for vision and growth, as well as the immune system. Vitamin A needs can be met by dietary intake of (1) preformed retinoids with vitamin A activity from animal products or (2) carotenoid precursors of vitamin A such as β-carotene and α-carotene from plant foods. The vitamin A activity in foods is currently expressed as retinol equivalents (RE). The definition of 1 RE is 1 μg of all-trans-retinol, 6 μg of all-trans-β-carotene or 12 μg of other provitamin α-carotenoids.

Recommended intakes. Recommendations for intakes of vitamin A are interpolated from infant and adult needs even though children

under age 5 are at greatest risk for vitamin A deficiency and this deficiency is most commonly due to a deficient dietary intake.[68] The recommendation for vitamin A intake for infants is based on the composition of human milk and the usual intake of healthy infants. Human milk contains 40 to 70 μg/dl of retinol and 20 to 40 μg/dl of carotenoids. Therefore the recommendation is set at 375 RE/day. The range of intake that supports normal growth is wide because infants have shown no signs of deficiency on one third of the recommended amount. After the first year of life vitamin A recommendations for children are extrapolated on adult needs and body weight. The recommended vitamin A intake is 400 RE at age 1 and increases to 700 RE by age 10 years. Table 2-29 indicates the recommendations for vitamin A intake by age. Intakes of greater than 10 times the RDA for age can cause toxicity over time.

Food sources. Pre-formed retinol is most abundant in liver and fish liver oils; significant amounts are also found in whole and fortified milk and in eggs. Active carotenoids are present

TABLE 2-30 *Selected Food Sources of Vitamin A*

Food	Household Measure	Vitamin A (μg RE)
Cow's milk, 2%	8 oz	150
Human milk	8 oz	178
Cheddar cheese	1 oz	90
Egg	1 large	84
Liver, beef	1 oz	3000
Butter	1 t	35
Apricots, canned	¼ c	79
Orange	1 medium	27
Peach	1 medium	47
Watermelon, diced	½ c	29
Carrots	¼ c	958
Acorn squash, baked, mashed	¼ c	22
Sweet potatoes, mashed	60 gm	256
Green peas	¼ c	27
Spinach, cooked	¼ c	399
Tomatoes, canned	¼ c	36
Margarine	1 T	140
Infant formula	8 oz	144
Beef	1 oz	0
Chicken	1 oz	2
Tuna	1 oz	5
Cheerios	½ c	150
Rice Chex	½ c	1
Oatmeal	¼ c	2
Infant rice cereal, dry	4 T	1
Kix	½ c	125

in carrots and dark, leafy, green vegetables. Foods fortified with vitamin A such as milk and margarine are also reasonable sources. Table 2-30 indicates reasonable sources of this nutrient for young children. Absorption of vitamin A is positively affected by dietary fat, protein, and vitamin E and negatively affected by oxidizing agents in food.

Vitamin D. Vitamin D (calciferol) is essential for skeletal formation. Ultraviolet light on skin is required to synthesize vitamin D_3 (cholecalciferol) from less active forms.

Humans can meet their vitamin D requirement from skin exposure to sunlight. Variables that affect the amount of vitamin D synthesized are amount of skin exposed; higher melanin content of skin, which requires a longer exposure; the angle of the sun; and the age of the individual. It has been suggested that 10 minutes of summer sun on face and hands will produce 400 IU or 10 μg of vitamin D_3.[69]

Recommended intakes. It is difficult to establish a recommended intake, since an individual can meet vitamin D needs through sun exposure alone. However, since many individuals require a dietary source to have adequate vitamin D, the recommendation is based on a level that will meet needs without sunlight. Since human milk has a questionable ability to meet the vitamin D needs of the infant without another dietary source, it is recommended that breast-fed infants who are not regularly exposed to sunlight receive vitamin D supplements of 5 to 7.5 μg/day. The appropriate nature of this recommendation is borne out in recent reports of rickets in infants who are exclusively breast-fed and whose mothers have a marginal nutritional status.[70] The recommendation for infants who receive formula is 7.5 μg/day. From 6 months of age through adulthood, that is, until peak bone mass is acquired, 10 μg vitamin D has been set as the recommendation. These recommendations are shown in table 2-29. Intakes of five times the RDA have demonstrated toxicity.

Although 2.5 μg/day cholecalciferol prevents rickets and ensures adequate absorption of calcium and normal mineralization of bone in the infant, better calcium absorption and some increase in growth have been noted with intakes of 10 μg cholecalciferol. Vitamin D can be formed by the action of sunlight on the skin. The amount formed depends on several variables, and amounts formed cannot be readily measured.

Food sources. Eggs, butter, and fortified margarine are recognized sources of vitamin D. Milk is supplemented with cholecalciferol to a level of 10 μg/qt as are infant formulas. The cholecalciferol content in breast milk is 0.63 to 1.25 μg/L.[71]

Vitamin E. Vitamin E functions as an antioxidant. It stabilizes cell membranes, regulates oxidation reactions, and protects polyunsaturated fatty acids (PUFA) and Vitamin A.

The most biologically active form of vitamin E is α-tocopherol, which is relatively inefficiently absorbed at 20% to 80%.

Recommended intakes. The recommendation for infants is 3 mg. The remaining recommendations are increased with increasing body size. Thus the recommendation is 4 mg α-TE for the remainder of the first year to 7 mg α-TE in childhood.

Defining appropriate intakes for vitamin E is complicated by large variations in the susceptibility to peroxidation of fatty acids in the diet and tissues. Requirements are related to the polyunsaturated fatty acid content of cellular structures. An assumption is made that requirements increase with body weight until maturity. An intake of 4 mg α-TE at 9 kg increasing to 10 mg α-TE at 45 kg of body weight should be satisfactory in diets providing 4% to 7% of energy as linoleic acid.

Newborns have low stores of vitamin E. If an adequate supply is not provided, a deficiency characterized by hemolytic anemia will occur. Newborns' diets should include a tocopherol content of 1 mg/gm of polyunsaturated fatty acids.[72]

Food sources. Vegetable oils provide tocopherol as do wheat germ and nuts. Vitamin E is vulnerable to loss in food processing, storage, and preparation.

Vitamin K. Since vitamin K functions in prothrombin formation, a prophylactic intramuscular dose of 0.5 to 1 mg of vitamin K is usually given to infants at birth as a protection against hemorrhagic disease of the newborn.[73,74] After receiving this dose, human beings are able to synthesize vitamin K from the bacteria in their gut. Infant formulas contain 4 μg/100 kcal. Since little is known about the vitamin K requirement, the RDA is set at 1 μg/kg/day or 5 to 65 μg/day depending on size. Vitamin K supplement is needed only for children who malabsorb fat.

Water-Soluble Vitamins

Vitamin C. Ascorbic acid functions in collagen synthesis, resistance to infection, and absorption of iron. An intake of 10 mg/day of vitamin C is adequate to prevent and cure scurvy in humans. It does not, however, provide for acceptable reserves. Breast-fed infants consuming 7 to 12 mg of vitamin C have been protected from scurvy.

Recommended intakes. An intake of 25 mg/day should provide an adequate margin of safety.[75] However, the RDA for infants is set at 30 to 35 mg/day. In relation to body weight, the vitamin C requirement of older children is higher than that of adults; thus the recommendation increases from 40 to 60 mg/day over time as shown in table 2-31.

Food sources. Fruits and vegetables are the primary sources of vitamin C in food patterns as indicated in table 2-32.

B Vitamins

Thiamin (vitamin B_1), riboflavin (vitamin B_2), niacin, pantothenic acid, and biotin are involved in intermediary metabolism. They are central to the metabolism of all cells and function as coenzymes in specific reactions along the glycolytic, tricarboxylic acid and pentose pathways.

Thiamin. This vitamin functions as a coenzyme used in energy metabolism; it also supports nervous system function. The requirement for thiamin is related to energy intake. Studies of thiamin requirements of infants are sparse. Those available suggest that the minimum requirement of infants is approximately 0.17 mg/day. For preadolescent children, 3 mg/1000 kcal was demonstrated as adequate.[76] Another study of 14- to 17-year-old males indicated that 0.4 mg/1000 kcal meets their minimum requirement.[77]

Recommended intakes. An intake of 0.3 to 0.4 mg of thiamin has been suggested for infants, and an intake of 0.5 mg/1000 kcal or 0.7 to 1.5 mg/day has been suggested as appropriate for children. These suggestions are reflected in the RDA (table 2-31).

Food sources. Thiamin is abundant in whole grains, brewer's yeast, pork, legumes, and nuts. Enriched bread and cereal products are also reasonable sources of this nutrient. Important thiamin antagonists are tea, coffee, and rice bran, which may increase requirements because they interfere with absorption and utilization of the nutrient.

TABLE 2-31   *Food and Nutrition Board, National Academy of Sciences—*
National Research Designed for the Maintenance
of Good Nutrition of Practically All Healthy People

Category	Age (Years)	Water-Soluble Vitamins						
		Vitamin C (mg)	Thiamin (mg)	Riboflavin (mg)	Niacin (mg NE)[a]	Vitamin B$_6$ (mg)	Folate (µg)	Vitamin B$_{12}$ (µg)
Infants	0.0–0.5	30	0.3	0.4	5	0.3	25	0.3
	0.5–1.0	35	0.4	0.5	6	0.6	35	0.5
Children	1–3	40	0.7	0.8	9	1.0	50	0.7
	4–6	45	0.9	1.1	12	1.1	75	1.0
	7–10	45	1.0	1.2	13	1.4	100	1.4
Males	11–14	50	1.3	1.5	17	1.7	150	2.0
	15–18	60	1.5	1.8	20	2.0	200	2.0
Females	11–14	50	1.1	1.3	15	1.4	150	2.0
	15–18	60	1.1	1.3	15	1.5	180	2.0

Modified from *Recommended dietary allowances,* ed 10, National Research Council, Washington, DC, 1989, National Academy Press.

[a]NE (niacin equivalent) is equal to 1 mg of niacin or 60 mg of dietary tryptophan.

TABLE 2-32   *Selected Food Sources*
of Vitamin C

Food	Household Measure	Vitamin C (mg)
Human milk	8 oz	12
Cow's milk	8 oz	3
Infant formula	8 oz	16
Broccoli, cooked	1 spear	22
Brussels sprouts	¼ c	18
Cabbage, raw, chopped	¼ c	11
Cabbage, cooked, wedge	¼ c	9
Cantaloupe, diced	½ c	34
Grapefruit	½	39
Orange	1 medium	70
Orange juice	½ c	48
Potato, boiled (2½ inch)	½	5
Strawberries	1 c	85
Tomato, raw, (2⅛ inch)	1	22
Tomatoes, canned	½ c	18
Tomato juice	½ c	22
Cheerios	½ c	6
Rice Chex	½ c	6

Riboflavin. This vitamin functions as part of the enzyme system used in energy metabolism; it also supports normal vision and skin health. Although signs of riboflavin deficiency are unusual, very low riboflavin intakes may interfere with growth.

Recommended intakes. Riboflavin needs are related to energy expenditure. A breast-fed infant is estimated to consume riboflavin at 0.26 to 0.48 mg/1000 kcal of energy/day. It is believed that riboflavin at 0.6 mg/1000 kcal of energy should be taken to meet the needs of all humans. The increase in body size translates into a recommendation of riboflavin at 0.4 to 0.5 mg/day for infants and 0.8 to 1.8 mg/day for children. These recommendations are shown in table 2-31.

Urinary excretion of riboflavin is low in adults and in children maintained on diets containing up to 0.5 mg/1000 kcal; it increases as riboflavin intakes increase. The minimum requirement is thought to be 0.85 mg/day.[72]

Food sources. Riboflavin is found abundantly in dairy products, meat, poultry, and fish as shown in table 2-33.

TABLE 2-33   *Selected Food Sources of Riboflavin*

Food	Household Measure	Riboflavin (mg)
Human milk	8 oz	0.09
Cow's milk	8 oz	0.48
Prepared infant formula	8 oz	0.16–0.24
Cheddar cheese	1 oz	0.11
Infant cereals, high protein	1 T	0.06
Infant cereals, rice	1 T	0.06
Farina	½ c	0.06
Oatmeal	½ c	0.03
Macaroni, enriched	¼ c	0.03
Broccoli	1 spear	0.03
Green peas	¼ c	0.04
Spinach	¼ c	0.09

Niacin. This vitamin is part of the enzyme system used in energy metabolism; it also supports health of the nervous and digestive systems, and skin. The niacin requirement is linked to tryptophan (an essential amino acid), thus the need for niacin equivalents. The fact that tryptophan is converted to niacin makes basic requirements for niacin difficult to determine. Sixty milligrams of tryptophan is equivalent to 1 mg of niacin and thus considered to be 1 niacin equivalent (NE). Minimum requirements appear to be 4.4 mg/1000 kcal.[72]

Recommended intakes. The niacin and tryptophan content in human milk is 1.5 mg/L and 210 mg/L, respectively, and the NE content is about 7 mg/1000 kcal. Little is known about the NE requirements of infants and children; therefore the recommendations are based on the adult level of 6.6 mg/1000 kcal. This translates to 5 to 6 mg/day in infancy and increases from 9 to 20 mg/day with increasing age and body size as shown in table 2-31.

Food sources. Meat contains both niacin and tryptophan and is a good source of the nutrient. In general, protein is about 1% tryptophan.

Vitamin B_6. Pyridoxine functions as part of the enzyme system used in amino acid and fatty acid metabolism. Since vitamin B_6 functions in amino acid metabolism, the requirement increases with increasing protein intake.

Recommended intakes. Dietary needs are roughly proportional to protein intake because of this nutrient's many roles in amino acid metabolism. The recommended intake of vitamin B_6 for infants is based on experience with proprietary formulas and an intake of 0.015 mg/gm protein or 0.4 mg/1000 kcal. An intake of 1.4 gm of vitamin B_6 with an intake of 60 gm of protein should be adequate. A generous intake for adolescents would be 2 gm/day.[72] The recommendation for infants is 0.3 to 0.6 mg/day and the recommendation from age 1 through childhood is 0.02 mg/gm of protein or 1 to 2 gm/day based on age and body size.

Food sources. Vitamin B_6 is found in chicken, fish, pork, eggs, oats, wheat, and peanuts. Milk and beef are poor sources of vitamin B_6. Foods as sources of vitamin B_6 are shown in table 2-34.

Folate. Folacin functions as part of the coenzyme used in new cell synthesis. The requirement for folacin in infancy is estimated to be 5 µg/kg of body weight.[78] For older children and adults, folacin needs are extrapolated from those of infants. Herbert believes 3.6 µg/kg to be an adequate intake from birth to 1 year, and 3 µg/kg is adequate for older children and adolescents.[78]

Recommended intakes. The folate content of human milk is used as the basis of the recommendation for folate intake for infants for the first year of life. The recommendation is for 3.6 µg/kg/day or 25 to 35 µg. The recommendation for children is interpolated from adult data and set at 50 to 200 µg based on size as shown in table 2-31.

Food sources. Folacin is found in a wide variety of foods. Yeast, leafy vegetables, legumes, and some fruits are particularly good sources of folacin.

Vitamin B_{12}. Cyanocobalamin functions as part of the coenzyme used in new cell synthesis.

Recommended intakes. The vitamin B_{12} allowance for infants is based on the content in the milk of lactating women with adequate vitamin B_{12} and a margin of safety, that is, 0.3 µg/day

TABLE 2-34 *Selected Food Sources of Vitamin B₆*

Food	Household Measure	Vitamin B₆ (mg)
Cow's milk	1 c	0.1
Human milk	1 c	0.03
Infant cereals, high protein	1 T	0.02
Infant cereals, rice	1 T	0.01
Infant dinners, vegetable and bacon	1 T	0.01
Infant dinners, vegetable and chicken	1 T	0.01
Strained beef	1 T	0.01
Strained chicken	1 T	0.03
Beef	3½ oz	0.27
Chicken	3½ oz	0.47
Peanut butter	1 T	0.06
Egg	1 large	0.07
Whole wheat bread	1 slice	0.05
White bread	1 slice	0.01
Green peas, canned	¼ c	0.03
Tomatoes, canned	¼ c	0.05
Squash, frozen	¼ c	0.04
Banana	1 medium	0.71
Orange juice	½ c	0.05
Strawberries	½ c	0.04

or 0.05 µg/kg body weight. For formula-fed infants the Committee on Nutrition of the American Academy of Pediatrics[79] recommends an intake of 0.15 µg/100 kcal. Herbert recommends an intake of 0.3 to 0.5 µg/day in infancy with gradual increases based on body size to 2 µg/day in adolescents.[80] The current RDAs are similar with a recommendation of 0.05 µg/kg body weight or a total intake of 0.7 to 2.0 µg/day.

Food sources. Animal products are the primary source of vitamin B₁₂ in diets.

Other Vitamins

Biotin. This vitamin functions as part of the coenzyme system used in energy metabolism, fat synthesis, amino acid metabolism, and glycogen synthesis. Biotin is essential for protein metabolism. However, there are no definitive data on biotin requirements; therefore the estimated safe levels of intake (10 to 15 µg/day in infancy) are based on observation and the content of human milk. The biotin in human milk, which is readily bioavailable, has been reported at levels up to 20 µg/L.[81]

Recommended intakes. Estimated safe levels for children are gradually increased with age from 20 to 100 µg/day. These recommendations are shown in table 2-31.

Food sources. Biotin is available from whole grains, liver, and yeast.

Pantothenic acid. This vitamin functions as part of the coenzyme used in energy metabolism. Although pantothenic acid has been demonstrated as metabolically important, deficiency has not been clinically recognized in humans.

Recommended intakes. Again, the provisional recommendation for safe intake is based on observation and measurements from human milk. Thus the safe intake has been set at 2 to 3 mg/day for infants and gradually increases from 3 to 7 mg/day with age.

Food sources. Meats, whole grains, and legumes are primary sources of pantothenic acid.

Usual intakes. Vitamins reported to be most often consumed in less than appropriate amounts by preschool and school-age children are riboflavin and vitamins A, C, and B₆.[82] Because goat's milk is folate deficient, attention must be given to that vitamin if infants are fed goat's milk.

Vitamin Supplements

The importance of appropriate vitamin supplementation of breast-fed infants is discussed in chapter 4. After infancy the percentage of children who are given vitamin supplements declines; however, over half of preschool and school-age children receive multivitamin-mineral preparations.

A survey found that for 10- to 13-year-old children 50% to 75% of the children had never taken vitamin supplements.[83] At age 13 years, 12% of the children were taking supplements. Children who could benefit most from supplements were not taking them. Those taking supplements often had dietary intakes that met the RDA from food alone. Breskin and others[84] noted no significant differences in biochemical indices with the exception of red blood cell folate of children who consumed supplements compared with those who did not, even though mean intakes of vitamin B_6 of the nonsupplemented group were 30% below the RDA. Many of the nonsupplemented children did not ingest two-thirds of the RDA of folate. All laboratory values were in the normal range of accepted standards.

The Committee on Nutrition of the American Academy of Pediatrics[73] defined four groups of children who are at particular risk and for whom vitamin supplementation may be appropriate: (1) children from deprived families, especially those who suffer from maltreatment; (2) children who have **anorexia,** poor and capricious appetites, or poor eating habits or who are on regimens to manage obesity; (3) pregnant teenagers; and (4) children who consume **vegan** diets.

Vitamin supplementation of diets of older children should be recommended only after careful evaluation of food intake. Diets of children who restrict their intake of milk because of allergies or fear of allergies, lactose intolerance, or psychosocial reasons should be monitored for riboflavin, vitamin D, calcium, and iron. Diets of infants and children receiving goat's milk should be carefully monitored for food sources of folacin. Diets of children who consume limited amounts of fruits and vegetables should be checked for sources of vitamins A and C.

Vitamin supplements, especially those that are colored and sugarcoated, should be stored in places inaccessible to young children so they are not confused with candy and ingested inappropriately.

Summary

The nutrient needs of individual children vary at any age depending on body size, patterns of activity, interaction of nutrients, and rates of growth. They are greatest per unit of body size in infancy and decline with age.

The recommended dietary intakes during childhood are extrapolated from needs of infants and adult males or are calculated on the basis of presumed energy or protein intake. Intakes of individual children should be evaluated not in relation to the total amounts listed on the RDA recommendations, but on the same basis the RDA was calculated.

Studies indicate that intakes of protein are generally adequate in North America. Nutrients most likely to be consumed in low or deficient amounts are calcium, iron, and vitamins A and C.

Children at risk for nutrient inadequacies are those from the following groups: deprived families; those who have an excessive appetite, poor eating habits, anorexia, or those on regimens to manage obesity; and those who consume vegan diets.

REVIEW QUESTIONS

1. Why is there such a wide range of acceptable energy intakes for infants and young children?
2. Why are the guidelines for protein, energy, vitamins, and minerals described as recommended intakes rather than requirements?
3. Under what circumstances are vitamin and mineral supplements appropriately recommended for infants? For young children?
4. Which factors most effect the bioavailability of absorption of iron?

SUGGESTED LEARNING ACTIVITIES

1. Calculate the energy intake of two children of the same age and gender whose heights are in the 10th and 90th percentile. Compare this with the RDA on the basis of total energy intake, kcalories per kilogram, and kcalories per centimeter.
2. Jocelyn is a 9-month-old infant who has been exclusively breast-fed. Her mother would like to have breast milk continue to be Jocelyn's primary source of nourishment. She is also interested in the addition of solids to Jocelyn's daily intake. Jocelyn is able to sit unsupported. She frequently puts toys into her mouth and sucks and chews on them vigorously.

   What specific foods would you suggest that Jocelyn's mother provide to her first? What nutrients are most important to provide from first foods?
3. Discuss the bioavailability of iron and zinc in foods acceptable to preschool children. How can one ensure an adequate intake?
4. Compare the content of a popular children's vitamin-mineral supplement with an adult vitamin-mineral supplement.

❖ ❖ ❖
CASE STUDY

Nourishment of a Preschool-Age Child

Joey is a 4-year-old boy. His weight is at the 10th percentile and his height is at the 50th percentile. Joey refuses to drink milk and will eat only small amounts of meat. Joey's pediatrician is concerned about the adequacy of Joey's calcium and iron intake as well as his overall nourishment. Joey's mom is concerned about his growth, though his growth channels are typical for him. Joey's mom has been asked to provide a four-day record of his food intake for your evaluation and recommendations.

1. What calcium intake would be appropriate for Joey?

What might you suggest as additional sources of calcium?
2. What intake of iron would you use as a guideline for assessment?
What additional information might you need to assess Joey's iron status?
What additional sources of iron might you recommend?
3. What additional information might you need to assess Joey's growth attainment?
4. What additional nutrients might be limited if Joey consistently refuses to drink milk?

5. William is a 13-month-old boy who weighs 8 kg and who was weaned from breast milk to infant formula at 11 months of age. His usual current intake is:

20–25 oz. milk-based infant formula
4–6 T infant rice cereal (dry)
¼ to ½ cup jarred chopped vegetable
¼ to ½ cup jarred chopped fruit
1 to 3 saltine crackers
4–6 oz. dilute (1:2) apple juice

Assess William's intake for: (1) total protein, (2) total energy, (3) calcium, and (4) iron.

Compare your assessment of William's nutrient intake with established guidelines. What is your evaluation of the adequacy of intake of the nutrients listed?
6. Compare the costs of meeting the RDA for vitamins with food or with vitamin-mineral supplementation.

REFERENCES

1. Food and Nutrition Board: Recommended dietary allowances, ed 10, National Research Council, Washington, DC, 1989, National Academy Press.
2. Whitehead RG: Dietary allowances: What to recommend, *Acta Paediatr Scand Suppl* 373:25–32, 1991.
3. Energy and protein requirements, Report of a Joint FAO/WHO/UNU Expert Consultation, Technical Report Series no. 724, World Health Organization, Geneva, 1985.
4. Recommended Nutrient Intakes for Canadians, Health and Welfare Canada, 1983.
5. How should the Recommended Dietary Allowances be revised? A concept paper from the Food and Nutrition Board, *Nutr Rev* 52:216–219, 1994.
6. Hildreth HG, Johnson RK: The doubly labeled water technique for the determinations of human energy requirements, *Nutr Today* 30:254, 1995.
7. Goran MI, Carpenter WH, Poehlman, ET: Total energy expenditure in 4 to 6 year old children, *Am J Physiol* 264:E706–711, 1993.
8. Butte NF, Moon JK, Wong WW, Hopkinson JM, Smith EO: Energy requirements from infancy to adulthood, *Am J Clin Nutr* 62:1047S–1052S, 1995.
9. Davies PSW, Ewing G, Lucas A: Energy expenditure in early infancy, *Br J Nutr* 62:621–629, 1989.
10. Lucas A, Ewing G, Roberts SB, Coward, WA: How much energy does the breast-fed infant consume and expend? *Br Med J* 295:75–77, 1987.
11. Prentice AM, Lucas A, Vasquesz-Velasquez, Davies P, Whitehead R: Are current dietary guidelines for young children a prescription for over-feeding? *Lancet* 2:1066–1069, 1988.
12. Ashworth A, Millward DJ: Catch-up growth in children, *Nutr Rev* 44:157, 1986.
13. White House Conference on Child Health and Protection: Growth and development of the child. III. Nutrition. Report of the Committee on Growth and Development, New York, 1932, Century House.

14. Hamill PVV and others: Physical growth: National Center for Health Statistics percentiles, *Am J Clin Nutr* 32:607, 1979.

15. Fomon SJ: *Nutrition of normal infants,* Mosby–Year Book, Inc. 1993.

16. Holt LE, Jr, Snyderman SE: The amino acid requirements of infants, *JAMA* 175:100, 1961.

17. Fomon SJ and others: Requirements for protein and essential amino acids in early infancy, *Acta Paediatr Scand* 62:33, 1973.

18. Fomon SJ, Filer LJ: *Amino acid requirements for normal growth.* In Nythan WL, editor: *Amino acid metabolism and genetic variations,* New York, 1967, McGraw-Hill.

19. Pineda OB and others: *Protein quality in relation to estimates of essential amino acid requirements.* In Bodwell CE and others, editors: *Protein quality in humans: assessment and in vitro estimation,* Westport, Conn, 1981, AVI Publishing.

20. Williams HH and others: *Nitrogen and amino acid requirements.* In *Improvements in protein nutriture,* Report of the Committee on Amino Acids, Food and Nutrition Board, National Academy of Sciences, Washington, DC, 1974.

21. Nakagawa I and others: Amino acid requirements of children: nitrogen balance at the minimal level of essential amino acids, *J Nutr* 83:115, 1964.

22. Fomon SJ: Requirements of recommended dietary intakes of protein during infancy, *Pediatr Res* 30:391, 1991.

23. Abernathy RP, Ritchey SJ: Position paper on RDA for protein for children, *Adv Med Biol* 105:1, 1978.

24. Committee on Nutrition, American Academy of Pediatrics: Commentary on breastfeeding and infant formula, *Pediatrics* 57:278, 1976.

25. Holman RJ, Caster WO, Weise HF: The essential fatty acid requirement of infants and the assessment of their dietary intake of linoleate by serum fatty acid analysis, *Am J Clin Nutr* 14:70, 1964.

26. Fomon SJ: Requirements of recommended dietary intakes of protein during infancy, *Pediatr Res* 30:391, 1991.

27. Healthy People 2000: Nutrition objectives, *J Am Diet Assoc* 91:1515, 1991.

28. Olson RE: The dietary recommendations of the American Academy of Pediatrics, *Am J Clin Nutr* 61:271–273, 1995.

29. Olson RE: The folly of restricting fat in the diet of children, *Nutr Today* 30:234–245, 1995.

30. Committee on Nutrition, American Academy of Pediatrics: Plant fiber intake in the pediatric diet, *Pediatrics* 67:572, 1981.

31. Barness LA: *Nutrition and nutritional disorders.* In Behrman RE, Kliegman RM editors: *Nelson's textbook of pediatrics,* ed 14, Philadelphia, 1992, WB Saunders.

32. Maller O, Desor JA: *Effect of taste on ingestion by human newborns.* In Bosma JF editor: *Oral sensation and perception,* Pub No (NIH) 73-546, Bethesda, Md, 1973, Department of Health, Education and Welfare.

33. Hey EN, Katz G: Evaporative water loss in the newborn baby, *J Physiol* 200:605, 1969.

34. Ziegler EE, Fomon SJ: Fluid intake, renal solute load, and water balance in infancy, *J Pediatr* 78:561, 1971.

35. Stolley H, Schlage C: Water balance and water requirement of preschool children, *Nutr Metab* 21 (suppl 1):15–17, 1977.

36. Arnaud SB and others: Serum parathyroid hormone and blood minerals: interrelationships in normal children, *Pediatr Res* 7:485, 1973.

37. Committee on Nutrition, American Academy of Pediatrics: Calcium requirements in infancy and childhood, *Pediatrics* 62:826, 1978.

38. Matkovic V: Calcium metabolism and calcium requirements during skeletal modeling and consolidation of bone mass, *Am J Clin Nutr* 245S–260S, 1991.

39. Christiansen C, Rodbro D, Neilsen CT: Bone mineral content and estimated total body calcium in normal children and adolescents, *Scand J Clin Lab Invest* 35:507, 1975.

40. Optimal calcium intake, NIH Consensus Statement 1994, Jun 6–8: 12(4):1–31.

41. Sheikh MS and others: Gastrointestinal absorption of calcium from milk and calcium salts, *N Engl J Med* 317:532, 1987.

42. Devlin J and others: Calcium intake and cow's milk free diets, *Arch Dis Child* 64:1183, 1989.

43. David L, Anast CS: Calcium metabolism in newborn infants, the interrelationship of parathyroid function and calcium, magnesium, and phosphorus metabolism in normal, "sick," and hypocalcemic newborns, *J Clin Invest* 54:287, 1974.

44. Harris L, Wilkinson AW: Magnesium depletion in children, *Lancet* 2:735, 1971.

45. Fomon SJ: Reflections on infant feeding in the 1970s and 1980s, *Am J Clin Nutr* 46:171, 1987.

46. Hallberg L and others: Menstrual blood loss—a population study, *Acta Obstet Gynecol Scand* 45:320, 1966.

47. Herbert V: Recommended dietary intakes (RDI) of iron in humans, *Am J Clin Nutr* 45:679, 1987.

48. Monsen ER and others: Estimation of available dietary iron, *Am J Clin Nutr* 31:134, 1978.

49. McMillan JA: Iron absorption from human milk, simulated human milk, and proprietary formulas, *Pediatrics* 60:896, 1977.

50. Committee on Nutrition, American Academy of Pediatrics: Iron-fortified infant formulas, *Pediatrics* 84:1114, 1989.

51. Dallman PR, Yip R: Changing characteristics of childhood anemia, *J Pediatr* 114:161, 1989.

52. Lozoff B and others: Long-term developmental outcome of infants with iron deficiency, *N Engl J Med* 325:687, 1991.

53. Krebs NF, Hambidge KM: Zinc requirements and zinc intakes of breast-fed infants, *Am J Clin Nutr* 43:288, 1986.

54. Cavan KR, Gibson RS, Grazioso CF and others: Growth and body composition of periurban Guatemalan children in relation to zinc status: a longitudinal zinc intervention trial, *Am J Clin Nutr* 57:344–352, 1993.

55. Gibson RS, Vanderkooy PD, MacDonald AC and others: A growth-limiting, mild zinc deficiency syndrome in some southern Ontario boys with low height percentiles, *Am J Clin Nutr* 49:1266–1273, 1989.

56. Hambidge KM and others: Zinc nutrition of preschool children in the Denver Headstart Program, *Am J Clin Nutr* 29:734, 1976.

57. Casey CE and others: Studies in human lactation: zinc, copper, manganese, and chromium in human milk in the first month of lactation, *Am J Clin Nutr* 41:1193, 1985.

58. Schlage C, Wortberg B: Zinc in the diet of healthy preschool and school children, *Acta Paediatr Scand* 61:421, 1972.

59. Picciano MF, Guthrie HA: Copper, iron, and zinc contents of mature human milk, *Am J Clin Nutr* 29:242, 1976.

60. Burt BA: The epidemiological basis for water fluoridation in the prevention of dental caries, *J Public Health Policy* 3:391, 1982.

61. Committee on Nutrition, American Academy of Pediatrics: Fluoride supplementation: revised dosage schedule, *Pediatrics* 77:758, 1986.

62. Taves DR: Dietary intake of fluoride ashed (total fluoride) v. unashed (inorganic fluoride) analysis of individual foods, *Br J Nutr* 49:295, 1983.

63. Krishnamachari, KAVR: *Fluorine.* In Mertz W, editor: *Trace elements in human and animal nutrition,* vol 1, San Diego, 1987, Academic Press.

64. Singer L, Ophaug RH, Harland BF: Dietary fluoride intakes of 15 to 19 year old males residing in the United States, *J Dent Res* 64:1302, 1985.

65. Leverett DH: Fluorides and the changing prevalence of dental caries, *Science* 217:26, 1982.

66. Butte NF and others: Macro- and trace-mineral intakes of exclusively breast-fed infants, *Am J Clin Nutr* 45:42, 1987.

67. Baker H and others: Vitamin profile of 174 mothers and newborns at parturition, *Am J Clin Nutr* 28:59, 1975.

68. Olson JA: Recommended dietary intakes of vitamin A in humans, *Am J Clin Nutr* 45:704, 1987.

69. DeLuca HD: Vitamin D: 1993, *Nutr Today* 28:6, 1993.

70. Feldman K and others: Inner-city babies susceptible to rickets, *Northwest Medicine* 7:28, 1991.

71. Tsang RC: The quandary of vitamin D in the newborn infant, *Lancet* 1:1370, 1983.

72. Horwitt MK: Interpretations of requirements for thiamin, riboflavin, niacin, tryptophan, and vitamin E plus comments on balance studies and vitamin B_6, *Am J Clin Nutr* 44:973, 1986.

73. Committee on Nutrition, American Academy of Pediatrics: Vitamin and mineral supplement needs in normal children in the United States, *Pediatrics* 66:1015, 1980.

74. Greer FR and others, Vitamin K status of lactating mothers, human milk, and breast-feeding infants, *Pediatrics* 88:751, 1991.

75. Olson JA, Hodges RE: Recommended dietary intakes (RDI) of vitamin C in humans, *Am J Clin Nutr* 45:693, 1987.

76. Boyden RF, Erikson SE: Metabolic patterns of preadolescent children: thiamine utilization in relation to nitrogen intake, *Am J Clin Nutr* 19:398, 1966.

77. Dick EC and others: Thiamine requirement of eight adolescent boys, as estimated from urinary thiamine excretion, *J Nutr* 66:173, 1958.

78. Herbert V: Recommended dietary intakes (RDI) of folate in humans, *Am J Clin Nutr* 45:661, 1987.

79. Committee on Nutrition, American Academy of Pediatrics: Commentary on breast-feeding and infant formulas, including proposed standards for formulas, *Pediatrics* 57:279, 1976.

80. Herbert V: Recommended dietary intakes (RDI) of vitamin B_{12} in humans, *Am J Clin Nutr* 45:671, 1987.

81. Heard GS and others: Distribution and bioavailability of biotin in human milk, *Fed Proc* 46:897, 1987.

82. Block G and others: Nutrient sources in the American diet: quantitative data from the NHANES II Survey. I. Vitamins and minerals, *Am J Epidemiol* 122:13, 1985.

83. Farris RP and others: Dietary studies of children from a biracial population: intakes of vitamins in 10- and 13-year olds, *J. Am Coll Nutr* 4:539, 1985.

84. Breskin MW and others: Water-soluble vitamins: intakes and indices in children, *J Am Diet Assoc* 85:49, 1985.

CHAPTER

3

Collecting and Assessing Food Intake Information

Peggy L. Pipes
Robin Pritkin Glass

+++

Objectives

After studying this chapter, the student should:

✔ *Be cognizant of all of the information that needs to be collected for a comprehensive evaluation of infants' and children's food intake.*

✔ *Be able to select the appropriate dietary methodology for any particular case or setting.*

✔ *Recognize the advantages and limitations of the various approaches to evaluating dietary intake.*

✔ *Be able to appropriately screen children who need evaluation of motor and psychosocial parameters that affect food intake.*

✔ *Be aware of the advantages and limitations of computer programs designed to calculate nutrient intake.*

Nutrition screening, evaluation, counseling, and education have become integral parts of many health care, public health, and supplemental food programs that serve infants and children. In addition, children perceived as having feeding problems, those who must consume modified diets, and those whose parents are concerned about the adequacy of their food intakes are frequently referred to a program for a team management approach. Plans for modifying food intake in childhood should be based on information more comprehensive than that which identifies excesses or deficits in energy and nutrient intakes and cultural food practices. Health care professionals must work jointly to synthesize information and develop programs that can be carried out by children or their parents. Goals for change in food intake should be identified and periodically reassessed. Therefore, it is imperative that health care professionals recognize the need for accurate data collection in relation to the nutrient intake from the food consumed, the developmental level of feeding behavior (oral motor screening), psychosocial issues that affect behavior, and parent-child interactions that affect food and nutrient intake.

Defining the energy and nutrient intake of individuals and populations is important not only for the clinical practitioner but also for those engaged in epidemiological studies of the relation of foods and nutrients to disease and in collecting information for program planning in public health. Much of the research attempting to assess the validity of approaches of securing and assessing food intake information has been directed toward food intake of large groups.

It is important to recognize that an assessment of food intake is not an *assessment* of nutritional status. The latter requires anthropometric data and biochemical and clinical evaluations as well as dietary intake data. Adequately collected food intake data can, however, provide information on which judgments of the adequacy of a child's current food intake can be made and plans for resolving concerns about food and nutrient intake can be designed and assessed. It is important for those who collect this information to be aware of the variety of methods of collecting food intake information and to develop skills for screening both oral motor feeding difficulties and psychosocial factors that may compromise a child's nutrient intake.

TOOLS FOR COLLECTING DIETARY INTAKE DATA

Health care professionals in clinical settings use a variety of tools for collecting dietary data, each tool having limitations and varying degrees of reliability. The choice of tool depends on the purpose of the interview, the time commitment of the professional, and the cooperation of the child or parents. Information sought will vary with the problem. For example, detailed documentation of an early feeding history may be important for counseling parents of young

children with feeding problems, whereas this would be inappropriate if the patient were an obese adolescent. Only one tool is used in some instances, whereas a combination of tools is appropriate at other times. It is important to recognize that valid methods for assessing the dietary intake of groups differ from those designed to collect information on one child for whom plans for nutrition education and counseling are to be developed. The tools most often used in the clinical setting are the 24-hour recall, the dietary history, and the 3- and 7-day food records. Food frequencies may be applicable in some circumstances.

The interview is the most important aspect of any of the tools used. The validity of the information obtained depends on the client's understanding of the reasons for the interview and the information sought, the client's comfort with the interviewer, and the interviewer's skills at probing for and validating information. Whether the child or parents should be interviewed depends on several developmental and psychosocial factors. Beal found that with few exceptions, girls under 12 years of age and boys under 13 to 14 years of age were unlikely to give reliable nutrition histories.[1] However, if there is considerable conflict between a preadolescent and the parents about food intake, it may be important to interview the child both individually and with the parents so that an appropriate counseling relationship can be established.

It must be remembered that assessment data are only as valid as the child's or parent's willingness to share information with the interviewer. It is important that they feel that it is important to provide the information requested and feel comfortable with the interview and the individual conducting the assessment. The interviewer should give a friendly greeting, a clear definition of the purpose of the interview, and the reasons for the questions asked, which aids in establishing rapport with the client. Providing an adequate diet for children is an important aspect of parenting. Parents may feel threatened when questioned about a child's food intake. In addition, the interviewer must have reasonable expectations for the respondent. The parent of several children cannot be expected to give information as precisely for one child as does a parent who devotes his or her time to an only child. A number of meals or snacks may be consumed outside the home in a daycare center or at school, and parents may not know what children eat in these settings.

During the interview the interviewer must be careful to avoid suggesting time, meals, food, or amounts consumed. For example, the question "When does your child first have something to eat or to drink?" is appropriate, whereas the question "When does your child first eat breakfast?" is inappropriate. The tone of voice is also important. Neither approval nor disapproval should be expressed verbally or nonverbally by facial expression. Food preferences of the interviewer should never be indicated. Silences must be accepted with comfort, and parents should be permitted time to formulate answers to questions and to ask questions of their own.

24-Hour Recall

The most common method used for collecting dietary data to characterize the nutrient intake of populations is the 24-hour recall, often used in combination with 1-, 3-, or 7-day food records. The 24-hour recall has also been used successfully to screen children at nutritional risk and can give some indication as to compliance with a dietary regimen during clinical follow-up. It cannot be substituted for more intensive methods when judgments regarding the adequacy of an individual child's food intake are to be made.

The child or the parents are asked to list, in portion sizes, every food that the child has consumed for the past 24 hours. Errors in the 24-hour recall have been reported to result from inability of the parents or children to remember exactly what was eaten, difficulties in estimating portion sizes, and lack of commitment of the individual being interviewed. Parents often are not aware of the foods consumed between meals. There is no assurance that the recall of the day selected is typical of other days. The accuracy with which portion sizes are reported can be increased by the use of food models and by skillful probing.

The 24-hour recall most often underestimates intake. Baranowski and others found that 17.7% of mothers underreported, whereas 10.4% overreported food intake of 3- to 4-year-old children compared with the recorded intake of observers.[2]

3- and 7-Day Food Records

The 3- or 7-day food record or a written diary of all food and beverages consumed is a tool commonly used to characterize current intakes of individual children (see Food Diary for Children, page 72, and Food Diary for Infants, page 71). Parents are instructed to measure or weigh portions of food offered and amounts not eaten and record the amounts consumed. Parents report that measuring and weighing pose no problems but that they find the rigidity of recording each time the child eats difficult. Sometimes they forget foods that are added to other foods; for example, catsup, butter, or jelly may be unintentionally omitted from the record. The differences between fruit-flavored drink and pure fruit juice may not be understood. Therefore careful instruction as to how to record food intake is important. Also, training with food models has been shown to be effective in improving the accuracy of the portions recorded for a week. Three-dimensional food models are especially useful with children.[3] Reviewing food records and verifying the information recorded can increase accuracy because brand names, portion sizes, and recipe ingredients are clarified.

No standard error has been found. Problems with both over- and underestimations of intake will be found.[4] Kavarvetti and others found that two days of records of food intake deviated from observed intakes by no more than 15%. Breakfast was the meal most accurately recorded. Cake was the food most frequently omitted.[5] Eight- to 10-year-old children, when adequately trained, appear to be able to accurately report on a tape recorder their food intake compared with their parent's written records.[6] Black and others found good agreement between mean energy intake calculated from weighed food records and energy expenditures from highly motivated normal weight volunteers. However, among randomly recruited individuals, underreporting was found. There were also indications that obese or previously obese individuals reported food intakes less than those observed.[7]

FOOD DIARY FOR INFANTS (BIRTH TO 1 YEAR)

Instructions

1. Record *all* formula, milk, and food that the baby consumes immediately *after* each feeding.
2. If your baby is breast-fed, record the time of day the baby is fed and how long the baby feeds.
3. If your baby is formula-fed, record the time of day the baby eats, the kind of formula the baby is fed, and the amount actually consumed.
   Infant formula preparation:
   Is the formula iron fortified?
   ☐ Yes   ☐ No
   Formula (brand name): _____
   _____ oz liquid *or*
   _____ T powder
   Water
   _____ oz
   Other (describe): _____
   _____ oz
   _____ T
   Total prepared formula
   _____ oz
4. If the baby spits up or vomits, estimate the amount.
5. Measure the amounts of any other foods carefully in terms of ounces of liquid (e.g., 2 oz apple juice), level T (e.g., 2 T dry rice cereal), or portions of commercially prepared or home prepared foods (e.g., ½ of a 4.7 oz jar or level T of strained peaches).
6. Does the baby take a vitamin supplement? ☐ Yes   ☐ No
   If yes, what kind? _____

Day 1

Date _____ Day of week _____

Most recent weight _____ on (date) _____

Time	Food or Formula	Amount	Time	Food or Formula	Amount

Modified from Food diary for infants, Center on Human Development and Disabilities, Seattle, 1994, University of Washington.

The number of days required for valid estimates of an individual's intake vary with the nutrient to be investigated. Investigations of the energy intake of children with the **Prader-Willi syndrome** indicate that 30 days of weighed food records were required for valid estimates of energy intake.

The provision of cassette recorders, which made it possible for individuals to record their intake on tape may facilitate and increase accuracy in recording.

Dietary History

Another method of reviewing dietary intake in retrospect is the research dietary history method developed by Burke[8] and modified and redescribed by Beale.[1] During an interview the investigator obtains an estimate of the frequency

❖

FOOD DIARY FOR CHILDREN

Instructions

1. Record all foods and beverages immediately after they are consumed.
2. Measure the amounts of each food carefully with standard measuring cups and spoons. Record meat portions in ounces or as fractions of pounds, e.g., 8 oz of milk; 1 medium egg; ¼ lb of hamburger; 1 slice of bread, white; ½ of small banana.
3. Indicate method of preparation, e.g., medium egg, fried; ½ c baked beans with a 2-inch slice of salt pork; 4 oz of steak, broiled.
4. Be sure to record any condiments, gravies, salad dressings, butter, margarine, whipped cream, relishes, e.g., ¾ c of mashed potatoes with 3 T of brown gravy, ¼ c of cottage cheese salad with 2 olives, ½ c of cornflakes with 1 t of sugar and ⅓ c of 2% milk.
5. Be sure to record all between-meal foods and drinks, e.g., coffee with 1 oz of cream, 12 oz of cola, 4 sugar cookies, 1 candy bar (indicate brand name).
6. If you eat away from home, please put an asterisk (*) in the food column beside the food listing.

Day 1

Date _____ Day of week _____ Weight _____

Time	Food	Amount	How Prepared

Modified from Record of food intake, Center on Human Development and Disabilities, Seattle, 1994, University of Washington.

and amounts of food and nutrient supplements consumed in a specified period, usually 1 to 6 months. Parents are questioned about the child's food likes and dislikes. If parent-child interaction or early feeding experiences are suspected to be factors in the nutrition concern, information is elicited on the early feeding history. The interview is often cross-checked with a 24-hour recall or 3-day record of food consumed and a food frequency questionnaire.

This method requires a skilled interviewer. The dietitian or nutritionist must gain the confidence of the parent or child, make good estimates, and judge whether the answers are reliable. The process is time consuming and cannot be adequately completed in less than 1 hour.

Several researchers have cautioned against using this tool as the sole source of data. One study compared the research-type dietary history with 10- to 14-day weighed food records for a group of subjects 6 to 16 years of age and found that no history agreed within 20% for all constituents; the greatest deviations were for vitamins A and D, energy, riboflavin, and thiamin. Other investigators compared dietary histories with 7-day food records and 24-hour recalls and found that dietary histories gave distinctly higher values than 7-day food records and 24-hour recalls for groups.

Food Frequency Questionnaires

Several researchers have developed food frequency questionnaires. Clients are asked to estimate the portion size and frequency with which they currently consume specified foods and mixed dishes. The format is computer compatible, so it can be keypunched and calculations are quickly returned. Advantages offered by the food frequency method include high response rates, minimal burden to the respondent, and the fact that they can be administered by nonprofessionals. They generally give higher estimates of intake than do food records.

Regardless of the method chosen to collect food intake information, one needs to be aware that limitations and biases exist in any method. The dietary history and food frequency methods probably overestimate while food records are likely to underestimate intake.[9,10] There also seem to be differences obtained by different interviewers. Some collect information that underestimates intake whereas the data collected by others on the same individual seem to overestimate intake. There are also client differences in the validity of answers to questions asked, adding another dimension to be assessed when evaluating the accuracy of information reported.

Using both the dietary history and a record of food intake is likely to add credibility to the assessment. The interviewer must, however, recognize the lifestyle demands of the respondent and negotiate a reasonable approach for both the client and health care professional. If parents are literate, concerned, and motivated, they may agree to keep the food records. Day-care workers and preschool teachers are generally agreeable about keeping records. However, it may be necessary to accept a 3-day, rather than a 7-day, record from a working mother with a large family. If the parents clearly do not want to keep the diet diary, the interviewer must be satisfied with the dietary history but recognize its limitations.

ASSESSING DIETARY INTAKE INFORMATION

When the dietary intake information has been collected, the adequacy of nutrients in the foods consumed is assessed. The choice of evaluation method and nutrients to be calculated is based on the precision and reliability of the information collected, the foods that appear in the dietary records, the interviewer's knowledge of foods as sources of nutrients, and the problem presented for evaluation.

In some instances intake data may be compared to food groups; other times, knowledge of foods that are present or absent in the dietary history as sources of nutrients may sufficiently indicate the presence or absence of problems of nutrient intake. If precise and complete information has been collected, hand or computer calculations of nutrients in the foods consumed may be compared with a reference intake.

When parents are unable or unwilling to give information that can be quantitated, such as when they report intake as bites of meat instead of one-fourth of a 2 oz hamburger patty or when cross-checks reveal inconsistencies, the analysis of food groups or foods as sources of nutrients seems appropriate. However, if the child is underweight or overweight or if food sources of a particular nutrient appear on the record only occasionally, calculations of nutrient intake are important.

Computer Programs

Well over 100 programs are available that assess nutrient intake using a computer database. The choice of the program that has a "best fit" is based on several important aspects of each program.

The best method of approach is to specifically identify the tasks appropriate to the setting. This is based on whether clients are outpatient or inpatient, whether analysis is for individual patient nutrient or screening intakes, and whether recipes and diaries are to be analyzed. The investigator should evaluate for the specific setting:

1. the most convenient hardware, e.g., personal or handheld computer;
2. the ease and speed with which items can be entered into a program;

3. the quality of the user's manual and help screens;
4. the ability to preview single food nutrients when entering food;
5. the ability to assign different volume or weight;
6. the data entry format (e.g., code numbers or selection from food groups); and
7. the presentation of the output data (e.g., tabular or graphic printouts).[11]

The database itself must be evaluated for the number of foods (databases vary from 250 to 5000+ foods), the number of nutrients calculated for each food (varies from 3 to 90 nutrients), and the number of missing values for each nutrient. It is necessary to understand the source of the nutrient data for the data and the capacity and availability of updating it.

Other considerations are features that may be desirable, such as comparison of the calculated intake data to comparative information (e.g., the RDA); emphasis on specific components (e.g., fats or amino acids); proposal of a menu based on specified restrictions; inclusion of food items especially used by infants and children such as formulas; and an activity analysis. It is also important that programs be periodically updated as new foods appear on the market and others disappear. It has been estimated that 13,000 new foods per year have been introduced during the 1990s.[11]

Although these programs need care in selection, maintenance, and periodic evaluation, they provide a time-efficient way of making calculations once the evaluator learns to use the programs. A much larger number of nutrients can be calculated by computer than is possible by hand (table 3-1).

Evaluating Intake Information

When calculations are complete, the data must be compared to recommended intakes for age, activity, and sex. All formulated recommendations are intended to be used to interpret data on groups of people and are not intended to be used for evaluating the adequacy of nutrient intakes of individuals.

Many of the computer programs compare nutrient intake to the RDA. These allowances for children are generally based on studies of adults from which extrapolations were made for children. A margin of safety above the average requirement is applied to each nutrient. This margin varies for each nutrient.

When interpreting the data one must be keenly aware of the **bioavailability** of the nutrients. In addition, changes in nutrient concentration of foods during storage and preparation must be considered.

Some programs define children at nutritional risk as those who consume less than two-thirds or three-fourths of the recommended daily dietary allowances of any nutrient, and include these children and their families in intensive nutrition follow-up. It may also be important for these children to have a more intensive nutrition evaluation, including biochemical evaluation of their nutritional status.

Anthropometry (height, weight, and skinfold measurements) can give indications of the appropriateness of the child's energy intake. If rates of weight gain are excessive or inadequate, calculations of the child's energy intake provide important data on which plans for adjustments in energy intake can be made.

SCREENING CHILDREN AT NUTRITIONAL RISK

The objective of screening is to identify infants and children who appear to have nutritional problems that require further investigation. The interview is brief, and information sought is qualitative. It is often performed by **paraprofessionals** (e.g., community health workers or nutrition aides), nurses, or other professionals who assume the role of case manager. The 24-hour recall screening questionnaires or questionnaires filled out by parents may be used (see Screening Questionnaire for Infants, pages 76–77 and Screening Questionnaire for Young Children, pages 78–79).

Screening programs are designed to reach as many individuals as possible at a minimum cost. Adequately nourished individuals may be mistaken as at risk; however, this is acceptable, since many others who are not adequately nourished will be identified.

TABLE 3-1 *Computer Report of One Day's Food Intake**

Quantity	Food	Gram	Energy (kcal)	Calcium (mg)	Total Protein (gm)	Vit C (mg)	Thiamin (mg)	Niacin (mg)	Riboflavin (mg)	Folate (µg)	Vit A (µg RE)	Vit D (µg)	Fe (mg)
1 large	Egg, whole, hardboiled	50.0	75	25	6.2	—	tr	tr	0.3	23	95.2	0.6	0.7
1 slice	White bread, enriched	25.0	67	31.5	2.0	—	—	0.9	tr	8.7	—	†	—
12 fl oz	Whole milk, fluid	366.0	225	437	11.7	—	—	—	0.6	18	138	3.8	—
0.25 c	Rice, white enriched	51.25	66	5.7	1.3	—	tr	0.7	—	1.7	†	—	—
57 gm (8/lb)	Frankfurter, Oscar Mayer, cooked	57.0	183	6	6.2	15	0.1	1.5	tr	2.0	†	0.5	0.6
1 c	Orange juice, fresh	248.0	112	21.9	—	96.5	—	0.5	tr	109	19.3	†	0.2
125 gm	Macaroni & cheese, Stouffer's	125.0	269	226	10.6	0.0	0.1	1.1	0.3	—	108	—	1.1
45 gm	Green beans, cut style, canned, solids drained	45.0	9	11.6	0.5	2.2	—	tr	tr	14.3	15.7	—	0.4
35 gm	Chicken drumstick, fried in veg. fat	35.0	85.8	4.2	9.4	—	tr	2.1	0.1	2.8	8.8	.19	—
1	Tortilla, wheat, baked/steamed	43.4	137	66.5	3.6	—	tr	1.4	—	†	.2	—	1.6
	TOTAL		1228	835	54	117	0.85	8.81	1.53	179	385	5.1	6.6

tr, Trace.

*Data are for a 2-year-old female child with a height of 82.4 cm and weight of 14.5 kg.

†Indicates there are no data on the item specified for that nutrient.

SCREENING QUESTIONNAIRE FOR INFANTS (BIRTH TO 1 YEAR)

	Yes	No
1. Is the baby breast-fed?	☐	☐
If yes, does he/she also receive milk or formula?	☐	☐

If yes, what kind? _____

	Yes	No
2. Does the baby receive formula?	☐	☐

If yes ☐ Ready-to-feed
      ☐ Concentrated liquid
      ☐ Other: _____

How is formula prepared (especially dilution)?

_____

_____

	Yes	No
Is the formula iron fortified?	☐	☐
3. Does the baby drink milk?	☐	☐

If yes ☐ Whole milk
      ☐ 2% milk
      ☐ Skim milk
      ☐ Other: _____

4. How many times does the baby eat each day, including milk or formula? ___

	Yes	No
5. Does the baby usually take a bottle to bed?	☐	☐

If yes, what is usually in the bottle? _____

6. If the baby drinks milk or formula, what is the usual amount in a day?
   ☐ Less than 16 oz
   ☐ 16–32 oz
   ☐ More than 32 oz

7. Please indicate which (if any) of these foods the baby eats and how often:

	Never or Hardly Ever (Less Than Once a Week)	Sometimes (Not Daily But at Least Once a Week)	Every Day or Nearly Every Day
Eggs	☐	☐	☐
Dried beans or peas	☐	☐	☐
Meat, fish, poultry	☐	☐	☐
Bread, rice, pasta, grits, cereal, tortillas, potatoes	☐	☐	☐
Fruits or fruit juices	☐	☐	☐
Vegetables	☐	☐	☐

8. If the baby eats fruits or drinks fruit juices every day or nearly every day, which ones does he/she eat or drink most often (not more than three)? _____

_____

9. If the baby eats vegetables every day or nearly every day, which one does he/she eat most often (not more than three)? _____

_____

	Yes	No
10. Does the person who cares for the baby have use of a		
Stove?	☐	☐
Refrigerator?	☐	☐
Piped water?	☐	☐

From Fomon SJ: *Nutritional disorders of children: prevention, screening, and follow-up,* Pub No 76-5612, Rockville, Md, 1976, Department of Health, Education and Welfare.

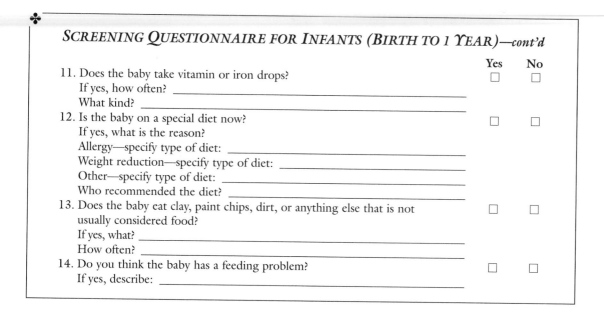

❖

SCREENING QUESTIONNAIRE FOR INFANTS (BIRTH TO 1 YEAR)—*cont'd*

	Yes	No
11. Does the baby take vitamin or iron drops?	☐	☐
If yes, how often? _____		
What kind? _____		
12. Is the baby on a special diet now?	☐	☐
If yes, what is the reason?		
Allergy—specify type of diet: _____		
Weight reduction—specify type of diet: _____		
Other—specify type of diet: _____		
Who recommended the diet? _____		
13. Does the baby eat clay, paint chips, dirt, or anything else that is not usually considered food?	☐	☐
If yes, what? _____		
How often? _____		
14. Do you think the baby has a feeding problem?	☐	☐
If yes, describe: _____		

Anthropometric data plotted on growth charts are also used in screening. In general, when children's growth patterns plot at less than the 10th percentile, when they are underweight or overweight for their lengths (see chapter 1), or when interviews show patterns of intake that indicate a nutrient consumed is in short supply, the children are referred for more intensive counseling.

From information on the screening questionnaire, parents of infants and children who need further evaluation or counseling can also be identified. A red flag could be raised when the infant screening questionnaire indicates that an infant was offered overdiluted or underdiluted formulas, if homogenized milk was offered to infants under 1 year of age, or if nonfat or 2% milk was offered any time in the first year. Other infants who may be identified as at risk include those who receive semisolid foods before 4 months of age and those who are bottle-fed as they go to sleep.

As the child ages, the quantity of milk consumed and the frequency in which the listed food groups are eaten can identify older children at risk.

All infants or children who require a modified diet to control chronic disease or whose parents perceive them as having a feeding problem need further assessment.

DIETARY ASSESSMENT

Parents and children referred for intensive evaluation of nutrient and energy intake should anticipate a more extensive interview. Even so, the dietitian/nutritionist should carefully explain the purpose of the questions to be asked and reasons for continuing "how much" and "how often" questions. Decisions regarding which tool will be used may be made after the parents and children arrive and express their concern or lack of concern.

The dietary history, in combination with a 7-day food record, is the preferred tool currently available for dietary assessment in a clinical setting. These procedures require a skilled nutritionist and are costly in time, and not all parents and children can respond with validity even though they may wish to do so.

SCREENING QUESTIONNAIRE FOR YOUNG CHILDREN (PRESCHOOL CHILDREN AND YOUNG SCHOOL-AGE CHILDREN)

Yes / No

1. Does the child drink milk? ☐ ☐
   If yes ☐ Whole milk
   ☐ 2% milk
   ☐ Skim milk
   ☐ Other: _____
   If yes, how much?
   ☐ Less than 8 oz
   ☐ 8–32 oz
   ☐ More than 32 oz
2. Does the child drink anything from a bottle (for children less than 4 years of age)? ☐ ☐
   If yes ☐ Milk
   ☐ Other: _____
3. Does the child take a bottle to bed? ☐ ☐
   If yes, what is usually in the bottle? _____
4. How many times a day does the child usually eat (including snacks)? _____
5. Please indicate which (if any) of these foods the child eats and how often:

	Never or Hardly Ever (Less Than Once a Week)	Sometimes (Not Daily But at Least Once a Week)	Every Day or Nearly Every Day
Cheese, yogurt, ice cream	☐	☐	☐
Eggs	☐	☐	☐
Dried beans, peas, peanut butter	☐	☐	☐
Meat, fish, poultry	☐	☐	☐
Bread, rice, pasta, grits, cereal, tortillas, potatoes	☐	☐	☐
Fruits or fruit juices	☐	☐	☐
Vegetables	☐	☐	☐

6. If the child eats fruits or drinks fruit juices every day or nearly every day, which ones does he/she eat or drink most often (not more than three)? _____
   _____
7. If the child eats vegetables every day or nearly every day, which ones does he/she eat most often (not more than three)? _____
8. Does the child usually eat between meals? ☐ ☐
   If yes, name the 2 or 3 snacks (including bedtime snacks) that the child has most often: _____
9. Does the person who cares for the child have use of a
   Stove? ☐ ☐
   Refrigerator? ☐ ☐
   Piped water? ☐ ☐

From Fomon SJ: *Nutritional disorders of children: prevention, screening, and follow-up,* Pub No 76-5612, Rockville, Md, 1976, Department of Health, Education and Welfare.

SCREENING QUESTIONNAIRE FOR YOUNG CHILDREN (PRESCHOOL CHILDREN AND YOUNG SCHOOL-AGE CHILDREN)—*cont'd*

	Yes	No
10. Does the child take vitamin or iron drops or tablets?	☐	☐

    If yes, how often? _____

    What kind? _____

| 11. Is the child on a special diet now? | ☐ | ☐ |

    If yes, what is the reason? _____

    ☐ Allergy—specify type of diet: _____

    ☐ Weight reduction—specify type of diet: _____

    ☐ Other—specify reason for diet and type of diet: _____

    Who recommended the diet? _____

| 12. Does the child eat clay, paint chips, dirt, or anything else that is not usually considered food? | ☐ | ☐ |

    If yes, what? _____

    How often? _____

13. How would you describe the child's appetite?

    ☐ Good

    ☐ Fair

    ☐ Poor

    ☐ Other: _____

Some programs use a food frequency questionnaire and 24-hour recall, a method that requires less time and is less taxing for the client but yields less valid and less useful information.

During this interview the nutritionist collects information about family interactions that affect a child's food intake (e.g., family members present at mealtimes, the use of food as rewards), the food budget and money spent for food, the frequency in which the family and children eat away from home, and the family's use of community resources that provide food or nutrition education (fig. 3-1).

The case of a 13-month-old girl referred for dietary assessment because of inadequate weight gain may clarify the process. The girl was the unplanned child of the second marriage of a couple who also had teenage children in their home. All medical reasons for failure to thrive had been ruled out. The interview with both father and mother proceeded as follows:

Interviewer: Let's begin with the early feeding history. Was the baby breast- or bottle-fed?

Mother: She was and still is breast-fed. I do not want her to drink formula or cow's milk. I have given her a little goat's milk from a cup.

Interviewer: Did she have any problems sucking at the breast?

Mother: None at all until she was 6 months. Then she wouldn't take much at a time but wanted to feed often. I want to breast-feed her as long as she wants to.

Interviewer: When was she introduced to foods other than milk?

Mother: I gave her cereal when the doctor told me to, about 5 months, then vegetables and fruits, and I think meat about 9 months. I made them for her from only fresh pure foods. I give her only "natural foods" now.

Interviewer: When did she begin finger-feeding?

Mother: About 6 months, I think. She feeds herself rice crackers.

Interviewer: When did she eat table foods that were not pureed?

Mother: I began mashing up vegetables and grinding meat when she was 8 months old.

FIG. 3-1   Nutritionist evaluates nutritional adequacy of preschooler's intake.

Interviewer: Does she drink from a cup?

Mother: She has a little goat's milk from a cup, but I have to help her hold it.

Interviewer: Does she try to feed herself?

Mother: She tries to get the spoon, but I can't stand the mess she makes so I feed her.

Interviewer: Now I would like for you to tell me how she lives her day with food. When does she first have something to eat or drink?

Mother: Well, she wakes about 3:00 or 4:00 in the morning and breast-feeds.

Interviewer: Then when does she have something to eat or drink again?

Mother: Well, she wakes again about 8:00, and I give her rice cereal from the health food store.

Interviewer: How much does she eat?

Mother: She's not too interested. Maybe ¼ cup.

Interviewer: Do you put anything on the cereal?

Mother: A little goat's milk.

Interviewer: How much?

Mother: An ounce or so.

Interviewer: Do you put anything else on the cereal?

Mother: Nothing else.

Interviewer: How often (out of 7 days) does she have rice cereal?

Mother: Oh, she has it 7 days at breakfast.

Interviewer: When does she have something else to eat or to drink?

Mother: She usually breast-feeds sometime in the morning.

Interviewer: How long does she stay at the breast?

Mother: About 10 minutes. She's learning to bite.

Interviewer: And when does she have something to eat again?

Mother: Between 11:00 and 12:00 I give her lunch. She likes yogurt and sardines. Sometimes I give her a cracker with sunflower seed butter on it, or if I have leftovers from the night before, I may give them to her.

Interviewer: What's next?

Mother: She usually breast-feeds after lunch and again midafternoon, and she has a bottle of pear juice some time in the afternoon.

Interviewer: How much pear juice does she drink?

Mother: Six or seven ounces.

Interviewer: How often does she have the juice?

Mother: Three or four times a week. If she doesn't have juice, she gets half of a small banana.

Interviewer: When does she eat again?

Mother: She eats with us about 7:00.

Interviewer: What does she usually eat?

Mother: I offer her fish, or yogurt, or cottage cheese, but she won't eat much. If we have turkey hot dogs or a vegetable she'll eat, I'll give her that.

Interviewer: How much does she eat?

Mother: About a tablespoon of two or three foods.

Interviewer: What do you do when she does eat?

Mother: I offer her more.

Interviewer: What do you do when she refuses to eat?

Mother: I try to find something else for her to eat or try to get her to eat another bite.

It became apparent during the interview that the *mother was unable to give information that could be quantitated, so a 7-day record of the child's food intake was requested,* which is shown in the box on the right. Quantitation of the 7-day food record showed an intake of 500 kcal/day or less in addition to the breast milk consumed. On this basis, inadequate energy and nutrient intake was diagnosed to be the cause of the infant's inadequate weight gain. *Therapy for this family involved much more than nutrition counseling. Psychosocial and parenting issues had to be dealt with as well.*

If children are overweight, activity patterns are explored. Discussions about the consumption of vending machine food and the effects of television on eating patterns may also provide important information.

It may be necessary to discontinue the detailed probing necessary for dietary history and use only a cross-check if parental tolerance for the continued questions is limited. It is also important to recognize that it may not be possible to obtain sufficient information during one interview; several follow-up clinic or home visits may be necessary to obtain a true picture of the child's feeding history and food intake.

Preschool teachers and public health nurses often provide information about a child's food intake at school and family food patterns.

When dietary data have been collected, an assessment is made of the following:
1. Parental knowledge of nutrition and appropriate foods for children
2. The adequacy of nutrients provided by the food offered to the child
3. The adequacy of the diet consumed by the child
4. Parental knowledge and use of community resources to improve the nutritional status of the child
5. Delays in feeding skills that affect food and nutrients consumed
6. Real or potential behavior patterns that can or do compromise a child's nutrient intake
7. The motivation of parents and the child to change the patterns of food intake

If this assessment indicates that adjustments need to be made only in the kinds of food or

---

❧
FOOD INTAKE RECORD

4:30 A.M.	Breast-fed
8 A.M.	Rice bran, 2 t
	Rice puffs, 1 T
	Goat's milk, ½ oz
9 A.M.	Breast-fed
10:15 A.M.	Banana, ¾ small
11:30 A.M.	Wheat grain crackers, ⅛
	Goat's milk, 2 oz
	Raw sunflower butter, 1 t
	Alfalfa sprouts, 1 t
	Mozzarella cheese, grated, 1 t
	Beets, 1 t
	Sardines, 3
	Goat's milk yogurt, 2 T
1 P.M.	Breast-fed
4:30 P.M.	Pear juice, 6 oz
5:30 P.M.	Sardines, 2
	Brown rice cracker, 1
	Sprouts, taste
7:50 P.M.	Goat's milk yogurt, 2 T
8 P.M.	Breast-fed

---

size of portions offered to and consumed by the child, or if a therapeutic diet is indicated, plans for modifying the child's food intake should be made with the child or parents. The counselor should be aware of community resources that help with the provision of food, such as the Supplemental Food Program for Women, Infants, and Children (WIC), the food stamp program, and school lunch programs. Clients may need help in contacting agencies that administer the programs. Plans for modifying food intake should be communicated to teachers, school lunch personnel, and others in the child's food environment.

If it appears that the child has delays in feeding skills or eating patterns or that parent-child interactions are also operative in problems presented, the nutritionist may need to screen for these specific problems so that appropriate referrals can be made.

EVALUATION OF ORAL MOTOR AND SWALLOWING FUNCTIONS

Children who are developmentally delayed or have abnormal muscle coordination may have difficulty with the various oral, swallowing, and fine motor skills needed for the process of eating. Failure to gain weight or eat appropriate foods for the child's age can be an early indication of a developmental or motor problem. Infants and children with these types of problems therefore may first be identified during a dietary intake interview and observation of feeding behavior. The nutritionist therefore needs a basic understanding of the development of normal oral skills so that early motor or oral motor difficulties can be identified and appropriate referrals can be made. Ideally, a knowledgeable pediatric therapist should be involved in the evaluation and planning of treatment for any individual with motorically based feeding problems.

Evaluation of Motor and Oral Motor Skills

Incoordination of **oral motor skills** or basic motor skills may be identified by an interview with the parents and by observation of the child's eating and drinking skills. The examiner should observe not only the level of the child's eating and self-feeding skills but also the level of assistance offered by the parent. Not only will this give the examiner information about the child's skill level, it may also give information about the relationship between the parent and child while eating.

The Screening of Eating Abilities form (pages 83–87) can be used by the dietitian or nutritionist during the dietary assessment when the child has not yet been seen by a skilled therapist. This screening tool was developed at the Child Development and Mental Retardation Center (CDMRC), now Center on Human Development and Disabilities (CHDD), of the University of Washington to provide comprehensive assessment of feeding behavior. Once the screening tool is completed, the evaluator should be able to determine whether the feeding difficulties are caused by abnormalities in overall motor and oral motor control or by developmental delay. Where age guidelines are mentioned, they are intended to be lenient in recognition of the normal range in acquisition of feeding skills. Many comprehensive evaluation tools are available for use in clinics, hospitals, and/or community centers.[12–17] Morris and Klein also provide a more detailed description of the normal oral motor sequence and many more examples of guiding questions that may be used during a parent interview.[12]

During the nutritional and oral motor assessment, the evaluator should not only observe the types of foods the child currently eats but, if developmentally appropriate, should also offer food textures at the next higher level. In this way, it can be determined whether the oral delays are caused by a lack of oral motor control or by lack of opportunity for more mature performance. For example, a child may demonstrate more mature lip, tongue, and jaw movements if foods are placed laterally between the gums or molars than if pureed foods are offered by spoon (fig. 3-2).

Difficulties in oral motor or swallowing control may be observed as a child moves to the next higher level of food texture, particularly when making the initial transition to solid food. The child may continue to use primitive oral patterns that were appropriate for the lower texture food until oral skills and familiarity are developed at the next level. Loss of food from the mouth, mild coughing or sputtering, or rejection of food should not necessarily be considered problems during this transition stage. Should these behaviors persist, however, more careful evaluation of oral motor control and responses to varied sensory stimuli should occur.

If the oral motor screen identifies delays in feeding behavior that do not appear to be secondary to abnormal motor control, changes in the diet can be suggested to support developmental progress as outlined in chapter 10. If abnormal oral and basic motor patterns are observed, however, referral to a specialized

Text continued on p. 88.

✤

SCREENING OF EATING ABILITIES

Child's name: _____ ID#: _____ B.D.: _____
Medical diagnosis, if known: _____
Name of evaluator: _____
Name of parent or caregiver: _____ Phone: _____
Other agencies involved: _____

I. Questions to ask of parent or caregiver
  A. What are your greatest concerns in regard to feeding?
  B. What are the food likes and dislikes of your child in relation to texture, temperature, color, and flavor?
  C. Are some foods more difficult for your child to eat than others?
  D. Are there any foods that your child cannot eat?
  E. Does your child take any medication or food supplements?
  F. When does your child have meals and snacks?
  G. Does your child eat with the family?
  H. Who assists at mealtimes (home, school, other)?
  I. How much assistance is given?
  J. What textures are usually eaten (thin liquid, thick liquid, soft spoon food, soft chewy food, ground food, chopped food, crunchy food—see list below)?

II. Tactile sensitivity
    These stimuli are applied toward the beginning of the evaluation before offering food, but after the child has had some opportunity to adjust to you as a stranger. Tell the child what you are going to do before applying the stimuli. Be cautious in overinterpreting inappropriate responses that may be social or behavioral and not necessarily tactile.

    First, lightly stroke the front and back of each of the child's hands. Then stroke the front aspect of the skin on each arm. Finally, stroke the face, lips, and gums with firm pressure of your fingertips.

Appropriate
Neutral or positive response to touch
  ☐ Hand, arm
  ☐ Face
  ☐ Gums, outside teeth, when stroked
    with a fingertip

Questionable appropriateness
Muscle tension, moving away from stimulus
  or vocal protest
  ☐ Hand, arm
  ☐ Face
  ☐ Gums, outside teeth, when stroked
    with a fingertip

Questionable appropriate responses may be caused by situational variables, but if the caregiver reports consistent negative responses, a therapy referral is indicated.

III. Food offered
    These foods are listed in sequence according to difficulty and are grouped into three levels of corresponding normal developmental skills. Ask the caregiver to first offer foods commonly eaten at home, then try some of the other textures at more difficult levels.

Modified from Carman P: *Screening of eating abilities,* Occupational Therapy Department, Center on Human Development and Disabilities, 1996, Seattle, University of Washington.

Continued.

❖

SCREENING OF EATING ABILITIES—*cont'd*

Watch carefully for amount of chewing, movement of food within the mouth, and tendency to choke. Small amounts of food are offered from each category appropriate to the child's developmental level so that satiation does not occur too quickly. Thin liquid is offered to every child, but soft spoon foods or soft chewy foods should be omitted when the child has demonstrated higher level skills. Thick liquid is offered only when thin liquids are difficult (evidenced by choking, liquid running out of mouth).

A. *Child less than 5 months of age developmentally* (needs head and trunk support while eating, e.g., needs to be held in adult's arms, infant seat, special support chairs).
   - ☐ Thick liquid (optional, offered when thin liquid is taken with difficulty): milkshake, thinned applesauce, thinned yogurt
   - ☐ Thin liquid: milk, water, fruit juice
   - ☐ Soft spoon food: applesauce, pudding, yogurt

B. *Child 5 to 12 months of age developmentally* (good head control, needs some trunk support while eating, sits upright in chair).
   - ☐ Soft chewy food, cheese, tuna fish
   - ☐ Crunchy food that dissolves readily: cracker, potato stick
   - ☐ Oblong finger food (easier to grasp): potato stick, green bean
   - ☐ Small finger food (harder to grasp): Cheerios, puffed cereal

C. *Child more than 12 months of age developmentally* (with good head and trunk control and tongue mobility, lateralization).
   - ☐ Hard crunchy food: melba toast, bread stick
   - ☐ Chopped table foods
   - ☐ Bite-sized table foods: raisins
   - ☐ Multitexture foods (solid plus liquid): apple, celery, soup
   - ☐ Chewy food: chicken, hamburger, small pieces of well-cooked meat
   - ☐ Hard foods that break into diffuse pieces: carrots, nuts (if older than 2 years of age)

IV. Observations of child eating

Caregiver is asked to feed the child in the usual way. Ask whether any particular equipment or furniture is used that may not be present for this observation.

Mark NA (not applicable) if child is younger than stated age. Asterisks indicate posture or movement that is always abnormal; other activity of questionable appropriateness may be caused by neurological immaturity or other factors.

A. *Positioning*

Appropriate
   - ☐ Held by caregiver (if younger than 1 year of age) within 30° of upright
   - ☐ Within 30° of upright, propped, or special seat (hips flexed 90° in usual sitting angle)
   - ☐ High chair
   - ☐ Other: _____

Questionable appropriateness
   - ☐ Held by caregiver (lying back, asymmetrical, or otherwise unusual)
   - ☐ Held by caregiver (older than 1 year of age)
   - ☐ Lying on flat surface
   - ☐ Other: _____

SCREENING OF EATING ABILITIES—*cont'd*

The health professional may wish to discuss alternative means of positioning if the usual method is questionably appropriate. If the child has abnormal muscle tone, appropriate positioning is much more difficult to achieve. Consultation with a physical therapist or occupational therapist should be obtained. Any of the following behaviors under the "questionable" column indicate need for a consultation or a therapy program.

B. *Posture and movement*

Appropriate

☐ Head in alignment with body
☐ Head control stable (expected by 4 or 5 months of age)
☐ Arms forward, hands midline (frequent by 4 to 6 months of age)
☐ Hands, legs, and feet move freely, without stiffness
☐ Hips flex easily for sitting, knees spread apart spontaneously for wide sitting base
☐ Trunk straight when sitting (expected by 5 to 6 months of age)

Questionable appropriateness

☐ Head frequently back or to one side, rotated to one side
☐ Lack of head stability, excess motions, floppy, pushes back, falls forward (older than 5 months of age)
☐ Arms frequently retracted at shoulders, hands do not come together (older than 4 to 5 months of age)
☐ Legs and feet seem stiff, seldom move, or move in stereotyped patterns
☐ Hips resist bending or intermittently extend; narrow sitting base, knees pull together
☐ Trunk tilted, slumped, rotated, or arched backwards (older than 5 months of age)

C. *Oral motor coordination*

JAW

Appropriate

☐ Jaw opens and closes easily, controlled to receive food
☐ Jaw stabilized with little movement
☐ Jaw moves up and down with slight lateral movements when chewing ("rotary")

Questionable appropriateness

☐ Jaw opens too wide or with tension
☐ Delayed jaw opening response to receive food
☐ Jaw moves up and down while drinking from a cup so liquid is lost (older than 12 months of age)
☐ Jaw clamps down intermittently (older than 2 years of age)
☐ Lack of up and down movement with solid food

TONGUE

Appropriate

☐ Tongue stays within mouth while drinking
☐ Tongue stays within mouth with foods
☐ Tongue lateralized, food placed at side (6 months of age); food placed midline (9 months of age)

Questionable appropriateness

☐ Tongue protrudes past border of lips while drinking
☐ Tongue protrudes with spoon foods
☐ Tongue moves forward and backward when solid foods are placed at side of mouth or presented midline, no lateral movement

Continued.

❖

SCREENING OF EATING ABILITIES—cont'd

LIPS

Appropriate
- ☐ Lips seal on nipple or cup rim
- ☐ Lips close on and clean spoon
- ☐ Lips move actively while chewing

Questionable appropriateness
- ☐ Liquids not retained well by lips with nipple, with cup (older than 24 months of age)
- ☐ Spoon foods not retained well by lips (older than 8 months of age)
- ☐ Passive lips while chewing

SWALLOW
- ☐ Swallows readily
- ☐ Swallows liquids, no choking
- ☐ Swallows solids, seldom chokes

- ☐ Delayed swallow, slows eating
- ☐ Chokes two or more times when drinking liquid from a cup
- ☐ Chokes two or more times when drinking liquids other than from a cup (bottle, etc.)
- ☐ Chokes two or more times when solids are fed

GAG REFLEX
- ☐ Normal **gag reflex** (readiness to vomit when pressure applied to pharyngeal wall, soft palate, posterior tongue)

- ☐ Gag reflex hyposensitive (slow or absent)
- ☐ Gag reflex hypersensitive (occurs to pressure on middle or front of tongue or at sight of certain food)

SALIVA CONTROL
- ☐ Swallows saliva (doesn't drool)

- ☐ Drools when not eating (older than 24 months of age) and when not teething

D. *Prehension*

Grasping of objects starts with a reflexive closing when the palmar surface of the hand is stimulated; the grasp becomes voluntary with maturity and is gradually refined to use of opposed fingertips. Any observations of questionable quality or prolonged primitive skill level should be cause for further evaluation.

Appropriate
- ☐ Reflexive grasp (fading by 3 months of age)
- ☐ Raking grasp, whole hand (by 6 months of age)
- ☐ Thumb to side of fingers (8 months of age and older)
- ☐ Thumb to fingertips of index and/or middle fingers

Questionable appropriateness
- ☐ Wrist flexed, hand often in awkward position
- ☐ Hand usually fisted (older than 3 months of age)
- ☐ Hand usually limp or grasp weak
- ☐ Grasps food too tightly
- ☐ Raking, use of whole hand (older than 12 months of age)
- ☐ Difficulty releasing grasp (older than 12 months of age)

❖

SCREENING OF EATING ABILITIES—*cont'd*

E. *Hand and arm movement*

A child must have head and upper trunk control before the hand can be used for purposeful reaching. At first the hand and arm movements appear to be random. Purposeful movements are first seen as a child brings the hands to the mouth and the hands together at midline. Reaching for toys and bringing them to the mouth precedes finger-feeding. As control of the trunk improves, arm and hand use matures. A child will usually grasp the spoon and help bring it to the mouth long before he or she is able to control it independently. The effort of holding a cup is seen initially as the cup is pushed tightly against the mouth to stabilize it; it is difficult at this stage to stop drinking and put a partially full cup back to the table without spilling. Abnormal muscle tone or lack of head and trunk stability interferes with the quality and effectiveness of hand use.

Appropriate

☐ Hand to mouth
☐ Hands to midline, hands together
☐ Hand touches object purposefully
☐ Toy to mouth
☐ Holds bottle or drinks from cup
  (hands may be on cup, adult controls)
☐ Self-feeds finger foods
☐ Helps with spoon
☐ Independent with spoon, spills
☐ Independent with spoon, no spills
☐ Holds cup with some assistance
☐ Independent with cup

Questionable appropriateness

☐ Arms tight, limited movement
☐ Hands usually fisted (older than 2 to
  3 months of age)
☐ Hand frequently misses object,
  overshoots (older than 6 months of age)
☐ No attempt to reach for food or spoon,
  even when hungry and food is within
  reach (older than 6 months of age)
☐ Uses spoon with much extraneous
  movement and spilling
☐ Other: _____

F. *Cooperation*

Appropriate

☐ Motivated to eat
☐ Accepts food passively
☐ Participates to best of ability
☐ Socially appropriate behavior

Questionable appropriateness

☐ Does not seem to care about eating
☐ Actively resists eating (turns
  mouth away or slow to open mouth)
☐ Physical skills not used to potential
  for self-assistance
☐ Socially disruptive, attention seeking

Any observations of questionable cooperation tend to reduce the validity of other observations. A more thorough evaluation of parent-child interaction during mealtime may be indicated and may be the primary area requiring assistance.

FIG. 3-2   Occupational therapist evaluates oral motor patterns of child with cerebral palsy.

♣
INDICATIONS OF SWALLOWING DYSFUNCTION

1. History of frequent upper respiratory infections or pneumonias of unknown etiology
2. Consistent coughing or choking during swallowing
3. Noisy or "wet"-sounding upper airway sounds after individual swallows, or noisiness that increases over the course of the feeding
4. Inability to handle own oral secretions
5. More than one swallow needed to clear a single bolus

pediatric occupational, physical, or speech therapist is necessary. Resources for names of treatment centers or private therapists may be available from individual state therapy associations, the local school district, or the nearest regional children's hospital. When specialized services are not immediately available, initial steps may be attempted to improve the quality of food intake by using the basic principles of positioning discussed in chapter 10.

The family's concerns, strengths, and resources are an important consideration in the development of any treatment program. The final feeding plan should be the distillation of the nutritionist's/therapist's goals and the family's goals. The rationale for suggested changes should be thoroughly explained and expectations for follow-through must be reasonable. It may take longer to feed a child in the desired position or when using therapeutic techniques, especially when they are first implemented. Implementing the new procedures at only a portion of the meal, or at the least stressful meal of the day, may ease the transition. Consideration of the client's and caregiver's comfort, feelings, and opinions is a key factor in developing an effective feeding program. Changes in motor or oral motor control may be slow to achieve. Changes in the feeding environment, however, may be easier to make and have significant impact on the long-term social, nutritional, and physical development of the individual.

Evaluation of Swallowing Function

Effective eating is not only the product of movements of the tongue, lips, jaw, and cheeks but also includes an efficient and safe swallowing mechanism. Since swallowing dysfunction can lead to aspiration, difficulties in swallowing function may influence children's food intake and thus their nutrition as well as affect their overall health. Therefore some assessment of the swallowing function should occur during a screening of the motor skills necessary for eating.

Typically, the swallowing function is divided into three phases: the oral phase, the pharyngeal phase, and the esophageal phase. The child's oral motor control is a reflection of the oral phase of swallowing. The oral phase sets the stage for the pharyngeal phase by forming the foodstuff into a cohesive bolus, moving it backward in the mouth, and propelling it into the pharynx at the appropriate time when the pharyngeal swallow is initiated. Thus oral motor difficulties may not only affect the type of food the child is able to eat, but also contribute to difficulties in swallowing.

The pharyngeal phase is what has typically been thought of as the swallow. During this phase the airway is closed and protected from aspirating food or liquid, and the bolus is propelled through the pharynx into the esophagus. Precise timing and closure of nasopharynx and larynx are needed to channel the bolus in the appropriate direction without aspiration. Although the clinician is able to make direct observations about the oral phase of swallowing, only inferences about the function of the pharyngeal phase can be made during clinical evaluation. The Indications of Swallowing Dysfunction box lists a number of clinical indications of swallowing dysfunction. If one or more of these indications are present, further detailed evaluation of swallowing is needed.

Several factors may impair the ability of children with cerebral palsy to swallow. Difficulties in oral motor control may impede the child's ability to form the foodstuff into an appropriate size bolus as well as interfere with propelling the bolus into the pharynx at the appropriate time as the swallow is initiated.[18] Aspiration may occur if parts of the bolus fall piecemeal into the pharynx before the swallow is initiated and the airway is closed. Children with cerebral palsy also have significant difficulty coordinating swallowing and breathing. Baseline respiratory rate is faster for children with cerebral palsy and tidal volume is less.[19,20] Children with cerebral palsy have difficulty timing and sustaining respiration during feeding and often swallow at variable times during the breathing cycle.[20] Inhibition of breathing in preparation for swallowing tends to occur when the food or liquid is visually presented and not just prior to the triggering of the swallow. Therefore, during feeding, ventilatory patterns are disrupted for a longer period of time in children with cerebral palsy, placing them at greater risk for aspiration due to poor coordination of swallowing and breathing.[21,22,23]

Detailed evaluation of the swallowing mechanism can be made only through a radiologic procedure. This test is known as the videofluoroscopic swallowing study (VFSS) or modified

FIG. 3-3   A child positioned for videofluoroscopy. The x-ray table is tilted vertically. A small child sits in a "Tumbleform" feeder seat. Wheelchairs or other adapted chairs may be used for larger children.

From Wolf LS, Glass RP: Feeding and swallowing disorders in infancy: assessment and management, Tucson, Ariz, 1992. Therapy Skill Builders.

barium swallow. The procedure is structured to simulate the child's typical feeding regimen in terms of seating, food types, and textures. Special devices may be needed to position the motor-impaired child for the procedure. Foods are mixed with barium, then feeding is viewed real-time with the fluoroscope and recorded on videotape for later review. The function and safety of the swallowing mechanism can be determined (fig. 3-3).[24]

This procedure is generally available only at tertiary-level hospitals. The personnel completing the study typically include a speech or occupational therapist and radiologist or radiology technician. These individuals should have a solid background in pediatric feeding processes to make the most reliable interpretation of the test results. This is a highly specialized procedure and may not be available in all locations. If, however, the child has significant nutritional, oral motor, and health problems, and swallowing dysfunction is a contributing factor, efforts should be made to obtain this radiologic evaluation of the swallowing function.

CONSIDERATION OF PSYCHOSOCIAL FACTORS

Whenever and wherever the nutrition of a child is discussed, consideration must also be given to factors that have no direct relationship on the feeding process. Eating behavior serves as a sensitive barometer of the general adjustment of child, parent, and family. For this reason intrapersonal and interpersonal factors that influence food intake should also be taken into consideration when collecting and assessing information.

Since parents are primarily responsible for providing infants and children with both food and the environment in which it is consumed, attention should be given to the parents' psychosocial well-being, adaptation to the parenting role, and general level of parenting skills. Because patterns of food intake, even in young children, can be altered by emotional status, screening should also consider the socioemotional development of the child. When appropriate food is available and there is no evidence of biological or organic problems in the child, it is not unusual to find that the cause of a disturbance in food intake is within the psychosocial/emotional category. Such problems can manifest themselves in a variety of ways, for instance, parent or child dissatisfaction with the feeding or mealtime situation, parental neglect or overconcern with food or feeding, anorexia or vomiting, and food aversions or food gorging.

Stress Level and Family Coping

Infants and children are sensitive to feelings and attitudes of parents, especially at feeding and bedtime. Younger parents, those who are dependent on relatives, those who have a history of unhappy childhoods, and those who are suffering from mental problems often have disturbed relationships with their children. These parental characteristics influence the eating behavior of children. It is reasonable to hypothesize that parents who are anxious or distressed somehow communicate these states to their babies and young children, which in turn affects eating behavior. Older children are also quick to identify tension or conflict between adults at the dinner table and to respond. Reality stressors such as job or financial worries, recent change of domicile, and illness or injury of child or parent are additional factors that can disrupt routines and can be associated with temporary symptoms related to food or feeding behavior. Personal problems of adult family members, for instance, marital discord, unresolved grief, depression, drug use, or lack of self-esteem, may also influence the feeding situation involving children. When the feeding problem appears to be nonorganic, it is appropriate to ask parents a few simple questions to determine the current and long-term emotional climate in the home. This can be done selectively in an interview or by using a questionnaire as a routine part of the assessment process (see the Screening Questionnaire for Family Stress).

Parental Feelings of Competence and Satisfaction

Clinical observations indicate that parental *feelings* of competence and satisfaction or dissatisfaction with the parental role are psychological factors that also have an influence on the food intakes and feeding behaviors of children. When an individual, for whatever reason, experiences minimal feelings of success in carrying out the activities associated with parenting, the opportunity for experiencing satisfaction decreases proportionately and the stage is set for problems in parent-child interaction. If the parent does not feel adequate in handling child-care activities outside of feeding, lack of confidence or feelings of incompetence can eventually be manifested in a problematic feeding situation. The mother who reported the following impressions was trying to deal with a 3-year-old boy whose diet consisted only of olives, avocados, and salmon:

I'll never forget what I felt like when he was 2 weeks old and I had to care for him completely on my own. It wasn't at all what I expected. I was scared to death and sure that every time he cried I must have done something wrong. There were half-filled bottles all over the house because I worried that the milk might spoil if Gary didn't drink it in 10 or 15 minutes. My mother-in-law didn't help. She is still always giving me suggestions for a better way to do something.

SCREENING QUESTIONNAIRE FOR FAMILY STRESS

	Yes	No
1. During the past year have any of the following occurred in your immediate family?		
Family moved?	☐	☐
Death, divorce, separation, loss of family member?	☐	☐
Marriage, reconciliation, pregnancy, new family member?	☐	☐
Serious injury or illness, problem with aging relative?	☐	☐
Loss of work, change of job, retirement?	☐	☐
Frequent or serious arguments or fights?	☐	☐
Money problems?	☐	☐
Drug or drinking problems?	☐	☐
Trouble with the law?	☐	☐
Some other serious problem?	☐	☐
If yes, what? _____		
2. During the past year:		
Has anyone in your family been seriously upset, depressed, or moody?	☐	☐
Have you been generally happy with your family's way of life?	☐	☐
Have you often felt lonely or cut off from other people?	☐	☐
Have you or your mate had serious differences that you feel may be related to differences in religion, race, nationality, or family background?	☐	☐
3. Have you and your children been separated for more than 1 day in the past year?	☐	☐
Do you have someone reliable to take care of your children when you need it?	☐	☐
Are your children cared for daily by someone outside the family?	☐	☐
If yes, has it been the same person for the past year?	☐	☐

Modified from Metz JR and others: *Pediatrics* 58:4, 1976.

In early infancy the close relationship to and dependence on the mother, in particular, often become linked with the feeding process. For this reason many individuals equate successful mothering with a well-nourished infant or child and a nonproblematic feeding situation. The comments of the mother of a toddler who has congenital heart disease and developmental delays, and who is still on a diet of pureed foods are illustrative:

I couldn't do anything about his heart, but I did pretty well at feeding him by that nasogastric tube. Nobody else could do it as well as I did. Now when he doesn't eat, I fix a special high energy pudding for him so that he doesn't lose weight. He really gobbles it down!

Factors like past experience, age, knowledge of child growth and development, and the input of significant family members or professionals are important determinants of parental feelings of competence. The standards of performance or values that parents hold for themselves, along with their more general feelings of self-esteem, are also related to perceptions of competence. But probably the most significant influence on parental feelings of success or satisfaction is the perceived responsiveness of the child; that is, does the child show developmental and social evidence of a positive response to parenting? With these determinants in mind the following questions can serve as guidelines for eliciting data on the adaptation to parenting and its associated emotional responses:

1. As you were growing up, did you observe or assist with the upbringing of younger children such as brothers or sisters, relatives, friends, or neighbors?
2. How would you rate your maternal feelings on a scale of 1 to 5, with 1 being very maternal and 5 being nonmaternal?
3. What has been the biggest surprise or thing you least expected about being a parent?
4. How satisfied are you with your child's physical growth and development?
5. How satisfied are you with your child's social adjustment?
6. How much influence does your spouse have on your ideas about childrearing? Do you usually agree or disagree on childrearing concerns?
7. Who or what has had the most influence on your ideas about childrearing? Books, magazines, or the media? Religion? Friends, neighbors, or relatives? Professionals? Formal education or parenting classes?
8. When you and your child are getting along as you usually do, how does your relationship with your child make you feel as a parent?
9. How satisfied are you with the way you handle your life in general?
10. How skillful do you feel as a parent?
11. How skillful a parent do you think you are *from the viewpoint of others* who know you well?
12. Before you had your own family, how did you feel about children?

Parent-Child Interaction

An integral component of assessment and data collection related to food intake is consideration of the interaction between child and parent. To have an indication of the effects of food and the feeding situation on the parent-child dyad, such data should be based on observation of both mealtime and nonmealtime situations. It is important to determine if food-related parent-child problems are situation specific or part of a more basic discord. Ideally, the assessment should be done in the home setting during mealtime *and* free-play situations. If this is not possible, every attempt should be made to simulate natural conditions in the clinic, office, or hospital environment.

Several research methods and standardized tools have been developed to evaluate parent-child interaction. Some practitioners may want to obtain training in the use of standardized assessment techniques; however, less formalized methods can also be helpful in collecting data. Using the concepts of **affectional ties, propensity to interact, feedback,** and **reciprocity** as organizers, it is possible to identify the essential elements of most interaction between parents and children.

I. **Affectional ties** (refers to the emotional attachment and degree of psychological involvement between parent and child)
   A. Appropriate interview questions
      1. Do you believe in unconditional parent love? Would you ever use such a term to describe your feelings about ____ ?
      2. How old was ____ when you really felt that he/she was *your* child?
      3. How does ____ know that you love and care about him/her?
      4. How do you know that ____ loves you?
      5. To whom or what is ____ most attached?
      6. Have you ever regretted the decision to become a parent? Occasionally? Frequently?
   B. Direct observation
      1. Attentiveness of parent to child's distress; physical comforting
      2. Use of expressions of love or special designations to refer to child *or* use of negative terms to refer to child; no reference to child by name
      3. Evidence of parental pleasure when child is complimented or comments are made regarding parent-child physical resemblances
      4. Evidence of strong mutual need for togetherness and a maximum avoidance of separation *or* parent or child tendency/preference for isolated activity

II. **Propensity to interact** (refers to the ability and desire of parent or child to give and receive communication)

  A. Appropriate interview questions
  1. When ____ is not around, do you ever find yourself thinking of something you want to do with him/her or something you want to tell him/her?
  2. Have you been (or are you ever) so preoccupied with adult worries or concerns that you don't have any energy left to interact with ____ ?
  3. Can you identify any person, thing, or situation that interferes with your relationship or communication with ____ ?
  4. How would you describe your relationship with ____ ?

  B. Direct observation
  1. Evidence of physical intactness (especially sensory and perceptual) of parent and child
  2. Evidence of emotional intactness of parent and child
  3. Presence or absence of reality stressors (as in the Family Stress Questionnaire, page 91)

III. **Feedback** and **reciprocity** (refers to chains of response between parent and child; activity of one that occurs as a direct result of stimuli from the other)

  A. Appropriate interview questions
  1. How does ___ let you know that he/she needs something or wants your attention? What is your usual response to this?
  2. Who or what usually initiates the interaction between you and your child?
  3. What do you do for ____ ? What does ____ do for you?

  B. Direct observation
  1. Efforts on the part of either parent or child to remain in touch (physically or verbally) that are successful
  2. Conversation, singing, laughing, or smiling that maintains an extended interaction (one partner answers the other, the latter responds in turn, and so on)
  3. Presence or absence of eye contact between parent and child
  4. Presence or absence of caregiving activity on the part of the parent in response to behavior (e.g., cry, yawn, request)
  5. Manner in which infant or young child is held
  6. Attention of parent to cues in the feeding situation (e.g., satiation, hunger, pacing)

When data indicate that a large part of a child's feeding or food intake problem is psychosocial, intervention must be planned accordingly. The primary focus of treatment is on strategies to alleviate stress and to support family coping abilities, on increasing parental knowledge and skill regarding childrearing, or on facilitating the parent-child relationship. In some situations these goals may be accomplished within the context of the feeding situation; however, in the majority of instances more specific treatment is indicated. Reality-based family needs demand rapid provision of concrete services to relieve situational demands. For this reason, referral to a public or private family service or social welfare agency may be appropriate. Those situations that require supportive counseling or education and anticipatory guidance may be handled in a variety of ways, for instance, with family therapy, enrollment in parenting classes, referral to a parent group, or one-on-one work with a qualified professional.

The variety of concerns presented about infants' and children's food intake clearly indicates that information sought must be based on problems presented and the health care professional's judgment. In some instances dietary intake data may provide sufficient information to design plans with parents and children to modify energy and nutrient intakes. In many cases, if plans are to be effective, the behavioral and psychosocial influences on a compromised food intake must be investigated. Parents of children with oral motor and self-feeding delays may need help in identifying specific foods to support developmental progress. Those with abnormal motor patterns need therapy.

Screening procedures may identify children with feeding problems of multiple causes, for whom an interdisciplinary assessment is appropriate. Factors that must be considered are adequacy of nutrient intake, structural abnormalities of the oral cavity, oral tissue health, medical status, speech development, living environment, social environment, and neurological integrity (including sensation). The collective data provide a base on which the cause of the problem may be determined, effective treatment plans may be designed, and progress may be assessed.

The team approach facilitates identification of priorities for treatment and use of a logical step-by-step approach. Periodic reevaluations of identified concerns indicate the effectiveness of programs designed.

Summary

Many studies have attempted to assess dietary methods. Most of these studies have found that children who provide information are not as reliable as adults. Even so, all methods have inherent limitations that should be recognized. The results of diet histories have not agreed with those of weighed food records when applied to individual children. Most studies have indicated that diet histories and food frequency questionnaires of children overestimate intake by individuals compared with 3- and 7-day food records. Children who have delays in feeding skills should be screened to determine whether the delays are because of abnormal motor patterns or an overall delay, which should determine the need for an occupational or physical therapy evaluation. Because many feeding difficulties in childhood are caused by parent-child interactions, it may be necessary to evaluate the family level of stress and coping and the interaction between parent and child.

REVIEW QUESTIONS

1. When is it necessary to collect dietary intake information?
2. Describe the advantages and disadvantages of the 24-hour recall.
3. How many consecutive days of food intake data are required for an accurate estimate of an individual's energy intake?
4. How does one identify the most appropriate computer program to use?
5. How does screening differ from assessment?
6. Under what circumstances is it important to screen children for oral motor difficulties when assessing food intake?
7. Why is it important to understand psychosocial factors that influence a child's food intake?

SUGGESTED LEARNING ACTIVITIES

1. Interview parents of a preschool child to collect a diet history. Assess the validity of the information collected.
2. Measure (in standard household measures) portions appropriate for children for 1 day; compare these with adult-size portions.
3. Keep a 7-day record of all food and beverages consumed. Assess the difficulty in keeping such a record.
4. Assess stress in the family of a preschool child whose parents consider the child to have a feeding problem.
5. Observe a comprehensive nutrition/feeding evaluation of a child who has oral motor feeding delays. Using appropriate tools, record dietary intake information, eating abilities, and level of family stress.

REFERENCES

1. Beal VA: The nutrition history in longitudinal research, *J Am Diet Assoc* 51:426, 1967.
2. Baranowski T, Sprague D, Baranowski JH, Harrison JA: Accuracy of maternal dietary recall for preschool children, *J Am Diet Assoc* 91:669, 1991.
3. Posner BM, Smigelski C, Duggal A and others: Validation of two-dimensional models for estimation of portion size in nutrition research, *J Am Diet Assoc* 92:738, 1992.
4. Mertz W: Food intake measurements: Is there a "gold standard"?, *J Am Diet Assoc* 92:1463, 1992.
5. Karvetti R, Lars-Runar K: Validity of the estimated food diary: Comparison of 2-day recorded and observed food and nutrient intakes, *J Am Diet Assoc* 92:580, 1992.
6. Van Horn LV and others: Dietary assessment in children using electronic methods, telephones and tape recorders, *J Am Diet Assoc* 90:412, 1990.

❖ ❖ ❖

CASE STUDY

Growth of a Male Infant with Down Syndrome

J. P. is referred for a nutrition evaluation.

J. P., a 14-month-old male with Down syndrome, who has been followed in a local pediatric clinic since birth, and his mother are referred for nutrition/feeding assessment and counseling. A videofluoroscopy and upper G.I. series performed at 3 months indicated no abnormalities. His cardiac status is considered

normal. He receives occupational/physical therapy twice a week.

J. P.'s weight and height have both declined in percentile on both the NCHS charts and Down growth charts since age 6 months, his weight more so than his height as shown in figure 3-4. He currently is 66 cm long and weighs 5.9 kg. His mother is concerned because J. P.

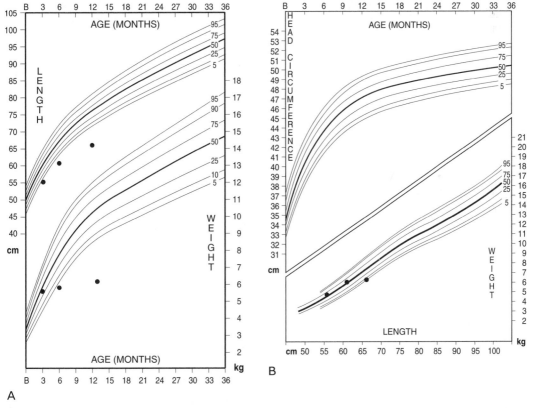

FIG. 3-4 Growth of a male infant with Down syndrome. **A.** Length and weight plotted on NCHS growth chart indicate decline since 6 months of age. **B.** Weight/length plotted on NCHS growth chart shows decrease in growth.

Continued.

✧ ✧ ✧

CASE STUDY

Growth of a Male Infant with Down Syndrome—cont'd

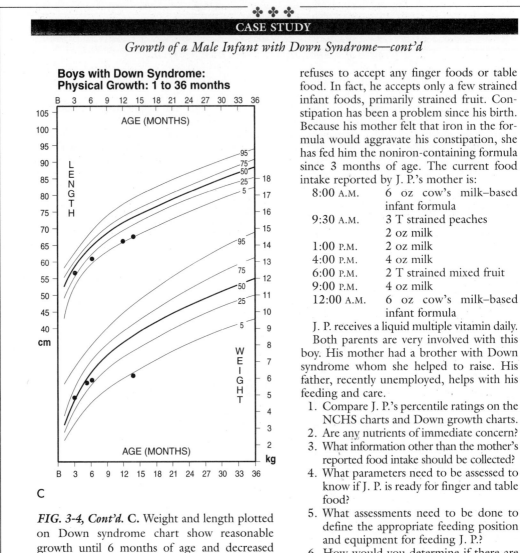

**Boys with Down Syndrome:
Physical Growth: 1 to 36 months**

C

FIG. 3-4, Cont'd. **C.** Weight and length plotted on Down syndrome chart show reasonable growth until 6 months of age and decreased weight gain at 15 months of age.

refuses to accept any finger foods or table food. In fact, he accepts only a few strained infant foods, primarily strained fruit. Constipation has been a problem since his birth. Because his mother felt that iron in the formula would aggravate his constipation, she has fed him the noniron-containing formula since 3 months of age. The current food intake reported by J. P.'s mother is:

8:00 A.M.	6 oz cow's milk–based infant formula
9:30 A.M.	3 T strained peaches 2 oz milk
1:00 P.M.	2 oz milk
4:00 P.M.	4 oz milk
6:00 P.M.	2 T strained mixed fruit
9:00 P.M.	4 oz milk
12:00 A.M.	6 oz cow's milk–based infant formula

J. P. receives a liquid multiple vitamin daily.

Both parents are very involved with this boy. His mother had a brother with Down syndrome whom she helped to raise. His father, recently unemployed, helps with his feeding and care.

1. Compare J. P.'s percentile ratings on the NCHS charts and Down growth charts.
2. Are any nutrients of immediate concern?
3. What information other than the mother's reported food intake should be collected?
4. What parameters need to be assessed to know if J. P. is ready for finger and table food?
5. What assessments need to be done to define the appropriate feeding position and equipment for feeding J. P.?
6. How would you determine if there are family stresses besides the father's current unemployment?

7. Black AE and others: Measurements of total energy expenditure provide insights into the validity of dietary measurements of energy intake, *J Am Diet Assoc* 93:527, 1993.
8. Burke BS: The dietary history as a tool in research, *J Am Diet Assoc* 23:1031, 1947.
9. Medlin C, Skinner JD: Individual dietary intake methodology: a 50 year review of progress, *J Am Diet Assoc* 90:1402, 1990.
10. Kaskoun MC, Johnson RK, Goran MI: Comparison of energy intake by semiquantitative food-frequency questionnaire with total energy expenditure by the doubly labeled water method in young children, *Am J Clin Nutr* 60:43, 1994.
11. Lee RD, Neiman D, Rainwater M: Comparison of eight microcomputer dietary analysis programs with the USDA nutrient data base for standard reference, *J Am Diet Assoc* 95:858, 1995.

12. Morris SE, Klein MD: *Prefeeding skills.* San Antonio, TX, 1987, Therapy Skill Builders.

13. Judd PL, Kenny DJ, Koheil R, Milner M, Moran R: The multidisciplinary feeding profile: A statistically based protocol for assessment of dependent feeders, *Dysphagia* 4:29–34, 1989.

14. Kenny DJ, Koheil RM, Greenberg J, Reid D, Milner M, Eng P, Moran R, Judd PL: Development of a multidisciplinary feeding profile for children who are dependent feeders, *Dysphagia* 4:16–28, 1989.

15. Jelm JM: *Oral-motor/feeding rating scale,* San Antonio, TX, 1990, Therapy Skill Builders.

16. Wolf LS, Glass RP: *Feeding and swallowing disorders in infancy: assessment and management,* Tucson, AZ, 1992, Therapy Skill Builders.

17. Glass RP, Wolf LS: Feeding and oral-motor skills. In Case-Smith J, editor: *Pediatric occupational therapy in early intervention,* Boston, 1993, Andove Medical.

18. Griggs CA, Jones PM, Lee RE: Videofluoroscopic investigation of feeding disorders of children with multiple handicap, *Dev Med Child Neur* 31:303–308, 1989.

19. Kenny DJ, McPherson KA, Casas MJ, Judd PL: Clinical Applications of Feeding Research. Presented at American Academy for Cerebral Palsy and Developmental Medicine Annual Meeting, Oct 3, 1992, San Diego, CA.

20. McPherson KA, Kenny DJ, Koheil R, Bablich K, Sochaniwskyj A, Milner M: Ventilation and swallowing interactions of normal children and children with cerebral palsy, *Dev Med Child Neur* 34:577–588, 1992.

21. Kenny DJ, Casas MJ, McPherson KA: Correlation of ultrasound imaging of oral swallow with ventilatory alterations in cerebral palsied and normal children: preliminary observations, *Dysphagia* 4:29–34, 1989.

22. Reilly S, Carroll L, Barnett S: Videofluoroscopy in the assessment of feeding disorders, *Dev Med Child Neur* 35:932–933, 1993.

23. Casas M, Kenny DJ, McPherson KA: Swallowing/ventilation interactions during oral swallow in normal children and children with cerebral palsy, *Dysphagia* 9:40–46, 1994.

24. Morton RE, Bonas R, Rourie B, Minford J: Videofluoroscopy in the assessment of feeding disorders of children with neurological problems, *Dev Med Child Neur* 35:388–395, 1993.

4 *Infant Feeding and Nutrition*

Peggy L. Pipes

❖❖❖

Objectives

After studying this chapter, the student should:

✔ *Recognize differences in human and other milks available for infants.*

✔ *Define the appropriate use of the various formulas and whole milk for infants.*

✔ *Recognize developmental landmarks during infancy that indicate a readiness for the infant to progress in feeding behaviors and a readiness for change in the varieties and textures of food that should be offered.*

✔ *Be aware of infant foods as sources of nutrients and appropriate use of foods to optimize the baby's nutritional status.*

✔ *Be aware of the variability among the personalities, growth patterns, and nutrient needs of infants at any age and the need to individualize what, when, how often, and how much each baby should be fed.*

At no time in the life cycle are as many changes in food and nutrient intake observed as during the first year of life. Influenced by a rapid but declining rate of physical growth, maturation of oral, fine, and gross motor skills, and relationships established with their parents, infants who are prepared at birth to suck liquids from a nipple are at 1 year of age attempting to feed themselves table food with culturally defined utensils. The need for nutrients and energy depends on the infant's requirement for maintenance, physical growth, and energy expenditure, whereas the foods offered to infants reflect culturally accepted practices. Infants' acceptance of food is influenced by both neuromotor maturation and their interactions with their parents. Because of the variability of the preceding parameters among infants, a variety of combinations of foods and milks are consumed by well-nourished children at any month during the first year.

PSYCHOSOCIAL DEVELOPMENT

Feeding is the fundamental interaction from which the relationship between parents and infants evolves and the infant's psychosocial development proceeds. Parents' responsiveness to the infant's cues of hunger and satiation and close physical contact during a feeding facilitate healthy psychosocial development. During the first year, being able to feed when hungry teaches babies a sense of trust and well-being, assurance that their needs will be met. For optimal development in early infancy, babies need to be fed as soon as they express hunger. As they grow older and learn to trust that their needs will be met, they can wait longer for the initiation of the meal. Tactile stimulation is also important. Babies need to be held and cuddled while they are fed. Some individuals believe that this skin contact facilitates bonding.

MATURATION OF DIGESTION AND ABSORPTION

The newborn is functionally immature. Although the normal neonate is well prepared to digest and absorb human milk, modified cow's milk formula, or soy formulas at birth, maturation of many of the enzyme systems occurs during and after the first year.

The stomach capacity of infants increases from 10 to 20 ml at birth to 200 ml by 12 months of age. The rate of stomach emptying depends on the size and the composition of the meal. During the first weeks after birth, gastric acidity decreases, and for the first few months it remains lower than in the adult.

Protein

Proteolytic activity of duodenal juice is as great in infancy as in adulthood. However, the total quantity of protein that can be digested per hour is less during infancy and childhood and increases with age.

Fat

A higher percentage of fat is absorbed in later life than in infancy. Younger infants lose a higher percentage of fat intake in their feces than do older infants. Cow's milk fat is not well absorbed by young infants. Vegetable oils mixed with commercially prepared infant formulas are well absorbed, although the reason for the degree of absorption of those containing oleo oil remains unclear. Absorption of fat begins to reach adult levels between 6 and 9 months of age.

Pancreatic lipase activity is low in the newborn, especially in the premature infant. The bile acid pool, although present, is reduced. When compared with an adult on the basis of body surface, the newborn, although able to synthesize bile, has a bile acid pool one-half that of the adult.

During infancy the position of the saturated fatty acid on the glycerol molecule influences absorption. Stearic acid is poorly absorbed in any position. Free palmitic acid hydrolyzed from positions 1 and 3 is poorly absorbed, whereas palmitic acid, which occupies position 2 on the glycerol molecule, remains as a monoglyceride and appears to be well absorbed.[1]

Carbohydrates

Maltase, isomaltose, and sucrase activity reaches adult levels by 28 to 32 weeks' gestation. Lactase, present at low levels at 28 weeks' gestation, increases near term and reaches adult levels at birth. Salivary and pancreatic **amylase** are low during the first months after birth. Concentrations of salivary amylase rise to adult levels between 6 months and 1 year of age, reaching two-thirds of adult levels by 3 months of age and full adult levels between 6 months and 1 year of age. Large variations in enzyme activity, however, have been noted among groups of infants. There appears to be no relationship between the activity of salivary amylase, the size of the infant, and intakes of starch-containing food before 3 months of age. Concentrations of pancreatic amylase increase from birth through the preschool years.

Most health care professionals believe that the introduction of infant cereal before 3 to 4 months of age is inappropriate.

RENAL FUNCTION

The newborn has an immature kidney. Functional development of the nephron is not complete until 1 month of age. The tubules are short and narrow and do not reach adult proportions until approximately 5 months. In addition, the pituitary gland produces only limited quantities of the antidiuretic hormone (ADH) vasopressin, which normally inhibits diuresis. These factors limit the newborn's ability to concentrate urine and to cope with fluid and electrolyte stress, that is, electrolyte-dense formula, limited fluid intake, diarrhea. By 1 month of age the normal infant can maintain water balance as efficiently as the adult.

Renal Solute Load

The major percentage of solutes presented to the kidney for excretion are the nitrogenous end products of protein metabolism: sodium, potassium, phosphorus, and chloride. If the elements were not utilized in new body mass or lost by nonrenal routes such as perspiration, they would have to be excreted in the urine. They are therefore referred to as the potential renal solute load. The potential renal solute load can be calculated by assuming all nitrogen is excreted, dividing dietary nitrogen by 28, and adding sodium, potassium, and chloride in the feeding expressed as milliosmoles, abbreviated mOsm.

These solutes must be concentrated in water derived from that pre-formed in the diet and formed from the oxidation of protein and carbohydrates. Each feed for typical infants yields approximately 95 ml of water per 100 ml consumed. Some water is utilized in new tissue and some is lost in the feces or by evaporation. The solutes are dissolved in the remainder. The concentrating capacity of some neonates has been reported to be as limited as 700 mOsm/L; of others as great as that of older children and adults, 1200 to 1400 mOsm/L. Human milk has a potential renal solute load of 93 mOsm/L; commercially available cow's milk–based formula, 133 mOsm/L; and soy formula, 177 mOsm/L.

Difficulties with the renal solute load are unlikely in typical infants fed human milk or a correctly prepared formula. Problems may occur when elevated environmental temperature or fever increase evaporative loss, when diarrhea occurs, and/or when infants consume a lesser volume of fluids.

MILK IN THE INFANT'S DIET

That human milk from adequately nourished lactating mothers offers nutritional, immunological, and psychosocial benefit to infants has never been questioned. However, the rates and duration of breast-feeding have decreased since 1984.

The incidence of breast-feeding is highest among mothers who are white, who have some college education, who have an average birth weight infant, and who are of increased maternal age. It is greater in the Pacific and Mountain regions, and least in the East and South Atlantic areas. Those who are less affluent, younger, and who have delivered their first child are least likely to breast-feed. Formula supplementation of breast-feeding has been consistently associated with a shortened breast-feeding duration.[2]

Interestingly, the decision to breast-feed is made before pregnancy by one-half to three-fourths of new mothers. Increased knowledge is associated with positive attitudes toward breast-feeding. Sources of influence about breast-feeding vary with ethnicity. Husbands or partners are most influential in the attitudes of white women, whereas mothers of Hispanics and close friends of blacks are most influential for those women. Reasons for rejecting breast-feeding include embarrassment, fear of pain, limitations on freedom and social life, and concern that the father would not be involved in feeding. Positive attitudes toward breast-feeding focus on healthy babies and convenience.[3]

Most typical full-term infants who are not breast-fed receive a cow's milk–based formula; very few receive fresh cow's milk. Milk-free formulas, including soy and hydrolyzed casein formulas, are fed to infants who do not tolerate milk.

Colostrum and Transitional Milk

For the first few days after birth, the breast-fed infant ingests a yellowish, transparent fluid called **colostrum.** Human colostrum contains more protein but less fat, carbohydrate, and energy than does mature human milk. Concentrations of sodium, potassium, and chloride are greater in colostrum than in later-produced milk. Between the third and sixth day colostrum changes to a milk that, compared with mature human milk,

TABLE 4-1   *Antiviral and Antibacterial Factors in Human Milk*

Factor	Shown in Vitro to Be Active Against
Secretory IgA	*Escherichia coli* (also pili and capsular antigens), *Clostridium tetani, Clostridium diphtheriae, Klebsiella pneumoniae, Salmonella* (6 groups), *Shigella* (2 groups), *Streptococcus, Streptococcus mutans, Streptococcus sanguis, Streptococcus mitis, Streptococcus salivarius, Streptococcus pneumoniae, Coxiella burnetii, Haemophilus influenzae* *E. coli* enterotoxin, *Vibrio cholerae* enterotoxin, *Clostridium difficile* toxins, *H. influenzae* capsule
IgM, IgG	*V. cholerae* lipopolysaccharide; *E. coli*
IgD	*E. coli*
Bifidobacterium bifidum growth z factor	Enterobacteriaceae, enteric pathogens
Factor binding proteins (zinc, vitamin B_{12}, folate)	Dependent *E. coli*
Lactoferrin	*E. coli*
Lactoperoxidase	*Streptococcus, Pseudomonas, E. coli, Salmonella typhimurium*
Lysozyme	*E. coli, Salmonella, M. lysodeikticus*
Carbohydrate	*E. coli* enterotoxin
Lipid	*Staphyloccocus aureus*
Ganglioside (GMI-like)	*E. coli* enterotoxin, *V. cholerae* enterotoxin
Glycoproteins (receptor-like) + oligosaccharides	*V. cholerae*
Analogues of epithelial cell receptors (oligosaccharides)	*S. pneumoniae, H. influenzae*
Milk cells (macrophages, neutrophils B and T lymphocytes)	By phagocytosis and killing: *E. coli, S. aureus, Salmonella enteritidis* By sensitized lymphocytes: *E. coli* By phagocytosis: *Corpus albicans, E. coli* Lymphocyte stimulation: *E. coli,* K antigen, tuberculin PPD Monocyte chemotactic factor production: PPD

From May JT: *Microbiol Sci* 5:42, 1988.   *Continued.*

has a high protein content. This is referred to as transitional milk. By the tenth day the breast-fed infant receives mature human milk.

Antiinfective Characteristics of Human Milk

In addition to nutrients, human colostrum and human milk contain antibodies, enzymes, and other factors that are absent or present in only minute amounts in cow's milk; factors that provide infants with protection against enteric infections.[4] Table 4-1 lists important antiviral and antibacterial factors present in breast milk.

Lactobacillus microorganisms in the gastrointestinal tract, whose growth depends on L-bifidus factor, produce acetic and lactic acids. The resulting acidic environment interferes with the growth of certain pathogenic organisms such as *Escherichia coli* and *Shigella* organisms and provides a medium in which lysozymes are stable. Lysozymes exert their effect by destroying bacterial cell membranes after the organisms have been inactivated by peroxides and ascorbic

TABLE 4-1   *Antiviral and Antibacterial Factors in Human Milk—cont'd*

Factor	Shown in Vitro to Be Active Against
Secretory IgA	Polio types 1, 2, 3, Coxsackie types A9, B3, B5, echo types 6, 9, Semliki Forest virus, Ross River virus, rotavirus, cytomegalovirus, reovirus type 3, rubella, herpes simplex virus, mumps virus, influenza, respiratory syncytial virus
IgM, IgG	Rubella, cytomegalovirus, respiratory syncytial virus
Lipid (unsaturated fatty acids and monoglycerides)	Herpes simplex; Semliki Forest virus, influenza, dengue, Ross River virus, Japanese B encephalitis virus, sindbis, West Nile
Nonimmunoglobulin macromolecules	Herpes simplex; vesicular stomatitis virus, Coxsackie B4, Semliki Forest virus, reovirus 3, poliotype 2, cytomegalovirus, respiratory syncytial virus, rotavirus
α_2-Macroglobulin (like)	Influenza hemagglutinin, parainfluenza hemagglutinin
Ribonuclease	Murine leukemia
Hemagglutinin inhibitors	Influenza, mumps
Milk cells	Induced interferon: virus or PHA
	Induced lymphokine (LDCF): phytohemagglutinin (PHA)
	Induced cytokine: by herpes simplex virus
	Lymphocyte stimulation: rubella, cytomegalovirus, herpes, measles, mumps, respiratory syncytial

acid also present in human colostrum and human milk.

Immunoglobulins (antibodies) to many different types of organisms, including pertussis, staphylococci, *E. coli,* and *Salmonella,* have been identified in colostrum and, in smaller amounts, in mature human milk. Since these immunoglobulins are not absorbed, they exert an effect only through the gastrointestinal tract. Infants who are breast-fed by mothers with high titers of antibodies to poliomyelitis are resistant to infection with orally administered polio vaccine. This effect is not believed to be operative after the infant is 6 weeks of age. Lactoperoxidase, an enzyme present in human milk and saliva, aids in killing streptococci and may act on other organisms.

Large amounts of lactoferrin and small amounts of transferrin (iron-binding proteins) in human milk exert a bacterial effect. Lactoferrin is less than 50% saturated with iron. It is bacteriostatic because it deprives bacteria of the iron-containing environment necessary for their normal cell growth.

There is no question that breast-feeding reduces infant mortality and morbidity in developing countries. The presence of the antiinfective and antiviral factors in human milk, in addition to the potential for unsanitary bottle-feeding, makes breast-feeding important for 1 to 2 years.[5] It has also become evident that the incidence of illness is less in breast-fed than formula-fed infants in industrialized societies.[6,7]

TABLE 4-2 Estimates of Concentrations of Nutrients in Mature Human Milk

Nutrient (Per Liter)	Amount in Human Milk[a]	Nutrient (Per Liter)	Amount in Human Milk[a]
	gm/liter ± SD[b]		µg/liter ± SD
Lactose	72.0 ± 2.5	Vitamin A, RE[d]	670 ± 200
Protein	10.5 ± 2.0		(2,230 IU[e])
Fat	39.0 ± 4.0	Vitamin D	0.55 ± 0.10
	mg/liter ± SD	Vitamin K	2.1 ± 0.1
Calcium	280 ± 26	Folate	85 ± 37[f]
Phosphorus	140 ± 22	Vitamin B$_{12}$	0.97[g,h]
Magnesium	35 ± 2	Biotin	4 ± 1
Sodium	180 ± 40	Iodine	110 ± 40
Potassium	525 ± 35	Selenium	20 ± 5
Chloride	420 ± 60	Manganese	6 ± 2
Iron	0.3 ± 0.1	Fluoride	16 ± 5
Zinc	1.2 ± 0.2	Chromium	50 ± 5
Copper	0.25 ± 0.03	Molybdenum	NR[i]
Vitamin E	2.3 ± 1.0		
Vitamin C	40 ± 10		
Thiamin	0.210 ± 0.035		
Riboflavin	0.350 ± 0.025		
Niacin	1.500 ± 0.200		
Vitamin B$_6$	93 ± 8[c]		
Pantothenic acid	1.800 ± 0.200		

Adapted from the Committee on Nutrition, Institute of Medicine: *Nutrition during lactation,* National Academy of Sciences, Washington DC, 1991, National Academy Press.

[a]Data taken from the Committee on Nutrition, 1985 unless otherwise indicated. The values are representative of amounts of nutrients present in human milk; some of them may differ slightly from those reported by investigators cited in the text.
[b]Standard deviation.
[c]From Styslinger L, Kirksey A: *Am J Clin Nutr* 41:21, 1985.
[d]RE, Retinol equivalents.
[e]IU, International units.
[f]From Brown CM, Smith AM, Piccino MF: *J Pediatr Gastroenterol Nutr* 5:278, 1986.
[g]From Sandberg DP, Begley JA, Hall CA: *Am J Clin Nutr* 34:1717, 1981.
[h]Standard deviation not reported; range 0.33 to 3.20.
[i]NR, Not reported.

Nutrient Compositions of Human Milk and Cow's Milk

Nutrients secreted in human milk vary and reflect individual biochemical variability among women, the diet consumed, the stage of lactation, and the length of time the mother has breast-fed. When milk is analyzed for nutrient content, the time of day the milk was expressed and whether foremilk or hindmilk is analyzed influence the results. Wide ranges of many vitamins and minerals have been reported. Table 4-2 lists estimated concentrations of nutrients in human milk.

Both human milk and cow's milk are complex liquids containing more than 200 components in the fat-soluble and water-soluble fractions. However, considerable differences in the quantity and availability of the nutrients in the two milks are evident. Differences are thought to reflect species' specific nutrient needs to support individual maintenance and growth needs of the offspring. This hypothesis is further supported by the fact that changes occur in the nutrient composition of human milk during lactation. For example, the concentrations of iron, copper, and zinc decline between 2 weeks and 5 to 9 months of lactation. Protein concentration decreases from the first week through 6 to 9 months of age and then rises slightly, reflecting the infant's declining needs during declining rates of growth.

Human milk provides similar amounts of water and approximately the same amount of energy as does cow's milk. The nutrient sources of the energy are, however, different. Protein supplies approximately 7% of the energy in human milk and 20% of the energy in cow's milk; the carbohydrate lactose supplies approximately 42% of the energy in human milk and 20% of the energy in cow's milk. The percentage of energy supplied by fat is similar in both milks.

The protein content of human milk is approximately 0.9 gm/100 ml compared with 3.5 gm/100 ml in cow's milk. Nonprotein nitrogen accounts for 25% of total nitrogen in human milk and 5% of total nitrogen in cow's milk. During lactation protein levels decrease.

Casein and **whey** constitute the protein in both human milk and cow's milk. Amounts of whey protein are similar in each. Cow's milk contains six to seven times as much casein as does human milk, and differences in the casein/whey ratios of the two milks are great. The casein/whey ratio of human milk is 40:60, whereas the casein/whey ratio of cow's milk is 82:18. β-Lactoglobulin, the dominant whey protein in cow's milk, is absent in human milk, in which α-lactoalbumin and lactoferrin are the dominant whey proteins.

During digestion in the stomach, the protein in milk mixes with hydrochloric acid. The result is the formation of curds from the casein and calcium and a liquid that contains whey. Because of its lower casein content, human milk forms a soft, flocculent, easy-to-digest curd in the infant's stomach. The increased casein content of fresh cow's milk causes it to form a tough, cheesy, hard-to-digest curd. Homogenization, boiling, and dilution of cow's milk modify the curd and prevent the formation of the hard curd in the stomach so that it is easily digested by the infant.

The amino acid composition of human milk meets the needs of the neonate with an immature enzyme system, whereas that of cow's milk may be inappropriate. The newborn has a limited ability to metabolize phenylalanine to tyrosine. Human milk has a low content of tyrosine and phenylalanine compared with cow's milk. The level of cystathionase, an enzyme that catalyzes the transulfuration of methionine to cystine, is low in the neonate. Taurine and cystine are present in much higher concentrations in human milk than in cow's milk.

The total fat content of human milk is similar to that of cow's milk. Saturated fatty acids predominate in cow's milk. The fatty acid pattern of human milk resembles that of the maternal diet. About 98% of the fat in human milk is triglycerides in which palmitic acid is in position 2, enhancing its absorbability. The average content of linoleic acid is 10% of fat, but ranges of 1% to 43% have been reported. Linoleic acid provides an average of 4% of the energy in human milk but only 1% of the energy in cow's milk. The cholesterol content of human milk averages 20 mg/100 ml, but there is considerable variability. Values up to 47 mg/100 ml have been reported. Cow's milk contains 7 to 25 mg/100 ml of cholesterol. Diurnal variations occur in human milk; the fat content is higher in early mornings, the short-chain fatty acid content is greater in cow's milk, and the fat content percentage of human hindmilk is higher than that of foremilk.

Both cow's milk and human milk contain lipoprotein lipase in the cream fraction that is stimulated by serum and inhibited by bile salts. Human milk contains an additional lipase that is stimulated by bile salts and contributes significantly to the hydrolysis of milk triglycerides. These enzymes contribute significantly to a higher percentage absorption of human milk fat as compared with butter fat.

The concentration of lactose is greater in human milk than in cow's milk. This nutrient is incorporated into galactolipids in the brain and spinal cord. Trace amounts of glucose, galactose, glucosamines, and other nitrogen-containing carbohydrates are also present in both milks. Human milk contains L-bifidus factor, a nitrogen-containing carbohydrate, in concentrations 40 times greater than that in cow's milk. This carbohydrate requires the *Lactobacillus* bacteria for growth.

Human milk from adequately nourished mothers is a reliable source of fat-soluble vitamins A and E and the water-soluble vitamins. The concentration of vitamin D in human milk has been shown to be influenced by maternal intake of vitamin D. The effect of sunlight on the infant is difficult to quantitate. However, vitamin D deficiency rickets continues to be identified in breast-fed infants and has occurred most often in infants with dark skin who have had little exposure to sunlight. Most breast-fed infants have exhibited normal growth and development without symptoms of vitamin D deficiency. A vitamin D supplement continues to be recommended for breast-fed infants, but evidence that supplements are necessary for infants with light skin is not convincing.[1]

Cow's milk is a reliable source of vitamin A and the B vitamins. It contains less vitamin E and more vitamin K than human milk. Most dairies fortify homogenized, 2%, and nonfat milk with vitamin D. Evaporated milk that is reconstituted with equal amounts of water is fortified with 400 IU/qt. Cow's milk is low in vitamin C.

Cow's milk contains four times as much vitamin K as human milk. In breast-fed infants the prothrombin level is 20% to 50% of that of the adult in the first few days. Hemorrhagic disease of the newborn may occur if vitamin K is not given. A prophylactic dose of 0.5 to 1 mg is usually given to breast-fed infants at birth.

Infants who are born at home and then breast-feed are at risk of vitamin K deficiency if they do not receive the supplement at birth. Women who plan to have home deliveries should be counseled before delivery about the infant's need for vitamin K.

Inadequate amounts of water-soluble nutrients in the maternal diet are reflected in milk produced for the infant. Infantile beriberi is well known in East Asians when maternal intakes of thiamin are inadequate. Vitamin B_{12} deficiency has been reported in breast-fed infants whose mothers adhered to vegan diets, had marginal intakes of vitamin B_{12}, or had a family history of pernicious anemia. Resolution of many of the neurological symptoms of the disorder followed treatment with vitamin B_{12}.[8]

The mineral content of cow's milk is several times greater than that of human milk. Cow's milk contains more than three times as much calcium and six times as much phosphorus as does human milk. The high phosphate load and calcium/phosphate ratio have been implicated as causes of late hypocalcemic tetany of the neonate.

The percentage of iron absorbed from human and cow's milk varies. The iron content of human milk declines between 2 weeks and 5 months from 0.5 to 0.3 mg/100 ml while that of cow's milk remains at 0.5 mg/ml. If infants continue to consume only breast milk after 4 to 6 months, they are at risk of negative iron balance and may deplete their reserves by 6 to 9 months.[9] Iron supplements are desirable for breast-fed infants.

Human milk contains less zinc than does cow's milk, although the bioavailability of zinc in human milk is much greater. In cow's milk zinc binds strongly to casein, but very little is bound to whey. The zinc-binding capacity of human milk protein is assumed to be minimal. Because stomach acid secretion is low in early infancy, ingested zinc may not be released from casein or its curd, making zinc from cow's milk inaccessible to infants. Studies suggest that the bioavailability of zinc in human milk is 59% and in cow's milk, 43% to 51%.

Plasma fluoride is poorly transferred to breast milk; thus breast-fed infants receive almost no fluoride. They should receive supplements of fluoride.

The high protein and mineral content of cow's milk places a much greater osmolar load on the kidney of the infant and obligates a greater amount of water for excretion. The margin of safety is smaller in cow's milk.

Antiallergenic Characteristics of Human Milk

The intestine of the newborn infant is permeable to macromolecules. Secretory IgA in human milk promotes closure of the gut and therefore decreases the permeability of **allergens.** Cow's milk protein β-lactoglobulin and serum bovine albumin are the most common allergens in infancy. Breast-feeding is the best prophylaxis for food allergy during infancy. Thus, it is apparent that if cow's milk is to be fed to infants, it must be modified.

NUTRIENT COMPOSITION REGULATIONS

Guidelines for energy and minimum and maximum levels of nutrients in formulas have been established by a number of groups, including the Committee on Nutrition of the American Academy of Pediatrics,[10] the European Society of Paediatric Gastroenterology and Nutrition, [11,12,13] a joint WHO/FAO commission,[14] and the Food and Drug Directorate in Canada.[15] In the United States, regulations regarding the composition of infant formula are established by the Food and Drug Administration.[16] Minimum levels for most nutrients and maximums for some have been established. It has been suggested that upper limits need to be established for nearly all nutrients.

MODIFIED COW'S MILK FOR INFANTS

Commercially manufactured formulas prepared from nonfat milk are available and generally used for feeding in infancy. (Table 4-3 lists nutrients in representative modified cow's milk formulas.) Three formulas are casein based utilizing fat-free milk as the protein source; three others are whey predominant. Combinations of vegetable oils, a high percentage of which are absorbed by infants, are added. Oleo oil also is added to one whey-based formula. Lactose is added to increase the energy concentration to approximately that of human and cow's milk.

Vitamins and minerals are added. Formulas are marketed both with and without ferrous sulfate in amounts that provide 12 mg per quart. Pediatricians encourage the use of formulas with iron.

Cow's milk formulas are prepared by modifying whole cow's milk to reduce the solute load by reducing the protein and mineral content. The curd tension is reduced through homogenization and heat treatment to produce an easily digested protein.

Hypoallergenic Formulas

The most commonly used products for infants with conditions that contraindicate the use of cow's milk are soy milks. The most frequently used formulas are constructed of protein isolated from soy meal fortified with methionine and corn syrup or sucrose, and soy or vegetable oils to which vitamins and minerals have been added. The trypsin inhibitor in raw soybean meal is inactivated during heat processing. The **goitrogenic effect** of soy is diminished by heating and by adding iodine.

Soy formulas are useful for potentially allergic infants but should not be used for infants with a documented allergy to cow's milk. Soy formulas are commonly used for infants who are recovering from diarrhea, and for children with galactosemia and lactase deficiency because these formulas contain no lactose.

Other formulas are marketed for infants who do not tolerate either soy or cow's milk. Nutramigen is prepared from a casein hydrolysate and corn oil, Pregestimil contains a casein hydrolysate and medium-chain triglycerides, and Alimentum contains free amino acids, medium-chain triglycerides, safflower, and soy oils. These formulas have an unpleasant odor and taste and are rarely accepted by infants if not introduced before 8 or 9 months of age. The composition of non-cow's milk–based formulas is given in table 4-4.

Goat's milk should be used with care during infancy. It is low in iron, folate, and vitamins C and D. It has a high solute load relative to cow's milk and may cause metabolic **acidosis** if fed in the first month of life. If goat's milk is used before 6 months of age, it should be diluted with water and carbohydrate should be added.

TABLE 4-3 Nutrient Content of Commercially Available Cow's Milk–Based Formula

Nutrient Source	Similac	Gerber Baby Formula	Enfamil	Good Start
Protein	Casein (evaporated skim milk)	Nonfat milk	Reduced minerals whey, nonfat milk	Reduced minerals whey, protein concentrate
Fat	Safflower, sunflower, coconut oils	Soy, coconut oils	Soy, coconut, palm olein, sunflower oils	Soy, palm olein, safflower, coconut oils
Carbohydrate	Lactose	Lactose	Lactose	Lactose, maltodextrin
Nutrient/100 ml (normal dilution)				
Energy (kcal)	68	67	67	67
Protein (gm)	1.45	1.5	1.5	1.6
Fat (gm)	3.65	3.6	3.3	3.4
Carbohydrate (gm)	7.2	7.2	6.9	7.4
Vitamin A (IU)	200	200	209	300
Vitamin D (IU)	40	40	43	60
Vitamin E (IU)	1.7	2	1.3	1
Vitamin C (mg)	5.5	6	5.5	8
Thiamin (μg)	65	67	53	60
Riboflavin (μg)	100	100	102	130
Niacin (mg equiv.)	.7	.7	.85	.75
Pyridoxine (μg)	40	40	43	15
Vitamin B$_{12}$ (μg)	.15	.16	.15	.2
Folic acid (μg)	10	10	10.6	9
Calcium (mg)	49.3	50	53	43
Phosphorus (mg)	37.8	39	36	24
Magnesium (mg)	4.1	4	5.3	4.5
Iron (mg)	1.2	Trace–1.2	Trace–1.2	1.0
Zinc (mg)	.5	.5	.5	.5
Copper (μg)	80	60	64	53
Iodine (μg)	9	5.4	4.1	5.6

Feeding infants formulas made from recipes that have not been proved to support adequate nutrition should be strongly discouraged. Malnutrition in infancy can result from the use of nondairy creamer to replace formulas, extended use of clear liquids after an episode of illness, and using recipes with little milk.

Formula Preparation

Manufacturers market formulas as liquid concentrates to be prepared for feeding by mixing equal amounts of the liquid and water. Ready-to-feed formulas that require no preparation are available in an assortment of sizes (4-, 6-, 8-, and 32-oz bottles and cans). Powdered formula

TABLE 4-4 *Nutrient Content of Soy Formulas and Other Special Formulas for Infants*

Nutrient Source	Prosobee	Isomil	Nutramigen	Progestimil	Alimentum	Gerber Soy	Next Step Toddler
Protein	Soy protein	Soy protein	Casein hydrolysate	Casein hydrolysate	Cystine, tyrosine, tryptophan	Soy protein	Soy protein
Fat	Soy oil	Coconut oil, soy oil	Soy, coconut, palm olein oils	Corn oil, medium-chain triglycerides, soy oils	Medium-chain triglycerides, safflower and soy oils	Soy, coconut oils, soy lecithin	Palm olein soy, coconut, sunflower oil
Carbohydrate	Corn syrup solids	Corn syrup solids, sucrose	Modified tapioca starch, sucrose	Corn syrup solids, modified tapioca starch	Sucrose, modified tapioca starch	Corn syrup	Corn syrup solids
Nutrients per 100 ML—normal dilution							
Energy (kcal)	68	68	67	68	68	67	67
Protein (g)	2.0	1.8	1.9	1.9	1.9	2.0	2.2
Fat (g)	3.6	3.7	2.7	3.8	3.7	3.6	3.0
Carbohydrate (g)	6.8	6.9	9.1	7.0	6.9	6.7	8.0
Vitamin A (IU)	210	203	210	256	304	203	203
Vitamin D (IU)	42.0	41.0	42.0	51.0	30.4	40	40
Vitamin E (IU)	1.4	2.0	2.1	2.5	2.0	2	1.4
Vitamin C (mg)	5.5	6.0	5.5	7.9	6.0	6	8
Thiamin (µg)	52.0	41.0	52.0	52.0	41.0	40	54
Riboflavin (µg)	63.0	61.0	63.0	63.0	61.0	61	61
Niacin (mg) (equiv.)	0.8	0.9	0.8	0.8	0.9	.7	.7
Pyridoxine (µg)	42.0	41.0	42.0	42.0	41.0	40	60
Vitamin B$_{12}$ (µg)	0.2	0.3	0.2	0.2		.3	.2
Folic acid (µg)	11.0	10.0	10.6	10.6	10.0	10	11
Calcium (mg)	63.0	71.0	63.0	63.0	71.0	64	78
Phosphorus (mg)	50.0	51.0	42.0	42.0	51.0	50	61
Magnesium (mg)	7.4	5.1	7.4	7.4	5.1	5.4	5.4
Iron (mg)	1.3	1.2	1.3	1.3	1.2	1.2	1.2
Zinc (mg)	0.5	0.5	0.5	0.5	0.5	.5	.8
Copper (µg)	63.0	51.0	63.0	63.0	50.7	50.7	50.7
Iodine (µg)	7.0	10.0	4.8	4.8	10.1	1.0	10.1

that is prepared by mixing 1 level tbsp of powder in 2 oz of water is also available. All of the formulas, when properly prepared and adequately supplemented, provide the nutrients important for the infant in an appropriate energy concentration and present a solute load reasonable for the normal full-term infant. Errors in dilution caused by misunderstanding the proper method of preparation, improper measurements, or the belief of the parents that their child should have greater amounts of nutritious food can lead to problems.

Result of Errors in Formula Preparation

Feeding dilute formula or water instead of formula can lead over time to undernutrition and/or water intoxication with symptoms of hyponatremia, irritability, and coma. Failure to appropriately gain in height and weight has been observed as a result of dilution of ready-to-feed formulas as if they were concentrates. Parents have also been known to add extra water to formula in the belief that a more dilute formula might reduce spitting up by their infants.

Use of undiluted formula is also dangerous to infants. Feeding undiluted concentrated formula increases energy, protein, and solutes presented to the kidneys for excretion and may predispose the young infant to **hypernatremia,** tetany, and obesity. Problems of improper formula preparation have most frequently been reported with the use of powdered formula and occur most often when an increased need for water caused by fever or infection is superimposed on consumption of an already high solute formula. Infants fed concentrated formula during such illnesses may become thirsty, demand more to drink, or refuse to consume more liquid because of anorexia secondary to illness. When the body is presented with more milk concentrated in the protein and solutes, the osmolality of the blood increases and hypernatremic dehydration may result.

Anticipatory guidance of parents of young infants should include information on the variety of formulas available to feed their infants, differences in methods of preparation of each product, and the dangers of overdiluted formula and excessive water intake.

PREPARATION OF FORMULAS

Because commercially prepared liquid formulas are sterile until opened and powdered formula is free of viable microorganisms of public health significance, sterilization is no longer recommended. Most parents prepare formula one bottle at each feeding and immediately feed the infant. It is important that the person preparing the formula wash hands carefully before proceeding. All equipment to be used during preparation, including the cans that contain the milk, the bottles, and the nipples, must be thoroughly washed and rinsed. Once opened, cans of formula must be covered and refrigerated. The formula is prepared immediately before each feeding. After the formula has been heated and the infant has been fed, any remaining milk should be discarded. Warm milk is an excellent medium for bacterial growth.

FORMULA AND MILK FOR OLDER INFANTS

One manufacturer markets a cow's milk–based formula for older babies. It is designed to accompany the feeding of semisolid foods and is higher in protein and lower in fat than formula for the younger infant. However, examination of the nutrient intakes of infants from 6 months to 1 year reveals intakes of nutrients completely adequate without the additional protein. There is no advantage in using this milk. Formulas prepared for younger infants are perfectly adequate for the first year.

Three manufacturers market formula for children over 1 year for whom whole cow's milk is inappropriate. One soy-based formula that includes corn syrup solids and sugar as carbohydrate and vegetable oils as fat is fortified with iron. There are also two elemental formula oral-feeding products for children over 1 year. These formulas are milk lactose and gluten free.

The use of whole milk in the first year is strongly discouraged. It has been noted to contribute to the incidence of anemia. Not only is there no iron in this milk, but it may cause a tiny blood loss from the intestinal tract. If a test of the baby's feces is done with paper impregnated with guiac solution or a fecal hemoglobin test is performed, small amounts of blood may be found.[17] Whole milk also contains inhibitors to iron absorption. Six- to 12-month-old infants fed whole milk and iron-fortified cereal (in which the percentage of absorption is known to be limited) have been found to be in negative iron balance and "at risk" for developing anemia.[18]

In addition to the concerns regarding the use of whole milk in the first year there are additional reasons for not feeding nonfat and/or 2% milk during the first year. Infants fed nonfat milk increase their intake and continue to gain weight but at a slower rate. They lose body fat, as evidenced by decreases in skinfold thickness, and lose energy reserves. Because milk solids are often added to 2% milk, it may increase the renal solute load. There is also concern that babies who consume the lower energy density milk will learn to eat more to reach satiation and that patterns of intake leading to obesity may be developed.[1] Even though one researcher has suggested that infants over 6 months of age can achieve adequate growth and nurture consuming this milk in combination with infant food, it is not recommended. Difficulties with using these types of cow's milk are greater in younger babies who depend primarily on formula for their energy and nutrient intake and have less mature gastrointestinal systems than older infants. As infants mature and after semisolid and other foods are introduced, the percentage of energy intake provided by milk decreases and feeding whole milk becomes less of a concern.

Substitute or imitation milks should not be offered to infants. These milks, defined by the Food and Drug Administration as nutritionally equivalent to whole milk or skim milk based on the content of only 14 or 15 nutrients, omit many nutrients recommended as components for infant formulas and are not appropriate for infants.

ECONOMICS OF INFANT FEEDING

Several attempts have been made to compare the economic impact of the provision of energy and nutrients to support human lactation with the use of prepared infant formula. Investigators have reported disadvantages both to breast-feeding and to formula-feeding.

It must be remembered that the numbers of foods that supply important nutrients for lactation are large. Therefore the economic impact can range from a minimal increase to a sizable increase over basic food costs.

The cost of commercially prepared formula varies with packaging. Concentrated formulas are the least expensive; ready-to-feed formulas are the most costly. The nutrient support for breast-feeding costs about 50% to 60% as much as the ready-to-feed formula.

Feeding the infant human milk can be less expensive or more expensive than commercially prepared formula depending on the parents' food purchasing practices and selection of foods. The many advantages of human milk far exceed any small monetary advantage for prepared formula. Parents may need help in the selection of appropriate low-cost foods, but breast-feeding should never be discouraged on an economic basis.

FOODS IN THE INFANT'S DIET

Although no nutritional advantage can be expected from the early introduction of semisolid foods, many families feed them to their infants in the first month of life. Semisolid foods are introduced by parents on the advice of physicians, neighbors, and friends and because parents think that it is time for their infants to eat foods other than milk. Some parents add semisolid foods in the hope that they will encourage their infants to sleep through the night, a commonly held belief that has been proved untrue. Other parents feed semisolid foods because they think that their infants are hungry, or because they consider the acceptance of these foods a developmental landmark.

Many infants receive table food by the time they can sustain a sitting posture. As infants begin to finger feed, increasing amounts of table food are included in their diets.

Semisolid Foods

The age of introduction of semisolid foods to infants in the United States declined from 1920,

TABLE 4-5   *Suggested Ages for the Introduction of Semisolid Foods and Table Foods*

Food	Age (Months)		
	4–6	6–8	9–12
Iron-fortified cereals for infants	Add		
Vegetables		Add strained	Gradually delete strained foods, introduce table foods
Fruits		Add strained	Gradually delete strained foods, introduce chopped well-cooked or canned foods
Meats		Add strained or finely chopped table meats	Decrease the use of strained meats, increase the varieties of table meats
Finger foods such as arrowroot biscuits, oven-dried toast		Add those that can be secured with a palmar grasp	Increase the use of small-sized finger foods as the pincer grasp develops
Well-cooked mashed or chopped table foods, prepared without added salt or sugar			Add
Juice by cup			Add

when these foods were seldom offered before 1 year of age, to 1960 to 1970, when they were frequently offered in the first weeks and months of life. Concern that this early introduction of semisolid foods predisposed infants to obesity and allergic reactions caused many health care professionals in the pediatric community to reexamine the appropriate age for the introduction of these foods. It is currently recommended that the feeding of semisolid foods be delayed until the infant's consumption of food is no longer a reflexive process, and the infant has the fine, gross, and oral motor skills to appropriately consume them (e.g., at approximately 4 to 6 months of age). Even so, many parents are reported to offer semisolid foods in the first month of life. Table 4-5 gives suggested guidelines for the introduction of semisolid foods to typical infants.

A vast number of commercially prepared canned and frozen foods are marketed for feeding the infant. The new parent may select organically grown products or products prepared from farms and vineyards that probably use fertilizers and insecticides. She will find single foods and juices, vegetables with meat dinners, and mixed juices in 2.5-oz, 4-oz, or 6-oz jars (first foods, second foods, and third foods). Juices are marketed in 4-oz, 8-oz, and 25.3-oz bottles; some juices are prepared from fresh fruit, others from concentrates. Some children may find toddler meals interesting.

Ready-to-serve single-grain dry cereals, such as rice cereal, are commonly the first food offered to infants because rice is considered the least allergenic of the cereal grains and because most cereals are fortified with electrolytic iron.

It appears to make little difference whether fruits or vegetables are introduced next. New foods should be added singly at intervals of no more than every three days. The introduction of nitrate-containing vegetables (e.g., carrots, beets, and spinach) is usually delayed until the infant is at least 4 months of age because the nitrate can be converted to nitrite in the stomach of the young infant. This can result in **methemoglobinemia.**

Infant's acceptance of semisolid foods. Parents report both immediate acceptance and rejection of semisolid foods, a fact that may relate to the parent's skill in feeding and attitudes and feelings about these foods. Some parents who believe that the use of semisolid foods is important add them to the formula, cut a larger hole in the nipple, and feed the infant semisolid foods in this manner. This practice increases the energy and nutrient composition of the formula and may deprive the infant of experiences that are important in the development of feeding behavior.

Parents are reported to mix milk with cereal until it is almost liquid and can easily be fed by spoon. Fruits are commonly reported as favorites. Vegetables appear to be accepted without problems. Yellow vegetables, green beans, and peas have been reported to be preferred vegetables; spinach and beets are often reported to be rejected. Strained meats are frequently rejected by infants. Parents state that the infants reject the sticky, granular texture rather than the taste of meats. Older infants are, as a result, often fed strained and junior vegetable and meat mixtures and high-meat dinners. Infants gradually accept new foods by increasing the quantity they consume. Breast-fed infants appear to accept greater quantities than do formula-fed infants.[19]

Food additives and fortification in semisolid foods. Concern that intakes of sodium in the first year might predispose infants to later **hypertension** has resulted in the deletion of salt from commercially prepared infant foods. Sugar is added only to desserts. All cereals are fortified with niacin, thiamin, riboflavin, calcium, and phosphorus. All dry infant cereals are fortified with electrolytically reduced iron.

Strained, jarred cereals with fruit are fortified with ferrous sulfate. High-meat and mixed dinners are prepared with rice or wheat flour or tapioca to increase shelf life. Modified corn starch or tapioca starch is included in some desserts. Fruits and fruit juices are enriched with vitamin C.

Home preparation of semisolid foods. It is both possible and economical for parents to prepare semisolid foods for their infants with a food grinder, blender, or strainer. The foods should be carefully selected from high-quality fresh, frozen, or canned fruits, vegetables, and meats and should be prepared so that nutrients are retained. The area in which the foods are prepared and the utensils used in preparation should be meticulously cleaned. Salt and sugar should be used sparingly, if at all. When the food has been cooked, pureed, and strained, it should be packaged in individual portions and refrigerated or frozen so that a single portion can be heated and fed without compromising the quality and bacterial content of the entire batch. Directions for preparation of infant foods are given in the box on page 000. Home-prepared infant foods have a greater energy content than commercially prepared foods, and many have a higher salt content. Parents who feed higher sodium intakes to infants probably add more salt to the infant's food than parents who offer lower sodium intakes.

Fruit juice. When a high percentage of infants were fed evaporated milk formulas, fruit juices containing vitamin C were commonly introduced in the first month of life; the widespread use of vitamin-fortified formula and vitamin supplements made this practice unnecessary. Because a sucrose-containing liquid consumed as infants go to sleep sometimes results in extensive dental caries (see pages 122–123), it is generally recommended that fruit juice not be given until the infant can drink from a cup. Juice intake should not replace more nutritionally dense foods.

Nutrients in semisolid foods. Ranges of nutrients found in any group of foods for infants are sizable (table 4-6).

Jarred cereals are fortified with ferrous sulfate, and dry infant cereals are fortified with electrolytically reduced iron. Absorption of electrolytically reduced iron is approximately 5% of that of ferrous sulfate.

Strained and junior fruits contribute one-third more energy, only a fraction of vitamin A, but twice as much vitamin C, as do vegetables when fed in equal amounts. Vegetables contribute small but important amounts of iron. Fruit juice is fortified with abundant amounts of vitamin C.

❖

DIRECTIONS FOR HOME PREPARATION OF INFANT FOODS

1. Select fresh, high-quality fruits, vegetables, or meats.
2. Be sure all utensils, including cutting boards, grinders, and knives, are thoroughly clean.
3. Wash your hands before preparing the food.
4. Clean, wash, and trim the foods in as little water as possible.
5. Cook the foods until tender in as little water as possible. Avoid overcooking, which may destroy heat-sensitive nutrients.
6. Do not add salt. Add sugar sparingly. Do not add honey to foods for infants less than 1 year of age.*
7. Add enough water so that the food has a consistency that is easily pureed.
8. Strain or puree the food using an electric blender, a food mill, a baby food grinder, or a kitchen strainer.
9. Pour puree into ice cube tray and freeze.
10. When food is frozen hard, remove the cubes and store in freezer bags.
11. Unfreeze and heat in serving container the amount of food that will be consumed at a single feeding (in water bath or microwave oven).

From Pipes PL: *Nutrition in infancy.* In Mahan LK, Escott-Stump S: *Food, nutrition, and diet therapy,* ed Philadelphia, 1996, WB Saunders.
*Botulism spores have been reported in honey, and young infants do not have the immune capacity to resist this infection.

Strained and junior meats contribute significant amounts of protein and iron. High-meat dinners contribute less than half as much protein as pure meat; vegetables and meat contribute less than one-fifth as much protein as pure meat. Strained and junior meats and high-meat dinners contribute similar amounts of iron; strained vegetables and meat contribute much less iron. Strained vegetables and meat provide slightly less than half as much energy as meat; high-meat dinners provide 75% as much energy as pure meat.

Strained and junior desserts are rich in carbohydrates and energy. A few are fortified with vitamin C. All have a sweet taste, and indiscriminate use of these items should be discouraged.

Infants receive table food soon after the introduction of supplemental foods. Most often the foods offered to infants are the same foods prepared for the remainder of the family. Between 7 and 12 months of age the energy intake from table food increases dramatically and that from commercially prepared foods declines. At 1 year of age over 50% of the energy

intake of infants is provided by table food. Little guidance has been provided for parents to determine appropriate table foods to feed their infants, and cases of choking and aspiration have occurred. Hot dogs, nuts, grapes, carrots, and round candies should be avoided (see the box "Appropriate Introductory Table Food for Infants").

Honey, sometimes used as a sweetener for home-prepared infant foods and formulas and recommended for use on pacifiers to promote sucking in hypotonic infants, has been implicated as the only food source of spores of *Clostridium botulinum* during infancy. These spores are extremely resistant to heat and are not destroyed by present methods of processing honey. **Botulism** in infancy is caused by ingestion of the spores, which germinate into the toxin in the lumen of the bowel. Honey should not be fed to infants less than 1 year of age.

Stages of development of feeding behavior indicate readiness to progress in textures of food and are discussed in the section on development of feeding behavior. The energy and nutrient

TABLE 4-6   *Ranges of Selected Nutrients per Ounce in Commercially Prepared Infant Foods*

Food	Energy (kcal)	Protein (gm)	Iron (mg)	Vitamin A (RE)	Vitamin C (mg)
Dry cereal	120	2.0–10.0	14.3	*	*
1st Foods™, 2nd Foods™, & 3rd Foods™ Foods fruits	12–29	0.0–0.3	0.0–0.1	0.3–34	*–6.3
1st Foods™, 2nd Foods™ & 3rd Foods™ vegetables	9–20	0.2–0.9	0.0–0.3	0.3–440	0.0–2.2
2nd Foods™ & 3rd Foods™ meats	28–37	3.8–4.4	0.2–0.4	*	*
2nd Foods™ & 3rd Foods™ dinners	12–22.4	0.5–1.1	0.1–0.2	0.3–341	*–5.3
2nd Foods™ & 3rd Foods™ desserts	19–25	0.0–0.5	0.0–0.1	*–10.5	*–4.0

*Quantity insignificant

© *1995 Gerber Products Company: Nutrient Values, Fremont, MI, Rev1294.*

1st Foods, 2nd Foods, and 3rd Foods are trademarks of Gerber Products Company.

TABLE 4-7 *Nutrient Content of Selected Table Foods Commonly Fed to Infants*

Food	Portion Size	Energy (kcal)	Protein (gm)	Iron (mg)	Vitamin A (IU)	Vitamin C (mg)
Cooked cereal (farina)	¼ c	26	0.8	Dependent on level of fortification		
Mashed potato	¼ c	34	1.1	0.2	10	5
French fried potato	3, 1″ to 2″	29	0.4	0.2		
Spaghetti	2 T	19	0.6	0.2		
Macaroni and cheese	2 T	54	2.1	0.2	107	
Liverwurst	½ oz	45	2.1	0.8	925	
Hamburger	½ oz	41	3.4	0.5	5	
Eggs	1 medium	72	5.7	1.0	520	
Cottage cheese	1 T	5	1.9		23.7	
Green beans	1 T	3	0.15	0.2	43	1
Cooked carrots	1 T	2.81			952	
Banana	½ small	40	0.5	0.35	90	5
Pudding	¼ c	70	2.2	Trace	102	
Lollipop	1 oz hard candy	109				
Saltine crackers	1	12	0.2			
Vanilla wafer	¼″ thick, 1¾″ diameter	18	0.2			
Cheese strips	¼ oz	28	1.78		92	

❖

APPROPRIATE INTRODUCTORY TABLE FOOD FOR INFANTS

Mashed potatoes
Well-cooked mashed vegetables (carrots, stringless green beans)
Soft, mashed fruits (bananas, peaches, pears)
Peeled, mashed vienna sausage
Well-cooked, *finely ground*, ground meats
Yogurt
Canned, drained tuna or salmon (no bones)
Mashed or refried beans

composition of foods offered must also be considered. Examples of table foods often offered and their contribution to an infant's dietary intake are given in table 4-7.

INTAKES OF INFANTS

Volume of intake and energy consumption is influenced not only by the infant's requirements for maintenance, growth, and activity but also by the parents' sensitivity to and willingness to accept cues of hunger and satiety, parental eagerness for the infant to feed, and the parents' skill at feeding. The energy concentration of the formula is also a determinant of the volume of intake, energy intake, and growth in early infancy.[1]

Infants feed differently and parents vary in their sensitivity to their child's cues. Mothers who spend more time stimulating their infants during feeding have infants who spend less time sucking during breast-feeding and consume less from bottles at feeding than infants of mothers who let the baby regulate pauses during feeding. Mothers who stimulate their infants during pauses between sucking prolong the pause and reduce the total consumption of food.

Growth Response to Feeding

Normal breast-fed infants regulate their milk intake to meet their needs for normal growth and development. Formula-fed infants have been reported to regain their birth weights more rapidly than breast-fed infants.

Exclusively breast-fed infants grow in length more slowly than formula-fed infants.

Energy intakes. Per unit of size, infants consume the greatest amount of energy between 14 and 28 days of age, a time known to many pediatricians as the hungry period. Mothers who are breast-feeding may find talking to a lactation counselor helpful when demands for milk suddenly increase. After this time, although total quantity and energy intakes increase, intakes per unit of size decrease. Infants consume greater amounts of food and nutrients at a decreasing amount per unit of body size as they grow older.

Wide ranges of volume of intake and energy consumption throughout the first year of life have been noted in both breast- and formula-fed infants by several researchers.[20,21,22,23] Formula-fed infants consume more energy per unit of body size than do breast-fed infants. Differences are significant after 3 months of age. Gains in weight are greater in formula-fed infants as are increases in body mass per gram of protein intake.[20,21] There is, however, no evidence of functional advantage in the more rapid growth.

Breast-fed infants consume less milk than bottle-fed infants. When semisolid foods are added to the infant's diet, they replace, rather than supplement, milk. This decrease in milk intake appears to be progressive as the intake of semisolid foods increases.

The energy concentration of the formula influences volume of intake during the first 41 days of life. Female infants who were fed formulas energy concentrated to 100 kcal/100 ml (30 kcal/oz) reduced their volume of intake but consumed a greater amount of energy, whereas those who were fed formulas diluted to 54 kcal/100 ml (16.5 kcal/oz) increased their volume of intake but consumed less energy, as compared with infants who were fed formulas of typical energy concentration. After this period, adjustments in volume of intake were sufficient so that energy intakes were similar for the entire 111-day study period. Infants who were fed the energy concentrated formula were, however, heavier for their lengths at 111 days of age than were infants who had been fed the energy dilute formulas.[1] Male infants who were fed formulas concentrated to 133 kcal/100 ml (40 kcal/oz) reduced their volume of intake but consumed a greater amount of energy during the first 84 days of life. They experienced supernormal rates of growth in both length and weight during the first 42 days of life compared with infants who were fed formulas providing 67 kcal/100 ml (20 kcal/oz).[1]

FEEDING BEHAVIORS

Defining developmental readiness for changes in textures of food and the acquisition of self-feeding skills is important in establishing realistic goals for normal and handicapped infants and children. Illingworth and Lister[24] have defined a critical or sensitive period of development in relation to eating, a time at which a specific stimulus, solid food, must be applied for the organism to learn a particular action, that of accepting and eating table food, which is more difficult to masticate. They point out that an infant learns to chew at about 6 or 7 months of age; thus, he or she is, at this point, developmentally ready to consume food. If solid foods are withheld until a later age, the child will have considerably more difficulty in accepting them.

In 1937 Gesell and Ilg[25] published observations of their extensive studies of the feeding behavior of infants. Their observations are as valid today as they were then. **Cineradiographic** techniques developed since then have permitted more detailed descriptions of sucking, suckling, and swallowing. More recently, physiologic studies have refined and clarified the original observation.[26]

Development of feeding behavior depends on the maturation of the central nervous system, which controls the acquisition of fine, gross, and oral motor skills, each of which influences the child's ability to consume food and the manner in which he or she suckles, sucks, chews, and swallows. Typical development proceeds in an orderly and predictable **cephalocaudal** sequence. Likewise, the sequence of acquisition of feeding skills occurs in a pre-dictable order influenced by the acquisition of function and behavior.

It is important to recognize that, even though the typical neonate is well prepared to suck and swallow at birth, the physical and neuromotor maturation during the first year alters both the form of the oral structure and the methods by which the infant extracts liquids from a nipple. Each of the parameters of change influences the infant's eating skills. At birth the tongue is disproportionately large in comparison with the lower jaw and essentially fills the oral cavity. The mandible is retruded relative to the maxilla, which protrudes over the mandible by approximately 2 mm. When the mouth is closed, the jaws do not rest on top of each other, but the tip of the tongue lies between the upper and lower jaws. There is a fat pad in each of the cheeks. It is thought that these pads serve as a prop for the buccinator muscle, maintaining rigidity of the cheeks during suckling. The lips of the neonate are also instrumental in sucking and suckling and have characteristics appropriate for their function at this age. A mucosal fold on the free edge of the gums in the region of the eyetooth buds of both jaws is instrumental in sealing off the oral cavity as the lips close around a nipple. The mucosal fold disappears by the third or fourth month when the lips have developed muscular control to seal the oral cavity.

The sucking, swallowing, and respiratory centers are located in close proximity within the brain stem. The rhythmic functions must be coordinated to allow for the crossing of the alimentary and respiratory pathways in the **pharynx.** Typical full-term newborn infants coordinate sucking, breathing, and swallowing. Newborn infants suck reflexively; they can breathe and suck simultaneously.

SUCKING

Cineradiographic studies led investigators to believe that processes of breast- and bottle-sucking were similar. More recent physiological studies have shown differences in the sucking pattern of breast- and bottle-fed infants.[26] In the initial phase of sucking the facial muscles constrict to form a seal around the nipple. The nipple is compressed against the palate by the tongue.

During breast-feeding the human nipple elongates to approximately twice its length; rhythmic movements of the tongue and lower lip during suck result in lowering of the mandible and protrusion of the tongue. Both positive and negative pressure create a suction. The bottle-fed infant creates a suction by pistonlike movements of the tongue, allowing for extraction of the milk.

At the beginning of a feed infants suck vigorously and continuously. This initial sucking is followed by a period when bursts alternate with periods of no sucking, or a pause. Sucking frequencies are relatively constant during bottle-feeding, but pressures vary markedly. There is considerable variability in milk flow within and among the types of nipples on the market, the most important determinant being the size of the nipple hole. Several factors influence the sucking pattern. Sweet solutions increase the continuity and speed of sucks. The infant's state of wakefulness influences the pressure and time between sucks. Near the end of a feeding there is a decrease in sucking pressure and an increase in the time between sucking clusters.

During swallowing, the food lies in a swallow preparatory position on the groove of the tongue. The distal portion of the soft palate is raised toward the adenoidal pad in the roof of the epipharynx. The tongue is pressed upward against the nipple so that the bolus of milk follows gravity down the sloping tongue reaching the pharynx. As the bolus moves downward, the posterior wall of the pharynx comes forward to displace the soft palate toward the dorsal surface of the tongue, and the larynx is elevated and arched backward. The bolus is expressed from the pharynx by peristaltic movements of the pharyngeal wall toward the back of the tongue and the larynx. The bolus spills over the pharyngoepiglottic folds into the lateral food channels and then into the esophagus.

The tonsils and lymphoid tissue play an important role as infants swallow; they assist in keeping the airway open and in keeping food away from the posterior pharyngeal wall as the infant is fed in a reclining position, thus delaying nasopharyngeal closure until food has reached the lower pharynx.

TABLE 4-8   *Sequence of Development of Feeding Behavior*

Age	Reflexes	Oral, Fine, Gross Motor Development
1–3 months	Rooting, suck, and swallow reflexes are present at birth Tonic neck reflex present	Head control is poor Secures milk with a suckling pattern, the tongue projecting during a swallow By the end of the third month, head control is developed
4–6 months	Rooting and bite reflexes fade Tonic neck reflex fades by 16 weeks	Changes from a sucking pattern to a mature suck with liquids Sucking strength increases Munching pattern begins Grasps with a palmar grasp Grasps, brings objects to mouth, and bites them
7–9 months	Gag reflex is less strong as chewing of solids begins and normal gag is developing Choking reflex can be inhibited	Munching movements begin when solid foods are eaten Rotary chewing begins Sits alone Has power of voluntary release and resecural Holds bottle alone Develops an inferior pincer grasp
10–12 months		Reaches for a spoon Bites nipples, spoons, and crunchy foods Grasps bottle and foods and brings them to the mouth Can drink from a cup that is held Tongue is used to lick food morsels off the lower lip Finger-feeds with a refined pincer grasp

Modified from Gesell A, Ilg FL: *Feeding behavior of infants,* Philadelphia, 1937, JB Lippincott.

As the infant grows older, the oral cavity enlarges so that the tongue no longer fills the mouth. The tongue grows differentially at the tip and attains motility in the larger oral cavity. The elongated tongue can be protruded to receive and pass solids between the gum pads and erupting teeth for mastication. Mature feeding is characterized by separate movements of the lip, tongue, and gum pads or teeth.

Sequence of Development of Feeding Behavior

The sequence of development of feeding behavior is given in table 4-8 and figure 4-1.

Newborn infants can neither focus their eyes nor direct their hands, yet they find nourishment. The **rooting** reflex, caused by stroking of the perioral skin including the cheeks and lips, causes an infant to turn toward the stimulus so

A

B

C

D

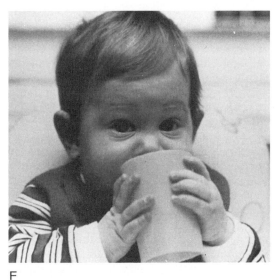

E

F

FIG. 4-1   Sequence of development of feeding behaviors. **A,** Infant sucks liquids. **B,** Five-month-old infant begins to finger-feed. **C,** Eight-month-old infant is fed table food. **D,** Eleven-month-old infant begins to feed himself. **E,** Eleven-month-old infant uses pincer grasp to finger-feed. **F,** Twelve-month-old infant drinks from cup.

that the mouth comes in contact with it. Stimulus placed on the lips causes involuntary movements toward it, closure, and pouting in preparation for sucking. These reflexes thus enable the infant to suck and receive nourishment. Both rooting and suckling can be elicited when the infant is hungry but are absent when the infant is satiated. During feeding, the neonate assumes a **tonic** neck position; the head is rotated to one side and the arm on that same side is extended while the other is fisted. The infant seeks the nipple by touch and obtains milk from the nipple with a rhythmic suckle. Semisolid foods, introduced at an early age into diets of many infants and fed by spoon, are secured in the same manner as is the milk, by stroking movements of the tongue with the tongue projecting as the spoon is withdrawn. Frequently, food is expelled from the mouth.

By 5 weeks of age the infant can focus the eyes on faces, and by 12 weeks of age the gaze can be shifted. At 10 weeks of age the infant is able to recognize the breast or bottle as the source of food.

4 to 6 months. By 16 weeks of age a more mature sucking pattern has become evident, with the tongue moving back and forth as opposed to the earlier up-and-down motions. Spoon-feeding is easier because the infant can draw in the lower lip as the spoon is removed. The tonic neck position has faded, and the infant assumes a more symmetrical position with the head at midline. The hands close on the bottle. By 20 weeks of age the infant can grasp on **tactile** contact with a palmar squeeze. By 24 weeks of age the infant can reach for and grasp an object on sight. In almost every instance the object goes into the mouth.

7 to 9 months. Between 24 and 28 weeks of age the beginning of chewing movements, an up-and-down movement of the jaws, occurs. This, combined with the ability to grasp, the hand-to-mouth route of grasped objects, and sitting posture, indicates a readiness of the infant to finger-feed. Infants at this age grasp with a **palmar grasp.** Therefore the shape of the food presented for the child to finger feed is important. Cookies, melba toast, crackers, and teething biscuits are frequently introduced at this stage.

Between 28 and 32 weeks of age the infant gains control of the trunk and can sit alone without support. The sitting infant has greater mobility of the shoulders and arms and is freer to reach and grasp. The grasp is more digital than the earlier palmar grasp. The infant is able to transfer items from one hand to another and learns to voluntarily release and resecure objects. The beginning of chewing patterns (up-and-down movements of the jaws) is demonstrated. The tongue shows more maturity in regard to spoon-feeding than to drinking. Food is received from the spoon by pressing the lips against the spoon, drawing the head away, and drawing in the lower lip. The infant is aware of a cup and can suck from it. Milk frequently leaks from the corners of the mouth as the tongue is projected before swallowing.

Critical stage of development. The introduction of soft, mashed (but not strained) foods is appropriate at this stage of development. In fact, it is at this stage of development that Illingworth and Lister believe it is critical to introduce the infant to harder-to-masticate foods.[24]

Between 6 and 12 months of age the infant gradually receives greater amounts of food from the family menu and less and less of the pureed and strained items. Foods should be carefully selected and modified so that they are presented in a form that can be manipulated in the mouth without the potential of choking and **aspiration,** as may occur with small grains of rice or corn. Many parents mash well-cooked vegetables and canned fruits and successfully offer them to their infants. Well-cooked ground meat dishes, such as ground meat in gravies or sauces, appear to be easily accepted, as is drained tuna fish. Custards, puddings, and ice cream soon become favorites.

Self-feeding. By 28 weeks of age infants are able to help themselves to their bottle in sitting postures, although they will not be able to tip the bottle adaptively as it empties until about 32 weeks of age. By the end of the first year they can completely manage bottle-feeding alone.

By 32 weeks of age infants bring their heads forward to receive the spoon as it is presented to them. The tongue shows increased motility and allows for considerably increased manipulation

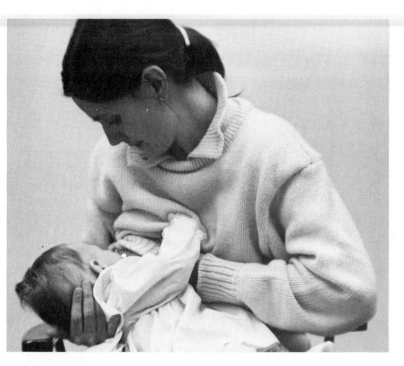

FIG. 4-2 Mother breast-feeds her 4-month-old infant.

of food in the mouth before swallowing. At the end of the first year, infants are able to manipulate food in the mouth with definite chewing movements.

9 to 12 months. During the fourth quarter of the first year, the child develops an increasingly precise **pincer grasp.** The bottle can be managed alone and can be resecured if it is lost. Infants at this age are increasingly conscious of what others do and often imitate the models set for them. By 1 year of age the patterns of eating have changed from sucking to beginning rotary chewing movements. Children understand the concept of the container and the contained, have voluntary hand-to-mouth movements and a precise pincer grasp, and can voluntarily release and resecure objects. They are thus prepared to learn to feed themselves, a behavior they learn and refine in the second year.

Infant feeding. Presented with the breast of an adequately fed, lactating mother or the nipple on a bottle of properly prepared formula, the hungry infant receives both biochemical and psychosocial nurturance. Most mothers warm the milk to body temperature. The infant held in a semireclining position who is offered the nipple sucks and receives the major portion of nourishment in 20 minutes. A flexible self-demand schedule is recommended. Newborn infants initially feed six to eight times a day at intervals of 2 to 4 hours and will consume 2 to 3 oz at a feeding (fig. 4-2).

Parents should recognize that infants are quite variable in their eating patterns. Not uncommonly they may want to eat at an interval of 2 hours, then wait 5 hours for the next feeding.

By 2 weeks of age most infants have increased the amount of milk consumed at a feeding and reduced the number of feedings to six. By 2 months of age, most infants are fed five times a day and sleep through the night. By 6 months of age, most consume three meals and four milk feedings a day.

Infants swallow air as well as formula during feeding. Holding the child in an upright position and gently patting the back encourages expulsion of swallowed air and prevents distension and discomfort.

Difficulties in infant feeding. During feeding, both the parents and the infant receive satisfaction and pleasure. The infant is pleased because hunger is satiated; the parents are pleased because they have fulfilled the needs of their newborn infant. Infants learn that they can trust their parents to feed them and that they please their parents by eating. Successful feeding provides the basis for the warm, trusting relationship that develops between infants and their parents.

Difficulties in feeding resulting from a weak suck, maternal difficulty in establishing adequate lactation, improper equipment such as firm nipples with small holes, or other causes are frustrating to both infants and their mothers. Hungry infants cry more frequently, demand to be fed more often, and may create anxiety in conscientious and concerned mothers.

Since infants have not yet learned to separate themselves from others in the environment, they perceive the feelings of others as their own immediate feelings in any particular situation. Thus they are easily susceptible to parental anxieties and may reflect these by crying and not eating well. When the infant does not eat well, parental anxieties may increase. Thus the cycle can begin. It is possible that such bottle-fed infants will feed more easily when presented the bottle by a less intense person. However, when the infant is successfully fed by another, the parents' feelings of inadequacy and anxiety may be increased.

To achieve successful parent-child feeding experiences, it is important to work directly with the parents. It may be necessary for the professional to determine any problems with equipment used and positioning, then to model a calm, relaxed feeding situation for the parents. Care should be taken not to usurp the parents' role, thus increasing their feelings of inadequacy. An approach that seems to be beneficial to all concerned is to (1) model a feeding, (2) sit beside the parents and talk them through a feeding while showing them how to use a relaxed position, (3) reinforce parenting behaviors, and (4) help them to become aware of cues from the infant that he or she is relaxed.

This method may need to be used for several feedings until the parent and infant can achieve a successful, relaxed experience. Even then, parents may need further support in their continuing efforts to create a relaxed and warm relationship with their infants during feeding.

Inadequate human milk. Cases of malnutrition and failure to thrive have been reported in breast-fed infants secondary to an inadequate milk intake, and thus an inadequate energy and nutrient intake. Feeding the baby at both breasts more frequently may help to increase the mother's milk supply. However, if weight gain continues to be less than adequate, the temporary use of supplemental feedings is appropriate.

It is important for parents to recognize that newborn infants demonstrate a pattern of crying in early life and that a crying infant is not a symptom of inadequate parenting. The amount of time an infant cries increases from 2 weeks of age to approximately 6 weeks of age, when it peaks. After this time crying decreases. The major concentration period is from 6 P.M. to 11 P.M. Other periods of crying occur in the morning from 4 A.M. to 7 A.M. and 9 A.M. to 11 A.M. By 10 weeks of age most infants become more quiet. Seldom is this crying a symptom of an allergy, and it is no indication for formula change.

Baby bottle tooth decay. Baby bottle tooth decay (BBTD), a characteristic pattern of tooth decay of all the upper and sometimes the lower posterior teeth, is often observed in children who are given sweetened liquids by bottle at naptime and nighttime as they go to sleep. As the children suck, the tongue protrudes slightly from the mouth, covering the lower front teeth. Liquids then spread over the upper and lower posterior teeth. Sucking stimulates the flow of saliva, which washes the debris from the teeth and promotes the secretion of compounds that buffer the acids in plaque. When babies are awake, they swallow the liquid quickly. However, if they fall asleep, sucking stops and the salivary flow and buffering are reduced. The sweetened liquid pools around teeth unprotected by the extended tongue, and bacterial plaque contacts the carbohydrate during the hours of sleep.[1]

Infant formulas, fruit juice, human milk, and cow's milk consumed when infants are falling asleep may cause decay. To prevent this dental destruction it has been suggested that infants be held when fed, burped, and put to bed without a bottle.

Colic. Parents of colicky babies—those who are otherwise healthy and well fed but who have an inconsolable agonizing cry for several hours each day, draw their legs onto the abdomens, and pass large amounts of gas—often request changes in the infants' formula. A number of psychosocial and dietary causes have been suggested as the cause of colic. Food allergy or intolerance is one of the causes in 12% to 15% of colicky infants. A 2- to 3-month trial of hypoallergenic formula such as Nutramigen may be warranted, but parents should not be led to believe that their colicky baby will have a lifetime of food allergy problems. Food intolerances or allergies in infants may be short lived. The response to the formula change may be to mechanisms other than allergy. It has been suggested that colic in some breast-fed infants be resolved by eliminating milk from the mothers' diets. Cruciferous vegetables, onion, chocolate, and milk in the mother's diet sometimes cause colic in the baby. Removing the offending foods from the diet of the mother of the affected baby resolves the problem.[27]

Spitting. Both spitting and regurgitation can occur in infants and usually cause concern for parents. During the early months of life some otherwise healthy infants spit a small amount of any milk or food ingested at each feeding. Although the infants do not fail to thrive, parents may seek help in resolving this situation. There is no therapy. The problem usually resolves itself by the time the infants can sustain sitting. Regurgitation, the effortless expulsion of gastric contents, is a symptom that demands medical evaluation. The most common cause of persistent regurgitation is gastroesophageal reflux, the result of decreased pressure in the lower esophageal sphincter. A prone position in contrast to a seated position increases sleep time and reduces crying time in these infants. There seems to be no difference between the prone or seated position regarding awake crying time. Surgery may be indicated.

Distractions. Some infants are easily distracted by noise or by other influences in the environment. Such infants feed more easily at the night feeding. Presentation of the bottle in a quiet, partially darkened room by a rested parent may promote successful feeding for both the parent and the infant.

Parental perception of feeding problems. Many parents perceive their infants as having feeding problems. Problems include refusal of a particular food because of taste or texture, dissatisfaction with amount consumed, spitting up, developmentally related problems such as refusing the bottle or refusing to be fed, and only finger-feeding. Such difficulties are usually of short duration and rarely compromise an infant's nutrient intake or physical growth. Parents, however, may need reassurance that their infant's development is normal and that their food-related behaviors are not of nutritional concern.

Recognizing Satiation Cues and Readiness to Progress

Successful infant feeding is generally regarded in our society as a measure of competent parenthood. As such, it is a reinforcing experience to parents. They must learn to recognize and to accept their infant's cues, since the infant uses a variety of cries and vocalizations to express needs. Parents, for one reason or another, cannot always discriminate their infant's cries. Consequently, they give food to satisfy all types of infant discomforts. The infant, in turn, may not learn to discriminate hunger from other discomforts and may learn to rely on eating to satisfy a wide variety of needs. Parents must learn to recognize satiation of hunger in infants and be willing to accept their infant's expressions of satisfaction, to set limits on amounts of food offered to eager eaters, and to decline the natural inclination to overfeed infants who please others by accepting more food. Satiety behaviors of infants are listed in table 4-9.

Parents who are eager for their infant to empty the bottle encourage excessive intakes of food and can reinforce eating to the extent that obesity may result. Infants may be offered food and formula by many people: parents, baby-sitters, aunts and uncles, siblings, and others.

TABLE 4-9   *Satiety Behaviors in Infants*

Age	Behavior
4–12 weeks	Draws head away from nipple
	Falls asleep
	When nipple is reinserted, closes lips tightly
	Bites nipple, purses lips, or smiles and lets go
16–24 weeks	Releases nipple and withdraws head
	Fusses or cries
	Obstructs mouth with hands
	Increases attention to surroundings
	Bites nipple
28–36 weeks	Changes posture
	Keeps mouth tightly closed
	Shakes head as if to say "no"
	Plays with utensils
	Hands become more active
	Throws utensils
40–52 weeks	Behaviors of above period typical
	Sputters with tongue and lips
	Hands bottle or cup to parent

From Pipes PL: *Health care professionals.* In Garwood G, Fewell R: *Educating handicapped infants*, Rockville, Md, 1982, Aspen Systems. With permission by Aspen Systems; modified from Gesell A, Ilg FL: *Feeding behavior of infants*, Philadelphia, 1937, JB Lippincott.

Parents who are dissatisfied with their infant's food intake may find that the infant has reduced the intake to compensate for food offered by others. Additional cues that parents must recognize are those that indicate the infant's readiness for increasingly independent feeding experiences. The infant's ability to put objects in his or her mouth and to chew on them indicates a readiness to use increasingly solid foods and to begin finger-feeding (fig. 4-3). Anticipatory guidance to parents during this period about developmental changes is an important factor in their acceptance of and adaptation to their infant's behavior.

Recognizing Nutrients and Energy Needs in the Infant's Diet

Most infants consume foods that provide nutrients in excess of recommended amounts, with the exception of iron. Human milk and formula provide the major source of protein and calcium and important sources of vitamin A and the B vitamins in early life. Breast-fed infants should receive supplements of iron, vitamin D, and fluoride. Iron-fortified formulas contribute appreciable amounts of iron in early infancy.

Most lactating mothers need to be away occasionally when it is time to feed their infant. It is therefore advantageous for the infant to have an occasional bottle with a rubber nipple after lactation is well established. Ready-to-feed formulas can be used, but many mothers prefer to express their own milk for such occasions. Manual expression is the choice of most mothers. However, manual and electric pumps are on the market and may be preferred by mothers who work and express for a day or more.

Once expressed, the milk must be stored so that it will be microbiologically safe with a minimal loss of nutrients. Freezing protects it from contamination with minimal change in milk composition. Immunoglobulin levels and nutritional properties are essentially unchanged. Milk should be refrigerated or frozen at once. It can be safely held in a refrigerator for 24 hours and in a freezer for up to 3 months.

Often breast-fed infants refuse a rubber nipple from their mother. They usually accept such a feeding from their father, a friend, or a baby-sitter.

Because of the great variability in energy and nutrients provided by foods offered to infants, selection of foods and the amounts offered should be based on the infant's rate of gain in height and weight as well as on nutrient needs. The introduction and acceptance of heme iron–containing foods before the time homogenized milk replaces iron-fortified formula or before iron

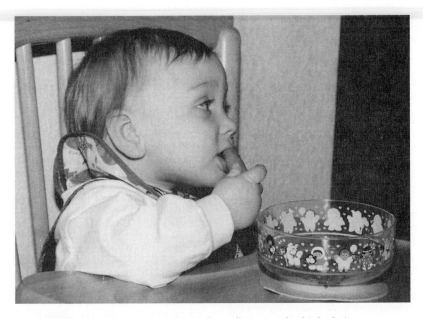

FIG. 4-3   Self-feeding may require a bowl that adheres to the high chair.

supplements are discontinued is important because the infant must continue to consume foods that provide this nutrient as it is deleted from milk or supplements. Fruit juice offers sources of vitamin C when vitamin-containing formulas are no longer consumed. It seems reasonable to encourage parents of infants whose gains in weight are more rapid than gains in length to feed the infants lower-energy infant foods such as vegetables and dinners. Parents of infants whose increments of weight gains are small should be encouraged to feed greater amounts of the higher-energy strained meats and fruits. Amounts of semisolid foods offered to infants should be adjusted to their appetites and rates of weight gain. Experiences with a variety of flavors and textures are thought to be conducive to acceptance of a variety of foods in later life.

Programs to Help Parents Optimize the Nutritional Status of Infants

Various federal and state programs include a component to improve the nutritional status of infants. State and local health departments have always considered nutrition services during pregnancy, lactation, and infancy an essential component of preventive health care. Nutritionists in these programs provide information about nutrition in infancy by preparing materials for public distribution, serving as a resource for other health workers, and participating in mother-infant and other classes.

Nutritionists provide nutrition education and individual counseling to parents in a number of federally funded programs designed to meet the needs of children at risk. Diagnostic clinics for infants and children also provide nutrition services, including nutrition screening, counseling, education, referral, and follow-up. Such clinics are included in programs funded to serve children, youth, and the developmentally delayed.

One program, the Special Supplemental Food Program for Women, Infants, and Children (WIC), provides specific food supplements to pregnant and lactating women and to infants and children up to 5 years of age who are at nutritional risk because of nutritional needs and inadequate income. The program provides only formula for the first 3 months,

✤ ✤ ✤

CASE STUDY

Nourishment of a Healthy Male Infant

The mother of Baby M. H., an 11-month-old male, feels that he is ready to drink whole cow's milk and to eat food from the table. She would like guidance in the selection of what to offer her baby and how to support developmental progress in feeding behavior.

Baby M. H. currently weighs 24 lb and 3 oz and is 31¾ in. long. His linear growth has plotted between the 90th and 95th percentile since 2 months of age, his weight between the 90th and 75th percentile. (See fig. 4-4.) His current weight/height plots in the 50th percentile.

He was breast-fed with only an occasional supplemental bottle until he was 5 months old. He was weaned from the breast at 9 months. At 8 months he was offered fruit juice by cup and was able to participate in drinking by holding the cup as his mother helped him elevate it.

At 5 months he was offered and willingly accepted applesauce. Other strained fruits and vegetables were introduced one at a time beginning a week later. He would willingly accept two spoonfuls at first but gradually increased both the quantity of a food he would eat. Between 6 and 9 months he was introduced to "2nd foods." He seemed to prefer these foods to the strained foods, especially enjoying macaroni and cheese, turkey dinner, sweet potatoes, and carrots. When he was offered strained meat, he clearly did not like it; he never closed his mouth but let the food slowly drool out.

At 6 months the baby began reaching out for objects to put in his mouth and was offered finger foods; he enjoyed mostly toasted bread, pieces of banana, canned fruit, and the commercially prepared meat sticks. He initially held the food with a palmar grasp. By 8 months he was using an inferior pincer grasp and enjoyed small pieces of food such as Cheerios. He would currently like to eat all his food by finger, including applesauce, and reaches for the spoon as it is offered.

The baby is fed in a high chair before his parents have their meal. He reaches for food that he sees them eating and has received a number of small bites. He chews with beginning munching rotary movements and has no problem with well-cooked soft vegetables and fruits. If he is given a small piece of fibrous meat such as a pork chop, he will chew on it and spit it out or squirrel it away in his jaw. It may be found there an hour or two later.

A two-day food record kept by the baby's mother is as follows:

Day 1

8:00 A.M.	8 oz whole cow's milk
8:30 A.M.	½ cup Cheerios
11:50 A.M.	2 oz "3rd foods"
	Vegetables and bacon
	½ graham cracker
	4 oz mixed fruit juice by cup
1:30 P.M.	8 oz cow's milk–based infant formula
4:00 P.M.	2 animal crackers
	1 slice peeled apple
8:00 P.M.	8 oz formula

Day 2

2:00 A.M.	formula
7:30 A.M.	8 oz whole cow's milk
9:00 A.M.	2 oz apples and blueberries
	½ cup Cheerios
10:00 A.M.	5 oz formula
11:45 A.M.	8 oz whole milk
3:00 P.M.	6 oz whole cow's milk
6:00 P.M.	6 oz turkey rice dinner
	¼ cup Cheerios
8:00 P.M.	8 oz formula
9:30 P.M.	10 Cheerios
	Bites of pork and vegetables from his parent's Chinese dinner

1. Calculate the food records kept by the mother. What percentage of M. H.'s energy intake is provided by milk? Will this change when he is offered more food from the family menu?
2. What food would you recommend for M. H. in making the transition from commercially prepared infant foods?
3. How skillfully will this child hold the spoon, his cup, and his food?
4. How much help will he need with using a spoon, drinking from a cup?

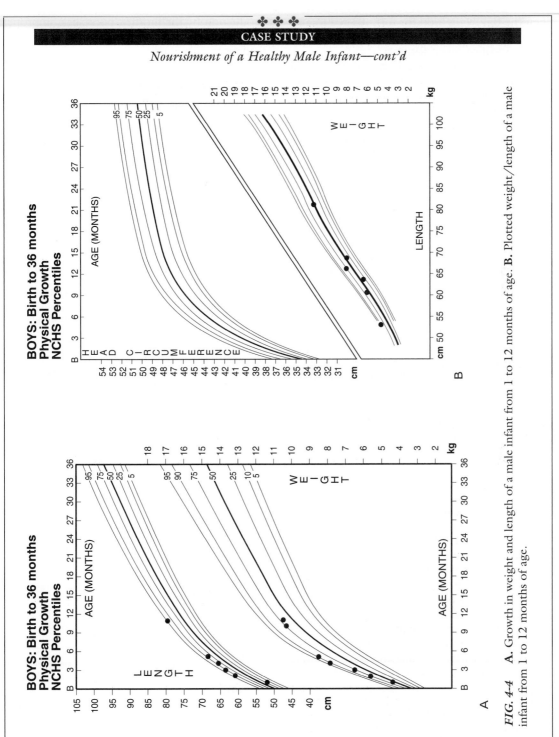

FIG. 4-4   **A.** Growth in weight and length of a male infant from 1 to 12 months of age. **B.** Plotted weight/length of a male infant from 1 to 12 months of age.

then the following food for formula-fed infants 4 to 12 months of age:

Iron-fortified infant formula

Infant cereal containing 45 mg iron/100 gm

Single-strength canned, frozen concentrated, or infant juices that contain a minimum of 30 mg vitamin C/dl

Mothers of breast-fed infants may be certified to receive the supplemental food themselves. Some breast-fed infants may be certified to receive partial food packages that include iron-fortified cereal and fruit juice.

It is important to recognize that the specific formulas, quantities of food provided, and the methods of implementation vary from state to state. Many states provide vouchers that can be redeemed at grocery stores for the specific foods; a few give the foods directly to the parents. Breast-feeding promotion and nutrition education are required components of this program.

Summary

Various combinations of milks, supplements, and semisolid foods can provide an adequately nourishing diet for infants. Maturation of the oral and fine motor skills indicate appropriate stages for the introduction of semisolid and solid foods. Current recommendations include breast-feeding by an adequately nourished mother, the introduction of semisolid foods at 4 to 6 months of age, and the introduction of finger foods when infants reach out, grasp, and bring items to their mouths.

If the mother is unable or unwilling to breast-feed, many properly constructed infant formulas are marketed that have been proved to support normal growth and development in infants. It is to the formula-fed baby's advantage to receive a formula with iron.

Infants should be permitted to establish their own feeding schedule and to be fed to satiety. When they develop a voluntary mature sucking pattern, the introduction of semisolid food is appropriate. When munching and rotary chewing begin, the introduction of soft-cooked table food is appropriate. Infants can begin to drink from a cup with help between 9 and 12 months of age.

Difficulties in infant feeding that indicate a need for intervention include inadequate milk production by the mother, poor suck, improper formula preparation, and parental anxiety about feeding their infants.

REVIEW QUESTIONS

1. Why are infants vulnerable to water imbalance?
2. List nutritional and other advantages of human milk.
3. Which formulas are suitable for infants allergic to cow's and soy milk formula?
4. Describe oral differences in the manner babies consume milk from the breast and from the bottle.
5. List developmental landmarks that indicate readiness for nonliquid milk foods.
6. How does a parent know if an infant has had enough to eat?

SUGGESTED LEARNING ACTIVITIES

1. Investigate the incidence of breast-feeding in the maternity unit of a local hospital.
2. Investigate local agencies in the community that provide support for the lactating mother.
3. Describe formula products available for feeding infants in the community.
4. Compare the cost of homemade and commercially available foods for infants.
5. Describe how useful parents find the nutrition information found on commercially prepared baby food container labels.
6. Observe infants feeding at 2, 4, 7, and 9 months of age, and describe changes in the way babies secure their food.
7. Describe appropriate therapy for breast-fed babies who are thought to be gaining weight too fast.

REFERENCES

1. Foman SJ: *Nutrition of normal infants,* St. Louis, 1993, Mosby.
2. Kurinij N, Shiono PH: Early formula supplementation of breast-feeding, *Pediatrics* 88:745, 1991.
3. Lasch M, Dungy CI, Russell D, Dusdicker LB: Impact of attitudes on maternal decision regarding infant breast feeding, *J Pediatr* 126:507, 1995.
4. May JT: Microbial contaminants and antimicrobial properties of human milk, *Microbiol Sci* 5:42, 1988.
5. Cunningham AS, Jeliffe DB, Jeliffe EFP: Breast feeding and health in the 1980s: a global epidemiologic review, *J Pediatr* 118:659, 1991.

6. Beaudry M, Dufour R, Marcoux S: Relation between infant feeding and infection during the first six months of life, *J Pediatr* 126:191, 1995.

7. Dewey KG, Heinig MR, Nommsen-Rivers LA: Differences in morbidity between breast fed and formula fed infants, *J Pediatr* 126:696, 1995.

8. Graham SM, Arvela OT, Wise GA: Long-term neurologic consequences of nutritional vitamin B_{12} deficiency in infants, *J Pediatr* 121:710, 1992.

9. Calvo EB, Galindo AC, Aspres NB: Iron status in exclusively breast-fed infants, *Pediatrics* 90:375, 1992.

10. Committee on Nutrition, American Academy of Pediatrics: Commentary on breast-feeding and infant formulas, including proposed standards for formulas, *Pediatrics* 57:279, 1976.

11. ESPGAN (European Society of Paediatric Gastroenterology and Nutrition), Committee on Nutrition: Guidelines on infant nutrition I. Recommendations for the composition of an adapted formula, *Acta Paediatr Scand* (suppl 262):1, 1977.

12. ESPGAN Committee on Nutrition: Comments on the composition of cow's milk based follow-up formulas, *Acta Paediatr Scand* 79:250, 1990.

13. ESPGAN Committee on Nutrition: Comments on the content and composition of lipids in infant formulas, *Acta Paediatr Scand* 80:887, 1991.

14. Joint FAO/WHO Alimentarius Commission: *Codex standards for foods for special dietary uses including foods for infants and children and related code of hygienic practice,* CAC/ Vol. 9 ed. 1, Suppl. 2, Rome, 1986, Food and Agriculture Organization of the United Nations/World Health Organization.

15. Food and Drug Directorate: *Food and drug regulations,* Division 25, Canada Gazette 124:73E, 1990.

16. Food and Drug Administration: *Rules and regulations. Nutrient requirements for infant formulas* (21 CFR Part 107) Fed. Reg. 50:45106, 1885.

17. Ziegler EE and others: Cow's milk feeding in infancy: gastrointestinal blood loss and iron nutritional status, *J Pediatr* 98:540, 1991.

18. Fuchs GJ, Farris RP, DeWier M and others: Iron status and intake of older infants fed formula versus cow milk with cereal, *Amer J Clin Nutr* 58:343, 1993.

19. Sullivan SA, Birch LL: Infants' dietary experiences and acceptance of solid foods, *Pediatrics* 93:271, 1993.

20. Hening MJ, Nommsen LA, Peerson JM: Energy and protein intakes of breast fed and formula-fed infants during the first year of life and their association with growth velocity: the Darling study, *Amer J Clin Nutr* 58:152, 1993.

21. Dewey KG, Henig MJ, Nommsen LA and others: Breast-fed infants are leaner than formula-fed infants at 1 yr. of age: the Darling study, *Amer J Clin Nutr* 57:140, 1993.

22. Butte NF, Smith EO, Garza G: Energy utilization of breast-fed and formula-fed infants, *Amer J Clin Nutr* 52:350, 1990.

23. Ernst JA, Brady MS, Rickard KA: Food and nutrient intake of 5 to 12 month old infants fed formula or cow milk: a summary of four national surveys, *J Pediatr* (suppl 117):586, 1990.

24. Illingworth RS, Lister J: The critical or sensitive period with reference to certain feeding problems in infants and children, *J Pediatr* 65:839, 1964.

25. Gesell A, Ilg FL: *Feeding behavior of infants,* Philadelphia, 1937, Lippincott.

26. Matthew OP: Science of bottle feeding, *J Pediatr* 119:511, 1991.

27. Lust KD, Brown JE, Thomas W: Maternal intake of cruciferous vegetables and other foods and colic symptoms in exclusively breast fed infants, *J Amer Diet Assoc* 96:46, 1996.

CHAPTER 5

Nutrition for Preterm and Low-Birth-Weight Infants

Joan Zerzan
Mary J. O'Leary

+++

Objectives

After studying this chapter, the student should:

✔ *Be aware of the reasons why the premature infant is at greater risk for nutritional problems than the full-term infant.*

✔ *Be aware of the vulnerability of the premature infant to a variety of medical problems that may limit nutrient and energy intake and complicate methods of feeding.*

✔ *Be aware of factors that determine whether the premature infant will receive parenteral or enteral feeds.*

✔ *Recognize that human milk from the infant's mother is an appropriate milk for the low-birth-weight baby.*

✔ *Know differences between formulas designed for the low-birth-weight baby and those designed for the full-term infant.*

Advances have been made in neonatal intensive care in recent years. New technologies, better understanding of pathophysiology, and regionalization of perinatal care have contributed to the increased survival of newborns requiring intensive care. Adequacy of postnatal nutrition affects the clinical course of critically ill babies and may influence their survival and long-term developmental outcome. This chapter describes current recommendations for nutrient intake, methods of nutritional support, and guidelines for nutritional assessment and management of preterm and low-birth-weight (LBW) infants requiring intensive care.

130

NUTRITIONAL SERVICES IN NEONATAL CARE

One hundred fifty thousand to 200,000 infants (or 4–6% of all newborns) are treated annually in neonatal intensive care units (NICU) in the United States. At least half of these infants are low birth weight.[1] The development and availability of neonatal intensive care as well as new technologies and subspecialties in care of the critically ill infant have been associated with increasing survival of the low-birth-weight infant, particularly the very-low-birth-weight (VLBW) and extremely low-birth-weight (ELBW) infant.[2] (See the accompanying box for definitions of these terms.) Practical considerations of limited economic, technical, and human resources prohibit the availability of intensive care facilities in all hospitals. A regionalized system of perinatal services has evolved over the past 20 years to ensure that all infants have equal access to the highest quality care. Elements of regionalization now include systems for identification of high-risk pregnancies and early referral to tertiary centers, structure and function of neonatal care units, formalization of arrangements with referring units, and transportation of sick neonates.

Delivery of Neonatal Care

The regional perinatal network encompasses three levels of neonatal care. Nurseries are classified as level I, II, or III, based on the type of care they are capable of providing.[3,4,5]

Level I nurseries provide uncomplicated neonatal care for healthy infants who are products of normal, full-term pregnancies. The personnel in these nurseries are trained in early detection of potential complications and use coordinated mechanisms for referral and transport of high-risk infants to level II or level III units. When problems arise, care provided in level I nurseries usually consists of stabilization until the infant can be safely transferred.

The personnel in level II nurseries provide a full range of services for healthy newborns. They also provide expertise in screening and referral of high-risk infants and are prepared to

---

❖

DEFINITION OF PRETERM OR LBW INFANTS	
Preterm	<37 weeks' gestation
Low birth weight (LBW)	<2500 gm or <5½ lb.
Very low birth weight (VLBW)	<1500 gm or <3⅓ lb.
Extremely low birth weight (ELBW)	<1000 gm or <2¼ lb.

---

care for moderately ill neonates or convalescing babies whose immaturity or medical risks preclude discharge.

Level III nurseries are specifically staffed and equipped to cope with the most serious types of neonatal illnesses and abnormalities. Increasing numbers of ELBW infants (<1000 gm) are being cared for in level III nurseries. A level III neonatal intensive care unit often assumes a leadership role within its region by setting standards of clinical care, developing educational materials, and providing consultative services to other nurseries. The nutrition specialist of such a unit may also have a similar opportunity and responsibility to serve as a regional resource for improvement in nutritional care of high-risk newborns.

Role of the Nutritionist

The National Research Council Committee on Nutrition of the Mother and Preschool Child has identified specific skills required to provide clinical services at each of the **three levels of neonatal care.**[6] These skills should enable the nutrition consultant to screen for various nutrition problems, monitor and assess nutritional progress, and develop and implement management plans.

Providing adequate nutrition to intensive care neonates is a challenge that requires the skillful input of several disciplines, including physicians, nurses, pharmacists, and occupational therapists. The nutritionist functions as a member of the health care team to facilitate nutritional support

---

❖

CLASSIFICATION OF INFANTS AS LGA, AGA, OR SGA

Large for gestational age (LGA)

Appropriate for gestational age (AGA)

Small for gestational age (SGA)

Birth weight > 90th percentile for gestational age

Birth weight between the 10th and 90th percentile for gestational age

Birth weight < 10th percentile for gestational age

---

of individual infants and to develop guidelines for safe and effective nutritional management of critically ill neonates.[7]

CHARACTERISTICS OF PRETERM AND LOW-BIRTH-WEIGHT INFANTS REQUIRING INTENSIVE CARE

Definition and Classification

Infants cared for in level III intensive care units typically include infants at high medical risk and critically ill babies with serious medical or surgical problems. Increasing numbers of preterm and LBW infants are being admitted to level III intensive care units (see the definition box on page 131). Although the medical status of larger babies may warrant intensive care, this chapter will focus on nutritional management of preterm and LBW infants who require intensive care.

Newborn infants may be classified by **gestational age,** birth weight, and weight/gestational age. Accurate assessment of gestational age is important in classifying an individual infant (see the accompanying box), and assessing intrauterine growth and maturity. An infant may be classified as large for gestational age (LGA), appropriate for gestational age (AGA), or small for gestational age (SGA), utilizing one of several intrauterine growth charts.[8,9] Classification of an infant as LGA, AGA, or SGA may have implications for early glucose tolerance, nutritional needs, and growth expectations. This information may be useful in establishing nutritional goals for individual infants and anticipating potential difficulties in meeting those goals in the immediate postnatal period.

Certain characteristics of preterm and LBW infants place them at immediate nutritional risk. Limited metabolic and nutrient reserves make these infants less prepared to maintain homeostasis immediately after birth and more vulnerable to nutrient deficiencies. Medical complications associated with prematurity may further compromise the nutritional status of these infants while metabolic and physiologic immaturity may complicate the provision of appropriate nutritional support.

Metabolic and Nutrient Reserves

Preterm and LBW infants have smaller metabolic and nutrient reserves and are physiologically less well prepared to maintain homeostasis immediately after birth than larger, full-term infants. Fat stores are limited because most fetal fat is deposited during the last six weeks of gestation. Fat contributes only 1% of the total body weight of the infant weighing 1000 gm. In contrast, 16% of the total body weight of the full-term infant (3500 gm) is fat.[10] Glycogen reserves of preterm infants are particularly small and are rapidly depleted. Babies who weigh 1000 gm have glycogen and fat reserves of approximately 110 kcal/kg.[10,11] Because basal metabolic needs are about 50 to 60 kcal/kg/day, these babies will rapidly run out of fat and carbohydrate fuel unless adequate nutritional support is established. Depletion time will vary between 2 and 4 days depending on the volume and concentration of IV dextrose that can be tolerated. Depletion time is even shorter for preterm or LBW infants who weigh less than 1000 gm.

It is often difficult to provide adequate nutrient intake during the first several days of life

TABLE 5-1 *Duration of Survival Expected in Starvation (H$_2$O Only) and Semistarvation (D$_{10}$W)*

Birth Weight (gm)	Estimated Survival Time (DAYS)	
	H$_2$O Only	D$_{10}$W
1000	4	11
2000	12	30
3500	32	80

From Heird WC and others: *J Pediatr* 80:351, 1972.[11]

because of immaturity of organ systems and severe medical problems. When adequate dietary intake cannot be achieved, fat and glycogen reserves will be depleted and the infant will catabolize vital protein tissue for energy. Even in the face of adequate energy, the infant will be in negative nitrogen balance without the provision of adequate protein. Heird and others[11] have theoretically estimated survival time of starved and semistarved infants assuming depletion of all glycogen and fat and about one-third of body protein tissue at a rate of 50 kcal/kg/day with and without exogenous energy as intravenous dextrose (table 5-1). The projected survival times are alarmingly short and occur at the expense of significant protein tissue catabolism. These numbers are estimates and lack empirical precision, but they do serve to demonstrate the disadvantage of the small infant when faced with inadequate nutritional support.

Because of limited protein and energy reserves, preterm and LBW infants are particularly vulnerable to the potential consequences of *protein energy malnutrition*.[12] Protein and energy malnutrition may have an impact on every organ system and may have long-term developmental consequences. In adult and animal studies, undernutrition is associated with diaphragmatic muscle atrophy, decreased respiratory muscle force, decreased ventilatory drive, and increased need for ventilatory support.[11,13] Apnea of prematurity has been attributed in part to muscle fatigue. Apnea has been noted more commonly in underfed neonates, and a reduction in apnea has been observed in neonates receiving glucose and amino acids compared with infants receiving only glucose.[13]

These studies suggest that undernutrition may further compromise the respiratory status of preterm infants with pulmonary disease. Animal and human studies also suggest that protein energy malnutrition at critical periods of rapid brain growth may result in irreversible impairment of brain growth and function.[14–19]

Two-thirds of the mineral content of the full-term infant is deposited in the last trimester. Infants born prematurely are deprived of this third trimester nutrient accretion. As a result, preterm infants are vulnerable to additional deficiencies. For example, preterm infants deplete iron stores at approximately 2 months of age and become dependent on dietary sources to prevent iron deficiency anemia. In contrast, full-term infants have sufficient iron reserves for 4 to 6 months of age. Calcium, phosphorus, and magnesium accretion increases in the fetus from 24 weeks, peaking at 34 to 36 weeks' gestation. Infants born prior to 36 weeks' gestation have lower bone mineral density than infants born at term and are at risk for osteopenia and rickets.

Medical Complications

Preterm and LBW infants may have a variety of clinical problems in the early postnatal period. These problems vary in type and severity depending on such factors as the intrauterine health of the fetus, the degree of prematurity, birth-related trauma, and functioning of immature or stressed organ systems. Although a wide range of medical problems may complicate the neonatal course of preterm and LBW infants, certain problems occur with such frequency that they can be considered typical problems of prematurity. Small, immature infants are at risk for the development of the problems listed in table 5-2. These problems may impact nutrient needs, and limit one's ability to provide adequate nutritional support. Treatment of these conditions may also have implications for nutritional management. For instance, treatment of respiratory or cardiac failure with fluid restriction may limit the provision of adequate energy. Medications

TABLE 5-2 **Examples of Problems Common to Preterm or LBW Infants**

System	Problem
Respiratory	Hyaline membrane disease, chronic lung disease (bronchopulmonary dysplasia)
Cardiovascular	Patent ductus arteriosus
Renal	Fluid and electrolyte imbalance
Neurological	Intracranial hemorrhage
Metabolic	Hypoglycemia, hyperglycemia, hypocalcemia, metabolic acidosis
Gastrointestinal	Hyperbilirubinemia, feeding intolerance, necrotizing enterocolitis
Hematological	Anemia
Immunological	Sepsis, pneumonia, meningitis
Other	ABCs (apnea, bradycardia, cyanosis)

TABLE 5-3 **Developmental Maturity and Nutritional Implications in Preterm Infants**

Functional Development	Nutritional Implication
• Immature suck-swallow-breathe coordination appears between 33–36 week's gestation	Impaired nippling ability and increased risk of aspiration
• Lower levels of lactase in infants < 34 weeks' gestation	Potential for some lactose malabsorption
• Lower lipase levels and bile acid pool	Potential for fat malabsorption (long chain fats)
• Reduced gastric volume	Volume intolerance
• Immature peristaltic and gastrointestinal motility patterns	Delays in gastric emptying, increased transit time, apparent feeding intolerance (e.g., residuals, regurgitation, abdominal distention), and constipation
• Alterations in renal and cardiac function	Fluid and electrolyte imbalance, alteration in protein tolerance (acidosis, azotemia, and hyperammonemia)

Adapted from Grant A, DeHoog S: *Nutritional assessment and support,* ed 4, 1991, Seattle.

to treat **bronchopulmonary dysplasia** (BPD) may negatively impact growth (steroids) and electrolyte balance (diuretics). These same medications may further impair bone mineral status. Nutritional management of these high-risk neonates, therefore, must take into account the occurrence and medical management of these problems, so that effective modalities of nutritional support can be employed.

Immaturity

Problems of metabolic and physiological immaturity may also complicate medical management and nutritional support. Although the fetal gut *structurally* resembles that of a newborn by 20 weeks' gestation, functional development is limited before 34 weeks' gestation. Immaturity of other organs also has implications for the nutritional support of preterm and LBW infants. Key developmental factors and their implications for nutritional support are listed in table 5-3.[20,21]

NUTRIENT REQUIREMENTS OF PRETERM INFANTS

The nutrient requirements of preterm infants are generally higher than those of full-term infants because of limited body stores, metabolic and physiological immaturity, and increased growth rates. Medical complications and treatment of those complications may further alter nutrient needs of individual infants by increasing needs or increasing losses.

Route of delivery also affects nutrient needs;[22] parenterally administered nutrients are delivered directly into the vascular system, thus bypassing the gastrointestinal tract, and are not subject to digestive and absorptive losses. However, parenterally administered nutrients may be lost through nutrient-nutrient interactions in solution, adsorption to delivery sets, **photodegradation,** and increased renal losses. Solubility may further limit the ability to provide adequate quantities of parenterally administered nutrients.

The exact quantities of nutrients required by preterm infants are still being defined. In the early 1980s, recommendations varied. In 1984 a consensus on vitamin and mineral requirements for preterm infants was established at a symposium convened by Dr. Reginald Tsang. In 1985 the Committee on Nutrition of the American Academy of Pediatrics (AAP) published recommendations, and in 1987 the European Society of Pediatric Gastroenterology and Nutrition (ESPANG) published a statement on the nutritional needs of preterm infants. These estimates, although initially established for predominantly larger and more mature infants, have been applied to ELBW infants in a clinical setting. This method has succeeded in extending the survival of small infants and producing growth without overt evidence of deficiencies.

With growing experience and research into the nutritional needs of extremely small and immature infants, a new consensus statement has recently been published. This statement takes into account gestational age and weight. Nutrient requirements are defined for three periods (initial, transition, and growth). Tables 5-4 and 5-5 list the consensus guidelines for vitamin and mineral intake for **parenterally** and **enterally** supported, stable, growing preterm infants.[23] A comparison of this consensus statement with AAP and ESPGAN recommendations can also be found in this text.[23]

Fluid and Electrolytes

Preterm and LBW infants are especially prone to disorders of fluid and electrolyte imbalance. Requirements are difficult to establish because of the many factors that can either increase or decrease losses. The goals of fluid and electrolyte

TABLE 5-4   *Parenteral Vitamin and Mineral Requirements of Preterm Infants*

Nutrient	Per kg/day
Fat-Soluble Vitamins	
Vitamin A	700–1500 IU
	1500–2800 IU w/lung disease
Vitamin D	40–160 IU (max 400 IU/day)
Vitamin E	3.5 IU (max 7 IU/d)
Vitamin K	8–10 µg
Water-Soluble Vitamins	
Vitamin C	15–25 mg
Thiamin	200–350 µg
Riboflavin	150–200 µg
Pyridoxine	150–200 µg
Niacin	4–6.8 mg
Pantothenate	1–2 mg
Biotin	5–8 µg
Folate	56 µg
B_{12}	.3 µg
Minerals	
Calcium	60–90 mg*
Phosphorus	47–70 mg*
Magnesium	4.3–7.2 mg*
Iron	.1–.2 mg#
Zinc	400 µg
Copper	20 µg^
Manganese	1 µg^
Iodine	1 µg#
Other Trace Minerals	
Selenium	1.5–2 µg ~
Chromium	.05–.2 µg
Molybdenum	.25 µg

*assumes fluid intake of 120–150 cc/kg/day
#see text for discussion of addition of iron and iodine to parenteral solutions
^omit with obstructive jaundice
~omit with renal failure
Adapted from *Nutritional needs of the preterm infant,* Tsang, R, editor, 1993, Williams & Wilkins.

TABLE 5-5 Enteral Vitamin and Mineral Requirements of Preterm Infants

Nutrient	Per kg/day
Fat-Soluble Vitamins	
Vitamin A	700–1500 IU
	1500–2800 IU
	w/lung disease
Vitamin D	150–400 IU (goal 400/day)
Vitamin E	6–12 IU (Max 25/day)
Vitamin K	8–10 µg
Water-Soluble Vitamins	
C	18–24 mg
Thiamin	180–240 µg
Riboflavin	250–360 µg
Pyridoxine	150–210 µg
Niacin	3.6–4.8 mg
Pantothenate	1.2–1.7 mg
Biotin	3.6–6 µg
Folate	25–50 µg
B_{12}	.3 µg
Minerals	
Calcium	120–230 mg
Phosphorus	60–140 mg
Magnesium	7.9–15 mg
Iron	2 mg*
Zinc	1000 µg
Copper	120–150 µg
Manganese	7.5 µg
Iodine	30–60 µg
Other Trace Minerals	
Molybdenum	.3 µg
Selenium	1.3–3 µg
Chromium	.1–.5 µg

*Some preterm infants may need additional iron secondary to blood losses in the neonatal period and inability to provide adequate iron during periods of medical instability. The AAP recommends 2 to 4 mg/kg/day continuing for 12 to 15 months of age.
Adapted from *Nutritional needs of the preterm infant*, Tsang, R, editor, 1993, Williams & Wilkins.

TABLE 5-6 Estimates of Water Losses and Requirements in LBW Infants

Source of Loss	Water Requirements
Evaporation	10–60 ml/kg/day
Fecal	10–15 ml/kg/day
Renal	2–5 ml/kg/hr
Growth	0–0.5 ml/kg/hr

management are to restore losses, allow normal postnatal fluid shifts to occur, maintain homeostasis, and allow for growth. Guidelines have been established but may need to be adjusted as individual clinical status dictates.

Estimates for fluid requirements include the sum of the predicted losses and the requirements for growth. Fluid losses include evaporative losses through the skin and respiratory tract, fecal losses, and renal losses. Evaporative losses are the most variable and can be substantial in the smallest, most immature infants secondary to increased skin permeability, larger body surface area relative to body mass, and greater skin blood flow relative to metabolic rate.[24–29] Estimates of fluid losses and requirements for growth are shown in table 5-6.

Several factors can either increase or decrease the fluid requirements of LBW infants by altering fluid losses. For example, radiant warmers and phototherapy lights markedly increase water requirements by increasing insensible fluid losses.[30,31] On the other hand, heat shields and thermal blankets help to decrease the evaporative water losses of LBW infants.[25,32] To determine total body requirements, the various factors that alter fluid losses should be taken into account and the appropriate adjustments should be made according to individual circumstances.

Because of the many variables affecting fluid needs, it is difficult to establish routine guidelines for fluid management of LBW infants. After initial administration of 80 to 140 ml/kg/day, subsequent needs are determined by clinical examination of the individual infant. Evaluation of weight changes, urine output, specific gravity, serum electrolytes, blood urea nitrogen, blood pressure, peripheral circulatory status, mucous membrane moisture, and skin turgor aid in individual fluid management. Fluids are gradually increased as tolerated to provide adequate nutrient intake. Many stable, growing preterm infants will tolerate 150 to 180 cc/kg/day.

Electrolyte requirements for preterm infants may vary depending on factors such as clinical status, renal function, and state of hydration. Initially, preterm infants may require little or no sodium to maintain normal plasma concentrations. During this time, ELBW infants are also at risk for hyperkalemia, and potassium may be withheld from intravenous fluids until homeostasis is achieved. Stable, growing VLBW and ELBW infants may require more sodium to prevent hyponatremia secondary to immature renal function and increased urinary losses. Medications such as diuretics may further alter electrolyte needs for individual infants.[37] Sodium intakes greater than 2 to 3 mmol/kg/day may be necessary to correct sodium deficits or replace increased losses. Electrolyte guidelines for preterm infants are shown in table 5-7.

TABLE 5-7   *Electrolyte Guidelines for Stable, Growing Preterm Infants*

Sodium	2–3 mmol/kg/day
Potassium	2–3 mmol/kg/day
Chloride	2–3 mmol/kg/day

(from Tsang, 1993)[23]

ENERGY REQUIREMENTS

Parenteral energy requirements differ from enteral requirements (table 5-8). Basal energy needs may be met with 50 to 75 kcal/kg/day. Increased energy is needed for growth. Preterm and LBW infants who are enterally fed require about 120 to 130 kcal/kg/day to grow while 70 to 90 kcal/kg/day supports growth in parenterally fed infants. A number of factors may alter the energy needs of preterm infants regardless of the method of nutritional support. These factors are summarized in table 5-9. The energy intakes of individual infants may need to be adjusted for appropriate growth to occur.

Parenteral

Studies of LBW infants generally show values for resting energy expenditure to be about 50 to 60 kcal/kg/day, provided that measurements are made under thermoneutral conditions and that the infants are relatively inactive. Provisions for 60 kcal/kg/day and adequate amounts of protein meet resting metabolic energy needs and allow nitrogen retention to occur.[33,34] Parenteral intakes of 70 to 90 kcal/kg/day with adequate protein allow for greater tissue protein synthesis and weight gain approximating intrauterine rates.[35,36]

Enteral

Sinclair and others[37] have estimated energy needs for maintenance and growth in enterally fed LBW infants as shown in table 5-10. Energy balance studies confirm total energy expenditure to be in the range of 44 to 88 kcal/kg/day

TABLE 5-8   *Energy Needs for Infants Receiving Parenteral Versus Enteral Support*

Type of Nutritional Support	Energy Needed for	
	Maintenance	Growth
Parenteral	50–60 kcal/kg/day	80–90+ kcal/kg/day
Enteral	75 kcal/kg/day	110–120+ kcal/kg/day

TABLE 5-9   Factors to Consider in Estimating the Energy Requirements of LBW Infants

Factor	Comment	Factor	Comment
Weight	Small babies may have: High heat losses secondary to a lack of subcutaneous fat insulation and a large body surface area High absorptive losses	Environmental stress	Energy needs may be increased by: Temperature instability Fluid losses (e.g., radiant warmers)
Classification	SGA infants may have: High basal metabolic rate Rapid growth rate	Feeding	Enterally fed infants require more kcalories for growth Inappropriate selection of a formula can increase absorptive losses
Postnatal age	Energy requirements may diminish with increasing postnatal age		In certain circumstances, continuous vs. bolus feeding may alter energy utilization Nipple-feeding may increase energy expenditure in some infants
Physiological stress	Energy needs may be increased by: High absorptive losses Hypermetabolic states (e.g., fever, sepsis) Malabsorptive problems (e.g., short bowel syndrome) Respiratory distress and chronic lung disease	Growth	Energy needs are increased when catch-up growth occur

with additional energy needed for growth and tissue deposition.[36] Many enterally fed preterm infants show appropriate growth on 120 to 130 kcal/kg/day. However, 130 to 150 kcal/kg/day may be required for adequate growth in some infants, particularly infants with severe respiratory distress, environmental stresses, or the need for rapid catch-up growth.

PROTEIN REQUIREMENTS

Protein needs of individual infants are influenced by the adequacy of energy intake and the quantity and quality of protein intake. Feeding studies corroborate the biochemical findings that preterm infants can digest and absorb an adequate quantity of protein for intrauterine rates of nitrogen accretion. Preterm infants have gastric, pancreatic, and intestinal enzymes necessary for protein hydrolysis, and there is active transport of amino acids in fetal life.[38,39] However, preterm infants have limited activity of some enzymes involved in amino acid metabolism, particularly cystathionase, tyrosine transaminase, and argininosuccinate synthetase.

These immaturities influence the specific amino acid requirements and the metabolic response of preterm infants given various types of protein. Preterm infants are susceptible to **hyperammonemia, metabolic acidosis,** and

TABLE 5-10 *Energy Requirements of LBW Infants*

Energy Used for (kcal/kg/day)		Energy Needed
Basal metabolic rate	50	
Activity	15	
Cold stress	10	
TOTAL MAINTENANCE		75
Specific dynamic action	8	
Fecal loss	12	
Growth	25	
TOTAL ADDITIONAL REQUIREMENTS		45
TOTAL ENERGY NEEDS FOR GROWTH		120

Adapted from Sinclair J and others: *Pediatr Clin North Am* 17:863, 1970.[37]

abnormal **plasma amino acid levels** when given proteins that differ in quality or quantity. Plasma amino acid patterns reflect protein quality as well as quantity in both parenterally and enterally fed preterm infants.[36,39]

Several methods have been used to determine protein requirements for preterm infants. The factorial approach utilizes the fetal model and calculates protein needs based on fetal accretion rates. Metabolic and balance studies have also been used to determine safe and adequate protein needs. Metabolic and balance studies demonstrate that with adequate energy, protein accretion increases linearly with increasing protein intake (2 to 4 gm/kg/day). Protein intakes above 4 gm/kg/day do not significantly impact protein gains and may contribute to the development of abnormal plasma amino acid patterns and metabolic acidosis. High protein intakes may have a negative impact on neurodevelopmental outcomes.[40]

Parenteral

Provision of 2.5 to 3 gm/kg/day of crystalline amino acids and adequate energy to meet basal metabolic needs, for example, 60 kcal/kg/day, promotes positive nitrogen balance in parenterally fed preterm infants. Provision of protein in excess of an individual infant's needs

or metabolic capability may result in metabolic acidosis, azotemia, and hyperammonemia and offers no apparent advantage. LBW infants are initially given a small amount of amino acids (.5 to 1 gm/kg/day) within the first 48 to 72 hours and the amount is gradually increased to 2.5 to 3 gm/kg/day.[41]

Enteral

One approach to estimating the protein needs of enterally fed preterm infants considers the goal to be intrauterine rates of protein accumulation (factorial approach). A reference fetus model is used to determine the amount of protein that would need to be ingested to match the quantity of protein that is deposited into newly formed fetal tissue.[42,43] To achieve these fetal accretion rates, additional protein must be supplied to compensate for intestinal losses and obligatory losses in urine and skin. Based on this approach, the American Academy of Pediatrics recommends 3.5 to 4.0 gm/kg/day of enteral protein.[44] Protein quality influences protein requirements, and whey-predominant proteins of high biological value, for example, human milk proteins, support growth in preterm infants at quantities less than 3.5 to 4.0 gm/kg/day. Preterm infants who ingest adequate energy and whey-predominant protein at 2.25 gm/kg/day show steady gains in weight and length although their rate of growth may be less than intrauterine rates of growth. Provisions of 2.9 gm/kg/day protein and 120 kcal/kg/day from human milk have been shown to support weight gain and nitrogen retention at intrauterine rates.[45-47]

The distribution of protein to nonprotein energy must also be considered. It is desirable that protein make up 7% to 16% of total energy. Feedings with less than 7% protein may limit growth; those with more than 16% may cause azotemia and acidosis.[48]

LIPID

The growing LBW infant needs an adequate intake of well-absorbed dietary fat to help meet the high energy needs of growth, to provide essential fatty acids, and to assist absorption of other essential nutrients such as fat-soluble vitamins and calcium. However, neonates in general and premature and SGA infants in particular are relatively inefficient in digestion and absorption of lipids.

The percentage of total energy as fat relative to carbohydrate and protein is another important consideration. Fat should constitute 40% to 55% of total energy in enterally fed infants. Because of limited clearance of intravenous fat, it is not practical to achieve this intake of fat in parenterally fed infants. Fat intakes greater than 60% of energy may lead to ketosis. Based on the fatty acid composition of human milk, linoleic acid should comprise 4% to 5% of energy and linolenic acid, 1%. Arachidonic acid and docosahexaenoic acid may be considered conditionally essential nutrients for some infants but the routine provision of these fatty acids remains controversial and long-term safety and efficacy need to be determined.[49]

VITAMINS AND MINERALS

Preterm infants are at risk for a number of nutrient deficiencies. Because fetal fat and minerals are deposited largely in the last trimester, the preterm infant is born with limited stores of many vitamins and minerals. Overt deficiencies have been documented in both parenterally and enterally fed preterm infants. For example, **osteopenia,** secondary to inadequate calcium and phosphorus intake; hemolytic anemia associated with vitamin E deficiency; and iron deficiency anemia have been extensively reported in this population.[48] Recommendations for vitamin and mineral intake for parenterally and enterally fed preterm infants have been made by several groups.[23,44,50,59] The consensus recommendations shown in Tables 5-4 and 5-5[23] take into account the increasing numbers of surviving ELBW and recommendations have been adjusted for weight.

NUTRITIONAL SUPPORT

Medical and metabolic instability in the immediate postnatal period may interfere with

TABLE 5-11 *Goals of Nutritional Support for Preterm Infants*

Phase	Goal
One: stabilization	Support fluid and electrolyte balance and glucose homeostasis
Two: maintenance	Prevent tissue catabolism and promote positive nitrogen balance
Three: transition	Promote tolerance to increase in nutritional support
Four: growth	Provide sufficient protein, energy, and other nutrients to support optimal growth

providing optimal nutritional support. The goals for nutritional support in this population may be divided into four phases (table 5-11). After initial stabilization, nutritional goals may be met with **total parenteral nutrition** (TPN), enteral feedings, or a combination of parenteral and enteral support. Transition from one phase to another depends on the individual infant's medical and metabolic status.

STABILIZATION

Immature preterm and LBW infants have an immediate need for fluid to replace ongoing water losses and rapidly become dependent on an exogenous source of glucose because of limited glycogen stores and decreased capacity for **gluconeogenesis.** To prevent hypoglycemia and to spare protein tissue, an IV solution containing dextrose is infused as soon as primary postnatal demands for resuscitation and stabilization have been met. In addition to fluid and glucose administration, sodium, chloride, and potassium are added in amounts to replace daily losses and maintain homeostasis.

TABLE 5-12   Guidelines for Glucose Load in LBW Infants

Birth Weight (gm)	Initial Glucose Load* (mg/kg/min)	Daily Incremental Increase (mg/kg/min)
<1000	4–6	1.5–2.0
1001–1500	6–8	1.5–2.0
1501–2000	8	As tolerated

Modified from O'Leary MJ: *Nutritional care of the low-birth-weight infant.* In Mahan LK, Arlin M: *Krause's food, nutrition and diet therapy,* Philadelphia, 1992, WB Saunders.

$$*\text{Glucose load} = \frac{\frac{\text{gm glucose}}{100 \text{ ml}} \times \underline{\quad} \text{ ml/kg/day} \times \frac{1000 \text{ mg}}{\text{gm}}}{1440 \text{ min/day}} = \frac{\%\text{dextrose} \times \underline{\quad} \text{ ml/kg/day}}{144} = \text{ml/kg/min}$$

Fluid

Fluid management of preterm infants should allow normal transition of body fluids from fetal to neonatal status during the first week of life. Weight loss typically occurs during this period as contraction of extracellular body water (ECW) and diuresis takes place. Preterm infants may lose up to 15% of their birth weight in the early neonatal period. After initial administration of 80 to 90 ml/kg/day, subsequent fluid needs are determined by clinical examination and accounting for factors that may increase or decrease fluid needs.

Lack of diuresis in the early neonatal period may complicate the course of respiratory disease in the preterm infant. Excess fluid may contribute to heart failure, edema, and persistence of an open patent ductus arteriosus. Excess fluid administration in the early postnatal period has also been associated with intraventricular hemorrhage. Inadequate fluid intake in LBW infants may result in dehydration, electrolyte imbalance, and hypotension.[51–58]

Glucose

Preterm infants are metabolically dependent on glucose in the immediate postnatal period and are susceptible to glucose intolerance secondary to immaturity and metabolic instability. These infants are at risk for both hypoglycemia and hyperglycemia. Glycogen stores and pathways for gluconeogenesis may not be completely developed. In addition, insulin production and function may be impaired.

Preterm infants initially receive glucose intravenously as dextrose (D glucose). In the early postnatal period, fluid volume and dextrose concentration is adjusted to avoid hyperglycemia and hypoglycemia. Hyperglycemia may lead to **glucosuria** and an **osmotic diuresis.** If these conditions are uncorrected, dehydration will occur. To prevent hyperglycemia and the consequences of dehydration, LBW infants should be started on amounts of glucose that do not exceed what the infant is able to metabolize. The amount of glucose administered is determined by its concentration and the rate of administration (glucose load). Calculation of glucose load and suggested guidelines for increasing glucose load are shown in table 5-12.

Electrolytes

During initial stabilization, preterm infants, particularly ELBW infants are at risk for electrolyte imbalance. Hypernatremia and hyperkalemia may occur during this period. Careful monitoring of serum electrolytes and fluid status dictate the early addition of sodium, potassium, and chloride to intravenous fluids. Initially sodium and potassium may be withheld until homeostasis occurs. Within the first 2 to 5 days electrolytes are added to the intravenous fluids (see table 5-7) to replace losses and meet the needs for growth.

PARENTERAL SUPPORT

Parenteral nutrition (the intravenous administration of a hypertonic solution of amino acids, carbohydrate, fat, electrolytes, vitamins, and minerals) can provide essential nutrients as the sole source of nutritional support. In this case the term *total parenteral nutrition,* or *TPN,* is used. Partial parenteral nutrition is used to supplement enteral feedings and is advantageous to preterm infants who are unable to tolerate full enteral feedings or who are being weaned from TPN to a program of complete enteral nutrition. Early provision of amino acids to preterm and LBW infants may prevent excess protein catabolism and improve glucose tolerance by stimulating insulin secretion.[60] LBW infants who are unlikely to tolerate adequate volumes of enteral feeding in the first week of life may be started on parenteral support by 48 to 72 hours of life.

Indications

Parenteral nutrition is indicated in these infants when the projected time to establish adequate enteral support exceeds the infant's metabolic reserves. Because malnutrition complicates the clinical course of these tiny infants, TPN may be indicated in preterm or LBW infants who are unable to receive enteral feedings in the first 2 to 3 days of life or who receive some enteral feedings in the first week of life, but in amounts insufficient to meet basal needs and promote positive nitrogen balance.[61]

Route of Administration

It is possible to support growth and positive nitrogen balance with parenteral nutrition by either **central** or **peripheral vascular routes.**[62] Selecting the peripheral versus the central route of administration involves several considerations that should be individualized according to the unique circumstances of each infant. The principal factors to be considered in choosing one technique over another are the energy and glucose needs, the projected duration of the need for parenteral support, and access.[62,63] Peripheral parenteral solutions are usually not as energy dense as central vein solutions. Peripheral veins are limited to dextrose concentrations of less than 10% to 12.5%. Blood flow through central vessels such as the superior vena cava is very rapid, and hyperosmotic fluids are quickly diluted. Central veins therefore may tolerate dextrose concentrations of 20% to 25%. This means that infants who receive parenteral nutrition through central veins can potentially receive more energy to promote positive nitrogen balance and growth. In the critically ill infant for whom prolonged parenteral therapy is projected, central vein nutrition is usually the treatment of choice (fig. 5-1).[64] If minimal stress is present, if vessel access is good, and if the anticipated duration of parenteral support is short, then the peripheral route of administration is often preferred.

Consideration of the advantages and disadvantages of either route of administration also plays a role in selecting the method of delivery in individual infants. In general, more serious technical and infectious complications are encountered in central delivery compared with peripheral delivery, but both routes have characteristic problems related to the method of administration. Although strict adherence to aseptic techniques and to established guidelines for catheter care and maintenance markedly decrease the incidence of these complications, neither method of delivery is benign.

Complications

Complications associated with parenteral nutrition may be **infectious, technical,** or **metabolic.** Table 5-13 lists the complications associated with parenteral support. The technical and infectious complications associated with parenteral support can be reduced by careful attention to aseptic conditions and judicious placement and maintenance of the catheters. Metabolic complications can be reduced by attention to solution composition, nutrient needs of individual infants, and monitoring nutritional tolerance. Development of new solutions to meet our growing knowledge of parenteral nutrition may further reduce the complications associated with parenteral support.[35,42,64]

FIG. 5-1 A central venous catheter has been surgically implanted in the superior vena cava. This type of catheter permits delivery of hyperalimentation by a central venous route.

Solution Composition

Parenteral nutrition solutions can provide essential nutrients to promote positive nitrogen balance and growth, but they must be tailored in their composition to meet the unique needs of each preterm and LBW infant. The theoretical and practical considerations involved in the management of pediatric parenteral nutrition have been summarized by Lebenthal.[64]

Carbohydrate. LBW infants are dependent on the availability of glucose. Glucose is provided as dextrose and is advanced as tolerated (see table 5-12). Glucose tolerance is monitored by serum glucose levels and evidence of glucosuria.

In some preterm infants, particularly those who are extremely immature, stressed, or septic, glucose intolerance may persist despite administration of conservative glucose loads. Persistent hyperglycemia may severely limit the provision of adequate energy. Increased energy intake has been reported with continuous insulin infusion in patients with persistent hyperglycemia.[65,66] Because of the difficulty in titrating insulin during infusion, there is concern that this therapy may result in extreme and precipitous fluctuations in serum glucose levels.

Efficacy and long-term consequences of insulin infusion will require further investigation. The early addition of amino acids to glucose infusions in preterm infants has the theoretical advantage of stimulating the infants' endogenous insulin secretion.

Protein. The first protein solutions available for IV use were hydrolysates of fibrin and casein, which have now largely been replaced by crystalline amino acid solutions. These solutions mimic the amino acid composition of naturally occurring proteins with high biological values, such as casein or egg albumin. Crystalline amino acid solutions show more efficient nitrogen utilization compared with protein hydrolysates.

Current amino acid solutions designed for adults support growth and positive nitrogen balance in LBW infants. In general, however, these solutions contain low or absent amounts of glutamate, aspartate, tyrosine, cysteine, and taurine and potentially excess amounts of methionine, glycine, and alanine. The plasma amino acid pattern of infants receiving parenteral nutrition reflect the amino acid composition of the solution.[67]

TABLE 5-13   *Complications Associated with Parenteral Nutrition*

Infectious	Sepsis
Technical	Cardiac or vascular thrombosis
	Pneumothorax
	Emboli
	Cardiac/thoracic/ peritoneal effusion
	Clotting of catheter
	Tissue necrosis
	Alteration in vascular perfusion
Metabolic	Fluid and electrolyte imbalance
Carbohydrate-related	Hyperglycemia/ hypoglycemia
	Fatty liver
Lipid-related	Hyperlipidemia
Protein-related	Metabolic acidosis
	Hyperammonemia
	Azotemia
	Abnormal plasma amino acid levels
Vitamin-related	Hypervitaminosis or hypovitaminosis
Mineral-related	Osteopenia rickets
	Hyperphosphatemia or hypophosphatemia
	Hypercalcemia or hypocalcemia
Other	Cholestatic jaundice
	Hepatic dysfunction

The impact of abnormal plasma amino acid levels on the premature infant is not clearly known. Glycine is a potent neurotransmitter inhibitor, and **hyperglycinemia** may have adverse effects on the developing central nervous system of premature infants. Premature infants receiving cysteine- or tyrosine-free diets demonstrate lower plasma levels of these amino acids and impaired nitrogen retention and growth.[68]

Low plasma levels of taurine have been noted in infants receiving taurine-free parenteral solutions. Taurine is involved in neural transmission and in retinal, cardiac, and muscle function.[70] Retinal changes have been noted in infants receiving long-term taurine-free parenteral solutions.

New amino acid solutions have been developed for the neonate and preterm infant.[69] Two solutions designed for use in pediatrics are commercially available: Trophamine (Kendall McGaw Laboratories), and Aminosyn PF (Abbott Laboratories). Compared with other solutions used for adults, the use of these pediatric solutions results in plasma amino acid profiles more like those of healthy infants fed with breast milk. These solutions are efficacious in normalizing plasma amino acid levels.

Lipid. Intravenous fat emulsions are used to meet essential fatty acid needs of preterm infants and to provide energy in a kcalorically dense, isotonic form. Preterm infants are at risk for developing essential fatty acid deficiency. A provision of 0.5 to 1.0 gm/kg/day of an IV fat emulsion will meet the essential fatty acid needs of these infants.[64,71,72]

Preterm infants receiving intravenous lipid are at risk for adverse changes in oxygenation, pulmonary function, and displacement of bilirubin from albumin.[64] Preterm infants also have limited lipoprotein lipase activity for hydrolysis of lipid to free fatty acids, and therefore have limited tolerance to IV lipids. Lack of exogenous carnitine may contribute to impaired lipid tolerance. Carnitine facilitates transport of fatty acids across mitochondrial membranes for oxidation and utilization as energy.[73-76]

Methods of improving lipid tolerance to meet the fatty acid needs of preterm infants are the subject of ongoing research. It has been suggested that heparin may improve lipid clearance by stimulating the release of lipoprotein lipase.[64,77] Carnitine supplementation has been shown to improve lipid clearance in some preterm infants.[74] It has also been suggested that alteration in the fatty acid profile of preterm infants receiving intravenous fat emulsions may improve lipid clearance. Haumont and others[78] noted that preterm infants receiving 10% Intralipid had higher triglyceride levels, higher cholesterol levels, and a higher percentage of low-density lipoproteins compared with infants receiving 20% Intralipid.[78] These solutions differ in the ratio of phospholipid to triglyceride. No specific recommendations, however, have yet been made related to carnitine supplementation, heparin infusion, or alterations in fatty acid composition of fat emulsions for IV use. Preterm infants are typically started on lipid to meet essential fatty acid needs (.5–1 gm/kg/day). Serum triglyceride levels are closely monitored and lipid is advanced as tolerated to 2.5–3 gm/kg/day. Infusion of lipid over a 24-hour period or at a rate less than .12 gm/kg/hr improves lipid tolerance.[79]

Vitamins and minerals. Vitamins and minerals are added to parenteral solutions according to guidelines.[23,50] The only IV multivitamin preparation currently approved for use in infants and children is MVI Pediatric (Armour Pharmaceutical Co). This product meets the 1979 recommendations of the Nutrition Advisory Group of the American Medical Association.[80] However, evidence suggests that LBW infants receiving this preparation often have low plasma vitamin A levels. Increasing the dose to provide higher intakes of vitamin A would result in excess intakes of water-soluble vitamins and vitamin E.[50] It has been recommended that the IV multivitamin preparation should be reformulated to meet the more recent guidelines.[50] The manufacturer of MVI Pediatric suggests that infants and children receive 5 ml MVI Pediatric, infants 1 to 3 kg receive 3.25 ml MVI Pediatric, and infants less than 1 kg receive 1.5 ml MVI Pediatric.

Minerals are added to parenteral solutions. Preterm infants have a higher requirement for calcium and phosphorus than full-term infants.[59] Because of insolubility, it is difficult to add enough calcium and phosphorus to parenteral solutions to meet these requirements. To prevent precipitation, calcium, phosphorus, and magnesium intakes may be described per liter and assume an average intake of 120 to 150 ml/kg/day.[50] Greene and others[50] suggest that these levels be used through a central venous line and not a peripheral line.

Trace elements are also added to parenteral solutions. Trace elements may be added individ-

ually, or as combinations. Several trace elements solutions are available for use in pediatric patients. Whereas zinc may be given to all LBW infants receiving parenteral nutrition, other trace elements must be provided according to expected duration of TPN, renal and hepatic function, and availability of trace element preparations.[50] Manganese and copper should be omitted when obstructive jaundice occurs. Selenium, chromium, and molybdenum should be omitted for infants with renal dysfunction. Iron is not generally added to TPN solutions because of concerns about possible adverse effects, as well as lack of an acceptable intravenous preparation and insufficient data on compatibility and pediatric usage.[50]

Nutritional Support and Monitoring

LBW infants who are unlikely to tolerate adequate volumes of enteral feeding in the first week of life may be started on parenteral support by 48 to 72 hours of life. Infants receiving parenteral nutrition should be monitored to determine the adequacy of nutrient intake and to detect and treat complications. Preterm infants have a small blood volume and the need for monitoring should take into account the relative probability that a particular complication will occur, the potential risks of monitoring, and the likelihood that the information provided will change clinical actions. A number of monitoring schedules have been proposed for infants receiving parenteral support.[81] These schedules often include electrolytes, acid-base status, serum glucose or Dextrostix, protein status (albumin and prealbumin), bone mineral status (calcium, phosphorus, and alkaline phosphatase), and liver function tests. Additional tests may be indicated in an individual infant, including white blood cell count (WBC) and culture, zinc, copper and iron, and lipid tolerance studies.

TRANSITION FROM PARENTERAL TO ENTERAL NUTRITION

Infants who receive TPN have relatively low digestive mass and delayed gastrointestinal growth compared with infants who receive enteral stimuli.[81] This is particularly true for infants who receive TPN for prolonged periods. Pancreatic hyposecretion, intestinal mucosal atrophy, and decreased parietal cell mass during TPN are, however, reversible on resumption of enteral feeding.[60,81]

It is desirable to initiate enteral feedings in LBW infants as early as possible. Even in small amounts, these feedings act to stimulate enzymatic development and activity, promote bile flow, and increase small intestinal villous growth. Small amounts of feeding may also contribute to maturation of peristaltic wave patterns in immature infants.[82–85] Early, minimal enteral feeds may improve growth and promote tolerance to later advancement to full enteral feeding.[86] Later, transition to total enteral nutrition may be easier for these infants.

When making the transition from parenteral to enteral nutrition, it is important to adjust both sources of nutrition to provide adequate intake for growth but avoid excessive intakes of any particular substrate. In general, when an infant is receiving optimal energy, protein, vitamins, and minerals from parenteral support, this is accomplished by slowly decreasing the volume of parenteral infusion as enteral intake increases. Intravenous fat emulsions may be decreased or discontinued when half to three-fourths of the intake is derived from an appropriate enteral feeding. When an infant is tolerating 75% of total feedings from an enteral source and continued advancement to full feeds is anticipated, parenteral support may be discontinued and the remainder of the infant's fluid volume may be provided by IV dextrose until full feeds are achieved.

ENTERAL NUTRITION
Initiation of Enteral Feedings

Decisions to initiate and advance enteral feedings involve many factors (see the box on factors to consider). The degree of prematurity, history of perinatal insults, current medical condition, medical and metabolic stability, and functioning of the gastrointestinal tract all influence the success and tolerance of enteral feeding. Optimal timing of the first feeding and advancement of subsequent feedings must be individualized.

❖
FACTORS TO CONSIDER BEFORE FEEDING A PRETERM INFANT BY AN ENTERAL ROUTE

- Perinatal
  Birth asphyxia
  Apgar scores
- Respiratory status
  Stability of ventilation
  Blood gases
  ABCs
- Medical status
  Vital signs (heart rate, respiratory rate, color, temperature, blood pressure, tone)
  Acute illness (sepsis)
- Gastrointestinal tract
  Anomalies (gastroschisis, omphalocele)
  Patency
  Functioning (bowel tones present, passage of stool)
  Risk of necrotizing enterocolitis
- Equipment/procedures
  Umbilical artery catheter
  Intubation/extubation
  Others

There is growing evidence that early initiation of small amounts of enteral feedings may be advantageous to preterm infants because it may stimulate the production and secretion of a number of gastrointestinal enzymes and hormones including **gastrin, enteroglucagon, motilin,** and **neurotensin,** which have **trophic** and **motility effects**.[82–84] Enteral feeding may contribute to maturation of motility patterns, improve glucose tolerance, increase bile flow, decrease hyperbilirubinemia, and improve calcium and phosphorus status.[85,89] Early enteral feeding may influence tolerance to subsequent feeding and improve growth.[86,87,88] Awareness of the potential benefits of enteral feeding, even in immature infants, has led clinicians to consider "nonnutritive feeding," which consists of feeding preterm infants small amounts to allow their gut to mature and adapt while supporting them nutritionally with parenteral infusions.

FIG. 5-2   A growing premature infant is being fed by oral gastric gavage.

FIG. 5-3   A mother feeds her premature infant during the transition from gavage to nipple.

Methods of Feeding

Once it has been decided that enteral feedings will be initiated, the optimal feeding technique must be selected. Preterm infants can be fed by gavage (tube) (fig. 5-2) or by nipple (fig. 5-3).[90,91]

Techniques. Gavage feeding is the choice for infants who are unable to coordinate sucking, swallowing, and breathing. Immature suck-swallow-breathe patterns are seen in infants less than 32 to 34 weeks' gestation. Respiratory distress and insults to the central nervous system may further impair suck-swallow-breathe coordination. Enteral feeding in these infants may be by orogastric or nasogastric gavage. Nasogastric tubes are more stable in their placement but may obstruct or irritate the infant's nasal passages. (This may be a problem for infants who must breathe through their noses or for infants with respiratory disease.) Orogastric feeding is preferred for infants with these conditions, but this method is associated with bradycardia and aspiration during tube placement, particularly in infants who are developing a cough and gag reflex. Nipple feeding may be attempted in infants who are greater than 32 to 34 weeks' gestation. The transition from gavage to nipple is often a complicated and slow process. Factors that can impede successful nipple feeding are shown in table 5-14.[92-94]

Composition of Feeding

Preterm infants can be fed human milk or formula. Selection of a milk with the following characteristics may facilitate tolerance to enteral feeding: (1) nutrient composition that is readily digestible and absorbable; (2) whey-predominant protein; (3) low renal solute load; and (4) iso-osmolality (300 mOsm/kg water). Human milk and premature formulas meet these criteria.

Human milk. Human milk has unique properties that benefit both full-term and preterm infants (see chapter 4).[95,96] Human milk contains growth factors that exert a trophic effect on the developing intestinal epithelium. The presence of enzymes such as lipase and amylase contribute to improved digestion and absorption of fat and carbohydrate. Human milk proteins are whey predominant, and their amino acid composition favors the needs of preterm infants. Human milk also contains a number of antiinfective factors that can provide protection against infection.

When preterm infants are fed their own mother's milk, they grow more rapidly than infants fed banked breast milk (mature milk). Some preterm infants can achieve intrauterine rates of weight gain when fed adequate volumes of their own mother's milk.[97] The more rapid weight gain observed in preterm infants fed

TABLE 5-14   *Factors Influencing Preterm Infants' Nippling Ability*

Factor	Significance
Poor coordination of suck-swallow-breathe	Risk of aspiration Decreased feeding efficiency Fatigue
Decreased or absent sucking pads	Decreased sucking strength and endurance
Decreased tone	Inability to maintain optimally flexed feeding posture
Diminished or absent gag and cough reflex	Increased risk of aspiration
Neurological and behavioral immaturity	More time is spent in sleep with short periods in quiet alert and awake states (which make feeding easier) Subtle cues of hunger, satiety, and distress (which alters infant-caregiver interactions) Difficulty maintaining an organized state (which can disrupt feedings)

Modified from Shaker CS: Nipple feeding premature infants: a different perspective, *Neonatal Network* 8:9, 1990, and Vandenberg KA: Nippling management of the sick neonate in the NICU: the disorganized feeder, *Neonatal Network* 9:9, 1990.

their own mother's milk has been attributed to differences in composition of milk from mothers delivering prematurely. Studies have reported that milk from mothers delivering prematurely is higher in protein, fat, energy, sodium, and some minerals.[97-102] Other investigators have shown no significant differences in the milk composition from mothers delivering prematurely; they suggest the differences seen are a function of lactogenesis and the volume of milk produced.

TABLE 5-15   Comparison of Premature Formulas and Standard Formulas

	Premature Formulas	Standard Formulas
	Designed and tested in preterm infants	Designed and tested in full-term infants
Energy concentration	24 or 20 kcal/oz	20 kcal/oz
Protein	Whey casein; 60:40	Whey casein; 60:40
Fat	Medium- and long-chain fats	100% long-chain fats
Carbohydrate	Lactose and glucose polymers	100% lactose
Vitamins and minerals	Fortified to meet the needs of preterm infants	Fortified to meet the needs of full-term infants
	Available with or without iron	Available with or without iron
Osmolality	Iso-osmolar	Iso-osmolar

Human milk does not meet the calcium and phosphorus needs of the rapidly growing preterm infant. Decreased bone mineralization, osteopenia, and rickets can occur in these infants when human milk is fed without calcium and phosphorus supplementation.[95,102–105] Human milk does not meet the protein, sodium, vitamin, and mineral needs of all preterm infants, particularly VLBW and ELBW infants. Fortification of human milk, however, can ameliorate the disadvantages of human milk feeding of preterm infants.

Formula. Formulas designed for full-term infants do not meet all of the nutrient needs of preterm infants. There are, however, specialized premature infant formulas that differ from standard cow's milk–based formulas for full-term infants. Table 5-15 summarizes these differences. Premature formulas support the special needs of preterm infants for growth and bone mineralization. These formulas are also well tolerated when fed in appropriate amounts.

Vitamin and mineral supplementation. Guidelines for vitamin and mineral intake established by experts serve as a reference in determining supplementation needs.[23,44,59] Premature infant formulas vary in nutrient composition, and therefore differ with respect to specific needs for vitamin and mineral supplementation. It is important to know the current nutrient content of premature formulas in order to make appropriate decisions regarding supplementation (table 5-16). Infants fed human milk also require supplementation. Human milk fortifiers are available that provide energy, protein, vitamins, and minerals. The amounts of calcium and phosphorus in these products promote optimal bone mineralization in preterm infants.

Stable growing preterm infants are likely to deplete their limited iron reserves by 2 months of age. A supplement of 2 to 4 mg/kg/day of elemental iron is recommended no later than 2 months of age for preterm infants fed either formulas or breast milk. The American Academy of Pediatrics recommends that supplementation continue until 12 to 15 months of age.[44]

Management of Enteral Feeding

The initial goal of enteral feeding is to facilitate normalization of gastrointestinal function and tolerance to the milk provided. Subsequent feedings should meet all the nutrient needs of growing infants. Human milk or premature formulas are usually fed to infants who weigh less than 2 kg. Infants greater than 2 kg may receive human milk or formulas designed for full-term infants.

Volume and Schedule

The amount of milk fed to preterm infants depends in part on their estimated stomach capacity. This varies with the size and postnatal age of the infant (for example, an 800 gm infant has an undistended stomach capacity of 2 to 3 ml). Preterm infants also have poor gastrointestinal motility, which may further limit volume

TABLE 5-16   *Select Nutrient Composition of Premature Formulas (Per 100 kcal)* *

	Similac Special Care (24 kcal/oz)	Enfamil Premature Formula 24 kcal/oz	NeoCare 22 kcal/oz
Protein			
Grams	2.71	3.0	2.6
% kcal	11	12	10%
Fat			
Source	MCT, soy, and coconut oil	MCT, soy, and coconut oil	Soy, High oleic % MCT, coconut oil
Grams	5.43	5.1	5.5
% kcal	47	44	49%
Carbohydrate			
Source	Lactose, glucose polymers	Lactose, corn syrup solids	Corn syrup solids, lactose
Grams	10.6	11	10.3
% kcal	42	44	41%
Vitamins and Minerals			
Calcium (mg)	180	165	105 mg
Phosphorus (mg)	90	83	62 mg
Sodium (mg)	43	39	33 mg
Vitamin A (IU)	680	1200	460 IU
Vitamin D (IU)	150	270	80 IU
Vitamin E (IU)	4.0	4.6	3.6 IU
Vitamin B_{12} (μg)	0.55	0.3	.4 μg
Vitamin C (mg)	37	35	15 mg
Folate (μg)	37	35	25 μg
Estimated Renal Solute Load (ERSL)	18.3	18.7	17.5
Osmolarity			
mOsm/L	250	260	260

*For complete and current nutrient composition of formulas, consult the most recent product information.

tolerance. Small, frequent feedings improve tolerance to milk feedings. Initial feedings should approximate the undistended stomach capacity (for example, 1 to 2 ml in the infant < 1 kg). Feedings may be initiated as either continuous drip or bolus feedings every 2 to 3 hours. Feedings are advanced as tolerated on an individualized basis. Many VLBW infants may not tolerate increases in total daily volumes greater than 20 ml/kg/day. Rapid advancement of enteral feedings has been associated with **necrotizing enterocolitis.**

ASSESSMENT AND MONITORING OF NUTRITIONAL SUPPORT

Both parenterally and enterally supported preterm infants are carefully monitored and nutritional status is assessed. Infants are monitored to determine tolerance to nutritional support and to prevent risks associated with the method of support. Nutritional status is assessed to determine efficacy of nutritional support (i.e., improvement of nutritional status or maintenance of appropriate nutritional status). Monitoring and assessment include clinical evaluation, laboratory assessment, and anthropometrics. Preterm infants have small blood volumes and the need for laboratory monitoring should consider the probability that a particular problem will occur, the potential risks of monitoring, and the likelihood that the information obtained will lead to a clinical intervention.

MONITORING

Preterm infants receiving parenteral nutrition are at risk for a number of metabolic complications associated with this method of nutritional support (see table 5-13). A number of monitoring schedules have been proposed for infants receiving parenteral support.[81,106] These schedules often include electrolytes, acid-base status, serum glucose, or Dextrostix. Monitoring of lipid clearance is often done by measuring serum triglycerides. Evidence of liver dysfunction is particularly important for infants on long-term TPN (>2 weeks). An increase in direct bilirubin is an early indicator of developing cholestasis.[107] Additional liver function tests may be obtained in infants showing evidence of hepatic dysfunction. Calcium, phosphorus, and magnesium are also included in many monitoring schedules. Additional tests may be indicated for an individual infant including white blood cell count (WBC) and culture, zinc, copper, and iron.

Tolerance to enteral feeding in preterm infants is primarily by clinical assessment (see box, p. 146). Indicators for feeding intolerance include gastric residuals, regurgitation, abdominal distention, changes in frequency

---

❖

POSTNATAL GROWTH PATTERNS OF PRETERM INFANTS

Weight loss	5%–15% of birth weight
Regain birth weight	1–2 weeks of age
Sustained growth	15 gm/kg/day weight gain and 0.5–1 cm/wk increase in length

and consistency of bowel movements, the presence of reducing substances or occult blood in the stool. These symptoms may be associated with necrotizing enterocolitis. These symptoms may also be associated with other changes in clinical status. The decision to reduce or discontinue enteral feeding takes into account not only the occurrence of one or more of these symptoms but also the overall clinical status of the individual infant.

ASSESSMENT OF NUTRITIONAL STATUS
Growth

All neonates have a growth pattern characterized by three phases: (1) weight loss; (2) regaining of birth weight; and (3) sustained growth. Postnatal weight curves are used to assess weight changes in the early neonatal period and depict this pattern. Two postnatal weight charts are currently available for clinical use with preterm infants. The Dancis, O'Connell, and Holt curves are based on data collected more than 40 years ago.[108] The postnatal weight curves by Shaffer and others are based on more recent data and demonstrate that infants currently lose less weight, regain birth weight sooner, and sustain a greater rate of growth (see the box entitled "Postnatal Growth Patterns of Preterm Infants").[109]

When an infant has regained birth weight and demonstrates a pattern of sustained growth, it is important to begin weekly measurements of body length and head circumference. Two growth curves are available that depict growth from 24 and 28 weeks, respectively, to 1 to 2 years corrected age.[110,111] These curves were generated from data collected in the 1960s and represent a cross-sectional sample of infants less than 40 weeks' gestation and full-term infants. Although these growth curves do not represent longitudinal reference growth curves, they are useful tools for evaluating patterns of growth in individual infants.

Growth curves have been printed that depict growth in weight, length, and OFC in a large group of preterm infants from 40 weeks to 1 year corrected age.[112] These curves are available for both sexes and have been divided according to birth weight less than 1500 gm and greater than 1500 gm (see appendix).

The NCHS curves for full-term infants can also be used to monitor growth after 40 weeks' gestation. When using these growth charts, age should be adjusted for prematurity until 1 to 2 years corrected age.

Laboratory Indices

Several laboratory measurements—such as serum proteins (albumin, transthyretin, transferrin, and retinol binding protein), serum vitamins (Vitamin D, retinol), and serum minerals (calcium, phosphorus)—have been used as indicators of nutritional status. Transthyretin, transferrin, and retinol-binding protein are more sensitive indicators of protein-energy status.[113] Albumin is more reflective of chronic protein energy status. Calcium, phosphorus, and alkaline phosphatase provide a means of monitoring bone mineral status. More accurate assessments of bone mineral content may be done but cost and practicality often limit the usefulness. X rays may also provide an indicator in infants with already demineralized bone.

Laboratory assessment of nutritional status in the preterm infant is often limited because reference ranges are often not available for this population. Serial measurements of certain laboratory indices may be useful in some preterm infants. These infants include those at risk for protein energy malnutrition, inadequate bone mineralization, inadequate intake, drug-nutrient interactions, increased losses, or malabsorption. Judicious ordering of blood tests and considera-

tion of risk versus benefit of taking a blood sample is advised in using laboratory indices for monitoring nutritional status. Laboratory monitoring must be streamlined to the individual infant's needs and clinical status.

OUTCOME

From the preceding discussion, it is apparent that it is possible to meet the metabolic and nutritional needs of premature and LBW infants in a manner sufficient to sustain life and to promote growth and development. With adequate nutritional support and advances in neonatal intensive care technology, more tiny immature infants are surviving than ever before.

During the past 10 years, survival rates for infants between 750 to 1000 gm have increased from 50% to 80%; for infants with birth weights between 500 to 750 gm, survival rates have increased from 10% to 50%.[114] Many of these small preterm infants have experienced complicated and prolonged hospitalizations and are discharged with ongoing medical problems and neurodevelopmental concerns. Studies are attempting to determine the long-term neurodevelopmental consequences and to delineate appropriate cognitive expectations for these vulnerable infants as well as appropriate growth expectations.

Neurodevelopmental Outcome

Surviving LBW infants are at increased risk for neurodevelopmental problems as they grow older. These problems range from minor motor and sensory impairment to severe handicapping conditions such as visual/hearing losses and cerebral palsy.[114-117] It is unclear what factors contribute to major and minor handicapping conditions in these vulnerable infants. Statistically, the ELBW infant (< 800 gm) has the greatest risk of morbidity. Neurodevelopmental evaluation during the first year may not be predictive of long-term developmental status or academic achievement.

Ongoing follow-up is crucial for detecting those infants with neurodevelopmental concerns and employing appropriate intervention

FIG. 5-4 A mother interacts with her premature infant who is 10 weeks old.

FIG. 5-5 Same child as in figure 5-4. Here she is healthy and 2½ years old.

strategies to further improve outcome (fig. 5-4). It is important to recognize that many preterm infants will not be impaired (fig. 5-5). Some larger LBW infants will develop and perform academically at the same level as healthy infants born at term.[117]

Medical Outcome

During the first few years posthospitalization, premature infants are at risk for ongoing medical problems (see table 5-17). Rehospitalization during the first year of life occurs more frequently in this population with VLBW infants having 4 to 5 times the increased risk. The risk of hospitalization is greatly increased in infants with bronchopulmonary dysplasia (BPD). BPD is a chronic lung disease that occurs in infants requiring oxygen or ventilatory support in the neonatal period. The incidence is inversely related to gestational age. BPD occurs in 6% to 24% of neonates requiring oxygen and ventilatory support. Rehospitalization in this group of infants is primarily secondary to respiratory tract infections, bronchiolitis, and pneumonia. Other medical complications that may occur in premature infants include gastroesophageal reflux, and anemia. Premature infants, particularly ELBW infants who were critically ill during their hospitalization, may have resolving conditions that need medical follow-up. Close medical follow-up may be arranged for infants with patent ductus arteriosus (PDA), BPD, nephrocalcinosis, cholestasis, osteopenia, or short-gut syndrome.

Growth

Intrauterine rates of weight gain (15 gm/kg/day) are often the goals during a premature infant's hospitalization. For the infant weighing 2000 gm (4.24 lb) or more, a weight gain of 30 gm/day reflects intrauterine rates of growth. Twenty to 30 gm/day weight gain between

TABLE 5-17 *Medical Conditions That May Require Monitoring and Follow-Up after Hospital Discharge*

Cardiovascular	PDA (patent ductus arteriosus)
Respiratory	BPD (bronchopulmonary dysplasia)
Renal	Nephrocalcinosis
Hepatic	TPN induced cholestasis
Hematologic	Anemia
GI	Short-gut syndrome, gastroesophageal reflux
Skeletal	Osteopenia, rickets
Other	Hernia, retinopathy of prematurity

40 weeks corrected age and 6 months allows the preterm infant to maintain a pattern of growth that parallels current growth curves. The growth velocity of term infants declines from 6 to 12 months of age. This may happen with some preterm infants. Continued weight gain at rates that exceed that of term infants of comparable age will allow for **catch-up growth** to occur (i.e., the infant who has fallen below the 5th percentile will gradually approach the 5th percentile and ultimately find his/her "own channel").

Preterm infants show different growth patterns than full-term infants even when corrected for gestational age. Although larger, stable preterm infants may demonstrate catch-up growth in the first 1 to 2 years of life, VLBW and ELBW infants are unlikely to show catch-up growth in the first 3 years of life.[119–121] Small size at 1 to 3 years of age in this group does not necessarily indicate small size at school age. Many of these infants achieve weights, heights, and head circumferences by 7 to 8 years of age that are similar to those of the reference population.[120,121,123]

Nutritional expectations. It is common practice to view the nutrient needs of preterm infants weighing 2 to 2.5 kg to be similar to the nutrient needs of full-term infants. The RDA is often used as a reference. This practice requires

validation, particularly for VLBW and ELBW infants. Recent evidence suggests that calcium and phosphorus needs may differ from full-term infants during the first year of life. For example, bone mineralization has been reported to be lower in preterm infants fed unfortified human milk during the first year of life. Monitoring of bone mineral status may be appropriate for preterm infants throughout infancy.[124,125]

The relationship between feeding practices and the growth patterns observed in this population after hospital discharge has not been clearly defined. Ernst[122] noted several feeding practices associated with lack of catch-up growth in VLBW infants. These practices included introduction of semisolids and cow's milk according to postnatal age (not corrected age), and the use of low fat milks.

Preterm infants fed a nutrient-enriched formula after hospital discharge were noted to have increased linear growth and weight gain when compared with infants fed a standard infant formula. The formula, designed for preterm infants after hospital discharge, was higher in energy, protein, calcium and phosphorus when compared with standard infant formula.[126,127]

During the first year of life, preterm infants will experience the gradual transition from predominant nipple feeding to solid foods. Many preterm infants will meet these feeding milestones according to corrected age and not chronologic age. Readiness for solid foods, therefore, may occur at 4 to 6 months corrected age. For the ELBW infant born at 24 weeks' gestation, for example, readiness for solids may not occur until 8 to 10 months' postnatal age. Appropriate assessment of developmental readiness for feeding transitions may facilitate the transition from infant to toddler feeding.

DISCHARGE AND FOLLOW-UP

Discharge and follow-up plans for preterm infants are individualized to the infants' needs. After successful transition at home, infants without ongoing medical problems may be followed at a frequency similar to term infants. Neurodevelopmental follow-up for preterm infants may

TABLE 5-18   Nutritional Risk Factors for Preterm Infants

Risk Factor	Comment
History of Risk	
*Prematurity and LBW	Especially ELBW, VLBW, and <32 weeks
*Small for gestational age	
*TPN >2 weeks	
*Medical complications of prematurity	BPD, heart disease, short-gut syndrome, neurologic impairment
*Inadequate nutrition or nutrition concerns	Inadequate growth, osteopenia, other documented nutritional deficits
*Feeding difficulties	GER, inadequate nippling, choking/ABCs with feeding, respiratory distress with feeding
Ongoing Nutritional Risk	
*Weight <6 lb at discharge	Limited reserves
*<37 weeks at discharge	Limited reserves, immaturity
*Feeding difficulties	GER, inadequate intake, choking/ABCs with feeding, respiratory distress with feeding, prolonged feeding times
*Home TPN or tube feeding	
*Medical conditions	BPD, heart disease, short-gut syndrome, neurologic impairment
*Documented nutritional deficits	Osteopenia, rickets, anemia

continue through school age to identify special needs and early intervention. Infants with medical problems, neurodevelopmental problems, or nutritional concerns will require more frequent monitoring and may require coordination of multiple health-care services.[128,129,130]

Preterm infants continue at nutritional risk after hospital discharge, particularly VLBW infants, ELBW infants, and infants with ongoing medical and neurological concerns.[131] *Identification of nutritional risk, assessment of nutritional status,* and *education and support* are part of the discharge and follow-up process for these infants. Critical times for nutritional evaluation include the immediate discharge period and key developmental stages of feeding. The latter include the introduction of semisolids at about 4 to 6 months developmental age, and weaning from the bottle to the cup and table foods at about 9 to 12 months developmental age. Assessment at these stages assists in evaluating

an infant's readiness for change, in selecting appropriate foods, in reassuring parents about growth and nutrition, and in preventing growth setbacks in infants with a history of slow growth and small size.

Identification of Nutritional Risk

Infants who are at nutritional risk include those who have increased nutrient needs, increased nutrient losses, difficulty ingesting adequate amounts of nutrients, or a history of inadequate intake and growth (table 5-18). Additional physical and environmental factors can also place preterm infants at nutritional risk. Assessment of risk factors identifies those infants who are at nutritional risk. Evaluation of growth, intake, and feeding of infants with nutritional risk factors will identify those infants with ongoing nutritional concerns. Infants with ongoing nutritional concerns should be monitored more frequently. Referral to other health subspecialties (nutrition, OT/PT, speech) may facilitate correction of the problem, and provide support and education to the family.

Growth Assessment

Periodic growth measurements are a part of follow-up nutrition assessment of preterm, LBW infants. Infants at nutritional risk should have more frequent growth assessment. Evaluation of individual growth patterns and growth velocity are useful indicators of nutritional status. Infants who remain smaller than term cohorts should have an established growth channel that parallels reference curves. Weight gains should be about 20 to 30 gm/day in the first 6 months of life but may decline to about 10 to 15 gm/day from 6 to 12 months of age. Length increases 1 cm/week until 40 weeks corrected age, 0.75 cm/week from 40 weeks to 3 months, and 0.5 cm/wk from 3 to 6 months of age. Weight to length should be proportional.[128–130]

In assessing growth, appropriate reference curves should be selected (see section on growth). When using the NCHS curves, growth should be plotted by corrected age until 1 to 2 years of age. Infants who are identified with ongoing growth concerns (i.e., rate of growth decelerates, failure to maintain adequate growth velocity, weight and length are not proportionate) should have further evaluation. Evaluation should include assessment of intake. Observation of a feeding may also provide valuable information.

Assessment of Intake. Normally the fluid intakes of preterm infants approximate 150 to 180 ml/kg/day (2.3 to 2.7 oz/lb) throughout the first year. This approximates 105 to 120 kcal/kg/day. Energy intake may need to be adjusted on an individual basis to support optimal growth. Initially preterm infants may take less than 24 oz of formula/day. Although this may meet fluid and energy requirements, a multivitamin supplement is necessary to meet vitamin requirements. Infants who are not meeting fluid requirements should have feedings assessed and intake needs adjusted to meet fluid needs prior to adjusting energy. Semisolids, cup, and table foods are introduced according

---

❖

CHECKLIST FOR ASSESSMENT OF INTAKE

_____ Fluid intake approximates usual intake (2.3 to 2.7 oz per lb)

_____ Fluid intake inadequate to meet fluid needs (<1.5 to 1.8 oz per lb)

_____ Caloric intake at or above usual intake for infant at current age and weight (100 to 120 kcal per kg per day)

_____ Caloric intake at or below 100 to 120 kcal per kg per day

_____ Infant receiving appropriate infant formula or breast milk

_____ Infant receiving multivitamin supplement if intake <24 oz per day

_____ Infant receiving iron by 2 months of age

_____ Semisolids introduced according to correct age and readiness (4–6 months corrected age)

_____ Weaning from bottle according to corrected age (12 months)

---

to developmental readiness and corrected age (see box on this page).

Education and support. Growth, developmental expectations, and early feeding experiences of preterm infants differ from term infants. Hospitalization alters the infant-caregiver feeding experience of preterm infants. These infants may have multiple feeders. Parental access to feeding may be limited. Adequate growth and feeding is often a final criterion for discharge, generating anxiety around these issues. After discharge, some infants may experience setbacks in feeding and growth. Provision of information regarding preterm feeding skills, nutritional needs of preterm infants, and growth expectations may facilitate the transition home and relieve parental anxiety. For the infant with ongoing growth and nutritional concerns, education and support may facilitate normal feeding transitions, appropriate food choices, and improved growth.

❖ ❖ ❖

CASE REPORT 1

Initial Stabilization and Parenteral Support

A 26-week, 980-gm infant was admitted to an NICU immediately after birth. The infant was intubated for respiratory distress and an exogenous surfactant was administered through the endotracheal tube. An umbilical artery catheter was placed to aid in ventilatory management. Fluid was initially infused through this line as D10 water at 80 cc/kg/day. Within the first 24 hours, the infant had problems with hypoglycemia and required several dextrose boluses. Over the next 24 hours, the infant became hypernatremic and required increased fluids secondary to increased insensible losses.

Because metabolic reserves are limited in an infant at this size and gestation and it was not expected that this infant would be advanced to full enteral feeds in the first week of life, the infant was started on parenteral nutrition at 48 hours of age.

The infant was started on a D12.5 solution containing amino acids (.5 gm/kg/day) and vitamins and minerals at 140 cc/kg/day. The infant also received a small amount of IVF to meet essential fatty acid needs (.5 gm/kg/day). Amino acids were gradually increased over 5 days to provide 3 gm/kg/day of protein. IVF was also slowly increased as tolerated to 2.5 gm/kg/day. Tolerance to IVF was monitored with serum triglyceride levels.

The infant continued to lose weight (12% of birth weight) and continued to have problems with hypernatremia. Fluids were increased to 160 cc/kg/day, but with increased fluids, the infant became hyperglycemic. Dextrose was decreased to D10 and glucose and electrolytes stabilized. By the end of this infant's first week of life, the infant was receiving 94 kcal/kg/day and 2.5 gm/kg/day of protein with appropriate amounts of vitamins and minerals. The infant was tolerating this regimen as ascertained with laboratory monitoring (acid-base status, triglycerides, electrolyte, and mineral levels). The infant was no longer losing weight and was in fluid balance.

❖ ❖ ❖

CASE REPORT 2

Transition from Parenteral to Enteral Support

Baby girl G was born at 26 weeks, weighing 960 gm (see case report 1). At day of life (DOL) 5, she was relatively stable on a ventilator (for respiratory support) and was receiving gradually increasing amounts of amino acids, calories and fat (84 kcal/kg/day and 1.6 gm/kg/day protein). Small amounts of enteral feedings (nonnutritive or gut-stimulation feeds) were started (see benefits of minimal enteral feeding). She was fed via gavage tube 1 cc q 3 hours either breast milk or a premature formula for 24 hours. After tolerating the small volume feeds, a slow advancement of enteral feeding was planned secondary to ELBW and respiratory instability. Feeds were advanced 20 cc/kg/day with continued parenteral support. The volume of the parenteral solution was decreased as enteral feedings were increased. Diuretics were started on DOL 8 secondary to a weight gain of 40 gm/day and changes in respiratory status. On DOL 11, she was at 80 cc/kg/day of breast milk (or ½ feeds on a total fluid volume of 160 cc/kg/day); IVF was decreased from 2.5 to 1.5 gm/kg/day and parenteral support was continued. On DOL 13, she was extubated. She was at ¾ feeds or 120 cc/kg/day (q3). Secondary to increased work of breathing, she was changed to q2 feeding. She was reintubated on DOL 14 and reached full feeds DOL 15. She tolerated full feeds at 160 cc/kg/day (q2) and the breast milk was fortified and vitamins were started. At this time, she was receiving 122 kcal/kg/day and 2.6 gm/kg/day and was gaining 12 gm/day (13/kg/day). Intake was increased to 133 kcal/kg/day and 3 gm/kg/day protein. The infant subsequently achieved a weight gain of 15 gm/kg/day.

❖ ❖ ❖

CASE REPORT 3

Enteral Feeding/Discharge Planning

Baby boy C was born at 25 weeks' gestation, weighing 760 grams (1.5 lb). Baby boy C's medical history includes BPD. He required ventilator support for the first 8 weeks of life. Following a 3-week course of steroids, he was successfully weaned from the ventilator at 11 weeks of age (postnatal age).

Baby boy C's nutrition and growth history was complicated. Initially he did not tolerate enteral feeding and required TPN for the first 3 weeks of life. Eventually he was able to tolerate gavage feeding of a premature formula but was unable to sustain optimal growth despite multiple dietary manipulations. He began nipple feeding at 35 weeks but was limited by his respiratory status and immaturity.

Baby boy C is now 41 weeks corrected age and weighs 2454 gm (5.4 lb). He is being discharged with BPD and continues to require oxygen. Feedings are breast milk (supplemented to 24 kcal/oz). He has been nippling all feeds for 2 weeks and gaining 20 gm per day. Fortification of breast milk was discontinued when he reached a weight of 2 kg (4.25 lb), and he currently receives a multivitamin supplement and iron. His mother plans on breast-feeding him.

At discharge, nutrition concerns included (1) history of inadequate growth and limited reserves, (2) immature feeding skills, which may continue to be compromised secondary to his respiratory status, (3) need for a higher energy feeding and dietary manipulation, and (4) transition to breast-feeding while maintaining and/or maximizing his weight gain.

Plans for discharge included (1) follow-up with his primary physician, to include a weight check four days post discharge, (2) follow-up for BPD at a pulmonary center to include nutrition assessment by an RD, (3) in-hospital and phone contact with a lactation consultant for transition to breast-feeding, (4) public health nursing referral, (5) follow-up at a developmental center for NICU graduates, and (6) home health nursing care. His parents had received instructions on formula preparation, expected intake, and signs of dehydration. Initial follow-up appointments were limited to the primary physician and in-home visits by the public health nurse. This was done to minimize disruption in his care and limit his potential exposure to infectious agents.

REVIEW QUESTIONS

1. List the major reasons why a premature infant is at greater nutritional risk than a full-term infant.
2. What are the major factors that determine whether a premature infant will receive parenteral or enteral feeds?
3. What are the differences between formulas designed for LBW infants and those for full-term infants?
4. Is human milk appropriate for the LBW infant?
5. How do the vitamin and mineral requirements of preterm infants differ from those of full-term infants?
6. How do parenteral protein and energy requirements differ from the enteral requirements for preterm infants?
7. How do parenteral requirements for vitamins and minerals differ from the enteral requirements of preterm infants?
8. Describe complications associated with parenteral nutrition.

SUGGESTED LEARNING ACTIVITIES

1. Review the medical record of an infant in a neonatal intensive care unit who is receiving total parenteral nutrition. Describe the conditions that made total parenteral nutrition the appropriate method of feeding. Calculate the energy and nutrient intake for the past 24 hours.
2. Describe how the transition is made from total parenteral nutrition to enteral feeding in a premature infant.
3. Discuss the advantages and potential problems of human milk as the sole feeding for a premature infant.
4. Describe appropriate vitamin supplementation for the premature infant on enteral feedings.
5. Investigate the long-term prognosis for growth and development of premature and LBW babies.

REFERENCES

1. Blackman J: Neonatal intensive care: Is it worth it? *Ped Clinics N Amer* 38:1497, 1991.
2. Hobar J, Lucey J: Evaluation of neonatal intensive care technologies, *The Future of Children* 5:139, 1995.
3. Committee on Perinatal Health: *Toward improving the outcome of pregnancy,* New York, 1976, The National Foundation—March of Dimes.
4. Committee on Fetus and Newborn: *Guidelines for perinatal care,* Evanston, Ill, 1983, American Academy of Pediatrics; and Washington, DC, 1983, American College of Obstetricians and Gynecologists.
5. Committee on Fetus and Newborn, American Academy of Pediatrics: Level II neonatal units, *Pediatrics* 66:810, 1980.
6. Committee on Nutrition of the Mother and Preschool Child, Food and Nutrition Board: *Nutrition services in perinatal care,* Washington, DC, 1981, Assembly of Life Sciences, National Research Council.
7. Poole RL, Kerner JA, Jr: Establishing a nutrition support team for an intensive care nursery, *Nutr Supp Serv* 3:35, 1983.
8. Lubchenco LO and others: Intrauterine growth as estimated from liveborn birth-weight data at 24 to 42 weeks of gestation. *Pediatrics,* 32:793, 1963.
9. Williams RL and others: Fetal growth and perinatal viability. *Obstet Gynecol,* 59:624, 1982.
10. Widdowson EM: *Growth and composition of the fetus and newborn.* In Assali NS, editor: *Biology of gestation,* vol II, New York, 1968, Academic Press.
11. Heird WC and others: Intravenous alimentation in pediatric patients, *J Pediatr* 80:351, 1972.
12. Ziegler EE: Malnutrition in the premature infant, *Acta Paediatr Scand Suppl* 374:58, 1991.
13. Van Aerde, JEE: Acute respiratory failure and bronchopulmonary dysplasia. In Hay W, editor: *Neonatal nutrition and metabolism,* St. Louis, 1991, Mosby.
14. Doelkel RD and others: Clinical semistarvation: depression of hypoxic ventilatory response, *N Engl J Med* 295:358, 1976.
15. Chandra RK: Immunodeficiency in undernutrition and overnutrition, *Nutr Rev* 39:225, 1981.
16. Abel RM and others: Malnutrition in cardiac surgery patients, *Arch Surg* 111:45, 1976.
17. Van Aerde JEE: *Acute respiratory failure and BPD.* In Hay WW, editor: *Neonatal nutrition and metabolism,* St. Louis, 1991, Mosby–Year Book.
18. Dobbing J: The later growth of the brain and its vulnerability, *Pediatrics* 53:2, 1974.
19. Rosso P, Hormazabal J, Winick M: Changes in brain weight, cholesterol phospholipid, and DNA content in marasmic children, *Am J. Clin Nutr* 23:1275, 1970.
20. Grand RJ, Watkins JB, Torti FM: Development of the human gastrointestinal tract: a review, *Gastroenterology* 70:790, 1976.
21. Lebenthal E, Leung, YK: Feeding the premature and compromised infant: gastrointestinal considerations, *Pediatr Clin North Am* 35(2):215, 1988.
22. Kerner JA, Jr: *Vitamin requirements.* In Kerner JA, Jr, editor: *Manual of pediatric parenteral nutrition,* New York, 1983, John Wiley & Sons.
23. Hansen JW: Appendix 1 and 2. In Tsang R, editor: *Nutritional needs of preterm infants,* 1993, Williams & Wilkins.
24. Kerner JA, Jr: *Fluid requirements.* In Kerner JA, Jr, editor: *Manual of pediatric parenteral nutrition,* New York, 1983, John Wiley & Sons.
25. Fanaroff M and others: Insensible water loss in low-birth-weight infants, *Pediatrics* 50:236, 1972.
26. Oh W: *Fluid and electrolyte management.* In Avery GB, editor: *Neonatology, pathophysiology, and management of the newborn,* Philadelphia, 1981, J.B. Lippincott.
27. Friis-Hansen B: Changes in body water compartments during growth, *Acta Paediatr Scand* 46 (suppl 110):1, 1957.
28. Bell EG, Oh W: Water requirement of premature newborn infants, *Acta Paediatr Scand Suppl* 305:21, 1983.
29. Hodson WA, Truog WE: *Parenteral nutrition.* In Hodson WA, Truog WA, editors: *Critical care of the newborn,* Philadelphia, 1983, WB Saunders.
30. Wu PYK, Hodgman JE: Insensible water loss in premature infants, *Pediatrics* 54:704, 1974.
31. Oh W, Karechi H: Phototherapy and insensible water loss in the newborn infant, *Am J Dis Child* 124:230, 1972.
32. Marks KA, Friedman A, Maisels MJ: A simple device for reducing insensible water loss in LBW infants, *Pediatrics* 60:223, 1977.

33. Anderson TL and others: A Controlled trial of glucose versus glucose and amino acids in premature infants, *J Pediatr* 94:115, 1981.

34. Zlotkin SH, Bryan MH, Anderson GH: Intravenous nitrogen and energy intakes required to duplicate in utero nitrogen accretion in prematurely born human infants, *J Pediatr* 99:115, 1981.

35. Heird, WC, Sudhe K: *Intravenous feeding.* In Hay WW, Jr, editor: Neonatal nutrition and metabolism, St Louis, 1991, Mosby–Year Book.

36. Bronstein, M: *Energy requirement and protein energy balance in preterm and term infants.* In Haw WW, Jr, editor: *Neonatal nutrition and metabolism,* St Louis, 1991, Mosby–Year Book.

37. Sinclair J and others: Supportive management of the sick neonate: parenteral calories, water and electrolytes, *Pediatr Clin North Am* 17:863, 1970.

38. Lebenthal E, Lee PC, Heitlinger LA: Impact of development of the gastrointestinal tract on infant feedings, *J Pediatr* 102:1, 1983.

39. Raissen D: *Amino acid and protein metabolism in preterm and term infants.* In Hay WW, Jr, editor: *Neonatal nutrition and metabolism,* St Louis, 1991, Mosby–Year Book.

40. Micheli JL, Schutz Y: *Protein in nutritional needs of preterm infants.* In Tsang R, editor: *Nutritional needs of preterm infants,* 1993, Williams & Wilkins.

41. Kerner JA, Jr: *Indications for parenteral nutrition in pediatrics.* In Kerner JA, Jr, editor: *Manual of pediatric parenteral nutrition,* New York, 1983, John Wiley & Sons.

42. Ziegler EE, Biga RL, Fomon SJ: *Nutritional requirements of the premature infant.* In Suskind RM, editor: *Textbook of pediatric nutrition,* New York, 1981, Raven Press.

43. Ziegler EE and others: Body composition of the reference fetus, *Growth* 40:329, 1976.

44. American Academy of Pediatrics, Committee on Nutrition: Nutritional needs of low-birth-weight infants, *Pediatrics* 75:976, 1985.

45. Gross SJ and others: Growth and biochemical response of premature infants fed human milk or modified infant formula, *N Engl J Med* 308:237, 1983.

46. Raiha NCR and others: Milk protein quantity and quality in low-birth-weight infants. I. Metabolic responses and effects on growth, *Pediatrics* 57:659, 1976.

47. Fomon SJ, Ziegler EE: Protein intake of premature infants: interpretation of data, *J Pediatr* 90:504, 1977.

48. Avery GB, Fletcher AB: *Nutrition.* In Avery GB, editor: *Neonatology,* Philadelphia, 1981, JB Lippincott.

49. Innis SM: Fat. In Tsang R, editor: Nutritional needs of the preterm infant, 1993, Williams & Wilkins.

50. Greene HL and others: Guidelines for the use of vitamins, trace elements, calcium, magnesium, and phosphorus in infants and children receiving total parenteral nutrition: report of the Subcommittee on Pediatric Parenteral Nutrient Requirements from the Committee on Clinical Practice Issues of The American Society for Clinical Nutrition, *Am J Clin Nutr* 48:1324, 1988.

51. Spitzer AR, Fox WW: Delivoria-Papadopoulos M: Maximum diuresis—a factor in predicting recovery from respiratory distress syndrome and the development of bronchopulmonary dysplasia, *J Pediatr* 98:476, 1981.

52. Bell EF and others: Effect of fluid administration on the development of symptomatic patent ductus arteriosus and congestive heart failure in premature infants, *N Engl J Med* 302:598, 1980.

53. Stevenson JG: Fluid administration in the association of patent ductus arteriosus complicating distress syndrome, *J Pediatr* 90:257, 1977.

54. Goldberg RN and others: The association of rapid volume expansion and intraventricular hemorrhage in the preterm infant, *J Pediatr* 96:1060, 1980.

55. Brown ER and others: Bronchopulmonary dysplasia: possible relationship to pulmonary edema, *J Pediatr* 92:982, 1978.

56. Harkavey KL: Water and electrolyte requirements of the very-low-birth-weight infant, *Perinatal Press* 6:47, 1982.

57. Constarino AT and others: Water as Nutrition. In Tsang R, editor: *Nutritional needs of preterm infants,* 1993, Williams & Wilkins.

58. Constarino AT and others: Sodium restriction vs daily replacement in VLBW premature neonates: A randomized blind therapeutic trial. *J Pediatr* 120:99, 1992.

59. Tsang RC: *Vitamin and mineral requirements in preterm infants,* New York, 1985, Marcel Dekker.

60. Micheli JL and others: Early postnatal intravenous amino acid administration in VLBW preterm infants. *Seminars in Neonatal Nutrition and Metabolism,* Vol 2, 1994.

61. Ziegler EE: Nutritional management of the premature infant, *Perinatology-Neonatology* July/Aug 11, 1985.

62. Winters RW: An historical review of the development of criteria for intravenous amino acid requirements, Clinical Conference on Pediatric Nutrition, *Acta Chir Scand* (suppl 517):7, 1982.

63. Ziegler M and others: Route of pediatric parenteral nutrition: proposed criteria revision, *J Pediatr Surg* 15:472, 1980.

64. Lebenthal E, editor: *Total parenteral nutrition,* New York, 1986, Raven Press.

65. Binder ND and others: Insulin infusion with parenteral nutrition in extremely low birth weight infants with hyperglycemia, *J Pediatr* 114:273, 1989.

66. Collins JW and others: A controlled trial of insulin infusion and parenteral nutrition in extremely low birth weight infants with glucose intolerance, *J Pediatr* 118:921, 1991.

67. Snyderman SE: *The protein and amino acid requirements of the premature infant.* In Jonxis JHP, Visser HKA, Troelstra JA, editors: *Metabolic process in the fetus and newborn infant,* Baltimore, 1971, Williams & Wilkins.

68. Gaull GE and others: Milk protein quantity and quality in low-birth-weight infants. III. Effects on sulfur amino acids in plasma and urine, *J Pediatr* 90:356, 1977.

69. Heird WC and others: Pediatric parenteral amino acid mixture in low-birth-weight infants, *Pediatrics* 81:41, 1988.

70. Gaull GE: Taurine in pediatric nutrition: review and update, *Pediatrics,* 83:3, 1989.

71. Friedman Z and others: Rapid onset of essential fatty acid deficiency in the newborn, *Pediatrics* 58:640, 1976.

72. Cooke RJ, Zee PL, Yeh Y-Y: Essential fatty acid status of the premature infant during short-term fat-free parenteral nutrition, *J Pediatr Gastroenterol Nutr* 3:446, 1984.

73. Christensen ML and others: Plasma carnitine concentration and lipid metabolism in infants receiving parenteral nutrition, *J Pediatr* 115:794, 1989.

74. Melegh B: Carnitine supplementation in the premature: metabolic problems of the newborn, *Biol of Neonate* 58(suppl 1):93, 1990.

75. Schmidt-Sommerfeld E, Penn D: Carnitine and total parenteral nutrition of the neonate: metabolic problems of the newborn, *Biol of Neonate* 58(suppl 1):81, 1990.

76. Helms RA and others: Enhanced lipid utilization in infants receiving oral L-carnitine during long-term parenteral nutrition, *J Pediatr* 109:984, 1986.

77. Zaidan H and others: Lipid clearing in premature infants during continuous heparin infusion: role of circulating lipases, *Pediatr Res* 19:23, 1985.

78. Haumont D and others: Plasma lipid and plasma lipoprotein concentrations in low birth weight infants given parenteral nutrition with twenty or ten percent lipid emulsion, *J Pediatr* 115:787, 1989.

79. Brans YW and others: Tolerance of fat emulsions in very-low-birthweight neonates, *Am J Dis Child* 142:145, 1988.

80. Nutrition Advisory Group: *Guidelines for multivitamin preparation for parental use,* Chicago, 1975, American Medical Association.

81. Kerner JA, Jr, editor: *Manual of pediatric parenteral nutrition,* New York, 1983, John Wiley & Sons.

82. Lucas A, Bloom R, Aynsley-Green A: Gut hormones and 'minimal enteral feeding,' *Acta Paediatr Scand* 75:719, 1986.

83. Aynsley-Green A: Plasma hormone concentrations during enteral and parenteral nutrition in the human newborn, *J Pediatr Gastroenterol Nutr* 2(suppl 1):S108, 1983.

84. Aynsley-Green A: Hormones and postnatal adaptation to enteral nutrition, *J Pediatr Gastroenterol Nutr* 2:418, 1983.

85. Berseth LL: Neonatal small intestinal motility: motor responses to feeding in term and preterm infants, *J Pediatr* 117:777, 1990.

86. Troche B and others: Early minimal feedings promote growth in critically ill premature infants, *Biol Neonate* 67:172, 1995.

87. Meetze W and others: GI priming prior to establishing enteral feeding, *J Ped Gastro and Nutr* 15:163, 1992.

88. Lucas A: Minimal enteral feeding, *Seminars in Neonatal Nutrition and Metabolism* 1:1, 1993.

89. Dunn L and others: Beneficial effects of early hypocaloric enteral feeding on neonatal gastrointestinal function: preliminary report of a randomized trial, *J Pediatr* 112:662, 1988.

90. Benda GI: Modes of feeding low-birth-weight infants, *Semin Perinatol* 3:407, 1979.

91. Hay, WW, editor: *Neonatal nutrition and metabolism,* St Louis, 1991, Mosby–Year Book.

92. Mathew OP: Science of bottle feeding, *J Pediatr* 119:511, 1991.

93. VandenBerg KA: Nippling management of the sick neonate in the NICU: the disorganized feeder, *Neonatal Network,* 9:9, 1990.

94. Shaker CS: Nipple feeding premature infants: a different perspective, *Neonatal Network,* 8:9, 1990.

95. Lebenthal E, editor: *Textbook of gastroenterology and nutrition in infancy,* ed 2, New York, 1989, Raven Press.

96. Steichen JJ, Krug-Wispe SK, Tsang RC: Breast-feeding the low birth weight preterm infant, *Clin Perinatol* 14:131, 1987.

97. Davies DP: Adequacy of expressed breast milk for early growth of preterm infants, *Arch Dis Child* 52:296, 1977.

98. Tyson JE and others: Growth, metabolic response, and development in very-low-birth-weight infants fed banked human milk or enriched formula. I. Neonatal findings, *J Pediatr* 103:95, 1983.

99. Gross SJ: Growth and biochemical response of preterm infants fed human milk or modified infant formula, *N Engl J Med* 308:237, 1983.

100. Jarvenpaa AL and others: Preterm infants fed human milk attain intrauterine weight gain, *Acta Paediatr Scand* 72:239, 1983.

101. Chessex P and others: Quality of growth in premature infants fed their own mothers' milk, *J Pediatr* 102:107, 1983.

102. Gross SJ: *Effect of gestational age on the composition of breast milk.* In Grand RJ, editor: *Pediatric nutrition,* New York, 1987, Raven Press.

103. Atkinson, SA, Radde IC, Anderson GH: Macromineral balance in premature infants fed their own mothers' milk or formula, *J Pediatr* 102:99, 1983.

104. Chan GM: Human milk calcium and phosphate levels of mothers delivering term and preterm infants, *J Pediatr Gastroenterol Nutr* 1:201, 1982.

105. Rowe J and others: Hypophosphatemia and hypercalciuria in small premature infants fed human milk: evidence for inadequate dietary phosphorus, *J Pediatr* 104:112, 1984.

106. Heird WC: *Total parenteral nutrition.* In Lebenthal E, editor: *Textbook of gastroenterology and nutrition in infancy,* ed 2, New York, 1989, Raven Press.

107. Vileisis, RA and others: Laboratory monitoring of parenteral nutrition-associated hepatic dysfunction in infants. *JPEN* 5:67, 1981.

108. Dancis J, O'Connell JR, Holt LE: A grid for recording the weight of premature infants, *J Pediatr* 33:570, 1948.

109. Shaffer SG and others: Postnatal weight changes in low birth weight infants, *J Pediatr* 79:702, 1987.

110. Babson SG: Growth of low-birth-weight infants, *J Pediatr* 77:11, 1970.

111. Gairdner D, Pearson J: A growth chart for premature and other infants, *Arch Dis Child* 46:783, 1971.

112. Casey PH and others: Growth patterns of low birth weight preterm infants: a longitudinal analysis of a large, varied sample, *J Pediatr* 117:298, 1990.

113. Polberger PE, Staffan KT and others: Eleven plasma proteins as indicators of protein nutritional status in very low birth weight infants. *Pediatrics* 86:916, 1990.

114. Hoffman EL, Bennett FC: Birth weight less than 800 grams: changing outcomes and influences of gender and gestation number, *Pediatrics* 86:27, 1990.

115. Bennett FC: *Neurodevelopmental outcome of premature/low-birth-weight infants: the role of developmental intervention.* In Guthrie RD: *Neonatal intensive care,* New York, 1988, Churchill Livingstone.

116. Collin MF, Halsey CL, Anderson CL: Emerging developmental sequelae in the "normal" extremely low birth weight infant, *Pediatrics* 88:115, 1991.

117. Resnick MB and others: Educational outcome of neonatal intensive care graduates, *Pediatrics* 89:373, 1992.

118. Bauchner H and others: Premature graduates of the newborn intensive care unit: a guide to followup, *Ped Clinic N Amer* 35:1207, 1988.

119. Casey PH and others: Growth status and growth rates of a varied sample of low birth weight preterm infants: a longitudinal cohort from birth to three years of age, *J Pediatr* 119:599, 1991.

120. Keith JK and others: Growth to age 3 among very low birth weight sequelae free survivors of modern neonatal intensive care, *J Pediatr* 100:622, 1982.

121. Georgieff MK and others: Catch-up growth, muscle and fat accretion, and body proportionality of infants one year after newborn intensive care, *J Pediatr* 114:288, 1989.

122. Ernst JA and others: Growth outcome and feeding practices of the very low birth weight infant (less than 1500 grams) within the first year of life, *J Pediatr* 117:S156, 1990.

123. Ross G, Lipper EG, Auld PAM: Growth achievement of very low birth weight premature children at school age, *J Pediatr* 117:307, 1990.

124. Abrams SA and others: Bone mineralization in former very low birth weight infants fed either

human milk or commercial formula: one-year follow-up observation, *J Pediatr* 114:1041, 1989.

125. Abrams SA, Schanler R, Garza C: Bone mineralization in former very low birth weight infants fed either human milk or commercial formula, *J Pediatr* 112:956, 1988.

126. Friel JK and others: Improved growth of very low birthweight infants, *Nutr Research* 13:611, 1993.

127. Lucas A and others: Randomised trial of nutrition for preterm infants after discharge, *Arch Dis Child* 67:324, 1992.

128. Bernbaum JC and others: Preterm infant care after hospital discharge, *Peds in Review* 10:195, 1989.

129. Swanson JA, Berseth CL: Continuing care for the preterm infant after dismissal from the neonatal intensive care, *Mayo Clin Proc* 62:613, 1987.

130. Hulseman, ML, Normal L: The neonatal ICU graduate: part II: fundamentals of outpatient care. *Am Family Phys* 45:1696, 1991.

131. Kelleher KJ and others: Risk factors and outcomes for failure to thrive in LBW preterm infants. *Pediatrics* 91:942, 1993.

CHAPTER

6

Food Pattern Development in Young Children

Miriam E. Lowenberg

❖❖❖

Objectives

After studying this chapter, the student should:

✔ *Recognize differences between hunger and appetite.*

✔ *Be aware of appropriate furniture and utensils for use when feeding young children.*

✔ *Be aware of the factors to consider when writing menus for young children.*

✔ *Know appropriate foods and methods of preparation for young children.*

✔ *Know common difficulties encountered by concerned parents when feeding young children.*

INTRODUCTION

This sixth edition of *Nutrition in Infancy and Childhood* is dedicated to Dr. Miriam E. Lowenberg, whose devotion to children and their nourishment was instrumental in shaping the direction of pediatric nutrition. Her passions were the study of the food likes and dislikes of children, how these preferences affect their food behavior, the role of cultural background on the development of food habits, and the impact of these factors on the nutritional status of children. She incorporated these principles into her work on improving the nourishment of children

in child care centers during World War II and later in working with children with developmental disabilities.

Miriam Lowenberg entered the University of Chicago in 1914 and enrolled in the Department of Household Art. Here she met Dr. Lydia Roberts, who inspired her to become a child nutritionist. She then moved to Iowa State University, where she received her master's degree in Child Nutrition and Child Psychology. For 12 years as the nutritionist at the Iowa State University Food Service, she observed children's food behavior at the nursery school lunch and

164

FIG. 6-1   Miriam E. Lowenberg, Ph.D. July 22, 1897–September 27, 1995.

worked with parents to monitor their children's food intake at home. During this time, she found that a menu that contained one crisp food, one soft food, and only one chewy food in the main course was the most popular with the children. She wrote *Food and Your Child* and *Your Child's Food* while at Iowa State University.

In 1943 while a doctoral student at the University of Iowa, she taught a course at the Vassar Summer Session on how to feed children in wartime day-care centers. After receiving her Ph.D. in 1944, she was asked to come to the Kaiser Shipyard Child Service Centers in Portland, Oregon, to feed the preschool children. This center served children between 18 months and 6 years of age. The program was so large that it employed 100 teachers and 26 kitchen staff in two centers. This experience deepened her commitment to the nourishment of children and enabled her to develop her culturally based view of child feeding and nourishment. In 1945,

when the Shipbuilding Center closed, Dr. Lowenberg joined Dr. C. Anderson Aldrich as Nutritional Supervisor for the Rochester Child Health Institute, which was associated with the Mayo Clinic. Here she designed a device called "Score Your Diet" to help pregnant women evaluate their diets and make adjustments for adequacy. She also provided nutrition counseling at all the Rochester Well Child Clinics. In addition, she worked with General Mills, Inc., to produce the film *Food as Children See It,* which was widely used as an educational tool in home economics classes and public health programs across the country.

In 1952 Dr. Lowenberg became head of the Department of Food and Nutrition of Pennsylvania State University. Dr. Lowenberg collaborated with Dr. Benjamin Spock on *Feeding Your Baby and Child,* published in 1955. These commonsense views on feeding infants and young children became the primary source of information for a generation of parents.

In 1963, after retirement, Dr. Lowenberg moved to Seattle and the University of Washington to become the Chief Nutritionist at the Child Development and Mental Retardation Center (CDMRC), which later became the Center on Human Development and Disabilities (CHDD). In the role of Chief Nutritionist she helped establish the training program for pediatric nutritionists with emphasis on nutritional intervention for children with developmental disabilities. Dr. Lowenberg's lifelong commitment to children and their families enabled her to establish a family-centered, culturally sensitive program long before these terms were in vogue.

Dr. Lowenberg and her colleagues Drs. E. Neige Todhunter, Eva D. Wilson, Moira C. Feeney, and Jane R. Savage wrote the celebrated *Food and Man,* published in 1968, which became *Food and People* in later editions.[1] This book focused on the role of culture in the development of food habits. In 1970 Dr. Lowenberg was honored by her professional peers when she received the Marjorie Hulsizer Copher award, which is the highest honor of the American Dietetic Association.

Dr. Lowenberg's nutrition work, intellectual integrity, and energy for living life to the fullest have influenced many nutrition professionals. We believe that this chapter summarizes her views about families and children. These views are as appropriate and useful today as when she expressed them. Dr. Lowenberg was an inspiration, mentor, and friend. We hope that her love of children and concern about their nourishment will continue to inspire those working with young children.

FOOD PATTERNS

Food patterns in the United States show distinct cultural characteristics that change as lifestyles change. Hurried small breakfasts, mid-morning coffee breaks, and light lunches followed by heavy evening dinners show modern adjustments to change. In the home, snacking is known to have increased as television has become an integral part of the day and night activities of the American family.

There are many different meal patterns in modern America. There are inner-city patterns of poor or rich families, suburban patterns, and rural patterns of nonfarm and farm families. The rich and the poor have throughout the ages had different food patterns. In fact, careful professional observers of young children eating in a group can often predict the home environment of an individual child.

The current enthusiasm for behavioral control of food intake points to a need to examine the day's program to learn when unneeded energy in food is consumed. Researchers now believe that what happens during the first year of life, as well as during the preschool years, is of paramount importance. During the first five or six years of life it is undoubtedly easier to learn to like all foods than it will be later.

At present the young child is introduced early to hamburgers and french fries when families eat out; attesting to this is one fast-food company's yearly sales—the highest in the restaurant industry. Eating out becomes a helpful respite for the young homemaker or working mother, and a pattern is established for the young child. When parents hope to establish a basic food pattern of meals enjoyed at home, they must deal with the child's desire to eat out, even if the child only knows about it because other children talk about eating out.

Goals for the development of food patterns are the following:

1. Children should be able to eat in a matter-of-fact way sufficient quantities of the foods that are given to them, just as they take care of other daily needs. Preschool children who truly enjoy most foods but are able to eat without fuss those they do not especially like will be fortunate later.
2. Children should be able to manage the feeding process independently and with dispatch, without either unnecessary dawdling or hurried eating.
3. Children should be willing to try new foods in small portions the first time they are served to them and to try them again and again until they like or at least willingly accept them.

Professionals interested in guiding parents or prospective parents must know which patterns produce healthy children and adults. We must also believe that it is possible to set up a home environment to foster the development of desirable food patterns in young children. Often an impersonal professionally trained outsider can point out to parents how they can set up such an environment. It must be understood that food patterns begin to be formed from the day of an infant's birth. This reminds me of a healthy, happy young mother who telephoned from her hospital room to report the birth of a daughter 4 hours before. She said with joy that her baby had already tried to nurse; this mother, although still tired from the birth process, had already enjoyed the process of even feeble breast-feeding.

Those who are concerned about obesity as our chief problem of malnutrition wisely point out that prevention, the preferred cure, should begin early in infancy. Parents who give their newborns the privilege of deciding that they have had enough food are well on the way to solving this problem. It is believed that when an individual forms a pattern of quitting to eat at the first indication of satiety, the food intake regulatory mechanism is encouraged to continue to function. Of course, food that produces the growth of good body tissues must be provided so that more than energy satiety is provided. This is an important part of early food patterning of a child.

The food patterns established in a home are reinforced by love of mother and father and therefore have far-reaching effects on lifetime patterns. No one has even phrased the functions of parents more aptly than did Aldrich and Aldrich[2] 40 years ago when they said:

According to nature's plan then parents are meant to enter the feeding situation for three reasons:

First, to provide the food,

Second, to support a child's progress from simple to mature methods of eating, and

Third, to make it easy for him to establish his own satisfying feeding habits.

Long ago I observed another principle that we need to emphasize with parents: it really is easier and quicker to change the food than it is to change the child. For instance, young children often have trouble swallowing dry food, and when extra milk is added to thin their mashed potatoes they seem thankful. Such methods are explained in detail later in this chapter.

To know what foods children like requires careful observations of young children while they are eating. Table 6-1 on pages 168–169 gives approximate amounts of foods that one can expect the average child to eat.* *In no way are these amounts to be used to force a certain amount of food on any specific child.* If any child, however, habitually eats less than the amount in the chart, the reasons should be determined. As always, a particular child's food dislikes, health condition, or specific family circumstances need to be considered.

CULTURAL PATTERNS

Many ethnic groups make up the population of the United States. Each ethnic food pattern, based on foods available and preferred, comes from the home country and is based firmly on tradition and often on long usage. Specific ways of cooking foods are always dependent on such factors as the fuel available, the time and the energy available for food preparation, and the interests and patience of the cook. For example, the generous use of rye breads and fish in the Scandinavian countries is a result of the cool and short growing season, the long coastlines, and the Scandinavian people's knowledge of successful fishing. Even after such countries are able to import other foods, the preferred foods are still used as tradition dictates. The cause for the abundant use by Polynesian peoples of the coconut, tropical fruits and vegetables, and fish that are abundant in tropical waters is obvious.

The history of a people is written in their preferred foods. This explains why schoolchildren in North Dakota and in Georgia react in radically different ways to rice used as a vegetable. For instance, rice, which grew well in the American south from early colonial times, has become a preferred food in that part of the country, yet when first used in lunches in some schools in North Dakota, rice was rejected as an unfamiliar food. Another vegetable of historic importance to the southern United States is okra. This vegetable is said to have been brought by slaves from Africa, and its popularity has even withstood the

---

*For 12 years I observed daily 20 nursery school children eating their noon meals. Later, for 2 years, the ideas generated by this observation were used in the daily feeding of 1000 children, mostly 18 months to 6 years of age, in two shipyard World War II nursery schools. My commission as chief nutritionist was to be in charge of feeding and nutritional development. Feeding for the 9 hours at nursery school was carefully planned, and mothers and fathers were also advised and helped to feed their children at home.

The knowledge gained while studying the eating patterns and food preferences of the nursery school children for 12 years was used to teach college students about feeding young children. All food was measured onto the child's plate before it left the kitchen serving area; second helpings and leftover foods were measured and recorded. For one school year, the adult who ate at a table with two or three children was asked

to record each child's reaction to each food and to the menu as a whole. They were to record: was a food too dry? too tough? too acid to be easily eaten? Were there other characteristics that made the food unsuitable? Were the combinations of foods acceptable and liked by the children? As these criticisms came in daily, corrections were made in the menus and recipes for the foods. During the following year the corrected menus and specific foods were again studied, and further corrections were made. During this study, each day a chart was made of the amounts of each food to be served to each child. The head teacher confirmed that when the children's appetites were closely studied a child's specific food intake could be accurately judged. Most thoughtful mothers can do this.

The advice in this chapter is based on the ideas gained from this meticulous study as well as on extensive tests of these ideas.

TABLE 6-1   *Food Pattern for Preschool Children**

Food	Portion Size	Number of Portions Advised	
		Ages 2 to 4 Years	Ages 4 to 6 Years
Milk and Dairy Products			
Milk†	4 oz	3 to 6	3 to 4
Cheese	½ to ¾ oz	May be substituted for one portion of liquid milk	
Yogurt	¼ to ½ c	May be substituted for one portion of liquid milk	
Powdered skim milk	2 T	May be substituted for one portion of liquid milk	
Meat and Meat Equivalents			
Fish§, poultry	1 to 2 oz	2	2
Egg	1	1	1
Peanut butter	1 to 2 T		
Legumes—dried peas and beans	¼ to ⅓ c cooked		
Vegetables and Fruits			
Vegetables		4 to 5 to include 1 green leafy or yellow‖	4 to 5 to include 1 green leafy or yellow
Cooked	2 to 4 T		
Raw	Few pieces		
Fruit		1 citrus fruit or other vegetables or fruit rich in vitamin C	1 citrus fruit or other vegetable or fruit rich in vitamin C
Canned	4 to 8 T		
Raw	½ to 1 small		
Fruit juice	3 to 4 oz		

*Diets should be monitored for adequacy of iron and vitamin D intake.
†Approximately ⅔ c can easily be incorporated in a child's food during cooking.
§Should be served once or twice per week to substitute for meat.
‖If child's preferences are limited, use double portions of preferred vegetables until appetite for other vegetables develops.

memory of those sad journeys to which those slaves were subjected. Blends in Creole dishes could only occur where Spanish, French, black African, and American Indian influences came together. During the latter part of the twentieth century most Americans have come to prize their cultural backgrounds, cultural foods, and cultural differences in food patterns.

In summary, two points should be emphasized. First, every ethnic diet must be based on **nutritional adequacy,** at least to some degree, for the group using it to survive. For example, the very poor and food-deficient Irish people of the nineteenth century, who had an extremely limited diet, could scarcely have chosen any two foods as nutritionally adequate as buttermilk

TABLE 6-1 *Food Pattern for Preschool Children*—cont'd*

Food	Portion Size	Number of Portions Advised	
		Ages 2 to 4 Years	Ages 4 to 6 Years
Bread and Cereal Grains			
Whole grain or enriched white bread	½ to 1 slice	3	3
Cooked cereal	¼ to ½ c	May be substituted for one serving of bread	
Ready-to-serve dry cereals	½ to 1 c		
Spaghetti, macaroni, noodles, rice	¼ to ½ c		
Crackers	2 to 3		
Fat			
Bacon	1 slice	Not to be substituted for meat	
Butter or vitamin A-fortified margarine	1 t	3	3 to 4
Desserts	¼ to ½ c	As demanded by energy needs	
Sugars	½ to 1 t	2	2

and potatoes. The nutritional adequacy for a desirable state of health may point, in some ethnic patterns, to a need for supplementation with some other foods. Adding needed foods to this basic diet is often much easier than changing the **staple food** of a group. This, however, means that it is desirable to maintain the basic pattern with only the needed supplementation. American Indian children who have been taught to like the wild greens that their families eat, for instance, should be encouraged to follow these food patterns. Second, children who learn the cues of ethnic food patterns at an early age should be allowed to make these patterns as permanent as possible in a new environment. Respect for differences in food patterns influences the way individuals view themselves and their worth.

POSITIVE REINFORCEMENT

Experience with helping young children form desirable feeding patterns shows that positive

reinforcement of desirable behavior is sound. (For further discussion of behavior modification, see chapter 8.) Some 40 years ago it was found that children developed desirable feeding patterns when they felt successful and when negative behavior was ignored. It is wise to find out why a child does not like or does not readily eat a certain food or combination of foods. Often it is easy to change the food or menu.

There are many ways to help children eat successfully. Portion size is of paramount importance. When children are presented with less food than they normally eat, they can accomplish the goal that the adult has set; they can then ask for second helpings. This allows them to receive adult approbation, which is a reward to them. If for some reason children cannot eat all the food that has been given to them, allowing them to set their own limit shows respect for them and lets them feel successful. However, when children restrict their food intake to much less than expected over a number of days, parents should investigate.

Improving an environmental situation often corrects this low intake of food (see pages 170–171 for specific suggestions).

HUNGER AND APPETITE

Food is taken into the body to satisfy the primal urge of **hunger.** According to physiologist Dr. Anton J. Carlson,[3] two unpleasant sensations are involved in what we call hunger. The first is a generalized weakness and restlessness all over the body, which is probably caused by a need for more sugar in the blood. The second is a definite localized sensation of pains of tension in the upper part of the stomach. These pangs of hunger are comparatively brief and are followed by periods when hunger pain is not felt. The infant and the young child are thought to have frequent and severe hunger pains. These sometimes are severe enough to cause an outcry as they awaken the infant from sleep. Infants' stomachs have been observed to show feeble hunger contractions 1 hour after nursing and strong hunger contractions 2½ to 3 hours after a feeding. The length of time the stomach shows in this way that it is ready for food varies with the individual infant. In the young child of 2 to 5 years of age these hunger pains are somewhat less frequent or pronounced than in the young infant, but they are still quite definite. Normally, food taken into the body gives immediate pleasure to a child when it eases the pain of hunger. If nothing else interferes, food is associated with the easing of pain, and pleasure results from eating.

Hunger is quite different from **appetite.** Most authorities agree that although hunger is an unpleasant sensation, appetite is a pleasurable experience. Appetite is usually defined as the pleasant association of a food with past experiences with that food. Appetite, associated with the sight and odor of food, stimulates the flow of digestive juices and is therefore a vital part of good digestion, as has often been demonstrated in the clinic and laboratory.

Many people have searched diligently and long for foods that taste like those mother used to cook when they were children. No doubt her foods were good, but they were probably not incomparable. The remembered foods were eaten at times when the child was thoroughly happy, and as a result, a strong appetite for them was created. As an individual grows older, the zest for the same food may be lessened. There is only the memory of or the appetite for the former food. Thus appetites for certain foods are undoubtedly built up in children not only from the flavor, color, and texture of the food itself, but also from the many associations with the food.

It is normal for a young child to be hungry. To be persistently nonhungry is decidedly abnormal. The child who is not hungry should be taken to a physician who will carefully assess his or her physical well-being (looking possibly for a chronic infection) and his or her daily habits. This child may not get enough brisk exercise in the open air or may need more sleep, a more regular diet pattern, sleep and rest, or a less stimulating environment.

If a child is in good health and is hungry, with a stomach calling urgently for food, food will be eaten to satisfy that urge rather than to satisfy whims. As has been so aptly said, hunger should control the child rather than the child control hunger. This fact may be taken advantage of in many ways. New foods in very small portions may be served at the time of the day when the child is hungriest. It should be remembered that for a young child a new food is a step in the dark; children are generally not as adventuresome as adults. If a child eats the new food when hungry, it will probably leave a pleasant sensation, and the next time this food is served it will be recognized as a friend. Children learn to like a food by tasting it time after time, even though the first tastes are but a few tiny bites.

SETTING UP A FOOD ENVIRONMENT

In helping parents to understand why children eat as they do, it is important to direct their attention to the fact that *behavior is caused.* When causes of behavior are understood, a food problem is on the way to being cured. Parents who understand why children eat as they do can usually set up an environment that promotes a healthy appetite. Often an outside professional person can help a parent to discover these causes and to restructure the environment. Preparental education in which specific appetite problems are discussed can help prevent them. Part of this education must emphasize the requirements of a good food environment.

How does a parent help a child develop desirable food patterns? The following are suggestions:

1. The parents, as "gatekeepers," must recognize that the kinds of food available to the preschool child in the home are what they buy and provide. Many parents need to be shown that, in this, they are *really in command*. In a well-child clinic, a mother complained that her 3-year-old child was eating too many potato chips, yet she admitted that she was the one who bought them. Of course, other family members must also cooperate in not having foods of this kind available.
2. Often parents must decide which of their own food patterns they want to pass on to their children. Some parents need to be assured that they can change their own food patterns; they may even need to be helped to do this.
3. Feeding programs for groups of preschool children have proven again and again that the eating habits of young children can be repatterned under skilled guidance. This should give parents added confidence.

DEVELOPMENTAL PATTERNS

Children develop for the most part in an orderly pattern—physically, emotionally, and psychologically.

Eating is always dependent on the abilities of the eater. For instance, when normal infants are born, they are able to root for a nipple and to suck vigorously to ingest milk. When infants are given a chance to satisfy their hunger in this manner, they attain their first success in eating. As parents discover the child's hunger patterns and provide foods to satisfy hunger, they set up the condition for successful eating.

DIFFICULTIES IN THE FORMATION OF GOOD FOOD HABITS AND WAYS TO AVOID THEM

When most infants are fed the first semisolid food, they often spit it out rather violently—not because they do not want the food but because they know only the sucking motion they have used thus far to ingest food (see chapter 4). Now they try this motion again, and the semiliquid cereal or food spatters everywhere. They must learn an entirely new feeding technique. If they fail in the first efforts, a parent may be spattered and naturally quite upset. The infants have met their first feeding disaster. To laugh at these efforts is unwise because the infant learns to do this to make parents laugh. Parents should prepare themselves in advance so that they can remain undisturbed by the incident.

Another difficulty enters into this situation—all the previous food has been liquid. Now, suddenly, here is a food with a new texture, as well as a new flavor that is different from the usual, mildly sweet milk. Difficulties may be avoided by giving the infant minute amounts of the new food, well moistened and thinned by the familiar milk, until the new food is easily accepted. **Weaning** begins at this time. The infant is being weaned away gradually from an exclusively fluid diet.

In this discussion weaning is used to mean a general process involving, as far as food is concerned, any change in food flavor, texture, consistency, temperature, or method of feeding. Many feeding difficulties arise because the changes are expected to take place too abruptly or because adults fail to realize how difficult some of these tasks are for the infant and the young child. A child can and will learn these new things, but neither the parent nor child should become upset over failures at first. Nor must the child learn to get attention by spitting food out or by refusing it. The problem can be avoided by demonstrating the technique for spoon feeding.

At approximately 6 months of age, even before the first tooth appears, most infants make chewing movements with their gums. At this time infants should be given foods such as small strips of oven-dried toast, which offer a chance for chewing at the same time as they soften to allow easy swallowing. It has been observed that when an infant is not given a chance to chew at this time, trouble in mastering this skill may occur later.

When the infant begins to gain the muscular ability to pick up small particles using the thumb and forefingers, particles of soft green beans or peas can be fed (see chapter 4 for a more detailed discussion of this). These efforts, along with reaching for the bottle and later holding it, are the infant's first efforts to learn to feed independently.

The stage of developing independence at 9 to 18 months of age can be either exciting or distressing for parents. If parents understand that exploring everything new is very important to an infant, they can encourage this exploration by providing new textures and flavors in foods; this allows an infant to discover what a food such as oatmeal feels like. At this stage many infants have learned to crawl out from their former sitting position or to walk. It is no longer satisfying to them to just look at something; they now want to examine it. Wise parents take advantage of this new learning by providing a wide variety of food. They should not be discouraged at first if the child only feels a food before chewing it.

During the first year an infant has tremendous adjustments to make, only one of which is learning new foods and new methods of eating. In helping this infant to form good patterns, we will be most successful if we provide thoughtful and understanding guidance in the following ways:

1. Introducing new textures and flavors gradually
2. Enlarging the child's experience with as many individual foods in as many different forms as possible
3. Feeding individual foods and not mixtures so that the infant may learn to appreciate foods for their own flavors and textures
4. Observing at what time of day the infant takes the new food most easily and giving it then
5. Being patient with the first efforts and allowing the infant to learn to feed himself or herself; offering help when the infant becomes too tired to finish the process easily
6. Being understanding of the infant's efforts in each new feeding process
7. Above all, securing the entire family's cooperation

The high level of nutritive need of the first year of life is superseded by a slower metabolic rate and a slower rate of growth; therefore the child does not need as much food per unit of body weight as before. What is eaten and how it is eaten are now more important than how much is eaten. To watch a young child grow increasingly independent in feeding himself or herself can be as thrilling for a parent as watching the taking of the first steps from chair to chair. Perhaps in no other area of development in young children is progress more individual. Each child should be allowed to try new skills over and over with no record of failures unless development is obviously too slow to show any progress.

When parents understand what children are telling them in the way they eat, rebellion against food can be lessened and future food refusals can be reduced. For instance, the realization that the 2-year-old child may have a sporadic appetite, which should not be the cause for undue alarm, may prevent the long-lasting influence of battles over food.

SPECIFIC SUGGESTIONS FOR SETTING UP A FOOD ENVIRONMENT

Perhaps no arrangements for eating are more important than those that afford physical comfort to a child. Children should always feel secure on a sturdy, well-balanced chair with their feet well supported on the floor or other structure. They should be able to reach their food easily without straining their muscles. This also provides a better opportunity to eat without spills, although wise parents also prepare table surfaces and floors for children's spills. Dishes and utensils as well as table arrangements can foster success in eating. It is desirable to give the child sturdy and as nearly unbreakable utensils as possible so that spills and breaking utensils will not give a sense of failure. Also it is important not to laugh at the child, because if parents laugh at a child's mistakes, the child may gain an undue feeling of being the center of attention.

When children's chairs are being purchased, these should be "tried on" as clothing is. Some chairs, for instance, are designed to fit a child's torso and are much more comfortable than are perfectly straight chairs.

Sometimes children, who for some months have eaten at the family table, may suddenly be happier eating at their own small table with a parent nearby. Some mothers even find it possible to eat a quiet noon meal with the child at a small table.

Colorful table arrangements intrigue young children and are worth the trouble to provide. When children have developed some skill in eating, they will appreciate eating from the family's best china. Parents who show confidence in a child's accomplishment are usually rewarded by the child's care in handling prized possessions. These children who have had help in gaining skill in successful eating are easy to recognize as one observes families eating together in restaurants.

Forks and spoons should be chosen for their suitability for young hands. The spoon, which is the first eating implement a child uses, should have a round shallow bowl and a blunt tip that allows the child to shove food from the plate into the mouth. A handle that is blunt, short, and easily held in the child's palm is desirable; at this age a child uses the hand as a mass of muscles. Only after 5 or 6 years of age is control of the finer muscles of the fingers accomplished. Forks with short, blunt tines are best adapted to the child's palm. Although some parents report that their children enjoy sharper tines with which they can spear food, sharp tines can be dangerous.

Glasses that sit firmly on the table and are small enough for children's hands to encircle are best for 2- to 4-year-old children. Small delicate handles on cups are difficult for small hands to maneuver.

The shape and weight of the dishes are also important. The young child delights in pouring his or her own milk. Interesting, squat pitchers

with broad handles from which the child can easily pour milk are recommended. Parents can be encouraged to experiment with dishes and utensils for their children and to look for those that satisfy children's needs.

FOOD LIKES

Patient observation and long experience in feeding young children, as well as in counseling parents, have given me an insight into what children want in their food. When this knowledge of children's preferences is combined with the knowledge of nutrients, children can be adequately and happily fed. The results of these observations are discussed on the following pages.

Menus

Simplicity in menus is important. At the same time there must be variety to allow young children to learn to know many foods, since variety in foods is a good foundation for an adequate diet.

The following outline gives a general meal pattern that should satisfy nutrient needs in a hungry preschool child.

A. Breakfast
 1. One high-protein food
  a. 1 egg *or*
  b. 2 oz muscle meat *or*
  c. ¾ c cereal, cooked, *or*
  d. 1 c dry cereal with 4 to 6 oz milk
 2. Bread with butter or margarine (1 slice whole grain or white enriched bread, plus 1 t butter)
 3. 6 to 8 oz milk
 4. Fruit—preferably one serving of citrus
  a. 4 oz orange juice *or*
  b. ⅓ to ½ medium-sized grapefruit *or*
  c. 1 medium-sized orange
B. Noon meal
 1. One high-protein food (see breakfast for list of high-protein foods)
  a. 1 serving thick soup or stew *or*
  b. 1 serving casserole dish of a protein food in a starchy base
 2. Vegetables
  a. 1 cooked (see table 6-1 for amounts)
  b. 1 raw (see table 6-1 for amounts)

3. Bread (1 slice whole grain *or* enriched white bread with 1 t butter)
4. 6 to 8 oz milk
5. Dessert
   a. Simple dessert based on a combination of milk, eggs, and fruit *or*
   b. Serving of fruit
C. Evening meal
  1. One high-protein food
    a. 2 oz meat *or*
    b. 1 oz cheese *or*
    c. 1 egg *or*
    d. Combinations of these and vegetables
  2. Vegetables
    a. 1 or 2 cooked *or*
    b. 1 raw
  3. Bread and butter (1 slice whole grain or enriched white bread with 1 t butter)
  4. 6 to 8 oz milk
  5. Dessert (see noon meal, dessert)
D. Snacks (between meals or at bedtime). These should provide some of the needed nutrients and be low in sugar and fat so that they do not interfere with the appetite for the following meal; use, for example, any of the following:
  1. Fruit juices with a cracker or a piece of bread *or*
  2. Small pieces of fruit *or*
  3. Small pieces of raw vegetables *or*
  4. Small pieces of cheese with a small piece of bread or cracker

Combinations of Food

Most children eat most easily those foods with which they are familiar. It is advisable that a very small portion of a new food be introduced with a familiar and popular food. If the child only looks at the new food or just feels or smells it at first, this is a part of learning to accept it.

Dry foods are especially hard for children to eat, as is discussed later in this chapter. In planning a menu, dry foods should always be carefully balanced with one or two moist foods. For instance, it is wise to put a slice of meat loaf (relatively dry) with mashed potatoes and peas in a little cream sauce.

Combinations of sharp, rather acid-flavored foods with mild-flavored foods are popular with young children.

Ease of Manipulation

The ease of eating food with the unskilled and seemingly clumsy hands of a young child is important. Many small pieces of foods such as cooked green peas or beans are difficult for a child to spoon up. These can be mixed with mashed potatoes for easier eating.

When a 2-year-old child eats a bowl of thin soup, many trials are made before it is finished. Although it is advisable to serve young children soups occasionally, one must realize that the process of spooning it is tiring. Two things may be done to make soup easier for a child to eat. It may be drunk from a cup, or the soup may be made slightly thicker so that it does not spill from the spoon easily. I suggested a two-way soup to a prominent soup company. The company promoted a canned soup that was to be thinned, preferably with milk, and then strained so that a child could spoon up the solid portion and drink the liquid. Soup for young children should be either spoonable or drinkable. Later, the child may have soup to be eaten with a spoon when he or she is able to manage a spoon without spilling its contents.

Many foods can be prepared so that a child can eat them with the fingers (fig. 6-2). Hard-cooked eggs may be served in quarters, cooked meat can be cut in small strips, and cooked green beans can be served as finger foods. Children have been observed to like oranges that have been cut in wedges (skin and all) much better than peeled and diced oranges. Young schoolchildren prefer simple pieces of raw vegetables with no salad dressing to mixed-up salads, which are much more difficult to eat. It is best to serve cottage cheese or similar foods separate from the lettuce leaf on a child's plate. Creamed foods served on tough toast are difficult for children to manage.

The size of pieces of food for children must be given serious consideration. Handling silverware and conveying food to the mouth at this early age is a greater task than many adults realize. Pieces of carrots that slide across the plate and are too small to remain on the fork

FIG. 6-2 Eighteen-month-old twins enjoy finger-feeding each other.

or cubes of beets so large that they must be cut into bite-size pieces exhaust the patience of a 2- or 3-year-old child. Most foods served to young children should be cut into bite-size pieces. When the child is 4 years of age and older, the skills to cut up some foods may have been developed. If, however, much difficulty in managing is noticed, small pieces should usually be served, accompanied by occasional encouragement to cut some foods. Canned pears and other soft fruits are usually easily cut into bite-size pieces.

Stringy spinach or tomatoes are a trial for anyone to eat. Much can be done with a handy pair of food shears in the kitchen to make these foods easier to eat. Finger foods, such as pieces of lettuce or toast, should be used in meals in which some of the foods are difficult to handle. Small sandwiches—that is, a large one cut into four squares—are popular with young children.

Texture

I have found it wise to serve one soft food (for easy eating), one crisp food (to allow easy chewing and enjoyment of the sounds in the mouth), and one chewy food (to use emerging chewing skills without having too much to chew) in each meal for young children.

Some children can fall into the habit of rejecting all foods of a certain texture; this limits the kinds of foods the child tries to eat (see pages 178–179 for suggestions on how to handle this problem).

Pieces of meat are hard for young children to eat because the teeth of 2- or 3-year-old children do not grind meat as easily as adult teeth do. This explains why children often prefer hamburgers or frankfurters and why thrice-ground meat is often popular with nursery school children. Most children's meat can be served as ground meat. When parents want a steak, a roast, or a pot roast, the mother can cook a small portion of ground meat from the freezer for the young child. Ground meat should be well cooked. It should not be allowed to become dry with a hard crust, which is hard for a child to eat.

Flavor

In general, young children reject strong flavors. Many children, however, do seem to like pickles, some spicy sauces, and beer, preferences that may seem to contradict this. In general, it has been found that children like food that is salted. Because some authorities now believe that all of us would profit by taking less salt, a good health habit to foster may be one of offering lightly salted or unsalted foods. In general, sharp spices such as pepper and acids such as vinegar should also be used sparingly on children's food.

Strong-flavored vegetables such as cabbage and onions are more popular with young children when served raw. If these vegetables are cooked, it is recommended that they be prepared in excessive amounts of water so that some of the strong flavor can be thrown away. Of course, water-soluble nutrients are lost if the water is discarded, but teaching children to eat these foods is most important at this time in their lives. A mild-flavored cream sauce also helps to make these vegetables more palatable. This was shown in a nursery school when some children asked for very mild-flavored creamed onions after they had eaten dessert.

Because young children often reject sharply tart fruits, such fruits should be diluted with those of mild flavor. Tart oranges were found to be popular when mixed with cooked peaches or bananas. The rule of one tart, one mild, and one crisp is good to follow. The crisp fruit may be small unpeeled pieces of apples.

In general, when helping children develop desirable food patterns, keep the natural flavor of the food so that only small amounts of sugar are needed. The use of a little honey is also recommended because it is sweeter than an equal amount of granulated sugar and less can be used.

Color

Children have a natural interest in color in their foods, and teaching them to appreciate the lovely fresh color of foods is a worthy aim. Young children are delighted when they may choose one of several different colored desserts. Green, orange, yellow, and pink are popular colors in food. Children in nursery schools rarely failed to comment on the food to which a tiny sprig of parsley had been added or to notice bits of hidden color such as tomato, carrot, or parsley in sandwiches.

Cakes, cookies, and candies containing molasses and dried fruits provide other nutrients in addition to energy. Natural fruit juices have more of the needed nutrients than sweetened, colored, and artificially flavored drinks. Because the water that fruit juices contain is also desirable for children, strong-flavored juices should be diluted, giving additional water to the child.

SPECIFIC FOOD PREPARATION

Children should be considered when the family plans meals. Many parents do, of necessity, vary their lifestyles when they are raising their families, so the importance of food-patterning during this period is emphasized. Young children can be taught that just as adults wear different clothes from children, so there are adult-type foods and drinks. Children often prefer an orange or a serving of another fruit to the cherry pie that is being served to adults.

Foods can be made soft enough in texture for young children by adding extra milk to a dry, starchy food.

If the parents prefer strong-flavored vegetables, a small portion for the young child can be rinsed under the hot water faucet before it is served.

A young child may prefer food served at room temperature. In fact, preschool children often appear frightened by hot food. They also often stir hard ice cream until it is soupy and less sharply cold.

While the father serves dinner at the table, the mother may prefer to dish the preschool child's food in the kitchen. This can serve two purposes: (1) young children's hunger makes them impatient participants at a meal, so rapid service of food is desirable, and (2) the mother can easily regulate the amount of food served or can make any sudden changes. Fathers sometimes have more difficulty serving small enough portions to a child than mothers do.

Table 6-1 has been devised from my many years of careful observations of how much the average child can eat easily. Some pediatricians who believe that children should not be forced to eat a specific amount of any food object to setting up such expectations in a chart. Yet mothers often need some help in the amount of food the *average* child can eat easily to get the needed nutrients. Such goals may also prevent mothers from expecting their children to eat more than their children want. These average portion sizes may be too large for a new food, for a disliked food, or for a nonhungry child. Of course, the hungry child can have extra servings.

FOOD DISLIKES

It is safe to allow every person to have at least one or two food dislikes. Unless a child is on a medically prescribed diet, no one food has to be eaten assuming that a family can afford a varied diet.

Some food dislikes, as has been previously discussed, have unusual causes. One woman reports that sugared oranges always have a flavor of castor oil to her, though she enjoys oranges without sugar. When she was young she was given doses of the then strong-flavored castor oil with sugared oranges to cover its flavor. Though she knows that she only imagines the castor oil flavor in the oranges, she says that even now she thinks, "What has been on my spoon, castor oil?" The association of sugared oranges and castor oil has survived with her over many years.

Substitutions for liquid milk, which children sometimes dislike, can temporarily be made. Powdered milk (4 T substituted for 8 oz of fluid milk) can be added to foods, and cottage or cheddar cheese can be used.

When children are in control of their appetite and hunger, they sometimes refuse all foods. This can be handled by structuring the environment in which they eat. One cold, winter day in a nursery school when we were weary of preparing food for nonhungry children, we decided to give the children a shock. On the usual array of dishes, we placed only 1 T of vegetable meat stew in the soup bowl. No other food was in evidence in the entire dining room, no baskets of sandwiches, no pitchers of milk, no trays of dishes of desserts. When the children took one look, they at once exclaimed,

"Where's our dinner? Is this all of our dinner?" Rather slowly, second servings were brought in from the kitchen. The food records showed that more food was eaten that day than any day for several weeks before.

Telling a child that we know he or she doesn't like boiled potatoes and can have more green beans often encourages a good appetite. However, when a child rejects many foods, for example, all vegetables or all meat, the parents should try to find out the reasons. Adequate substitutions may need to be made. For instance, in hot summer weather, fruits can replace cooked vegetables in a child's diet if the family budget can tolerate the extra cost. This serving of fruit sometimes stimulates failing appetites.

At times parents may need to seek professional help from someone who understands children both from closer observation of many children eating and from knowing the findings of research in the area. My observation and research have shown me the importance of the following:

1. Belief that changes can occur in a child's eating patterns is of primary importance. Eating is one of the pleasures of life. The individual who likes the foods he or she needs to eat for the adequate nutrition of the body is fortunate.

2. The goals set by someone counseling parents about children's eating should be easy to accomplish. Success in following the advice of professional people promotes confidence and positively reinforces the child who succeeds in eating what is presented. When a food dislike is firmly established before the parent seeks help, it will probably not disappear suddenly; only gradual correction can be expected. Progress may not be consistent, and temporary failures to reach the goal must be expected. Often the best methods of correction are progressive. For instance, to help a child learn to eat food with texture, a mother can gradually add coarser textured food to those that are usually eaten.

3. Parents should accept a child's strong dislike for a particular food and should

substitute another food that provides the same nutrients. Often a temporary release of pressure concerning eating a specific food causes the child to try it later. A mother who was looking at her 3-year-old son's noon meal food consumption record in a nursery school said, "But he never eats eggs at home and this noon he had seconds!" That is exactly the reason that a parent enrolling a child is not asked about the child's food dislikes, but only about the foods that make the child ill. Another mother said to her son as she looked at the school records, "But you don't like turnips!" Whereupon her son answered, "Yours are black. They are white at nursery school. I like them white!"

4. Children are good judges of well-prepared food. Sometimes classes in food preparation for parents or prospective parents would be the best approach to handling children's food dislikes.

5. Sometimes the war over children's eating becomes so sharp that withdrawing one of the combatants is the only solution. Someone other than the parent feeding the child temporarily may be a solution to the problem.

6. Because children are usually rhythmic in all they do, the satisfaction of their hunger should also be kept rhythmic. This means that meals served at the same time each day generally promote a good appetite. Fatigue, the most defeating factor in children's appetites, is thus avoided. I have found again and again that starving a child to get the child to eat does not promote good eating.

COMMON PROBLEMS

Healthy, hungry children will eat if they are given a calm atmosphere in which to eat. This is the first and most important consideration.

One of the most common problems, that of fatigue, has just been discussed. Sympathy should be extended to the child who, eating at a tearoom in a large store after a morning of shopping, just looks at the food and cries when

urged to eat. The child probably needs to rest more than he or she needs to eat.

When a child is regularly more hungry at a certain time of day than at other times, this should be accepted. Perhaps the greater hunger at the evening meal is caused by having rested while watching a favorite television program before dinner. Sometimes healthy outdoor running followed by a quiet rest restores a lagging noontime appetite. It was found that nursery school food costs increased when the children played outdoors in a warm Iowa March after a cold and confining February.

Some of the earliest eating skills learned by a young child are those of chewing and swallowing. Each of these is accomplished to a great extent by trial and error. Some impatient parents worry over this slow progress.

Swallowing seems to be difficult for some children. They tend to swallow only after the food is thoroughly chewed and finely ground. In fact, some children hold food in the cheeks like chipmunks, and some children eat their dessert and still have the vegetable in their cheeks. The fact that some children apparently gain more enjoyment from filling their mouths full of food than from taking small mouthfuls makes learning to chew and swallow a bit complicated for them. These children may almost appear helpless as they sit with packed mouths. Encouraging them to take small bites and to chew and swallow each mouthful has been successful in some cases.

No discussion of children's food problems would be complete without a discussion of the so-called vegetable war. Sometimes this may be created at first by a generally disgruntled parent who really wants to have the child reinforce his or her own belief that all vegetables are horrible. Perhaps a father associates cooked vegetables with his mother with whom there was always a clash. Histories of American colonial times tell of husbands who refused their wives the money to buy seeds for green leafy vegetables because they considered these foods fodder. This was, of course, in the "previtamin days." This idea of fodder appears too often in the history of food patterns. Yet we also find in these histories stories of gathering wild greens for use during the so-called hunger weeks of spring when the food preserved for winter was either all gone or too spoiled to be used. It is also interesting to observe in tropical countries of Asia and Africa the vast array of what are to us strange-looking green leafy vegetables that are bought eagerly from native markets.

The rejection of some kinds of foods can easily be passed down from parents to their children. Sometimes a dislike for the usually popular milk can be directly accounted for in this way. The labeling of salads as "women's food" may also have caused some boys to reject them.

All of these influences, although subtle, are definitely effective in the development of food prejudices. Being branded as someone who does not like carrots often prevents a child who would later like to try them from doing so. When we begin to understand the basis of a food prejudice, we are on the way to counteracting it.

However, many children do like vegetables. Some raw vegetables are preferred, but well-cooked vegetables are accepted also. Of course, I am assuming here that strong acrid odors and unpleasant flavors are not present in these cooked vegetables. When a person, coming in from outdoors and the fresh air, smells unpleasant cooking odors in a poorly ventilated kitchen, a prejudice may precede the actual meal. Sometimes better selection at the market of tender young root vegetables is necessary to prevent the unpleasant "woodiness" in root vegetables.

Another specific food problem concerns the child who is exceptionally fond of sweet foods; often parents who are very fond of such foods have patterned the child to be overfond of them. Sweet foods used as rewards or as special treats also reinforce the child's desire for sweets. The use of cake for a birthday celebration is too well grounded in American tradition to be uprooted, but we should recognize that a wonderful birthday cake reinforces the value of a sweet food. One child asked whether fruit cake (always served in his home at Christmas time) was Christ's birthday cake.

Summary

In no other area are family influences stronger than in food preferences. The association of mother's food and her love lasts over years and may supersede all outside influences. Studies have shown that of all meal patterns, Sunday dinner meal patterns change most slowly when a family moves to a new country. A father's influence on a child's food preferences was shown in one study in which children were found to dislike the foods that the father disliked.[4] The principal reason was that since mothers did not serve the food fathers disliked, these foods were unfamiliar to the children and they refused them when they were served later.

Modern parents, buffeted by their children's faith in television advertisements for food as well as by the sweets offered in vending machines at school, sometimes lose faith in their role as the "home gatekeeper." They may need professional bolstering to reinforce their faith in themselves so that they actually do control the food in their homes and in their children's lives.

To assist children to develop desirable food patterns, I recommend the following:

1. All foods should be well prepared and attractive in color, flavor, and texture, so that the child will approach the meal and eat it happily. Children appreciate and enjoy an attractive plate and often comment on foods being "pretty"; they eat with greatest enthusiasm when there is a variety of flavors and textures in the meal.

2. The environment for eating should be suited to the abilities and comfort of the young eater. This includes appropriate tables and chairs as well as suitable dishes and implements.

3. A child should be expected to have a good appetite and to be hungry when in good physical and emotional health.

4. Appetite will be fostered if the child is hungry and happily excited over the fact that it is mealtime.

5. Pleasant associations with the food are fostered if the meal can be eaten successfully with reasonable effort. Fatigue often defeats children's desire for food. They should come to the meal rested, and the eating process should not be tiring.

REVIEW QUESTIONS

1. What is the difference between hunger and appetite?

2. How does one help an infant to accept new foods?
3. Describe dishes and utensils appropriate for preschool-age children.
4. How can foods be prepared so that they are easy for the child to eat?
5. How can tastes and textures of food be combined to make a meal pleasing for the young child?

SUGGESTED LEARNING ACTIVITIES

1. During observation of a preschool feeding program, identify food preferences of the children.
2. Describe factors in the environment that, at mealtimes, influence children's food acceptance.
3. Discuss appropriate portions for 2- and 5-year-old children.

4. How can parents facilitate a child's acceptance of new textures?
5. Describe appropriate tables, chairs, and utensils for feeding young children.

REFERENCES

1. Lowenberg ME and others: *Food and people,* New York, 1979, John Wiley & Sons.
2. Aldrich CA, Aldrich MM: *Feeding our old-fashioned children,* New York, 1946, Macmillan.
3. Carlson AJ: *The control of hunger in health and disease,* Chicago, 1916, University of Chicago Press.
4. Bryan MS, Lowenberg ME: The father's influence on young children's food preference, *J Am Diet Assoc* 34:30, 1958.

7 Factors Shaping Food Patterns in Young Children

Cristine M. Trahms

✦✦

Objectives

After studying this chapter, the student should:

✔ *Understand the development of taste preferences of infants and young children.*

✔ *Understand the role of adult and peer influences on children's food acceptance.*

✔ *Recognize social and cultural influences on food patterns of children.*

✔ *Understand the effect of television on food preferences and intake of children.*

✔ *Understand the role of learning in the development of food preferences, regulation of food intake, and ability to distinguish between food and inedible substances.*

We all developed our own unique set of food habits without necessarily understanding the factors that shaped our individual patterns and choices. Nutrition professionals and educators have long been curious about the forces that shape food habits and consequently health status. It is generally accepted that patterns of food choices are developed early in life and that parents are influential in shaping food-related behaviors. The traditional manner of counseling parents has been to provide nutrition information and to hope for a concomitant increase in knowledge and change in attitudes and behaviors related to nutrition and food choices. Guidance on shaping food-related behaviors has been primarily based on observation and common-sense principles.

This chapter is a sequel to Dr. Lowenberg's discussion (chapter 6) of the practical aspects of the development of the food habits of young children. It describes some of the research that has helped us begin to understand the interactions of environmental factors that shape food-related behaviors. It is difficult to define in a measurable manner those terms related to food behavior, such as food choices, food preferences, dawdling, and coaxing. It is equally difficult to measure the intervening and confounding variables that may affect food behavior. Parents no longer, if they ever did, have the sole significant impact on the food choices of their young children.

The interaction of factors that shape food choices is currently being evaluated. These factors include the nutrition attitudes and knowledge of parents and child-care providers, economic and social status of the family, ordinal position of the preschool child, siblings and peers, and media advertising.

It is difficult but necessary to begin to incorporate both an assessment of individual nutritional adequacy and an evaluation of food patterns in an effort to assess the effect of food preferences on long-term health status.

Factors that have been evaluated for the young child are texture, taste, familiarity of food, preferences of the child compared with those of parents and other significant adults, and interaction patterns of parents and children around food. The limitations of these reports are those frequently encountered when dealing with a complex set of interacting factors. However, these reports indicate a direction for clinical practice and suggest important considerations in developing multidimensional research models that build a solid base for that practice.

PHYSIOLOGICAL BASIS OF TASTE

In 1825, Brillat-Savarin observed in *The Physiology of Taste,* "It is not an easy matter to determine the precise nature of the organ of taste. It is more complicated than it would appear at first sight."[1] The nature of taste is still largely unknown. It is an essential part of our lives, influencing our food choices and our willingness to consume enough of specific foods to provide

adequate nourishment. Some aspects of taste are believed to be innate to the human organism, whereas others are dictated by genetics, and still others are believed to be developed by physical maturation and experience. Willingness to ingest food is affected by a series of factors that include the sensory attributes of food, immediate hunger, nutritional status, prior experience with the food, environment, and beliefs and feelings about food. Recent work with infants and young children has endeavored to measure these almost immeasurable aspects of taste.

The infant's primary method of learning in the first few months of life is through the mouth. Activity in and around the mouth of the infant is geared toward developing oral motor skills necessary for nourishment and survival. Breast milk is possibly a source of flavor experiences for the young infant because some of the flavors in foods consumed by the lactating woman are transferred to human milk. It is not known whether these early flavor experiences through breast milk affect later food acceptance.

It is believed that preference for sweet tastes is innate to the infant.[2] However, this preference may be modified in early life. Sugar water must be offered to the infant to maintain the newborn level of preference for sweetness. Without this exposure in the early newborn period, the relative acceptance of this beverage diminishes.[3]

Aversion to bitter tastes appears at an early age (fig. 7-1). Reactions to salty tastes are initially neutral.[2] This indifference for the taste of salt shifts to relative preference for salt at about 4 months of age when this taste interacts with other tastes in foods. Younger children and infants prefer a saltwater solution. However, preschoolers reject this solution, favoring instead relatively high levels of salt in foods that are usually associated with a mildly salty taste. For example, preschoolers prefer a much higher level of salt in soup than do most adults.[4]

The genetic makeup of an individual affects basic taste responses, which in turn affect food acceptance. The classic genetic difference is capability to be a "taster" for 6-N-propylthiouracil (PROP) or a "nontaster" for the compound. Tasters to PROP are more sensitive to

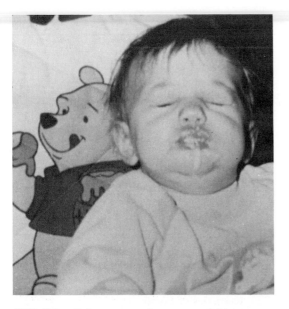

FIG. 7-1 Infants recognize sour and bitter tastes and make their feelings known.

bitter taste. However, only recently has the link between genetics of taste and food preference been explored for young children. The young children who were nontasters preferred cheese and milk more than the tasters.[5] The implication for selecting foods as sources of nutrients based on the genetic status of taste is noteworthy and warrants further evaluation.

DEVELOPMENT OF FOOD PREFERENCES

Innate tastes are only one aspect of food preference. Factors that influence the food habits of young children are listed in table 7-1. Infants and young children often favor foods because they are offered or because their parents and peers enjoy them. For preschool children, sweetness and familiarity are primary enhancers of choice (fig. 7-2); familiarity becomes less important with older children.[6] (See table 7-2.)

FIG. 7-2 Familiarity is an important determinant of food preferences. Children learn to like the foods they are offered.

TABLE 7-1   Factors Shaping Food Choices

**Characteristics of Parents
and Child Care Providers**
Nutrition knowledge
Nutrition attitudes
Personal food choices
Personal eating style (e.g., pace and frequency
    of eating)
Nonnourishment uses of food

Characteristics of Family
Family composition
Economic status
Social status
Educational level of adults
Occupation of adults
Ordinal position of child
Number and age of children in home

Characteristics of Peers and Siblings
Food preferences
Nonnourishment uses of foods
Nutrition attitudes

Characteristics of Child
Age
Genetics of taste
Conditioned responses
Activity level
Stage of growth
Developmental stage

Interactions with Adults around Food
Satiety cues respected
Pace and frequency of eating that adults expect
    from the child
Social interaction and communication patterns
    around food
Type of food offered
Benefit versus threat contingencies

Characteristics of Foods
Texture
Taste
Familiarity
Sweetness
Appearance

Media
Foods advertised
Promotion of foods for nonnourishment capabilities
Promotion of desired body shape
Purchase—influence efforts at supermarket

Preference rankings made by preschool children are highly correlated with consumption,[7] and the preferences of children can be strongly influenced by their peers. Fear of a new food can be diminished by increasing exposure to the food.[8] Rejection of a food can be turned into acceptance by repeated exposure to the food. However, often a food must be offered 10 to 15 times before a young child is willing to accept the food. Parents are often discouraged by repeated refusals and discontinue offering the new food. A food must be tasted for exposure to

*TABLE 7-2   Acceptance of New Foods
               by Young Children*

Child's Age	Rate of Acceptance of a New Food
2-year-olds	70% refused to try a new food
5-year-olds	100% tried a new food
	**Most Important Factors
in Acceptance of a New Food**
3-year-olds	Familiarity and texture
4-year-olds	Sweetness and familiarity

TABLE 7-3 *Adult Influence on Children's Eating*

Parents and providers influence children's eating by:
- Verbal prompting at mealtime
- Nonverbal influences (food purchases and presentation of food)
- Their own eating behavior
    - Children are more likely to eat a food when they see an adult eating it
    - Pace of eating: children will imitate parent's pace of eating
    - Timing of eating: children will learn to eat meals or to snack during the day
- Using food for nonnourishment purposes

the food to be effective in changing refusal to acceptance; just looking at the food is not enough.[10]

It would also seem that the food preferences of young children would be significantly influenced by the adults who provide their care and thus their food (table 7-3). Child-parent preference associations would be expected to be strong because of intimate social contact inside the family. However, the evidence is contradictory. One study suggests that both the mother and the father influence a child's food preferences equally, possibly because of the high priority given to the father's preferences in the family menu.[9] Another study shows that unrelated adults of the same subcultural group, such as day-care teachers, exert an influence equal to that of parents in development of food preferences.[11]

The increasing role of day care in the development of the food behavior of young children needs examination. Parents and providers need to work together to provide a consistent series of prompts that support the development of appropriate, healthful food behaviors.

In a comprehensive evaluation of family resemblance in food patterns, mother-child choices were similar, whereas father-child choices had no relationship. Parent–older child similarities in food choices were stronger than

parent–younger child similarities. The food preferences of young children were more similar to those of their siblings than to those of their parents,[12] perhaps because children in a given family generally accept a narrower range of foods than the adults accept (fig. 7-3).

Even though the family constellation has changed with increasing numbers of single-parent and blended families, the relationship between gender and food roles appears not to have changed much.[13] Women are still the primary "purchasers and preparers" of foods brought into the home. The change has been in the frequency of meals eaten away from home by children—at day care, preschool, school breakfast or lunch, or fast-food restaurants.

While it would appear that roles in the home have not changed much, many women are preparing food less often for their young children. However, the report of the Continuing Survey of Food Intakes of Individuals (CSFII) indicates that changes in maternal employment appear to have no detrimental effect on the nutritional adequacy of the diets of young children. In fact, reported intakes of total fat, saturated fat, cholesterol, and sodium did not increase with maternal employment.[14] The impact of these changes in food choices on nutrition and long-term health is not understood.

LEARNED RESPONSES THAT AFFECT FOOD INTAKE

The role of learning in the process of regulation of intake, food preferences, and differentiating food from nonfood substances is important. Young children must learn to differentiate food from nonfood substances. It has been demonstrated that the young child learns by experience to place "items" into edible foods and inedible categories, such as disgust (feces), danger (poisons), inappropriate (grass, sticks), and unacceptable combinations (catsup on cookies). The youngest children had a high to moderate level of acceptance of all categories of food and nonfood items offered. Fortunately, the acceptance of dangerous and disgusting

FIG. 7-3   Siblings exert influence on food preferences.

substances decreased with age. However, almost all of the children accepted combinations that were unacceptable to adults (e.g., a hot dog with chocolate sauce).[15]

Young children must also learn to differentiate hunger from other cues, since the failure to learn to discriminate among various cues can lead to inappropriate eating and perhaps intake regulation disorders. Birch and Deysher[16] found that young children show clearer evidence for energy compensation than adults. Nearly all of the children studied (95%) ate less at lunch following a high-energy density preload than a low-energy density preload. Only 60% of the adults had this same pattern (fig. 7-4).

A significant learned food behavior is the response to the parent's admonition to eat specific foods "or else!" (fig. 7-5). A preschool child usually knows that foods presented as the means in the contingency are the ones that are usually disliked (e.g., "Eat your spinach before you can have more french fries"). When a food is placed as the "means component," or food to be

consumed to receive the reward, of a contingency to increase the consumption of a particular food, the consumption of that food increases while the contingency is in effect. However, the consumption of the food is actually reduced after the contingency is removed.[17] Birch speculates that this system reinforces the innate drive for sweetness.[10] Food used as a reward in a noncontingent manner with adult attention appeared to enhance preference toward that food.

Young children responded in a more positive manner to nutrition guidance that was presented in a benefit appeal rather than a threat appeal format. The benefit appeal stresses the positive aspects of changing practices and the threat appeal presents the consequences of not changing practices.[18] Accenting the positive aspects of healthy food choices appealed to young children. This learning style needs to be more fully evaluated for long-term effect.

Nutrition awareness is a component of development of long-term food habits. How parents communicate with children about foods sets a

FIG. 7-4   Taste rather than appearance is an important factor in the development of food preferences of young children.

FIG. 7-5   Young children have their own ideas about when and how to eat.

baseline for development in this area. The nutrition messages from parents to children could be categorized as general nutrition, specific nutrition, encouragement, passive and nonverbal, example, authoritarian, bribe and rewards, and positive or negative messages in each category. The children responded to positive messages that were general but frequent (this food will make you strong) and to specific nutrition messages (milk gives you strong bones) from parents.[19]

EXTERNAL CONTROLS OF FOOD PREFERENCES

"Attempts to externally control the child's intake reflect an implicit assumption that children are incapable of self-regulation and the attempts at control often have effects counter to those intended."[16] External control strategies may lead the young child to see that external cues, such as the amount of food remaining on the plate, rather than the internal cues of hunger and satiety are important to the regulation of food intake.

Satiety is specific to particular foods and influences both the choice of a food and the amount of a food that is eaten; this specificity can lead to a greater intake when a variety of foods is available. Food intake in humans increases as the variety of foods offered at a meal increases.[20] Children who are not exposed to coercive parenting strategies (e.g., have a safe, comfortable eating environment), are able to modify their intake based on the energy content of their diets. Children were offered a fixed volume as a first course of either high or low energy content and then allowed to choose foods as desired. These children chose less after the high energy content fixed volume and more after the low energy content fixed volume of food (fig. 7-6).[16]

Davis,[21] supported by recent work of Story and Brown[22] and Birch and others,[23] documents the differing roles of parents and children in facilitating and making appropriate food choices and eating on the development of food patterns. Primary guidelines to the role differentiation are

- to offer foods of highest nutritional value; and
- to recognize the appetites of young children are a *reliable* guide to the amount of food that needs to be consumed.

To offer our children nonnutritional foods and to override their ability to respond to hunger and satiety cues is to do a grievous disservice.

SOCIAL INFLUENCES ON DEVELOPMENT OF FOOD HABITS

Social influence is one of the most important aspects of food acceptance and rejection. An estimated 50% of all people have conditioned

FIG. 7-6 "All done." Children express satiety clearly and in a variety of ways.

taste aversions. The relationships between food rejection and other personality variables such as anxiety, instability, and poor self-concept have been questioned. Mothers of 2- to 7-year-old children were asked, "Is there anything about your child's current eating behavior that bothers you?" The most frequent response was finicky behaviors; the most common food listed was vegetables. Mothers were also concerned about eating habits, especially dawdling and messiness. Even with cautious interpretation there was a relationship between the feeding problems score and psychological-behavioral problems. For example, greater acting-out, toileting problems, and fearfulness were reported for children who had higher feeding problems scores.[24]

The effect of disordered parental eating on the food-related behaviors of young children needs to be further addressed. It would seem that parents who have a distorted perception of their body size and have taught themselves to not respond to hunger or satiety cues would teach some of these misperceptions to their children. The parenting skills and awareness of child development of mothers with eating disorders were compared with a control group. Mothers with eating disorders (both anorexia nervosa and bulimia nervosa) reported more problems with lactation, the adherence to a fairly rigid feeding schedule for their infants, and more frequent behavior problems with their children than control mothers.[25] Mothers of children with nonorganic failure to thrive described higher levels of dietary restraint for themselves than control mothers. Despite the diagnosis of failure to thrive, these mothers believed their children to be of normal weight or only slightly underweight. Further, they restricted their child's intake of foods they considered to be too sweet, fattening, or unhealthy.[26]

Evidence suggests that the adolescent preoccupation with dieting and body shape may actually begin in elementary school. By age 7 years, children appear to have adopted the adult cultural values of attractiveness. In a survey children always ranked the drawings of obese children the lowest[27] Of children in grades three to six, nearly half wanted to be thinner, and most of these children had already tried to lose weight. The boys and girls were nearly equally preoccupied with body shape.[28] This indicates the need to better understand the development of eating behavior and attitudes of children.

CATEGORIZATION OF FOODS

How children categorize foods is a facet of food choice that has been only recently evaluated. Children 5 to 11 years of age were asked to separate food into groups by whatever criteria they chose to use.[29] The children, regardless of age, used some common characteristics to divide foods into categories, such as sweet versus nonsweet foods, meal entrees versus drinks or breakfast foods. None of the children used nutrient terminology to classify foods into groups (e.g., protein foods), nor was dislike of a particular food used as a basis for classification. The cognitive stage of the children indicated the ability of the child to sort foods into groups and to follow guidelines established by Piaget.[30]

The younger children who are classified as preoperational in Piaget's terminology used concrete features to classify foods (e.g., sweet versus bitter taste or liquid versus solid). They also used the occasion of eating as a basis for classification (e.g., meal entrees versus breakfast foods). As cognitive development increased, so did the basis for food classification. Those children in Piaget's concrete operational category were able to classify foods in more than one category and by more than one characteristic (e.g., both amount of processing and plant or animal origin). All of the children formed a sweets group, 50% a fruits group, 50% a vegetable group, about 50% a drinks group, about 25% a dairy group, and 20% a breads and cereals group.[29] It may be reasonable to use these spontaneous notions about food groups as the basis for nutrition education even when the goal is to foster a more sophisticated understanding of nutrition.

NUTRITION KNOWLEDGE OF CAREGIVER

Nutrition knowledge of parents and other caregivers is an important factor to consider in the shaping of the food preferences of children. The degree to which knowledge of nutrition is incorporated into family meal planning appears to be related to positive attitude toward self, problem-solving skills, and family organization (fig. 7-7).[31] The ordinal position of the preschool child in the family appears to influence choices of specific foods regardless of equivalent knowledge of nutrition of mothers.[32] When preschool children were the youngest children in a family, mothers were found to be less susceptible to children's requests for new products. They were willing, however, to accommodate that preference when the preschool-age child was the oldest child in a family.

Day-care teachers would presumably also have an impact on the development of food preference in young children. In a survey, day-care teachers reported that they knew little about nutrition, but they thought it was important.[33] Since young children are responsive to early influences, the role of the day-care teacher in shaping positive food-related attitudes needs to be strongly supported by the nutrition community. Day-care providers readily acknowledged that they need more information and guidance on developing good food habits and planning meals for preschool children.[34]

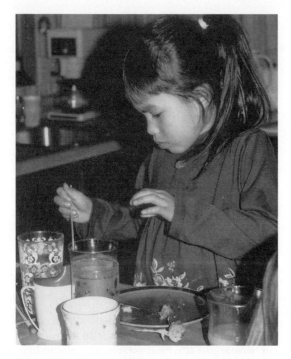

FIG. 7-7 Young children learn food acceptance and food preparation skills by observing adult modeling of these behaviors and practicing themselves.

INFLUENCE OF FAMILY

Hertzler[35] has encouraged the development of a broader conceptual framework for studying children's food behavior and urged that the family unit be included in the research model. The influence of the family unit on changing food-choice patterns to manage obesity has been reviewed.[36] Families can provide the appropriate role models and reinforcements that are most likely to bring about appropriate food habit changes. Mealtime companionship is important to young children. The food intake and consequently nutrient intake were determined to be more adequate for those children who had positive adult companionship at meals.[37]

The child-parent interactions have an important influence on food consumption. There appeared to be differences between the interactions of thinner children and their mothers and fatter children and their mothers in both food and nonfood situation.[38] The thinner children and their mothers talked more with each other, ate less food, ate more slowly, and in general had a more positive, supportive relationship than the fatter children and their mothers. This type of study begins to look at the broader construct of family units as related to food and eating and needs to be further researched.

Mothers of obese 3- to 4-year-old children reported that they exercised less control over the foods the child ate and were less satisfied with the child's food choices than the reports from the parents of average weight children.[39] These parents of obese children were also dissatisfied with the amount of food the child consumed between meals. These parents controlled time, frequency, and type of food eaten by their children, but not the amount of food eaten. The location and activity at meals were reported as managed by the parent. However, this same management did not extend to snacks while watching television. All parents reported that children's food preferences were considered when making food purchases. Sweets were offered frequently after children had eaten a "good meal." Average weight children were offered sweets only after a good meal was eaten more often than obese children. Parents of obese children felt that their children ate too much food between meals. Many of these parents felt that their own food behavior influenced the children's food behavior. Time of eating, types of foods liked or disliked, location of eating, and watching television were the parental habits that by their report influenced the children's behavior. The parents did not feel that the amount of food they ate influenced the amount of food their children ate. However, these parents felt that the influence their personal food habits had on the children's food behavior decreased as the amount of time the parent spent working outside the home increased.

Obviously children respond to the social environment when they make food choices for themselves. It has been demonstrated that preferences for foods were enhanced when foods were offered as a reward or with brief positive social interactions with adults.[40] Parenting behaviors that have been recognized as related

TABLE 7-4   *Nonnourishment Uses of Foods*

Use	Foods Most Frequently Used
As a reward for good behavior	Sweets, desserts, baked goods, fruits
Withheld as punishment for inappropriate behavior	Desserts, sweets
As a pacifier	Baked goods, juice
As the instrumental component of a contingency	Sweet foods, desserts

to increased nutritional adequacy of the intakes of young children are
- allowing the child enough time to eat;
- asking the child to help prepare food or set the table;
- allowing the child to make decisions about the type of food eaten; and
- giving small portions when introducing a new food.[37]

When parents overtly monitored or only said they would monitor the food choices of children, the children adjusted the foods they selected. In general, they chose foods lower in sugar than when supervised.[41]

Hertzler[42] discussed the negative influences of development of inappropriate choices, which are primarily too much stimulation and attention at meals and negative or inappropriate parenting. When surveyed, more than half of the parents interviewed promised foods as a reward and also withheld foods as a punishment (table 7-4).[37] Parents are more likely to prompt a child to eat after the child refuses a food than after the child requests a food. Greater attention to a child's food refusals may result in less desirable eating behaviors and support a decreased preference for those foods.[43]

NUTRITION EDUCATION

The overt shaping of food choices and food behaviors by educational strategies happens less specifically than we would like for optimal nourishment. Results suggest that healthy snack choices increased in school in the training setting. However, without a strategy for promoting generalization of healthy snack choices such as cueing, little generalization across settings occurred even at school. Furthermore, general-ization to healthy snack choices at home was achieved only when individualized procedures to program at-home choices were organized and implemented. Unfortunately, even with cueing, the change was not permanent. After withdrawal of the reinforcement procedures snack choices eventually returned to baseline levels.[44] It is obvious that knowledge of healthy eating alone is not sufficient to change children's eating behavior. Parental involvement in the nutrition education programs has been more successful in changing food choices and eating behaviors. Kirks and Hughes[45] demonstrated that the diets of young children whose parents concomitantly received nutrition education were better than those of children whose parents were not directly involved (fig. 7-8).

Efforts have been made to teach young children to consume diets lower in total fat. When children were asked, "What does it mean to be healthy?" 82% responded, "Eat the right foods." All of the children thought it was important to be healthy. The right kinds of foods were described as foods from the fruit and vegetable group. Unhealthy foods were listed as foods high in sugar. Most children defined health in a positive fashion.[46]

Parents of fourth graders felt that the schools should have a significant role in nutrition education, but were not overly eager to participate themselves. The goals the parents wanted achieved were to learn about nutrition and to learn label reading. Parents felt that barriers to good nutrition in the home were

- differing likes and dislikes of family members;
- children's desire for foods that are advertised;
- the difficulty of "breaking" faulty habits; and
- lack of time to prepare nutritious meals.[47]

FIG. 7-8   Food patterns are influenced by nutrition education activities such as making bread.

In contrast, it has been documented that changes in behavior and knowledge of nutrition implemented at school do not necessarily carry over at home. Nutrition education with parents as part of the program is more effective than without parents' participation.

Recent work with innovative techniques (e.g., open ended questions and concept maps), to assess nutrition knowledge and beliefs of young children indicate that young children are intellectually ready to learn more about food, nutrition, and positive health habits than previously believed (fig. 7-9).[48] These types of innovative techniques warrant more exploration.

INFLUENCE OF MEDIA ON THE FOOD BEHAVIORS OF YOUNG CHILDREN

In addition to the many familial, cultural, and psychosocial influences on children's food habits, mass media affects children's requests for and attitudes toward food. Of the forms of mass media, television has the greatest impact on children because it reaches many children before they are capable of verbal communication. Children spend more time watching television than they spend at school and more than they spend in any activity other than sleeping. Children from low-income families watch more television than do children from moderate- to high-income families.[49] It has been estimated that, as a group, children watch television for 26 hours per week from preschool to junior high school.[50] This means that the average child watches 3 hours of television advertising per week and 19,000 to 22,000 commercials per year.

Children often are unable to separate commercials from the program and frequently explain them as part of the program especially if a host-selling format is used. Slightly older children (7 to 8 years of age) were more favorably influenced by the host-selling format than younger children.[51] School-age children (11 to 12 years of age) are conscious of the concept of

FIG. 7-10   Children who are distracted during mealtime may not learn to appreciate the flavor, appearance, and taste of foods; the distraction may interfere with appreciating satiety.

FIG. 7-9   Play activities help young children explore and develop food preparation skills.

commercials, the purpose of selling, and the concept of sponsorship and are less likely to accept advertisers' claims without question. They perceive that television commercials are designed to sell products rather than entertain or educate.

It has been pointed out that certain attributes of food are promoted as superior to others. The main characteristics presented positively are sweetness, chocolateyness, and richness.[52] Many food manufacturers, in other words, deemphasize the physiological need for nutrients and encourage selection on the basis of sweet flavor. Exposure to such messages may distort a child's natural curiosity toward other characteristics of food, such as the fresh crispness of celery or apples.

In the past 10 years little has changed in terms of the kinds of foods advertised with programs targeted at young children, e.g., Saturday morning cartoons. In a recent survey 71% of the commercials were for food products and 80% of those were for foods of low nutritional value.[53] The foods most frequently advertised contained amounts of energy, fat, and sodium high enough to be noteworthy.[54]

There is an ongoing concern about the influence of television on the growth and health of young children (fig. 7-10). It has been demonstrated that television influences the eating habits and thus the nutritional status of children in three significant ways:

- television advertising influences family food purchases and the snacking patterns of young children;
- the use of food as depicted by television programs shows food being used for many activities other than the satisfaction of hunger; and

- the few overweight children used on television programs suggests that inappropriate use of foods has no impact on health or nutritional status.[55]

Dietz and Gortmaker[50] outline other aspects of television watching and television advertising that are of concern:

- the relationship between increased television watching and increased snacking;
- the relationship between consumption of foods advertised on television and viewing time; and
- the relationship between increased viewing time and the number of attempts by the young child to influence the food purchases of the parent.

The foods advertised on weekend children's programming are usually high-energy density foods that if purchased and consumed without an increase in activity, can lead to inappropriate weight gain and poor eating habits. The larger intake of highly concentrated sweet and fat foods plus the decrease in activity that is associated with excess television watching has led to an increase of obesity among children in the United States.

Parents must set limits on their children's requests for advertised food and may need support in their efforts to do so. They may need guidance in principles of behavior modification (see chapter 8) and reassurance that it is to the child's advantage to learn that not all advertised products are a part of every child's meal pattern.

Other advertising also influences children's food requests. Prize offers lead to increased demand for and consumption of certain foods.

The influence of media, especially television, cannot be overemphasized. Children are susceptible, vulnerable, and responsive to carefully crafted messages of consumption.

Summary

The feeding relationship between the child and the parent or caregiver is an important one. The tempo of parent-child interaction gives the child cues on how much and how fast to eat. The shaping of this tempo and pattern ultimately affects nutritional status and overall well-being. Young children are shaping patterns for a lifetime. They are developing a sense of food as nourishment, as well as an appropriate sense of food's uses in comfort, sociability, and satisfaction.

The child has innate taste. Adults are responsible for enhancing the sense of taste or defeating it by setting the tone of the interaction around food. Clearly adults must be mindful of the nutrient needs of children. Satter[56] states that the parent or caregiver is responsible for what is offered; the child is responsible for how much to eat. Although there are still many unanswered questions about the formation of food preferences, it is clear that preferences are a major determinant of food selection. If allowed free choice, children select sweet foods over nonsweet, more nutritious foods. Giving children free access to highly preferred but nutritionally weak foods encourages the development of nutritional problems during childhood and beyond.

Parents who are responsive to the developmental aspects of food-related behaviors will assist their children in developing food-related behaviors that support healthy growth and development (table 7-5).

To exert a maximum influence on the health and well-being of young children, nutrition educators must attend to the influences that shape the food preferences and eating patterns of young children. These influences are dynamic and multidirectional. Figure 7-11 indicates one approach to describing these influences. Young children are shaped by their family in significant ways. Effective nutrition work with young children and their families requires nutrition educators to forge strong ties with social scientists and continue to work together even though research on the influences on eating behavior of children is methodologically difficult because food-related behaviors are influenced by a complex series of interacting effects, and these effects are dynamic, not static, for the child.

TABLE 7-5   *Progress with Food Behaviors*

The Behavior	As Your Child Sees It	As You See It	What to Do
Refusal of new foods	It's something new. Your child is curious but probably distrustful of the unknown.	You want your child to learn to eat and enjoy a variety of nourishing foods.	Introduce only one new food at a time. Offer a small amount at first, at the beginning of a meal. Allow time for the child to look at and examine the food. New foods are refused when a child doesn't feel well or is tired and irritable. If the food is refused, do not make a fuss; rather, offer the food again a few days later.
Food dislikes	Your child is asserting independence by rejecting a food that does not immediately appeal. Or your child may not like the taste of the food.	You want your child to overcome the dislike and accept the food.	Refrain from making an issue of the dislike as this will make the child more determined to avoid the food. Try combining the food with other favorites. Offer small portions. Prepare the food in a different way. A vegetable might be served raw instead of cooked. Do not use the food as part of a contingency, "If you eat your 'X,' you may have dessert." This strengthens the dislike of the food. Set an example. Remember, children are entitled to a few dislikes.

Continued.

TABLE 7-5   Progress with Food Behaviors—cont'd

The Behavior	As Your Child Sees It	As You See It	What to Do
Refusal to eat a meal	Your child may be asserting independence or may not feel like eating because of a previous snack or tiredness.	You feel that your child needs nourishment and should eat at meals.	If this happens occasionally and your child appears to be well, remove the food until the next meal. No bribes or punishment and no meal replacement or snacks until the next mealtime. A skipped meal will not damage a healthy child. If your child appears ill, consult your doctor. Few well children starve themselves unless food becomes a weapon against parents.
Dawdling or playing with food	Your child may not be hungry or may be trying to attract attention.	You may become irritable and feel that you should take over and help your child to speed up eating.	Allow a reasonable amount of time. Offer help if needed. Explain that you will remove the food when your child is finished. Refrain from making a "scene." This may be what your child was looking forward to. Once the food is removed, there is no more until the next meal.
The same food is requested meal after meal	A food or combination of foods appeals, and your child requests it often.	You feel that variety is important and also are tired of preparing the same foods again.	It is not unusual for a child to have a preference for a food or food combination. It is fine to accommodate for a few days; usually these strong preferences do not last long if an issue is not made of it.

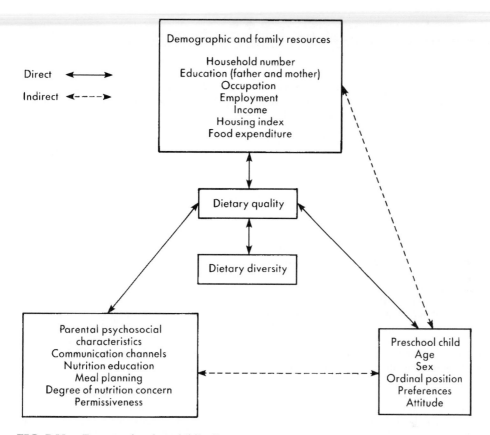

FIG. 7-11   Factors related to child's dietary status.
(From Caliendo MA, Sanjur D: *J Nutr Educ* 10:69, 1978.)

REVIEW QUESTIONS

1. Which factors are most important in determining food preferences for young children?
2. How do developmental stage and age of the young child affect food preferences?
3. What is the role of the media, especially television, in the food preferences of young children?
4. What role do parents and other caregivers play in the development of food habits?
5. How does social interaction shape food choices for young children?

SUGGESTED LEARNING ACTIVITIES

1. Ask a group of 3-year-old children and a group of 4-year-old children to separate a group of edible and nonedible items from two containers. Describe the differences of food choices by age groups.
2. Describe the effectiveness of food contingencies in getting a child to accept a specific food.
3. Plan and implement a 30-minute nutrition education program for children 5 to 6 years old.
4. Watch children's television for 1 hour and describe the food commercials presented during that hour.

✦ ✦ ✦

CASE STUDY

Factors That Shape Food Patterns

Stephanie is a single parent with three young children: Megan, age 3; Travis, age 6; and Ryan, age 7. The boys are out of bed early on school mornings and have bowls of cereal with milk for breakfast at about 7 A.M. Their favorite cereals are those promoted especially for children and feature cartoon characters, bright colors, and varied shapes. Megan eats a quick breakfast in the car between home, when her brothers are dropped at school, and before she arrives at day care. Her current favorite breakfast is a toaster pastry.

Megan receives her morning snack, lunch, and afternoon snack at day care. Travis and Ryan receive lunch at school and an afternoon snack at after-school care.

Stephanie stops by the day care for Megan at about 5:30 and must hurry to meet the boys before 5:45 when after-school care closes. The children are usually hungry and tired and Stephanie realizes that to avoid conflict among the children, she must have dinner prepared within 30 minutes of arriving home. Sometimes she offers them crackers or cookies to stave off fighting and crying. She usually prepares microwave individual meals because the children's food preferences are so dissimilar. Megan will eat only macaroni and cheese; Travis likes only potato and meat dishes; and Ryan will eat chicken and hot dogs. Stephanie and the children usually have ice cream and cookies before they prepare for bedtime and stories.

The family is referred to you by their pediatrician at the Well Child Clinic. The primary concern is Travis, whose rate of weight gain has increased. His stature continues at the 25th percentile for age, and his weight has increased from the 50th percentile to the 90th percentile for age.

Stephanie is appropriately concerned about Travis's weight and is willing to work with you to try to make appropriate changes. However, she also is concerned about these issues:

1. Similar weight gain patterns for Ryan and Megan;
2. Megan's refusal to expand the variety of foods she is willing to eat;
3. Travis and Ryan's limited variety of food acceptance at home and at school;
4. Dealing with the children's demands for foods they see advertised;
5. The amount of money she spends on groceries each week.

Outline a strategy that you might negotiate with Stephanie to address the referral from the pediatrician and the concerns she has raised.

---

5. If you were asked to provide a diet of 1000 kcal/day for a very overweight 2-year-old boy (weight: 40 pounds, greater than 95th percentile; height: 90th percentile, NCHS), what factors would you need to consider in relation to the family unit and eating environment?

6. If you were a nutrition consultant to a preschool that provides morning and afternoon snacks for the children and provides milk at lunch although children bring their own lunches: a. What easy, nourishing snacks that can be linked to activities for the children would you recommend? b. What basic concepts do you consider important in developing guidelines or inservice education for parents who prepare their children's lunches?

REFERENCES

1. Brillat-Savarin A: *The physiology of taste,* New Haven, Conn. Leete's Island Books.
2. Lawless H: Sensory development in children: research in taste and olfaction, *J Am Diet Assoc* 85:577, 1985.
3. Beauchamp GK, Cowart BJ: Congenital and experimental factors in the development of human flavor preferences, *Appetite* 6:357, 1985.
4. Cowart BJ, Beauchamp GK: The importance of sensory context in young children's acceptance of salty tastes, *Child Dev* 57:1034, 1986.
5. Anliker JA and others: Children's food preferences and genetic sensitivity to the bitter taste of 6-n-propylthiouracil (PROP), *Am J Clin Nutr* 54:16, 1991.

6. Birch LL: Dimensions of preschool children's food preferences, *J Nutr Educ* 11:77, 1979.

7. Birch LL: Preschool children's food preferences and consumption patterns, *J Nutr Educ* 11:189, 1979.

8. Pelchat ML, Pliner P: "Try it. You'll like it." Effects of information on willingness to try novel foods, *Appetite* 24:153, 1995.

9. Burt JV, Hertzler AA: Parental influence on the child's food preference, *J Nutr Educ* 10:127, 1978.

10. Birch LL, McPhee L, Shoba BC, Pirok E, Steinberg L: What kind of exposure reduces children's food neophobia? looking vs. tasting, *Appetite* 9:171, 1987.

11. Birch LL:The relationship between children's food preferences and those of their parents, *J Nutr Educ* 12:14, 1980.

12. Pliner P, Pelchant ML: Similarities in food preferences between children and their siblings and parents, *Appetite* 7:333, 1986.

13. Schafer RB, Schafer E: Relationship between gender and food roles in the family, *J Nutr Educ* 21:119, 1989.

14. Johnson RK and others: Effect of maternal employment on the quality of young children's diets: the CSFII experience, *J Am Diet Assoc* 92:213, 1992.

15. Rozin P and others: The child's conception of food: differentiation of categories of rejected substances in the 16 months to 5 year age range, *Appetite* 7:141, 1986.

16. Birch LL, Deysher M: Conditional and unconditional caloric compensation: evidence for self-regulation of food intake in young children, *Learning and Motivation* 16:341, 1985.

17. Birch LL, Marlin DW, Rotter J: Eating as the "means" activity in a contingency: effects on young children's food preferences, *Child Dev* 55:431, 1984.

18. Lawatsch DE: A comparison of two teaching strategies on nutrition knowledge, attitudes and food behavior of preschool children, *J Nutr Educ* 22:117, 1990.

19. Anliker JA and others: Parental messages and the nutrition awareness of preschool children, *J Nutr Educ* 22:24, 1990.

20. Rolls BJ: Experimental analysis of the effects of variety in a meal on human feeding, *Am J Clin Nutr* 42:932, 1985.

21. Davis CM: Self selection of diet by newly weaned infants: an experimental study, *Am J Dis Child* 36:651, 1929.

22. Story M, Brown JE: Do young children instinctively know what to eat? The studies of Clara Davis revisited, *N Engl J Med* 316:103, 1987.

23. Birch LL and others: The variability of young children's energy intake, *N Engl J Med* 324:232, 1991.

24. Pelchant ML, Pliner P: Antecedents and correlates of feeding problems in young children, *J Nutr Educ* 18:23, 1986.

25. Evans J, leGrange D: A comparative study of the attitudes of mothers towards their children, *Inter J Eating Disorders* 18:39, 1995.

26. McCann JB, Stein A, Fairburn CG, Dunger DB: Eating habits and attitudes of mothers of children with non-organic failure to thrive, *Arch Dis Child* 70:234, 1994.

27. Feldman W and others: Culture versus biology: children's attitudes toward thinness and fatness, *Pediatrics* 81:190, 1988.

28. Maloney MJ and others: Dietary behavior and eating attitudes in children, *Pediatrics* 84:484, 1989.

29. Michela JL, Contento IR: Spontaneous classification of foods by elementary school-aged children, *Health Educ Q* 11:57, 1984.

30. Bybee RW, Sund RB: *Piaget for educators*, ed 2, Columbus, Ohio, 1982, Charles E Merrill.

31. Swanson-Rudd J and others: Nutrition orientations of working mothers in the North Central region, *J Nutr Educ* 14:132, 1982.

32. Phillips DE, Bass MA, Yetley E: Use of food and nutrition knowledge by mothers of preschool children, *J Nutr Educ* 10:73, 1978.

33. Gillis DEG, Sabry JH: Day-care teachers: nutrition knowledge, opinions, and use of food, *J Nutr Educ* 12:200, 1980.

34. Dirige OV and others: An assessment of the nutrition education needs of day-care providers, *J Am Diet Assoc* 91:714, 1991.

35. Hertzler AA: Children's food patterns—a review. I. Food preferences and feeding problems. II. Family and group behavior, *J Am Diet Assoc* 85:551, 1983.

36. Hertzler AA: Obesity—impact on the family, *J Am Diet Assoc* 79:525, 1981.

37. Stanek K and others: Diet quality and the eating environment of preschool children, *J Am Diet Assoc* 90:1582, 1990.

38. Birch LL and others: Mother-child interaction patterns and the degree of fatness in children, *J Nutr Educ* 12:17, 1981.

39. Seagren JS, Terry, RD: WIC female parents' behavior and attitudes toward their children's

food intake—relationship to children's relative weight, *J Nutr Educ* 23:223, 1991.

40. Birch LL, Zimmerman SI, Hind H: The influence of social-affective context on the formation of children's food preferences, *J Nutr Educ* 13:115, 1981.

41. Klesges RC and others: Parental influence on food selection in young children and its relationship to childhood obesity, *Am J Clin Nutr* 53:859, 1991.

42. Hertzler AA: Review of nutrition education programs for preschoolers, *Top Clin Nutr* 5:35, 1990.

43. Ray JW, Klesges RC: Influence on the eating behavior of children, *Annals New York Academy Sciences* 669:57, 1995.

44. Stark LJ and others: Using reinforcement and cueing to increase healthy snack food choices in preschoolers, *J Appl Behav Anal* 19:367, 1986.

45. Kirks BA, Hughes C: Long-term behavioral effects of parent involvement in nutrition education, *J Nutr Educ* 18:203, 1986.

46. Perry CL and others: Modifying the eating behavior of young children, *J Sch Health* 55:399, 1985.

47. Crockett SJ and others: Nutrition intervention strategies preferred by parents: results of a marketing survey, *J Nutr Educ* 21:90, 1989.

48. Singleton JC and others: Role of food and nutrition in the health perceptions of young children, *J Am Diet Assoc* 92:67, 1992.

49. Reid LN, Bearden WO, Teel JE: Family income, TV viewing, and children's cereal ratings, *Journalism Q* 57:327, 1980.

50. Dietz WH, Gortmaker SL: Do we fatten our children at the television set? Obesity and television viewing in children and adolescents, *Pediatrics* 75:807, 1985.

51. Kunkel D: Children and host-selling commercials, *Comm Res* 15:17, 1988.

52. Gussow J: Counternutritional messages of TV ads aimed at children, *J Nutr Educ* 4:48, 1972.

53. Cotuga N: TV ads on Saturday morning children's programming—what's new? *J Nutr Educ* 20:125, 1988.

54. Windhauser MM and others: A nutritional evaluation of food and beverage products as advertised to children on Saturday morning television, *J Am Diet Assoc* 91:A-83, 1991.

55. Palumbo FM, Dietz WH: Children's television: its effect on nutrition and cognitive development, *Pediatr Ann* 14:793, 1985.

56. Satter EM: The feeding relationship, *J Am Diet Assoc* 86:352, 1986.

8 Managing Mealtime Behaviors

Sally M. O'Neil
Peggy L. Pipes

❖❖

Objectives

After studying this chapter, the student should:

✔ *Be aware of behavior management as a therapeutic approach to changing food patterns of children.*

✔ *Understand one approach to the analysis of behavior.*

✔ *Recognize the need to individualize reinforcers.*

✔ *Understand when it is appropriate to use food as a reinforcer.*

✔ *Be aware of methods used to teach children self-feeding.*

Parent-child interactions are important determinants of children's acceptance of food and attitudes toward eating. They contribute to the development of typical eating patterns, as noted in chapter 7. They are also responsible for difficulties that are presented to health care professionals. Parents, anxious about their children's nutrient intakes, sometimes urge, nag, or pressure children to eat, and children often assume control of the feeding environment. The battle for control may become so intense that the children's nutrient intakes may be compromised. The conflict may result in a variety of problems including failure to thrive and obesity.

Parent-child interaction is a complex reciprocal process in which each response to an action can become the cause of future behaviors and in which both parents and children learn new behaviors. This interaction continuum includes parents' expressions of attitudes, values, interests, beliefs, and their caregiving behavior, as well as children's individual growth patterns, learning potential, and ability to incorporate increasingly complex experiences into their current stages of thinking and functioning. Behavior is both the cause and effect of other behaviors. All parent-child interactions are both elicited by the child and influence the child. For instance, the cries of a hungry infant can become the stimulus for the mother to respond by feeding the infant.

Behavior modification is a therapeutic tool that is often used as a system of analysis and intervention for a wide variety of child development

201

problems.[1-3] It is also commonly used as a therapeutic tool to manage weight problems (such as
obesity), to extinguish socially unacceptable feeding behaviors (such as throwing food), and to
increase a child's acceptance of a variety of foods
or to teach self-feeding.[4,5] Sometimes nutritionists and dietitians work jointly with behaviorists
in establishing and monitoring such programs.
Often, nutritionists and dietitians apply behavior
management concepts themselves. Concepts and
methods of behavior modification are presented
in this chapter.

BASIC CONCEPTS IN BEHAVIOR ASSESSMENT AND MANAGEMENT

Behaviorists have determined that behaviors
are increased, maintained, or decreased by the
consequences that immediately follow them.[6]
These consequences can be reinforcing or punishing. Since **reinforcers** and **punishers** are
defined from an individual's point of view, what
may be reinforcing to one person may not be to
someone else; the determination of what is reinforcing or punishing depends on the effect of a
particular consequence on the behavior that
preceded it. To be a reinforcer, a consequence
must increase the behavior that it follows.

Reinforcers are of two types: positive and negative. Positive reinforcement is a consequence in
which something desirable to the subject is
added or applied to his or her environment as a
result of a specific behavior. A smile, a hug,
praise, food, and money are examples of positive
reinforcers. Negative reinforcement, on the
other hand, is a consequence in which something unpleasant is removed or terminated. For
example, a person who is annoyed by loud static
on the radio may turn down the volume or turn
off the radio.

The silence, or absence of static, is a negative
reinforcer for turning off the sound, and the person is likely to do it again if static recurs. All reinforcers must increase the behavior that they follow. The important distinction between these two
concepts is that in positive reinforcement something pleasant is added as a consequence and in
negative reinforcement something unpleasant is
removed as a consequence.

Punishers decrease the behaviors that they follow. They are defined operationally in two ways.
Punishment involves consequences in which
something averse is added or applied, such as a
spanking. **Extinction** involves those consequences in which a positive reinforcer is removed.
For example, the withholding of adult attention
(ignoring) during a child's temper tantrum or
withholding eye contact when someone else is
talking should decrease negative behaviors.

Interaction Processes Between Positive and Negative Reinforcement and Punishment

To examine positive and negative reinforcement and punishment as interactive processes, it
is important to analyze the various parts of interaction. Peterson[7] has suggested that one way to
do this effectively is to consider interaction in
terms of A (antecedent events), B (behavior),
and C (consequences). Consider the following
example in which the **ABC analysis** is used. A
mother takes her preschool son into a grocery
store. The child immediately begins to ask for
candy, then whines and cries when the mother
refuses to give him any. After several minutes of
loud crying and repeated looks from other shop-
pers, the mother gives the child a piece of candy.
The child immediately stops crying. A diagram-
matic analysis of this situation is presented below.

A (antecedent)	B (child's behavior)	C (consequence)
1. Enters store	2. Asks for candy	3. Mother refuses
	4. Cries and yells	5. Mother gives candy
	6. Stops crying	

In giving her child candy the mother reinforced
her child for crying. Also, because he was reinforced, it is highly likely that the child will repeat
this behavior during future trips to the grocery
store. The mother received negative reinforcement because the crying ceased after the mother
gave the child the candy. By giving candy, she terminated something that was aversive to her—the
child's crying. In this interaction both mother and
child were reinforced for their behaviors. The
child was positively reinforced (candy was added)
for crying, and the mother was negatively reinforced (crying was removed) for giving the candy.
Both are likely to repeat their behaviors next time.

What if, in a similar situation, the mother decided to ignore the child? What would the mother's consequences be if ignoring stopped the crying? As before, she is negatively reinforced if she successfully stops the crying. Because the mother will be negatively reinforced for whatever she does that stops the crying, she may be reinforced for being inconsistent: giving candy one time, ignoring the child the next, and perhaps spanking another time.

It is easy for parents to become trapped in their responses to their children's behaviors and thus become unable to see those aspects of their interactions that are ineffective for both of them. It becomes important for parents to consider how they would like to respond most consistently to their child in the light of the behaviors they would like their child to learn. Parents have to consider their child's stage of development and reinforcers that fit his or her particular stage and personality. In addition, they have to be aware of the effects of the child's behavior on themselves. This is no small task, and it seems to become especially important around mealtimes. Since nutrition, socialization, and intense family interactions converge in this event, it is no wonder that so many clinical issues arise around mealtime behaviors.

Assessment of Mealtime Behaviors

Initial assessment consists of identifying the patterns of parent-child mealtime behaviors. The observation checklist (see the box on page 204) is a useful recording guide that pinpoints both problem behavior and desirable behavior. This tool can be used by professionals who are recording their direct observations or by parents who are recording the mealtime behaviors of themselves and their children. Behaviors can be tallied for each meal.

Once problem behaviors are identified, the most frequent eating and noneating behaviors and their consequences can be identified in ABC sequences. Parents are helped to first identify those behaviors they wish to foster in their children, and then those they wish to change. The next step is to determine appropriate consequences for all the behavior categories.

As noted earlier, parents generally behave toward their children (reinforce, punish, or ignore) in certain ways because of the reinforcement they receive from their children. For instance, they may reinforce a crying child with a cookie because they know this will stop the crying. Thus the parent is negatively reinforced for giving the child the cookie. Frequently, to help parents change the consequences they provide their children, it is necessary to look at the reinforcers parents are getting for their own behavior. One way to do this is to help them identify the subsequent child behavior step to the ABC pattern. For parents to alter their antecedent cues to the child, they must be aware of these behaviors and their part in the entire ABC pattern. The brief case studies that follow illustrate a variety of parent-child ABC patterns that relate to mealtimes.

1 Laura refuses to drink milk.

A (mother)	B (child)	C (mother)
1. Pours milk into glass	2. Starts crying	3. "Drink your milk."
	4. Cries	5. Removes milk and gives child soda
	6. Stops crying and drinks soda	

In this instance the mother was negatively reinforced. She successfully terminated the crying by giving the child soda, which, in turn, positively reinforced the child's crying when milk was presented to her.

2 Billy, a toddler, writes his own menu.

A (mother)	B (child)	C (mother)
1. Presents applesauce to Billy in highchair	2. Cries and whines, points to refrigerator	3. "What do you want?"
	4. Cries, points to cupboard	5. "Do you want a cracker?"
	6. Cries, points to refrigerator	7. "What do you want?
	8. Cries, points to refrigerator	9. "No, you can't have ice cream."
	10. Child screams	11. "OK, here is some ice cream."
	12. Stops crying	

CHILD BEHAVIORS AT MEALTIME

Meals Observed

Noneating behaviors	1	2	3	4	5	6
Arguing						
Complaining						
Crying						
Hitting						
Noncomplying						
Not sitting at table						
Teasing						
Yelling						
Pouting						
Whining						
Moving hands nonpurposefully						
Talking back						
Throwing food or utensils						
Spitting						
Gagging						
Refusing certain foods						

Eating behaviors	1	2	3	4	5	6
Using fingers for finger foods						
Using utensils appropriately						
Sitting at table						
Accepting variety of foods						
Socializing as appropriate						
Complying to requests						

PARENT BEHAVIORS AT MEALTIME

Meals Observed

Antecedents to child behaviors	1	2	3	4	5	6
Commanding						
Requesting						
Questioning						
Prompting verbally						
Physically assisting						
Interrupting						
Positioning child appropriately						
Presenting food appropriately						
Presenting appropriate utensils						

Consequences of child behaviors	1	2	3	4	5	6
Commenting positively						
Commenting negatively						
Ignoring						
Touching						
Spanking						
Yelling						
Arguing						
Laughing						
Using same tone of voice						
Talking in distracting ways						

In this situation the child keeps his mother going in circles in an effort to stop his crying. A management plan was developed with her in which she would leave the room and when the child would stop crying she would return and praise him for eating so nicely. The ABC looked like this:

A (mother)	B (child)	C (mother)
1. Presents applesauce to Billy in highchair	2. Cries, points to cupboard	3. Leaves room (can see child, but he can't see her)
	4. Slowly stops crying, starts eating applesauce	5. Returns and says "My, what a big boy!"
	6. Child laughs and keeps on eating	

3 John, a school-age child who has a hearing impairment, wanders at mealtimes.

A (parents)	B (child)	C (parents)
1. Announce dinner	2. Sits at table with parents	3. Talk to each other, ignore John
	4. Gets up and wanders around house	5. Yell, "Come back here!"
	6. Approaches dining room	7. Ignore John
	8. Wanders away from dining room	9. "Come here, John," Father goes and leads him to table
	10. John sits and looks at food	11. Ignore John

When counselors discussed this ABC with John's parents, the parents decided that they had been reinforced by John's absence at the table since, before that time, he had had tantrum behavior at the table. They believed that he should eat with them, but it was more comfortable to eat without him and to feed him later. A management program was developed with them in which they agreed to reinforce him for sitting

at the table, using signing as well as verbal praise, and to try to include him in the general conversation. A subsequent ABC looked like this:

A (parents)	B (child)	C (parents)
1. Announce dinner	2. John sits at table, starts eating	3. Talk and sign to John
	4. Leaves table	5. Ignore John
	6. Approaches table	7. Talk and sign to John, discussing day's events
	8. Sits down, starts to eat	9. Eat, yet continue to socialize with John
	10. John talks, signs, eats, and remains seated during meal	

The importance of antecedents. Although consequences are important in maintaining behaviors, the antecedent events frequently tell a child or parent that certain behaviors will be reinforced. As discriminative stimuli, antecedents set the occasion for reinforcers. For example, when the mother in case 1 poured the milk, the child knew that if she cried at that time she would be likely to get soda instead.

Frequently, in an attempt to get control of such a situation this parent may have suggested as she poured the milk, "You have to drink milk, you will not get soda this time." However, the child cries anyway, even louder and longer than before. To terminate the crying the parent generally gives in and replaces the milk with soda. Instead of discouraging the child, the parent has only made the discriminative stimulus even stronger by adding the verbal reminder when pouring the milk.

Another example of important antecedents is demonstrated in case 4.

4 Suzi was a preschooler with a handicapping condition that caused blisters on her esophagus. She vomited often, which caused her mother great anxiety. In her anxiety, she actually inadvertently cued Suzi's behavior. Suzi, in turn, used these cues to control her mother's responses.

A (mother)	B (child)	C (mother)
Meal 1		
1. Presents food	2. Eats	3. Sits with book, does not talk to child
Meal 2		
1. Presents food	2. Gags and spits up food	3. Fusses over Suzi, cleans her up, then finishes feeding her the meal

In assessing this situation, it was found that Suzi did not vomit at every meal. Yet somehow she was getting cues about when to vomit. In an attempt to further identify these cues, the mother's meal preparation was observed as part of the antecedent behavior. Surprisingly, the typical ABC pattern for vomiting and nonvomiting meals looked like this:

A (mother)	B (child)	C (mother)
Vomiting meal		
1. Preparing lunch, says, "Suzi, you have carrots today. I hope you don't vomit them."	2. Starts eating, then gags and vomits carrots	3. Attends, cleans up child, and feeds her the rest of the meal
Nonvomiting meal		
1. Preparing lunch, says "Oh good, Suzi, you have macaroni today."	2. Eating well	3. Sitting with book, ignoring Suzi

For the vomiting meal, mother was cueing Suzi to the fact that if she vomited she would get attention, be cleaned up, and be fed her lunch. For the nonvomiting meal no such cue was given, so Suzi ate her lunch as expected. These ABC patterns were discussed with the mother, and a strategy was developed in which she would not read at mealtime, would reinforce Suzi for eating by talking with her at mealtime, and would only provide antecedent verbal cues such as in the nonvomiting meal. A later ABC pattern looked like this:

A (mother)	B (child)	C (mother)
1. "Suzi, we have carrots today."	2. Eats, smiles, and talks to mother	3. Attends to Suzi by smiling and conversing

USE OF FOOD AS A REINFORCER

The success of any behavior management program depends on the appropriate selection of the reinforcer for the individual child. Not infrequently, those concerned about the quality of the child's food intake have expressed concern over the use of food for reinforcement. It is important to recognize that the decision to use food as a reinforcer is made only after a careful assessment process in which a variety of reinforcers are tried. In some instances food is the only reinforcer with which a child can learn appropriate behaviors. If this is the case, food should be used and other reinforcers (e.g., affection and praise) can be paired with it until they also become reinforcing for the particular individual and food no longer needs to be used.

When it has been determined that food will be the most effective reinforcer for a child, several considerations are important. The first factor to be considered is the food to use. In many instances potato chips and candy are used when foods that would supply nutrients, such as raisins or cheese, might be just as effective. In any case, any food used as reinforcers must be considered as part of the total nutrient and energy intake.

Another factor to consider is the timing of food reinforcers. If one is concerned that the child eat adequate meals, training programs that use food reinforcers should not immediately precede a meal. Likewise, if success in the training program is important, a program using food reinforcers should not directly follow a meal. Any individual may become satiated by food unless adequate time has elapsed between intervals of food intake.

Satiation can also occur when too much of the same food is given to ensure maximum effectiveness of the reinforcer. Particular foods used during a training program should not be available to the child at any other time of the day. For instance, a child may be given a dish of ice cream daily at home. If a decision is made to use a dish of ice cream in a program at school, the ice cream should no longer be available at home.

Consistency is also important when applying reinforcers. As children learn an increasing variety of behaviors, they learn about new and different reinforcers. Food and feeding habits may be incorporated into behavioral repertoires designed to gain adult attention. Throwing utensils or food may cause a variety of interesting adult reactions. A parent may laugh at one such incident, respond with anger at another, and at a third may feed the child in exasperation. In the effort to keep up with the child, parents may respond inconsistently, depending on their mood at the time. Consistency means that desirable behaviors generally are reinforced, whereas undesirable behaviors are not reinforced and may even be punished. The child should know what desirable behaviors are expected by his or her parents and, in turn, what consequences can be expected for certain behaviors.

TEACHING SELF-FEEDING BEHAVIORS

In addition to the use of reinforcement, **shaping** and **fading** techniques are useful for teaching new behaviors and skills. Both of these procedures are used by parents and professionals for teaching feeding behaviors.

Shaping is the reinforcement of successive approximations to a desired behavior. In this procedure the behavior is broken down into its component steps. The types and number of steps are determined by the task to be learned. The first step is reinforced; when that step is learned, the next step is added and the reinforcement is shifted to the second step in the chain of responses that lead to the desired behavior.

Teaching Spoon-Feeding by Shaping

1. Desired behavior: independent spoon-feeding
2. Changing steps in child responses
   a. Child looks at spoon
   b. Child moves hand toward spoon
   c. Child touches spoon
   d. Child picks up spoon
   e. Child puts spoon in dish
   f. Child scoops food
   g. Child brings food to mouth
   h. Child takes food off spoon
   i. Child returns spoon to dish
3. Reinforcement: bites of food or other reinforcers as each step is accomplished

Fading is a different procedure in that the entire behavior is used each time for reinforcement. Instead of requiring the child's responses to proceed through several steps, the trainer's cues are changed as the child's skill develops. For example, the trainer holds the child's hand around the spoon and puts the child through the motions of scooping food onto the spoon, bringing the spoon to the mouth, and returning the spoon to the dish. As the child gradually assumes independent movement, physical assistance is decreased and the trainer only provides assistance as needed to complete the task. The number and type of trainer cues needed depends on the task to be learned and the abilities of the child.

Teaching Spoon-Feeding by Fading

1. Desired behavior: independent spoon-feeding
2. Steps:
   a. Holding child's hand around spoon, scoop food, and bring arm, hand, and spoon to mouth. Allow child to take food off spoon in mouth, then (still holding child's hand around spoon) return spoon to dish.
   b. Holding child's hand around spoon, bring it toward mouth and allow child to complete movement to mouth if possible. Assist through rest of cycle.
   c. Assist child in holding spoon and scooping food. By touching arm slightly, provide cues that assist child in completing movement to mouth. Also by touches, assist child in returning spoon to dish.
   d. Provide only as much assistance as child needs to pick up spoon, scoop food, move spoon to mouth, and return to dish.

The actual number of steps delineated for any given individual depends on the developmental level and skill that the individual possesses before using either of these procedures.

Using the Behavior You Want to Extinguish as a Reinforcer

Anytime the actual behavior can be used as a reinforcer, it becomes under your control and can be changed. Annie was a child with severe handicaps whose meals were given in liquid form in a bottle. At almost every meal she was offered food on a spoon, but when she refused it, she was given her bottle to hold for herself and was left alone. Thus, she was being continuously reinforced for refusing food on a spoon.

A plan was devised in which her bottle would be used as a reinforcer for Annie taking food in any other way. Because she was reinforced for refusing food from a spoon, it was decided to start with teaching her to drink from a cup with a cover and spout. Accordingly, every 4 to 5 swallows Annie took from the cup, she was reinforced with 4 to 5 swallows from her bottle. At first, much of the cup food was spit out, but by the second meal Annie got the idea, and she began to swallow the food from the cup.

In addition to the bottle as a reinforcer, she received positive attention for drinking from the cup. By the sixth meal, Annie was drinking her whole meal from the cup, with just a bit of food as "dessert" from the bottle.

Then it was decided to try spoon-feeding again, this time using the cup as a reinforcer. The bottle would be given only occasionally with juice. The same procedures were repeated, only this time for every mouthful of thickened food taken by spoon, a drink of milk was given from the cup.

At first the spoon with a bit of food on the end was touched onto her lips, followed by a drink from the cup. As soon as she accepted this (by the third spoonful), food on the spoon was introduced further into her mouth, until by the end of the meal she was accepting half-full spoonfuls. By the next meals she was reinforced with the cup for several spoonfuls of food.

This type of program, using one behavior to reinforce and strengthen another, was a very effective method of learning for Annie. She learned to accept a variety of soft table food, some of which she was learning to chew. She learned to hold a cup by herself, and she was beginning to learn to feed herself with a spoon.

GENERAL CONSIDERATIONS IN THE USE OF BEHAVIOR MANAGEMENT TECHNIQUES

Behavior modification is generally easy to use as a method of therapeutic intervention. The process of values clarification steps parents go through to identify those behaviors they want to foster in addition to those they want to eliminate can take time. The main difficulty lies in the behavioral analysis, which is necessary to pinpoint the specific behaviors and their consequences. Frequently, the relationships between behaviors and their consequences (particularly when two or more persons are involved) are difficult to discover, and care must be taken to delineate them with accuracy and reliability. Behavior is never simple, and it becomes increasingly complex when viewed within a framework of human interaction. Yet to try to remedy behaviors in isolation is to treat them outside the context of their everyday occurrence. This, in turn, leads to unsuccessful programs.

The preceding examples have been assessed by direct observation of mealtime behaviors, yet there are more complex situations that might preclude direct observation or that could be greatly altered by the presence of an observer. In-home videotaped recordings frequently work well for these situations. Parents are usually willing to allow several meals to be videotaped to pinpoint difficulties. These tapes are analyzed according to their ABC patterns. Important segments of tape are then played back to the parents, who frequently are able to discover the problems themselves. Frequently, this is an impetus for them to discuss their feelings and concerns about the situations and to generate alternative ways of behaving with their children. The combination of media and behavioral approaches to parent training for children with behavioral and developmental disabilities are considered to be effective means for dealing with a variety of child development issues.[8,9] Professionals must consider all the possible effects of the techniques before implementing them and should secure assistance while learning the procedures involved. Collaboration of nutritionists, nurses, and professionals from other disciplines helps continually refine observation and recording techniques and management procedures. The role of each discipline in the analysis, program design, and implementation must be well defined to make the program successful.

During nutrition and feeding evaluation, observations of parental and child behaviors by professionals from two or more disciplines help to identify more reliably the cause of a specific problem. Programs should be designed jointly with parents by one team member who is skilled in behavior management. Changes in physical growth, nutrient intake, and behavior should be monitored on an interdisciplinary basis to direct attention to both psychosocial (behavioral) and physical parameters.

Summary

Feeding and nutrition problems during childhood may result from inappropriate parent-child interactions. Behavior management programs when adequately implemented can resolve these problems. Observations of parent-child interactions give clues as to the antecedent to the behavior and the reinforcers that cause it to continue. Reinforcers used in behavior management programs must be individualized for each client. If food is used as a reinforcer, the program and nutrient intake should be carefully monitored to ensure that it does not compromise the child's nutritional status.

REVIEW QUESTIONS

1. Define positive and negative reinforcers.
2. Why are antecedents important when analyzing behavior?
3. What food behaviors are most often modified with behavior modification?
4. Why does one collect ABCs?
5. How does one teach self-feeding using behavior modification techniques to a developmentally delayed child?

SUGGESTED LEARNING ACTIVITIES

1. Observe a child eating a family meal. What cues do parents give the child to eat? Identify positive and negative reinforcers parents consciously or unconsciously use.
2. How would you identify appropriate foods and reinforcers for a child who needs a behavior management program?
3. Describe feeding problem behaviors for which a behavior management program would be appropriate.
4. Define factors that should be monitored to ensure that a child's nutritional status is not compromised when a behavioral management program is planned to change a child's feeding behavior.
5. Design a behavior management program to effect an increase in textures of food acceptable to a developmentally delayed child.

REFERENCES

1. France KG, Hudson SM: Behavior management of infant sleep disturbance, *J Appl Behav Anal* 23(1):91, 1990.
2. Rostain AL: Attention deficit disorders in children and adolescents: difficult diagnoses in pediatrics, *Pediatr Clin North Am* 38:3, 1991.
3. Selinske JE, Greer RD: A functional analysis of the comprehensive application of behavior analysis to schooling, *J Appl Behav Anal* 24:107, 1991.
4. Epstein LH and others: Ten-year followup of behavioral, family-based treatment for obese children, *JAMA* 264:19, 1990.
5. Finney JW: Preventing common feeding problems in infants and young children, *Pediatr Clin North Am* 33:4, 1986.
6. Cooper, JO, Heron TE, Heward WL: *Applied behavior analysis,* Columbus, Ohio, 1987, Merrill.
7. Peterson LW: Operant approach to observation and recording, *Nurs Outlook* 15:28, 1967.
8. Dauz-Williams P, Harrison-Elder J, Hill S: Media approach to family training in behavior management: two families, *Issues Comp Pediatr Nurs* 9:59, 1986.
9. Van Hasslet VB, Sisson LA, Aach SR: Parent training to increase compliance in a young multihandicapped child, *J Behav Ther Exp Psychiatry* 18:3, 275, 1987.

9
Vegetarian Food Patterns for Infants and Children

Cristine M. Trahms

✦✦

Objectives

After studying this chapter, the student should:

✔ *Be aware of the effect of vegetarian and vegan food patterns on the nutritional status and growth of infants and children.*

✔ *Understand nutritional and growth parameters that should be monitored for children who follow vegetarian food patterns.*

✔ *Understand which combinations of foods provide adequate energy, protein, and all other nutrients for children who follow vegetarian food patterns.*

✔ *Be able to provide guidance for texture modification of foods for young children on vegetarian food patterns.*

✔ *Understand appropriate ways to counsel children and families who have chosen to follow vegetarian food patterns.*

Using plant foods as the primary source of nutrients in the food pattern, for example, a vegetarian diet, is both a traditional and a recent dietary pattern. Many religious groups have traditionally advocated a meat-free food pattern, and this practice continues today. The people of many countries have also historically been vegetarian or near vegetarian, not necessarily by choice, but because of limited food availability.

In the United States the early vegetarian movement in the nineteenth century believed that morality was directly related to physiology and nutritional well-being. Movement leaders such as Sylvester Graham (graham crackers, graham flour) and John Harvey Kellogg (breakfast cereals) were both fanatical in their beliefs and more interested in the moral implications of the vegetarian diet than the nutritional ones.[1] Though they left a legacy of foods they originated, the vegetarian pattern of eating and nutritional merits was overshadowed by the attachment to moral issues. Only recently has objective evaluation of vegetarian nutrition been approached in the United States.

Currently, many people are choosing a nonmeat food pattern; in 1985 it was estimated that 6.5 million people in the United States were vegetarian; by 1995 that number had increased to 12.4 million people.[2] Families and individuals are making this choice for a variety of religious, ecological, philosophical, and health reasons. Thus the nonmeat food pattern may be prescribed by the organized group or based on the personal choices of the individual. The generally accepted definitions of nonmeat food patterns are shown in table 9-1. Many people who describe themselves as **vegetarians** may eat meat as often as once a week or twice a month, while other vegetarians may choose rigid food patterns that forbid them even yeast and honey. More than half of all vegetarians are **lacto-ovovegetarians,** and less than 10% adhere to a **vegan** food pattern. Few of those interviewed had parents who were also vegetarian, but most expected their own children to continue the vegetarian food pattern. About one-fourth of these vegetarians were affiliated with traditional religious groups.[2] Since individuals seldom make their personal food choices based on these descriptive categories, it is reasonable to evaluate foods as sources of nutrients rather than to impose labels on individual food patterns. This method of evaluation also provides an appropriate basis for nutrition education.

The practice of eating meat does not inherently ensure good health, just as the practice of omitting meat does not ensure poor health. The interrelationships of nutritional needs, food choices, health practices, religious convictions, and social mores are complex. The exclusion of one food or group of foods does not necessarily swing the pendulum of health or nutritional adequacy in either the positive or the negative direction. Dissimilar food and health practices among groups often make it difficult to interpret reported data. Therefore when discussing vegetarianism—the concept of not eating meat—one must carefully consider all other factors.

TABLE 9-1   *Food Choice Patterns*

Vegetarian Type	Eating Pattern
Vegetarian	eats no poultry, meat, fish
Lacto-ovovegetarian	eats eggs, dairy products
Lacto-vegetarian	eats dairy products
Vegan	"strict," "pure," or "total" vegetarian; eats no animal products
Macrobiotic vegetarian	food or beverage restrictions in addition to most animal products; may use supplements, advocate fasting

HEALTH ADVANTAGES AND DISADVANTAGES

It is important to understand that there are adequate and inadequate vegetarian and vegan diets. Among the health advantages of a nonmeat food pattern for adults are decreases in cholesterol, triglycerides, and other blood lipid constituents.[3] Although there is disagreement on the specific dietary factors that support these changes, the vegetarian food pattern, both in long-term and short-term evaluations, appears to exert a positive effect on blood lipids. For adult African Americans a vegetarian diet has been shown to be associated with lower cardiovascular disease risk factors than a meat-containing diet.[4] A vegetarian food pattern also seems to reduce the incidence of obesity,[5,6] hypertension,[7,8] coronary artery disease,[9] diabetes,[10] gallstones,[11] cancer,[12] osteoporosis,[13] ischemic heart disease;[14] has improved outcome management of patients with renal disease,[15] and has maximized endurance performance.[16]

These reports are evaluations of adults in industrialized countries who have made other lifestyle changes in addition to omitting meat from their food patterns. Lifestyle factors, such as abstinence from smoking and alcohol use, a high level of exercise, or seclusion from the rest of society, must be considered potential intervening or modifying variables in the impact of the vegetarian diet on long-term health. The critical variable may not be meat at all but a complex set of relationships involving eating habits, activity, stress, body fat, and alcohol and tobacco use.[8] Nonvegetarians may achieve the benefit of a vegetarian diet by eating a carefully planned meat-containing food pattern with increased fruit, vegetables, and fiber.[17]

Many of the reports that indicate nutritional disadvantages to a vegetarian food pattern have been conducted in developing countries where the total amount of food and food choices available are limited. In these situations, lack of food to provide adequate energy and nutrient intakes determines nutritional status rather than a conviction to be vegetarian. A negative impact of a vegetarian food pattern for adults has also been reported in the United States. Young adults have become overzealous in following specific teachings or omitting specific foodstuffs from their food patterns. One example is the Zen **macrobiotic** followers who felt that tea and brown rice were the way to purity. Even the leaders of the group warned against this extreme practice and encouraged a more moderate food intake pattern that included grains, legumes, fruits, and vegetables. Iron status appears to be problematic even for adults who carefully plan their vegetarian food pattern. All iron consumed by the vegetarian group was nonheme; the nonvegetarian group consumed 10% of their iron as heme iron. Both male and female vegetarians had lower ferritin concentrations than nonvegetarians even though iron intake was higher.[18] Adolescent women, however, had low iron intakes and iron stores regardless of vegetarian/nonvegetarian status.[19]

In general, the more restricted the pattern of food choices, the more likely the individual is to be at high nutritional risk. Young children and pregnant women, who are generally considered to be at high nutritional risk, are thought to be particularly vulnerable to food intake patterns that limit both the quantity and the kinds of food consumed.

Growth of Children

Birth weight. There appear to be no detrimental effects on the offspring of the vegetarian or vegan mother if she chooses a food pattern that provides the required nutrients in appropriate quantities to support the pregnancy. No differences in birth weights between the vegetarian infants (both extensive and limited food group avoidances) and the control infants were noted.[20] Infants born to vegan mothers on "The Farm" (a collective community in Tennessee) had weights comparable to the U.S. average.[21] Birth weight was 180 gm lower for macrobiotic than for control group women; however, increasing birth weight was associated with increasing maternal weight gain and frequency of consumption of dairy products and fish by macrobiotic women.[22,23] Birth weight appears to be affected by maternal serum zinc status. Women with low serum zinc levels were more likely to have infants of low birth weight regardless of vegetarian status.[24]

Infants

Growth success and growth failure have been reported for children on vegetarian and vegan food patterns as shown in table 9-2. Similar patterns of growth for infants have been described for the Dutch and Boston children, for whom weight and length were within the normal limits for the first 6 to 8 months of life.[25,26] In general, infants who receive an appropriate quantity and quality of breast milk or formula grow well. Vegetarian and vegan women tend to breastfeed their infants until the end of the first year, which supports growth in early infancy.

Growth rate declined fairly rapidly in late infancy and then reached its nadir by 18 months of age.[22,25] Weaning is a time of nutritional vulnerability for all children. This vulnerability is demonstrated by changing growth patterns. Weaning from breast milk to foods of a lesser energy density and biological value of protein can negatively affect the growth of young children, regardless of whether they are vegan or vegetarian. Weaning poses a problem to vegetarian and vegan infants if the biological value of protein and energy density of foods are reduced when breast milk is discontinued and dairy foods are omitted when solids are added. Growth for all of the children was improved if they consumed some dairy products.

TABLE 9-2 *Selected Reported Weight and Height of Vegetarian and Vegan Children*

Report, Year	No. of Subjects	Mean Age	Food Pattern	Growth Reference	Size of Children
Brown, Bergan 1975[39]	10	1–6	Zen macrobiotic (vegan)	—	Mean weight and height = 40%
Shull and others, 1977[20]	72	< 5 yr	Vegetarian	Harvard	Greater than 2 years of age, subjects are the same as control for weight and height; less than 2 years of age, subjects are shorter, lighter than control
			Macrobiotic (vegan)		Slightly lower size attainment than vegan (not significant)
Dwyer and others, 1978[27]	119	2.33 yr	Vegetarian extensive vs. limited food group avoidances	Harvard	Adjusted for mid-parent height, 61% < 10th percentile, the difference is more pronounced with increased avoidances
Fulton and others, 1980[46]	48	3.8 yr	Vegan "The Farm"	HANES	Mean height and weight less than mean of HANES; height more affected; 83% had height < 50th percentile
Dwyer and others, 1982[45]	39	4 yr	Vegetarian	NCHS	Height, weight within normal limits
Dwyer and others, 1983[26]	142 + controls	0–6 yr	Macrobiotic vegetarian	NCHS	Length more affected than weight; macrobiotic children are shorter than vegetarian; females shorter for age than males
van Staveren and others, 1985[30]	92	1–3 yr	Vegetarian macrobiotic (vegan)	Dutch	Height and weight for age shorter and lighter; weight for length OK

Continued.

TABLE 9-2   Selected Reported Weight and Height of Vegetarian and Vegan Children—cont'd

Report, Year	No. of Subjects	Mean Age	Food Pattern	Growth Reference	Size of Children
Rona and others, 1987[32]	7103	Primary school age	Vegetarian	British	Weight for height, TSF is similar to nonvegetarian
Sanders, 1988[47]	37	1–6 yr	Vegan	British	Girls < 50% for weight Boys < 50% for height and weight
van Staveren, 1988[25]	300	0–8 yr	Macrobiotic	Dutch	Growth delay after 5 months, height and weight for age are shorter and lighter but within reference limits
Dagnelie and others, 1988[22]	243	0–8 yr	Macrobiotic	Dutch	0–8 months = normal growth; 8–18 months = growth lag; 2–4 years = catch-up for weight and skinfolds, not height
Dagnelie and others, 1989[42]	53 + controls	4–18 mo	Macrobiotic	Dutch	Weight gain less for macrobiotic infants, after 14 months growth stabilized at 10th percentile
O'Connell and others, 1989[21]	404	4 mo– 10 yr	Vegan "The Farm"	NCHS	1–3 year olds were shorter; by age 10 height for age, weight for age, and weight for height were in the 25th to 75th percentiles
Tayter, Stanek, 1989[41]	17 + controls	10–12 yr	Lacto-ovovegetarian	NCHS	Boys height > 50th percentile, weight > 30th percentile Girls height = 45th percentile, weight = 50th percentile
Sabate and others, 1990[31] Sabate and others, 1991[40]	2272 + controls	6–18 yr	Lacto-ovovegetarian (SDA)	NCHS	Average height and weight > 50th percentile: boys taller than controls, girls no different; both boys and girls leaner than controls

Preschool Children

Deficits in height and weight have occurred among young children on vegan diets.[25-28] Young vegan children were significantly shorter and lighter than were age- and gender-matched vegetarian children and control children.[29] Some catch-up growth has been demonstrated between 2 and 4 years of age.[21,22,28]

After adjustment for midparental height, 61% of 119 preschool vegetarian children were in less than the 20th percentile (Harvard) for height.[27] Nearly half of the children had parents who consumed macrobiotic food patterns; the remaining children were almost equally members of yoga groups, Seventh-Day Adventists, or without group affiliation. Almost all (96%) of the children had been breast-fed. The vegetarian children younger than 2 years of age showed mean weight and length velocities that were lower than the reference charts, whereas those of the older vegetarian children were comparable with reference charts.[20] This pattern of growth was also reported for Dutch children.[30]

School-Age Children

When growth patterns of vegetarian and nonvegetarian schoolchildren were compared, both groups of children demonstrated growth patterns that were compromised[26] or appropriate.[31,32] It appeared that the more limiting the food choices were, the more growth was affected. In general, length was more affected than weight, although measurements were generally within normal limits. Evaluation of food intakes suggested that protein intakes for vegetarian children were adequate, and energy intakes were below the accepted recommendations.

The availability of adequate nutrients to the child was a more significant factor than the beliefs of the parents and the concomitant prescribed food pattern. The more restrictive the food choices and quantities of food available, the greater the negative effect on growth. However, the lower relative weight of the well-nourished vegetarian schoolchildren may provide health advantages in adulthood.

Nourishment

Nutrients of concern. Young children consuming diets consisting only of plant foods seem to be at greater risk for nutritional inadequacies. The most commonly reported low dietary intakes are in protein, calcium, total energy, essential fatty acids, riboflavin, iron, zinc, folate, and vitamins B_{12} and D. A summary of reported nutrient intakes of vegan and vegetarian children is shown in table 9-3. The wide range of nutrient intake—whether generous, adequate, or inadequate—reflects differing philosophies of childrearing, beliefs about properties of foods, and economic resources of the groups evaluated.

Factors Influencing Children's Intakes

The young child depends on caregivers to provide adequate foods as sources of nutrients. The young infant being exclusively breast-fed by a mother who has a marginal or deficient vitamin B_{12} intake may have an increased risk of deficiency.[33] Older children who consume diets restricted in animal foods may also be at risk for vitamin B_{12} deficiency if the choices of foods available to them are severely restricted and exclude all animal foods. The adequacy of nutrient intake may also be affected by food preferences, which are demonstrated early in life. The older infant and toddler with rigid food preferences may be at risk for deficits of protein, energy, calcium, iron, zinc, and vitamins D and B_{12} despite adequate food availability. Table 9-4 lists situations that adversely affect the growth and nutritional well-being of the young child on a restricted food pattern.

Infants who are breast-fed but whose food patterns are not appropriately supplemented with additional foods may suffer adverse nutritional and growth effects, especially if they are weaned to a cereal gruel or other form of predominantly vegan food pattern.[28,34]

Limitations in nutrient availability may be in part related to family food choices and to the individual preferences of the child, who may not eat foods that are offered. An example of nutritional risk caused by limited food choices is the young child who was offered a grain beverage

TABLE 9-3 **Selected Reported Mean Nutrient Intakes of Vegetarian and Vegan Children**

Report, Year	No. of Subjects	Mean Age (yr)	Food Pattern	Energy (kcal)	Protein (gm)
Brown, Bergan 1975[39]	10	1–6	Zen macrobiotic (vegan)	1002–1267	34.4–41
Fulton and others, 1980[46]	48	3–8	"The Farm" vegan, boys	1580–2141	52–62
			"The Farm" vegan, girls	1509–2249	49–65
Dwyer and others, 1982[45]	39	4	Vegetarian	103/kg	3.3/kg
van Staveren and others, 1985[30]	92	1–3	Vegetarian	1020 (84–98/kg)	36 (2.8–3.5/kg)
			Macrobiotic (vegan)	1010 (85–92/kg)	31 (2.2–3.3/kg)
Sanders, 1988[47]	37	1–6	Vegan (British)	30% kcal from fat	10% kcal
Dagnelie and others, 1988[22]	50 + controls	10–20 mo	Macrobiotic (Dutch)	—	—
Taytor, Stanek, 1989[41]	17 + controls	10–12	Lacto-ovovegetarian (SDA)	Boys = 2315 Girls = 1650 (28%–31% kcal from fat)	67 56.5 (↓ than controls)
Dagnelie and others, 1989[42]	53 + controls	4–18 mo	Macrobiotic	(↓ than controls)	80% of rec (↓ than controls)
RDA, 1989*		1–3		1300	16
		4–6		1700	24

*Recommended Dietary Allowances, 1989.

TABLE 9-4 **Factors Affecting Appropriate Intake for Young Children**

Breast-feeding mother who has marginal/deficient vitamin B_{12} intake

Breast-feeding without supplemental foods after 6 months of age

Child who refuses groups of foods (beans, whole grains, most vegetables)

Texture of foods not modified for chewing and self-feeding skills of child (well-cooked grains, cooked mashed beans)

Volume of foods required to meet needs is too large (½ c milk vs. 1 c cooked broccoli for calcium)

Child has small appetite; meals and snacks are not offered at regular intervals

consisting of rice, sesame seeds, and oats in a reasonable protein complement. However, the quantities that the child was willing to consume did not provide adequate nutrients to support normal growth.

The young child on a diet composed totally or primarily of plant proteins may have problems obtaining an adequate intake of energy if the volume of food required to meet energy needs is large.

In addition to volume, texture may influence the adequacy of the intake of the young child (fig. 9-1). Many foods that contain adequate quantities of protein and are rich sources of nutrients must be texture modified for the young child; for instance, beans must be well cooked and mashed or pureed. Even rice must

Calcium (mg)	Iron (mg)	Vit D (µg)	Vit B$_{12}$ (µg)	Fiber (gm)
359–402	0.1–11.9	—	—	—
323–426	18–25	—	10.8–19.2	—
296–340	14–16	—	10.9–15.8	—
685	12–16	1.3–9.9 (51–395 IU)	0.6–4.4	—
783	7.1	0.5	—	16
345	10.8	0.3	—	24.9
52% of rec	142% of rec	Sunlight	280% of rec	—
	15% iron deficiency	—	Significantly less than controls	—
1400	17	—	—	5
1040 (↑ than controls)	10.7 (↑ than controls)	—	—	4.5 (similar to controls)
280 (↓ than controls)	5.1 (↑ than controls)	↓ than controls	0.3 (↓ than controls)	—
800	10	10 (400 IU)	0.7	—
800	10	10	1.0	—

be mixed with liquid and mashed for the infant. The young child may not chew whole grain breads well, and consequently the nutrients may not be well absorbed. The same is true for nuts, seeds, dried fruits, and some vegetables.

Cases of kwashiorkor (protein and energy deficiency) among infants whose parents were vegetarian[35,36] and poor weight gain in children fed cereal-based formulas[37–39] have been described. The infants were fed restricted quantities of kokoh (a grain milk) and other foods. The children were rehabilitated on appropriate vegetarian or near vegetarian food patterns within a few months. In all of these reports the number of children evaluated was small, and long-term observations on growth, cognitive development, or nutrient intake were not available. More recent reports do not support this degree of neglect or lack of knowledge about provision of adequate nutrients and energy to young children.

The school-age, Seventh-Day Adventist vegetarian children ingested less junk food and dairy products, but more starchy foods, protein products, fruits, and vegetables than nonvegetarian peers.[31,40] Girls had lower intakes of energy, protein, and fat, and boys had greater carbohydrate and iron and less protein intakes than nonvegetarian peers.[41] For school-age children, the more restrictive the food pattern, the shorter the child and the more compromised the intakes of energy, protein, vitamin D, and iron.[32]

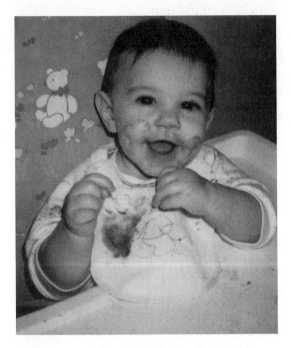

FIG. 9-1   Young children thrive when nutrients are provided in foods of appropriate texture.

Nutrient Intakes

There are adequate and inadequate vegan, vegetarian, and meat-containing food patterns. Because of rapid growth, children are at greater risk than adults for manifestation of nutrient deficiencies. Analysis of nutrient intake was completed on macrobiotic infants breast-fed until about 13 months of age, and then given solids consisting of porridge, vegetables, sesame seeds, and legumes, but no fruits or animal products. The food patterns for these infants were calculated to contain less energy, protein, fat, cholesterol, calcium, riboflavin, and vitamin B_{12} and greater amounts of fiber, iron, and thiamin than for control infants.[42,43]

Calculation of nutrient intakes of preschool children has shown that children whose food patterns excluded all animal foods consumed significantly less total protein, fat, calcium, and riboflavin than did vegetarian children and control children.[43,44] Intakes of iron and calcium were also calculated at lower than acceptable

levels. Recently the intakes of a small number of children (mean age of 4 years) consuming different types of vegetarian food patterns were evaluated. The findings suggested that these food patterns met the dietary goals for the United States for carbohydrate, fat, protein, sodium, and cholesterol. Some children had intakes limited in iron and in vitamins D and B_{12}.[45,46] Young children who received some appropriate nutrients, for example, 142% of the British recommendations for iron from whole meal bread, 280% of the recommendations for vitamin B_{12} because of supplementation, and 10% of energy from protein, but only 52% of calcium all from nuts and legumes, were shorter and lighter than their peers.[47] The limitation of nutrients in vegetarian or vegan food patterns is contingent on the foods offered or restricted and the food preferences and appetite of the child. The nutrients of concern and the probable reasons for the limitation of intake are summarized in table 9-5.

Vitamin D. Vitamin D deficiency rickets has been reported in breast-fed infants of vegan and vegetarian mothers. All of the infants had hypocalcemia, and three-fourths had **tetany** or convulsions.[48] Rickets has been identified in infants who do not receive a vitamin D supplement, whether breast- or formula-fed[49] or whether vegetarian or not.[50]

Clinical identification of rickets has recently been reported in older infants who demonstrated the classic symptoms: growth failure, listlessness, delayed motor development, and abnormal gait.[51] Bone deformity was evident on further investigation. The children received little or no cow's milk or formula and no vitamin D supplements. Not all of the children were vegetarian or vegan, again demonstrating the need to evaluate food patterns for specific nutrients.

Healing, however, occurred with dietary changes in all cases. Of 52 children on macrobiotic food patterns, 88% had vitamin D intakes of less than 100 IU/day compared with vegetarian children, of whom only 18% had vitamin D intakes this low.[52] Although five children had pathological findings related to bone mineralization, roentgenograms did not indicate rickets. Clinically, only three children demonstrated

TABLE 9-5 *Nutrients of Concern for Young Children on Restricted Food Patterns*

Nutrient	Reason for Concern
Vitamin D	Fortified dairy foods or fats may not be offered
Calcium	Highly bioavailable calcium from dairy foods or vegetables higher in calcium may not be offered or accepted
Vitamin B_{12} (cobalamin)	Vitamin B_{12} not found in plant foods; supplement may not be offered
Zinc	Whole grains or fortified cereals may not be offered or accepted
Iron	Nonheme iron is less bioavailable than heme iron; bioavailability may not be enhanced
Fiber	Whole grains may not be well cooked or well chewed by the child for maximum break down and utilization of nutrients
Energy	Volume of "bulky" high-fiber foods required to meet energy needs may be too much
Protein	High-quality protein from dairy foods, eggs, fortified soy foods may not be offered or accepted
Fat	25–30% of energy from fats may not be offered

signs (bowed legs) that could possibly be attributed to vitamin D deficiency. The serum calcium and serum phosphorus levels of the children on both macrobiotic and vegetarian food patterns were within normal limits. Eight of the children on macrobiotic food patterns and two of the vegetarian children had elevated serum alkaline phosphatase levels.

Calcium. Calcium deficiency and osteomalacia in the presence of an adequate intake of protein and energy further emphasize the need to evaluate all of the nutrient components of a food pattern.[53] In the presence of vitamin D, calcium is absorbed at about 30% to 35%; without vitamin D, this rate decreases to about 10%. It is challenging to provide adequate dietary calcium without dairy products or calcium fortified drinks.[54]

Vitamin B_{12}. Vegan women who do not take vitamin B_{12} supplements may have low vitamin B_{12} levels in their milk, and their infants may demonstrate compromised metabolic status.[55] Case reports cite growth failure and other clinical signs of vitamin B_{12} deficiency in infants who were breast-fed by vegan women.[56] Apparently these infants required more vitamin B_{12} than could be supplied by breast milk of women with marginal vitamin B_{12} stores. The more restricted the food pattern, the greater the risk for deficiency for vitamin B_{12}.[57,58]

Zinc. The status of zinc nutriture for vegan and vegetarian children has not been fully evaluated. It would seem that zinc intake may be limited in some restricted food patterns. A combination of increased fiber intake, calcium, and phytic acid plus low bioavailable zinc led to decreased serum zinc levels in adults.[59]

The trace element content of vegetarian diets may be similar or higher than that of nonvegetarian diets. However, the bioavailability of the trace elements may be compromised.[60] Children who are vegetarian may be more vulnerable to suboptimal zinc status.

Iron. Vegan and vegetarian food patterns rely on nonheme iron from plant sources to meet iron needs for growth and development. The absorption of nonheme iron is increased when ingested in the presence of ascorbic acid, whereas calcium inhibits iron absorption. There is also an important dose-effect relationship between iron absorption and the phytate content of the food pattern. Fermentation (e.g., bread with yeast) breaks down the phytate components and increases the availability of the iron in whole grains.

Children who consume very restricted diets have iron deficiency; about 15% of young macrobiotic children were iron deficient. Children who consume a balanced lacto-vegetarian or vegan diet have an iron status similar to children who eat meat.[61]

Fiber. Absorption of nutrients may be a problem if the fiber content of the infant's or young child's food pattern is high. High fiber intakes render intakes less energy dense and are believed to decrease intestinal transit time, lead to malabsorption, and bind iron, calcium, zinc, and other trace metals. Recent recommendations for fiber suggest "age plus 5 grams" for children over age 3 years. This recommendation is for most American children whose intakes of fiber are often low and for vegetarian children whose intakes are often high.[62]

Energy. The volume of food required to meet the energy needs of young children may interfere with adequate intakes. This is especially true for children who are offered bulky foods without texture modification. A model proposed by Payne[63] suggests that an adequate, safe protein/energy ratio in young children is close to 5% of total energy from protein. Since most cereal grains seem to provide protein levels close to this, energy deficit rather than protein deficit may be the cause of protein/energy malnutrition in children. Energy intake should be adequate to promote acceptable growth.

Protein. Protein utilization is affected by a variety of factors, including quality and quantity of ingested protein, percent of energy as fat, total energy intake, biological variation of the individual, and growth and maintenance needs (e.g., age and nutritional state).[64] Protein utilization among young children has been evaluated and is successful in terms of the ability of vegetable protein to maintain growth and nitrogen balance for young children. Commercially formulated legume products and combinations of grains, legumes, and milk solids promote rehabilitation from malnutrition.[65-67] In the United States few if any children must exist on a single food that in turn must supply all or the majority of nutrients. The young breast- or formula-fed infant is the exception. Infant food must be chosen carefully to meet the rigorous nutrient requirements for supporting normal growth and development.

Fat. Fat absorption in young children depends on levels of dietary protein intake.[68] Low protein intakes, even with adequate energy intakes, are detrimental to maximum fat absorption and may ultimately increase total energy requirements. Children on diets containing 5% or more of total energy as protein (FAO/WHO recommendation) showed improvement of fat absorption as protein intakes increased.

Choosing Foods for Young Children

Protein. It is important that the protein sources offered to children be appropriately combined so that the pattern of amino acid intake will be adequate to support normal growth.

Combining proteins. In combining plant proteins, not only must foods that supplement the most limiting amino acids be combined, but they should be combined in proportion for the most efficient utilization of protein. This ratio becomes of little concern when adequate quantities of protein and energy are available to the young child. Appetites of young children fluctuate widely on a day-to-day basis, making it important that all foods eaten provide nutrients rather than only energy.

Careful attention to combining plant proteins in the best proportion for optimal utilization is a must, especially for the child of a vegan family. Some combinations that are practical and acceptable to young children are shown in table 9-6.

Preschool-age children are in the process of developing individual food patterns and are not amenable to eating foods because they are good sources of protein. It is often difficult to persuade children to eat foods in a proportional relationship or to eat a sufficient volume of legumes, grains, seeds, and nuts in a form they can easily digest. Therefore it is difficult to provide sufficient quality and quantity of proteins and an adequate amount of energy to support normal growth for young children without a concentrated source of high–biological value protein such as dairy foods or eggs in their food pattern.

Meeting the Nutrient Needs of Vegetarian Children

Examples of recorded food intakes of vegan, vegetarian, and nonvegetarian children that show the variety of foods and general quantities needed to provide reasonable intakes of nutrients are given in table 9-7. Calculated

TABLE 9-6 *Table Foods Appropriate for a Vegetarian Toddler*

Yogurt, cottage cheese	Macaroni and cheese
Cooked, mashed beans	Toasted whole grain
Cooked rice with	breads, bagels
vegetables	Soy-based meat analogs
Cooked cereal with	Crackers with cheese
fruit	Legume-vegetable
Peanut butter on bread	soups
Pieces of peeled fruit	Cut up bean/cheese
Pieces of cooked	enchiladas
vegetable	English muffin pizza
Sauteed tofu with	with cheese
vegetables	Tortilla with refried
Fruit muffins made	beans
with yogurt	Hummus with pita
Peanut butter on apple	wedges
wedges	Scrambled eggs with
Oatmeal cookie with	toast wedges
milk	Cottage cheese with
Peanut butter cookie	fruit
with milk	Vegetable patty pieces
Spaghetti with tomato	Vegetable stir fry with
lentil sauce	tofu
Cornbread with	Beans and rice with
vegetable soup	tortilla

nutrient intakes from these food records are shown in table 9-8.

Child 1 was provided a vegan food pattern without dairy foods or eggs. The intake was limited in protein, energy, vitamin C, vitamin B_{12}, zinc, calcium, iron, and fat. Some of these limitations resulted from the vegan food pattern and some resulted from the unwillingness of the child to accept certain foods. No vitamin or mineral supplements were provided. Growth of this child was less than the 5th percentile for weight and length, and the 25th percentile for weight for length. Growth and size were compromised because of an inadequate intake of foods to provide energy, protein, fat, and essential nutrients.

Child 2 was also offered a vegan food pattern. This child was offered and consumed a greater variety of foods. Total protein, energy, and iron intakes were more appropriate than Child 1. Fiber intake was high and potentially compromised utilization of nutrients. Calcium intake was inadequate because no readily concentrated and bioavailable source of calcium was ingested. No vitamin or mineral supplements were provided. This child was at the 10th percentile for weight and length, and the 25th percentile for weight for length.

Child 3 was offered a vegetarian food pattern that included milk. Intakes of protein, calcium, and fat were generous; other components were at or above recommended levels. No vitamin or mineral supplements were provided. Growth and size were appropriate. Weight, length, and weight for length were at the 50th percentile.

Child 4 consumed a food intake pattern that included meat and provided a generous intake of protein, energy, and calcium. Calculated intake of iron from food was less than the current recommendations. A supplement was provided. Fiber, zinc, and vitamin C intakes were at less than the current recommendations for age. Fat intake was at the current recommended level of percent of total energy intake. Growth and size were appropriate. Weight, length, and weight for length were at the 50th percentile.

Special attention needs to be paid to providing adequate sources of vitamins, minerals, and trace metals in a form that is bioavailable in the food patterns of young children. Factors that interfere with absorption of nutrients and ways to enhance absorption are shown in table 9-9. Commercially prepared and fortified soy-based infant formulas are appropriate sources of all of the critical nutrients for young children. Other sources of nutrients that are of concern for young children are shown in table 9-10. Nutrient values of foods common to nonmeat food patterns and generally accepted by young children are shown in table 9-11.

Zinc. Although the information on zinc intakes of children is limited, it is known that zinc intakes are at risk for inadequacy in a vegan food pattern. Phytate in cereal is known to bind zinc and decrease its availability. It has been suggested that foods highest in zinc and lowest in fiber, such as tofu (soy cheese) and hard cheeses,

TABLE 9-7   Recorded 1-Day Intakes of Young Children

Food	Portion Size	Food	Portion Size
Child 1 (age 12 months)—Inadequate Vegan Intake		**Child 3 (age 13 months)—Vegetarian Intake**	
		Milk, whole	9 oz
Oatmeal, cooked	½ c	Cereal mixture	
Raisins	1 t	Cornmeal, dry	¼ c
Yellow squash, cooked	½ c	Wheat germ	3 T
Apple	1 medium	Milk, whole	¼ c
Oatmeal, cooked	1 c	Apple	1 T
Yams, cooked	½ c	Soybeans, cooked	1 c
Pudding		Apricot, dried	2 halves
Apple cider	1 c	Apple	½ medium
Arrowroot flour	1 t	Potato, baked	½ small
No supplements		Tomato	1 small
		Cheddar cheese, grated	¼ c
		Soy oil	2 t
Child 2 (age 14 months)—Better Vegan Intake		Milk, whole	9 oz
Kokoh (cereal mixture)	1¼ c	Milk, whole	9 oz
Rice	½ c	No supplements	
Sweet rice	¼ c		
Whole oats	⅛ c		
Sesame seeds	⅛ c	**Child 4 (age 12 months)—Nonvegetarian Intake**	
Wakame (sea weed)	½ t	Peach, canned	½
Squash, baked	⅛ c	Link sausage	2
Whole wheat noodles	½ c	Toast, white	½ slice
Miso soup		Margarine	½ t
Miso (fermented soy)	1 t	Egg yolk	1
Scallions	1 t	2% Milk	8 oz
Onion	1 t	2% Milk	8 oz
Kokoh	1¼ c	Veal	50 gm
Nori (sea weed)	1 piece	Cracker	1
Cauliflower	¼ c	Rice, cooked	½ c
Adzuki beans, cooked	⅛ c	Tomato	¼ medium
Watercress	1 sprig	2% Milk	8 oz
Brown rice pudding	1¼ c	2% Milk	8 oz
Squash, cooked	¼ c	Supplement: Poly-vi-sol	6 ml/day
Apple, baked	2 T		
Raisins	1 t		
No supplements			

be emphasized in the vegetarian food pattern to maintain an adequate intake of this nutrient.[69] Miso, wheat germ, legumes, nuts, and sprouts are also reasonable food sources of zinc.[70]

Vitamin B$_{12}$. Since animal foods are the primary sources of vitamin B$_{12}$, care must be taken

to avoid vitamin B$_{12}$ deficiency for the infant and young child by ensuring adequate maternal stores during lactation and by providing overt sources for the young child. These sources may be supplemented brewer's yeast, vitamin B$_{12}$ tablets, dairy foods, or eggs. Recent data

TABLE 9-8   *Calculated Nutrients in Recorded Intakes of Young Children*

Nutrient	Child 1 Inadequate Vegan	Child 2 Better Vegan	Child 3 Vegetarian	Child 4 Nonvegetarian	RDA* 1–3 Years
Protein (gm)	11.3	36.4	67.3	56.5	16
Energy (kcal)	547	1105	1323	1961	1300
Dietary fiber (gm)	9.4	25.7	13	1.8	—
Vitamin A (RE)	383	599	667	746	400
Vitamin D (μg)	0	0	10	11	10
Vitamin C (mg)	27	31	45	26	40
Vitamin B_{12} (μg)	0	0	3.3	5.2	0.7
Zinc (mg)	2.3	8.3	8.5	7.4	10
Calcium (mg)	80	490	1422	1335	800
Iron (mg)	4	12.9	9.9	3.9	10
Fat (gm)	5	24.5	61.7	33.6	—
%kcal as fat	8	20	42	31	30

*Recommended Dietary Allowances, 1989.

TABLE 9-9   *Factors that Influence Utilization of Nutrients*

Factor Limiting Utilization	To Enhance Absorption
Phytate (binds zinc)	Use cooked or leavened grain products, include dairy foods
Fiber (binds iron, calcium)	Cook legumes well
Nonheme iron	Consume with ascorbic acid–rich foods
Bulk	Modify texture and offer concentrated sources of energy (e.g., nut butters, dried fruit spreads, avocado)
Oxalate (binds calcium)	Offer milk

suggest that vitamin B_{12} from algae and other plant foods is not bioavailable.[71,72]

Vitamin D. Vitamin D needs may be met via exposure to sunlight, fortified milk or soy formula, vitamin D supplements, or cod liver oil.

No one is sure how much sunlight a person needs to make vitamin D because it depends on exposure, time, and the angle of the sun. However, children who are exposed to sunlight on a regular basis do not demonstrate vitamin D deficiency.

Calcium. Calcium is readily available from cow's milk or a commercially prepared and fortified soy formula. Dark, green leafy vegetables and legumes are also reasonable sources as is firm tofu that has been precipitated with calcium sulfate instead of magnesium (e.g., 115 mg vs. 13 mg calcium/100 gm tofu).[73] A calcium supplement may be needed if adequate food sources are not ingested.

Iron. Iron deficiency anemia is a common occurrence in childhood regardless of food choice patterns. The most bioavailable sources of iron are muscle meats. The bioavailability of plant sources of iron is variable and less than that of heme sources.[74] However, nonheme iron bioavailability is improved if ascorbic acid–rich foods are consumed at the same meal. Guidelines for enhancing the nutrient levels of diets of children with macrobiotic food patterns have been proposed (table 9-12). Macrobiotic food patterns are strictly proscribed because of religious or moral tenets and are generally not completely

TABLE 9-10   *Sources of Nutrients of Concern for Young Children Consuming Vegetarian Diets*

Nutrient of Concern	Sources
Iron: plant foods do not contain heme iron	Legumes, green leafy vegetables, whole grains, fortified cereals, dried fruits, blackstrap molasses
Vitamin B_{12}: plant foods do not contain vitamin B_{12}	Eggs, dairy foods, vitamin B_{12}–fortified foods such as nutritional yeast, breakfast cereals, soymilks, meat analogues, and supplements (not miso, tempeh, sea vegetables)
Vitamin D: limited sunlight exposure	Regular exposure to sunlight, or source of vitamin D from fortified milk, supplement, or cod liver oil. Infants should receive a vitamin D supplement.
Calcium: without dairy foods, bioavailable calcium intake may be limited	Dairy foods, fortified soy formulas, legumes, tofu processed with calcium sulfate, almonds, sesame seeds, low-oxalate green leafy vegetables
Zinc: without meat and dairy foods, zinc may be limited	Legumes, hard cheeses, whole grain breads and cereals, wheat germ, fortified cereals, tofu, miso, nuts

vegetarian. These guidelines were developed with the support of the macrobiotic group in the Netherlands who have participated in research on the nutritional adequacy of this food pattern.[23]

Counseling the Vegetarian Family

The word *vegetarian* has a specific nuance or value system attached to it for all persons who have chosen to apply that label to themselves. Health care professionals in the counseling role should carefully examine their own biases and, whether they are negative or positive, try to approach the family or household as open mindedly as possible.

It seems reasonable that one should first ask the family to describe the foods regularly included and excluded in the family's food pattern and the individual's food pattern (see chapter 2). A survey of women in Seattle indicated the importance of this approach.[75] Less than 50% of the persons who described themselves as vegetarians never ate meat, 30% ate meat once or twice per month, and nearly 10% ate meat as often as once per week.

Every food pattern that a person chooses has positive aspects that should be defined and reinforced (fig. 9-2). Clinical experience indicates that a counseling and supportive role is much more effective than a directive or argumentative approach. People can, in fact, adequately meet their nutrient needs in a variety of ways, and the individual variability of nutritional needs is wide.

SPECIAL CONCERNS FOR INFANTS AND CHILDREN

For the infant and young child, linear growth and rate of weight gain can be used as indices of appropriate energy intake. It is appropriate to ask the mother of an exclusively breast-fed infant to describe her own intake. All the usual guidelines regarding adequate fluid, protein, calcium, and energy to maintain health and support lactation are appropriate.

It is necessary to ensure that the breast-fed infant receives adequate supplies of iron and vitamins B_{12} and D. Iron in breast milk is well

TABLE 9-11 *Nutrient Values of Selected Foods Providing Nutrients of Concern for Vegetarian Children*

Food	Amount	Protein (gm)	Energy (kcal)	Ca (mg)	Fe (mg)	Zn (mg)	B_{12} (µg)
Baby cereal, dry	4 T						
Mixed		1.2	36	68	7.2	.44	
Oatmeal		1.2	40	72	7.2	3.6	
Rice		.8	36	80	7.2	2.0	
Baby vegetables, strained	1 jar, 128 gm						
Green beans		1.7	32	49	.96	.26	0
Carrots		1.1	34	29	.47	.2	0
Peas		2.8	68	16	.72	.5	0
Squash		1.1	30	30	.38	.18	0
Meat analogues:							
(Loma Linda)							
Chicken, frozen	2 sl, 57 gm	10	160	25	1.1	.63	2.0
Ocean fillet, frozen	1, 47 gm	11	130	45	.9	.66	2.0
Vege-burger, canned	½ c, 108 gm	22	110	32	2.7	1.1	2.0
Sizzle franks, canned	2, 70 gm	10	170	49	1.6	.78	2.0
Sandwich spread, canned	3 T, 48 gm	4.0	70	21	.7	.62	2.0
Vege-scallops	6 pc, 78 gm	14	70	17	1.1	1.1	2.0
Stew pac, canned	2 oz, 57 gm	10	70	17	.73	.62	1.0
(Millstone)							
Meatless loaf	1 oz	9.9	90	67	2.2	.46	
Vege-burger	½ c, 108 gm	20	110	12	1.1	2.7	
(Worthington)							
Choplets	2, 92 gm	19.1	105	11	1.9		
Cereals, cooked							
Cream of Rice	¾ c	1.6	95	6	.3	.29	
Cream of Wheat	¾ c	2.9	100	38	7.7	.24	
Farina, enriched	¾ c	2.5	87	3	.88	.12	
Oatmeal	¾ c	4.5	108	15	1.2	.86	
Cereals, ready-to-eat, fortified							
Cheerios	½ c	2.1	55	24	2.2	.29	.75
Corn Chex	½ c	1	55	1	.9	.06	.75
Crispy Rice	½ c	.9	56	2.5	.35	.23	.4
Kix	¾ c	1.2	55	17.5	4	.14	.75
Wheat Chex	⅓ c	1.4	50	5.5	2.2	.37	.75
Cheese							
Cheddar	1 oz	7.1	114	204	.19	.88	.23
Cottage	1 T	3.5	29	17	.7	.2	.18
Cream cheese	2 T	2.1	99	23	.34	.15	.12
Mozzarella, part skim	1 oz	7.8	79	207	.7	.89	.26
Parmesan, grated	1 T	2.1	23	69	.5	.16	
Ricotta, part skim	¼ c	7.2	85	168	.27	.83	.18
Swiss	1 oz	8.1	107	272	.5	1.11	.48

Continued.

TABLE 9-11   *Nutrient Values of Selected Foods Providing Nutrients*
of Concern for Vegetarian Children—cont'd

Food	Amount	Protein (gm)	Energy (kcal)	Ca (mg)	Fe (mg)	Zn (mg)	B_{12} (µg)
Egg, large	1, 50 gm	6.1	79	28	1.04	.72	.66
Dairy products							
Milk, whole	8 oz	8	150	288	—	1.0	1.34
Lowfat, 2%	8 oz	8.1	121	297	.12	.95	.89
Yogurt, whole	8 oz	7.9	139	274	.11	1.34	.84
Infant formulas							
Mead Johnson							
Enfamil	8 oz	3.2	160	112	3.04	1.28	4
Prosobee	8 oz	4.8	160	152	3.04	1.28	4.8
Ross Labs							
Similac	8 oz	3.2	160	120	2.88	1.2	4
Isomil	8 oz	4.0	160	168	2.88	1.2	7.2
Soy products							
Soy milk	1 c	6.6	79	10	1.38	.54	0
Soy meal, defatted	¼ c	15	103	74	4.2	1.5	0
Miso	¼ c	4.1	71	23	.9	1.1	—
Tempeh	¼ c	3.9	41	19	.5	.4	—
Tofu, raw, firm	¼ c	4.9	46	65	3.3	.5	0
Grains							
Masa harina de maiz	⅓ c	3.5	137	77	2.93	1	0
Whole wheat flour	¼ c	4	100	12.2	1	—	0
Wheat germ, toasted	1 T	2.1	27	3.2	.6	1.2	0
Tortilla, corn	1, 30 gm	2.1	67	42	.57	.43	0
Brown rice, cooked	1 c	4.9	232	23	1	—	0
Nut butters							
Almond butter	1 T	2.4	101	43	.59	.49	0
Cashew butter	1 T	2.5	83	6	.72	.73	0
Peanut butter, creamy	1 T	4.6	95	5	.29	.47	0
Sesame butter, tahini	1 T	2.6	89	64	1.34	.69	0
Legumes, cooked							
Adzuki beans	¼ c	4.3	73	16	1.2	1	0
Black beans	¼ c	3.8	57	12	.9	.5	0
Garbanzo beans	¼ c	3.6	67	20	1.2	.6	0
Black eye peas	¼ c	3.3	49	11	1.1	.5	0
Kidney beans	¼ c	4	55	29	1.3	.4	0
Split peas	¼ c	4.1	58	6.5	.6	.5	0
Pinto beans	¼ c	3.5	59	21	1.1	.5	0
Miscellaneous							
Molasses, blackstrap	1 T	0	43	137	3.2	—	—
Brewer's yeast	1 oz	11	80	60	4.9	—	—
Torula yeast, dried	1 oz	13.5	99	100	6.4	3.6	.17

TABLE 9-11   *Nutrient Values of Selected Foods Providing Nutrients of Concern for Vegetarian Children—cont'd*

Food	Amount	Protein (gm)	Energy (kcal)	Ca (mg)	Fe (mg)	Zn (mg)	B_{12} (µg)
Fruits and vegetables							
Orange juice, frozen	8 oz	1.7	112	22	.24	.13	0
Apple juice	8 oz	0.2	116	16	.92	0.7	0
Tomato juice	6 oz	1.4	32	16	1.06	.26	0
Avocado	½ med	1.8	153	9.5	1	.36	0
Beet greens, cooked	½ c	1.9	20	82	1.37	.36	0
*Broccoli, cooked	½ c	2.3	23	89	.89	.12	0
*Collards, cooked	½ c	1.5	18	74	.39	.61	0
Spinach, cooked	½ c	2.7	21	122	3.21	.69	0
Chard, cooked	½ c	1.7	18	10	.18	—	0
*Kale, cooked	½ c	1.2	21	47	.59	.15	0
*Mustard greens, cooked	½ c	1.6	11	52	.49	—	0
*Turnip greens, cooked	½ c	0.8	15	99	.57	.1	0
Bamboo shoots, cooked	¼ c	.47	4	6	1.2	—	0
Dried fruit							
Apricots	5 halves	.7	46	8	.8	.13	0
Currants, zante	¼ c	1.8	102	31	1.17	.23	0
Dates	5	.8	114	13	.48	.12	0
Figs	1	.57	57	27	.44	.11	0
Raisins, seedless	⅓ c	1.6	150	48	5	.15	0
Prunes	2	.44	40	15	.41	.09	0
Sprouts							
Alfalfa, raw	10 gm	.1	1	1	.03	.03	0
Lentils, cooked	10 gm	.9	10	1.4	.3	.15	0
Mung beans, cooked	¼ c	.7	7	3.54	.2	.14	0
Soy, cooked	¼ c	2	19	14	.3	.25	0

*Low-oxalate green leafy vegetables.

TABLE 9-12   *Adaptation of Macrobiotic Diet for Young Children*

If fortified food products and supplements are considered unacceptable:

Provide 25–30% of energy intake from fat, using oil as necessary

Provide ~1.3 µg vitamin B_{12} and ~3 µg vitamin D per day by including 20 gm fatty fish/day

Provide calcium, protein, and riboflavin in 1 serving/day of dairy products

Reduce fiber intake of children <2 years of age by sieving cereal foods

Dagnelie and van Staveren, 1994[23]

absorbed by the infant.[76] Well-nourished lactating women who are following a vegetarian food pattern have adequate supplies of nutrients in their breast milk.[77,78] However, vitamin B_{12} may be a concern, especially if the mother's levels are low or if she has chosen a vegan food pattern. A supplement or additional food choices may be necessary to provide adequate quantities of vitamin B_{12}. Usually, if the need for a particular nutrient can be clearly documented, parents are willing to reexamine their philosophical basis for making food choices, and a reasonable decision or compromise can be reached for the ultimate nutritional welfare of the child.

FIG. 9-2 A young child who enjoys a variety of foods and is healthy and well-nourished on a nonmeat food pattern.

When breast-feeding is not feasible, the infant needs to receive adequate quantities of a properly prepared infant formula. This can be a soy or a cow's milk infant formula, but it must provide adequate quantities of critical nutrients such as protein, calcium, iron, energy, and vitamins B_{12}, A, and D. Fortified soy infant formulas do promote normal growth and development in infants.

Home-prepared infant formulas made with cow's milk, goat's milk, or soy base and supplemented with calcium, yeast, lactose, and other vitamin and mineral preparations are not advised. These types of formula are susceptible to errors in measurement and dilution; thus they put the infant at risk of excess or deficiency of specific nutrients and potential renal solute problems.

A tool has been developed for screening of potential nutritional problems of vegetarian infants and young children in the clinical setting. Aspects of growth, size, and foods as sources of nutrients are rated. Nutritional risk areas are highlighted by use of the checklist. Infants and young children whose nutrient intake appears to be at risk for low or deficient intake can then be referred for more detailed nutrition evaluation and counseling (table 9-13).

SPECIAL CONCERNS FOR ADOLESCENTS

Many adolescents and young adults who choose vegetarian or semivegetarian food patterns are concerned with their own health and the nutrition that is basic to it. Often their food choices are based, at least in part, on political and philosophical convictions. These young people need information and supportive counseling to make sound health decisions while they continue to make the political or philosophical statement of their choice.

Young adolescents who are not yet emancipated from the nuclear family may use food selection as a means of establishing independence. In this situation parents must remain flexible, tolerant, and interested in the adolescent's convictions regarding food choices.

TABLE 9-13   *Nutrition Worksheet for Children Who Are Vegetarian*

Infants

Yes   No

☐   ☐   Is infant's weight gain appropriate? (>5 percentile wt/length)
☐   ☐   Is overall infant development appropriate for age?

If infant is **breast-feeding:**
☐   ☐   Does mother's food pattern contain adequate fluid, protein, calcium, vitamin B_{12}? (Use Foods as Sources of Nutrients assessment form below)
☐   ☐   Is the infant supplemented with vitamin D (10 µg/day)?
☐   ☐   Is the infant receiving a supplemental source of iron (1 mg/kg/day)?
☐   ☐   Is the infant receiving a supplemental source of vitamin B_{12} (0.3 µg/day)?

If infant is **formula-fed:**
☐   ☐   Is a commercial cow milk or soy-based iron-fortified infant formula offered to the infant?
☐   ☐   Is an appropriate volume consumed? (>24 oz/day)?
Fortified or unfortified soy milk, goat milk, skim cow's milk, or any other "milks," such as tofu milk, rice milk, and nut milk, should not be used as the primary milk source during the first two years of the infant's life.

Children

Growth

Is following channels?	☐ Weight	☐ Height	☐ Head circumference
Is decreasing across channels?	☐ Weight	☐ Height	☐ Head circumference
Is increasing across channels?	☐ Weight	☐ Height	☐ Head circumference

Appropriate benchmarks for a toddler who is offered a vegetarian food pattern:
☐   Typical growth
☐   Source of high-quality protein (milk or soy-based infant formula, dairy foods, fortified soy milk, eggs)
☐   Foods are appropriate in texture (well-cooked, mashed beans; cooked vegetables)

Foods as Sources of Nutrients:
For Infants and Young Children

Energy
Adequate energy intake is reflected in adequate growth

Protein
Adequate is >25 gm/day
- 1 serving = ½ c milk or soy-based infant formula, milk, yogurt, fortified soy milk, ¾ oz cheese, 1 egg, or ½ portion meat analog
  1 serving = 4 gm protein × _____ servings = _____ gm protein
- 1 serving = ¼ c cooked soy, ⅛ c cooked red, white, or black beans, ¾ TB peanut butter
  1 serving = 2 gm protein × _____ servings = _____ gm protein
- 1 serving *whole grains* = ½ slice bread, ¼ c rice or cereals
  1 serving = 1 gm protein × _____ servings = _____ gm protein

    Total grams protein/day = _____

Developed by Cristine M Trahms, MS,RD
University of Washington, 1997

Continued.

TABLE 9-13   Nutrition Worksheet for Children Who Are Vegetarian—cont'd

Calcium

Adequate intake is >800 mg/day

- 1 serving = ½ c milk-based infant formula, dairy foods, soy-based infant formula or fortified soy milk
  1 serving = 150 mg calcium × _____ servings = _____ mg calcium
- 1 serving = ½ slice whole-grain bread or ¼ c rice or cooked cereal or ¼ c cooked dark green, leafy vegetables
  1 serving = 35 mg calcium × _____ servings = _____ mg calcium
- 1 serving = ½ c *calcium*-fortified fruit juices
  1 serving = 150 mg calcium × _____ servings = _____ mg calcium

           Total mg calcium/day = _____

Vitamin D

Daily intake of:

☐   Milk or soy-based infant formula, fortified milk or soy milk, other dairy foods
☐   Daily outdoor exposure to sun
☐   Supplement
☐   Fortified margarine
☐   None

Vitamin C (Ascorbic acid)

Daily intake of:

☐   Citrus juices, fruits, tomato, strawberries, cantaloupe, dark green leafy vegetables
☐   None

B-carotene, which is converted to vitamin A

Daily intake of:

☐   Milk or soy-based infant formula, fortified milk or soy milk, other dairy foods
☐   Fortified ready-to-eat cereal
☐   Broccoli, carrots, dark green leafy vegetables, sweet potatoes, tomatoes, winter squash
☐   None

Zinc

Daily intake of:

☐   Whole-grain breads, cereals
☐   None

Iron

Daily intake of:

☐   Whole-grain breads, cereals
☐   Well-cooked legumes
☐   Milk or soy-based infant formula, fortified soy milk, meat analogs
☐   Dark-green leafy vegetables
☐   Fortified ready-to-eat cereal
☐   Supplement
☐   None

TABLE 9-13   Nutrition Worksheet for Children Who Are Vegetarian—cont'd

Vitamin B$_{12}$ (Cobalamin)
Daily intake of:
☐   Milk or soy-based infant formula, dairy foods, fortified soy milk, eggs, meat analogs
☐   Fortified ready-to-eat cereal
☐   Supplement
☐   None

Risk Assessment

Based on the information above, check areas of concern.
☐   Growth has increased or decreased across channels since last visit
☐   Limited high-quality protein foods in diet
☐   Dairy foods not in diet or no calcium supplement
☐   Few fruit or vegetables or no vitamin and mineral supplement
☐   No source of vitamin D
☐   No whole-grain breads, cereals, or legumes in diet
☐   No source of vitamin B$_{12}$
☐   No source of iron

Plan
If any concerns are checked above; request a detailed food record for evaluation and refer for nutritional counseling. Also, evaluate hematocrit, hemoglobin status, and other biochemical parameters as needed.

When there is little understanding, the food pattern can quickly become another point of intense family conflict. It must be remembered that an unusual food pattern is not necessarily a harmful food pattern. The parents and the adolescent need guidance to discern the difference. Any direct criticism of food choices may be considered personal criticism, so counseling must be supportive. It should reinforce the positive aspects of the chosen food pattern and consider the energy and nutrient needs required for growth, development, and physical activity. Nonjudgmental discussion of alternatives and a mutual decision-making process among the health care professional, the adolescent, and the parent can guide adolescents in making healthful and responsible food choices.

Nutrient needs can be met by careful planning and by including foods that are equivalent sources of specific nutrients. Figure 9-3 defines foods as sources of nutrients and the foods that can be exchanged to provide the equivalent nutrients. This scheme may be used not only by vegetarians but also by those who have specific food likes and dislikes or by those who for some other reason feel the need to restrict the variety of choices in their food intake patterns.

Guidance for Families

In addition to the food guide (table 9-14), the following point should be kept in mind when counseling a family that has chosen to become vegetarian: The goal of the health care professional is the same as when counseling a nonvegetarian family, that is, to promote good health through reasonable food choices.

Table 9-15 reflects the responsibilities of the nutrition counselor, who may not be vegetarian, in counseling an adolescent or family who has chosen or who is choosing a vegetarian food pattern.

If you **exclude** these foods	then you **limit** these nutrients	so you **replace** with these foods
Meat Fish Poultry	Protein, iron, energy, vitamin B$_{12}$, essential fatty acids, zinc	Dairy foods, grains, legumes, fortified soy milk
Milk/ Dairy foods	Protein, riboflavin, vitamin D and B$_{12}$, calcium, zinc	Legumes, fortified soy milk, dark green vegies
Grains	Protein, iron, calcium, zinc	Legumes, dairy foods
Legumes	Protein, iron, zinc, calcium	Whole and fortified grains, dairy foods, dark green vegies, nuts, miso, tofu

*Consider supplementation of nutrients in low supply for young children: vitamins D and B$_{12}$ and iron.

FIG. 9-3   Thoughtful food choices provide all *key nutrients* for a nonmeat food pattern. (From Trahms CM: *Body Basics* 4(5), 1991, University of Washington.)

Summary

The more restrictive food choices become, the more difficult it is to plan a nutritionally adequate food pattern. Dietary inadequacy is more likely to occur in children than in adults. Vegetarian food patterns that include prudently chosen plant foods and a reasonable amount of dairy foods are adequate to support normal growth and development for people of all ages, including young children and pregnant and lactating women. These recommendations are supported by a position paper from the American Dietetic Association,[79] as well as others.[80-84] General recommendations to support an adequate nutritional intake for young children who are vegetarians and vegans are shown in table 9-16.

Becoming Vegetarian,[85] *The "New" Laurel's Kitchen,*[86] and *Jane Brody's Good Food Book*[87] are helpful manuals that include nutrition information as well as recipes for those who choose nonmeat food patterns.

It should be noted that these recommendations for an appropriate vegetarian food pattern are in accord with the Healthy People 2000 Objectives[88] for lower fat, higher complex carbohydrate food choices for all people.

REVIEW QUESTIONS

1. Why are infants of vegan mothers susceptible to vitamin B$_{12}$ deficiency?
2. List the nutrients most likely to be present in marginal or deficient amounts of (a) vegetarian and (b) vegan diets for children.
3. Describe an adequate food intake pattern for a vegetarian child.
4. What are the most likely nutritional problems for a vegan child?
5. What bioavailable sources of protein, energy, zinc, and vitamins B$_{12}$ and D would be most reasonably suggested for a vegan child?

TABLE 9-14 Vegetarian Food Guide

Food Group	Portion Size	Number of Daily Portions		
		Pregnant	2 to 3 Years	4 to 6 Years
Breads, cereals, pasta	1 slice bread ⅓ c granola ¾ c cooked cereal 1 biscuit, muffin 1 T wheat germ ¾ c cooked rice	6	3	3
Protein foods				
Legumes, meat analogues	1 c cooked beans ¼ c peanut butter 6 oz tofu	¾	⅛	¼
Nuts and seeds	3 T	1	⅛	¼
Dairy products, milk	1 c milk, yogurt 1 oz cheese 4 T cottage cheese	4	2–3	2–3
Eggs		1½	1	1
Fruits and vegetables	1 c, raw ½ c, cooked ½ c juice	5–6	2	3
Extra foods	No recommendation			

Modified from Smith EB: *J Nutr Educ* 7:109, 1975.

TABLE 9-15 Nutrition Counseling Strategy for Vegetarian Family or Individual

Support	Evaluate	Encourage
Support individuals and families in every positive aspect of their chosen food pattern • Be nonjudgmental about the stated reasons for specific food choices • Recognize the wide variety of food choices that are appropriate to maintain good health • Understand the self-selected food taboos and food preferences and the reasons for them	Evaluate the food intake of a specific family member, identifying possible nutrients at risk for a deficient intake because of food choices or food preparation methods • Help the family recognize the differing needs of infants, young children, adolescents, adults, pregnant women, and sedentary individuals • Work with individuals to identify food as sources of nutrients	Encourage family members to purchase foods that provide the most nutrients for the money • Encourage the evaluation of foods for their nutrient content, packaging, and processing • Encourage the use of simple foods, whole grains, fresh fruits, and vegetables • Encourage the use of cooking methods that conserve nutrients • Encourage all family members to evaluate personal food choices based on the time available for food purchase and preparation, the effort and skill required for food preparation, the money available for food purchase, and values related to these choices

TABLE 9-16   *General Recommendations for Vegetarian Food Pattern*

- Use an appropriately supplemented milk or soy-based formula for infants and toddlers who are not breast-fed
- Use a variety of fruits and vegetables
- Use whole-grain breads and cereals
- Provide nutrient-dense foods to meet energy and nutrient needs
- Provide adequate energy to support normal growth for each individual (infant, child, adolescent)
- Based on age and activity, limit high energy, low nutrient density foods (chips, high fat snacks, salad dressings)
- Provide adequate bioavailable quantities of limiting nutrients (iron, calcium, zinc, vitamin B_{12}, vitamin D) by either appropriate foods, fortified foods, or supplements
- Modify texture of foods to fit the developmental skills of the child
- Use dairy foods to promote appropriate growth in older infants and children

❖ ❖ ❖

CASE STUDY

Assessment of Growth and Nutrient Intake of an Infant

You are presented with a referral that contains the following information:

- First Well Child Clinic visit for Maya, who is a 7-month-old girl. She comes with her mother, 3-year-old sister, and 4-year-old cousin who mother cares for during the day.
- History: Normal term pregnancy. No maternal smoking, drugs, or illnesses. Maternal weight gain of 27 lb. Uncomplicated vaginal delivery. Infant birth weight of 3.7 kg (75th percentile). No infant jaundice. Infant breast-fed; no supplemental bottles offered. Birth weight regained by first pediatric visit at 10 days of age.

By 6-week visit, Maya's weight gain had slowed; she weighed 3.8 kg (10–25th percentile). Length continued at the 50th percentile. Pediatrician suggested formula feeding; mom agreed to supplement breast-feeding with infant formula feeds. Mom had surgery when Maya was 4 months old and discontinued breast-feeding.

- Diet: Family is vegetarian. Presently Maya is offered cooked cereal, yogurt, and spinach. She drinks 26–28 oz infant formula/day. Mom reports that Maya has frequent, loose stools.
- Social: Mother and father are both unemployed. Mom reports that this is stressful.

Dad is hopeful of employment soon. Both parents and sister are healthy.

- Immunizations: Up-to-date by mother's report.
- Weight: 6 kg (≤5th percentile); Length: 66.9 cm (50th percentile); OFC: 43.3 cm (50th percentile).
- Physical exam: Skin clear, no dentition, neck supple, no adenopathy, chest clear, abdomen soft, no hepatosplenomegaly, no muscular wasting, normal neurological exam.
- Language: Age appropriate—babbles, turns to voice, imitates sounds.
- Motor: Age appropriate—sits without support, bears weight on legs, takes 2 cubes, transfers hand to hand, rakes raisin.

1. What are your concerns about the growth of this infant?
2. Do you need additional information from the family about food preferences and beliefs?
3. What would you recommend as a nutrition plan for this infant?
4. What table foods would you suggest be added to provide nourishment and energy to support growth?
5. What milk would you suggest for this infant after transition from formula?

SUGGESTED LEARNING ACTIVITIES

1. Plan a menu for a 2-year-old vegetarian boy who weighs 10 kg. He is unwilling to consume beans of any kind. His mother is unwilling to offer more than 1 cup of milk or yogurt per day.

2. Outline teaching objectives and a food pattern for a young woman with a 6-month-old infant who is at the 25th percentile for length and weight. The mother prefers to avoid all animal products. The infant is totally breast-fed. The mother plans to continue breast-feeding until the infant is 1 year of age.

3. Mikaela is a 4-year-old girl enrolled in the Head Start Program. She has been labeled "anemic" on the entrance physical examination. Her weight/stature is at the 10th percentile. Her mother is strongly opposed to all supplements. The family is vegan. Outline a plan for the family and for the classroom.

4. A mother of two young children (5 and 6 years of age) has recently become vegetarian and is adjusting her cooking habits and the family food pattern. Her children are picky eaters in both the variety and quantity of food they are willing to consume. She feels that they may have lost weight on the vegetarian food pattern. Suggest how she can provide appropriate intakes for her children.

REFERENCES

1. Whorton JC: Historical development of vegetarianism, *Am J Clin Nutr* 59:1103S, 1994.
2. Johnson PK: Vegetarians among us: implications for health professionals. *Top Clin Nutr* 10:1, 1995.
3. Masarei JRL and others: Vegetarian food patterns, lipids and cardiovascular risk, *Aust NZ J Med* 14:400, 1984.
4. Melby CL, Toohey ML, Cebrick J: Blood pressure and blood lipids among vegetarian, semivegetarian, and nonvegetarian African Americans, *Am J Clin Nutr* 59:103, 1994.
5. Slattery ML and others: Meat consumption and its associations with other diet and health factors in young adults: the CARDIA study, *Am J Clin Nutr* 54:930, 1991.
6. Mäenpää P and others: Effects of low-fat lactovegetarian diet on health parameters of adult subjects, *Ecol Food & Nutr* 25:255, 1991.
7. Sacks FM, Kass EH: Low blood pressure in vegetarians: effects of specific foods and nutrients, *Am J Clin Nutr* 48:795, 1988.
8. Beilin LJ: Vegetarian and other complex diets, fats, fiber, and hypertension, *Am J Clin Nutr* 59:1130S, 1994.
9. Resnicow K and others: Diet and serum lipids in vegan vegetarians: a model for risk reduction, *J Am Diet Assoc* 91:447, 1991.
10. Snowdon DA: Animal product consumption and mortality because of all causes combined, coronary heart disease, stroke, diabetes, and cancer in Seventh-Day Adventists, *Am J Clin Nutr* 48:739, 1988.
11. Dwyer JT: Health aspects of vegetarian diets, *Am J Clin Nutr* 48:712, 1988.
12. Swarner J: The vegetarian diet and cancer prevention, *Top Clin Nutr* 10:17, 1995.
13. Hodgkin GE: Osteoporosis and vegetarian diets, *Top Clin Nutr* 10:34, 1995.
14. Whitten C: Vegetarian diets and ischemic heart disease, *Top Clin Nutr* 10:27, 1995.
15. Pagenkemper J: The impact of vegetarian diets on renal disease, *Top Clin Nutr* 10:22, 1995.
16. Nieman DC: Vegetarian dietary practices and endurance performance, *Am J Clin Nutr* 48:754, 1988.
17. Nair P, Mayberry JF: Vegetarianism, dietary fibre and gastro-intestinal disease, *Dig Dis* 12:177, 1994.
18. Alexander D, Ball MJ, Mann J: Nutrient intake and hematological status of vegetarians and age-sex matched omnivores, *Eur J Clin Nutr* 48:538, 1994.
19. Donovan UM, Gibson RS: Iron and zinc status of young women aged 14–19 years consuming vegetarian and omnivorous diets, *J Am Coll Nutr* 14:463, 1995.
20. Shull MW and others: Velocities of growth in vegetarian preschool children, *Pediatrics* 60:410, 1977.
21. O'Connell JM and others: Growth of vegetarian children: the Farm study, *Pediatrics* 84:475, 1989.
22. Dagnelie PC and others: Do children on macrobiotic diets show catch-up growth? *Eur J Clin Nutr* 42:1007, 1988.
23. Dagnelie PC, van Staveren WA: Macrobiotic nutrition and child health: results of a population based, mixed-longitudinal cohort study in the Netherlands, *Am J Clin Nutr* 59:1187S, 1994.
24. Neggers YH and others: A positive association between maternal serum zinc concentration and birth weight, *Am J Clin Nutr* 51:678, 1990.
25. van Staveren WA and others: Food consumption, growth, and development of Dutch children fed alternative diets, *Am J Clin Nutr* 48:819, 1988.
26. Dwyer JT and others: Growth in "new" vegetarian preschool children using the Jenss-Bayley curve fitting technique, *Am J Clin Nutr* 37:815, 1983.

27. Dwyer JT and others: Preschoolers on alternate lifestyle diets, *J Am Diet Assoc* 72:264, 1978.

28. Dwyer JT and others: Size, obesity and leanness in vegetarian preschool children, *J Am Diet Assoc* 77:434, 1980.

29. Trahms CM and others: Restriction of growth and elevated protoporphyrin in children deprived of animal protein, *Clin Res* 25:179, 1977.

30. van Staveren WA and others: Food consumption and height/weight status of Dutch preschool children on alternative food patterns, *J Am Diet Assoc* 85:1579, 1985.

31. Sabate J and others: Anthropometric parameters of school children with different life-styles, *Am J Dis Child* 144:1159, 1990.

32. Rona RJ and others: Vegetarianism and growth in Urdu, Gujarati, and Punjabi children in Britain, *J Epidemiol Community Health* 41:233, 1987.

33. Specker BL: Nutritional concerns of lactating women consuming vegetarian diets, *Am J Clin Nutr* 59:1182S, 1994.

34. Poskitt EME for Nutrition Standing Committee of the British Paediatric Association: Vegetarian weaning, *Arch Dis Child* 63:1286, 1988.

35. Chase HP and others: Kwashiorkor in the United States, *Pediatrics* 66:972, 1980.

36. Shinwell ED, Gorodisches R: Totally vegetarian diets and infant nutrition, *Pediatrics* 70:582, 1982.

37. Robson JRK and others: Zen macrobiotic dietary problems in infancy, *Pediatrics* 53:326, 1974.

38. Roberts LF and others: Malnutrition in infants receiving cult diets: a form of child abuse, *Br Med J* 1:296, 1979.

39. Brown PT, Bergan JG: The dietary status of "new" vegetarians, *J Am Diet Assoc* 67:455, 1975.

40. Sabate J and others: Attained height of lacto-ovovegetarian children and adolescents, *Eur J Clin Nutr* 45:51, 1991.

41. Tayter M, Stanek K: Anthropometric and dietary assessment of omnivore and lacto-ovovegetarian children, *J Am Diet Assoc* 89:1661, 1989.

42. Dagnelie PC and others: Nutritional status of infants aged 4 to 18 months on macrobiotic diets and matched omnivorous control infants: a population-based mixed-longitudinal study. II. Growth and psychomotor development, *Eur J Clin Nutr* 43:325, 1989.

43. Sanders TAB, Reddy S: Vegetarian diets and children, *Am J Clin Nutr* 59:1176S, 1994.

44. Trahms CM, Feeney MC: Evaluation of diet and growth of vegans, vegetarian, and nonvegetarian preschool children, *Fed Proc* 34:675, 1975.

45. Dwyer JT and others: Nutritional status of vegetarian children, *Am J Clin Nutr* 35:204, 1982.

46. Fulton JR and others: Preschool vegetarian children: dietary and anthropometric data, *J Am Diet Assoc* 76:360, 1980.

47. Sanders TAB: Growth and development of British vegan children, *Am J Clin Nutr* 48:822, 1988.

48. Hellebostad M and others: Vitamin D deficiency rickets and vitamin B_{12} deficiency in vegetarian children, *Acta Paediatr Scand* 74:191, 1985.

49. Dagnelie PC and others: High prevalence of rickets in infants on macrobiotic diets, *Am J Clin Nutr* 51:202, 1990.

50. Inner-city babies susceptible to rickets, *Northwest Med* 7:28, 1991.

51. Rudolf M and others: Unsuspected nutritional rickets, *Pediatrics* 66:72, 1980.

52. Dwyer JT and others: Risk of nutritional rickets among vegetarian children, *Am J Dis Child* 133:134, 1979.

53. Marie PJ and others: Histological osteomalacia due to dietary calcium deficiency in children, *N Engl J Med* 307:584, 1982.

54. Weaver CM, Plawecki KL: Dietary calcium: adequacy of a vegetarian diet, *Am J Clin Nutr* 59:1238S, 1994.

55. Specker BL and others: Vitamin B_{12}: low milk concentrations are related to low serum concentrations in vegetarian women and to methylmalonic aciduria in their infants, *Am J Clin Nutr* 52:1073, 1990.

56. Higginbottom MC and others: A syndrome of methylmalonic aciduria, homocystinuria, megaloblastic anemia and neurologic abnormalities in a vitamin B_{12} deficient breast fed infant of a strict vegetarian, *N Engl J Med* 299:317, 1978.

57. Dagnelie PC and others: Increased risk of vitamin B_{12} and iron deficiency in infants on macrobiotic diets, *Am J Clin Nutr* 50:818, 1989.

58. Miller DR and others: Vitamin B_{12} status in a macrobiotic community, *Am J Clin Nutr* 53:524, 1991.

59. Bindra GS and others: [Phytate] [Calcium]/[Zinc] ratios in Asian immigrant lacto-ovovegetarian diets and their relationship to zinc nutriture, *Nutr Res* 6:475, 1986.

60. Gibson RS: Content and bioavailability of trace elements vegetarian diets, *Am J Clin Nutr* 59:1223S, 1994.

61. Craig WJ: Iron status of vegetarians, *Am J Clin Nutr* 59:1238S, 1994.

62. Dwyer JT: Dietary fiber for children: how much? *Pediatrics* 96:1019, 1995.

63. Payne PR: Safe protein-calorie ratios in food patterns: The relative importance of protein and energy intake as causal factors in malnutrition, *Am J Clin Nutr* 28:281, 1975.

64. Young VR, Pellett PL: Plant proteins in relation to human protein and amino acid nutrition, *Am J Clin Nutr* 59:1203S, 1994.

65. Graham GG and others: Dietary protein quality in infants and children. IX. Instant sweetened corn-soy-milk blend, *Am J Clin Nutr* 26:491, 1973.

66. Bressani R and others: Protein quality of a soybean protein textured food in experimental animals and children, *J Nutr* 93:349, 1967.

67. Knapp J and others: Growth and nitrogen balance in infants fed cereal proteins, *Am J Clin Nutr* 26:586, 1973.

68. MacLean WC and others: Effect of the level of dietary protein intake on fat absorption in children, *Pediatr Res* 11:774, 1977.

69. Freeland-Graves JH and others: Zinc and copper content of foods used in vegetarian food patterns, *J Am Diet Assoc* 77:648, 1980.

70. Truesdell DD and others: Nutrients in vegetarian foods, *J Am Diet Assoc* 84:28, 1984.

71. Dagnelie PC and others: Vitamin B_{12} from algae appears not to be bioavailable, *Am J Clin Nutr* 53:695, 1991.

72. Herbert V: Vitamin B_{12}: plant sources, requirements and assay, *Am J Clin Nutr* 48:852, 1988.

73. Poneros AG, Erdman JW: Bioavailability of calcium in tofu, tortillas, nonfat dry milk and mozzarella cheese in rats: effect of supplemental ascorbic acid, *J Food Sci* 53:208, 1988.

74. Lynch SR and others: Iron absorption from legumes in humans, *Am J Clin Nutr* 40:42, 1984.

75. Johnston PK: *Infant feeding among Seventh-Day Adventists,* master's thesis, Seattle, 1979, University of Washington.

76. Saarinen UM, Siimes MA: Iron absorption from breast milk, cow's milk, and iron supplemented formula, *Pediatr Res* 13:143, 1979.

77. Finley DA and others: Inorganic constituents of breast milk from vegetarian and nonvegetarian women: relationships with each other and with organic constituents, *J Nutr* 115:772, 1985.

78. Finley DA and others: Breast milk composition: fat content and fatty acid composition in vegetarians and nonvegetarians, *Am J Clin Nutr* 41:787, 1985.

79. American Dietetic Association: Position of the American Dietetic Association: Vegetarian Diets, *J Am Diet Assoc* 93:1317, 1992.

80. Haddad EH: Meeting the RDAs with a vegetarian diet, *Top Clin Nutr* 10:7, 1995.

81. Haddad EH: Development of a vegetarian food guide, *Am J Clin Nutr* 59:1248S, 1994.

82. Truesdell DD, Acosta PB: Feeding the vegan infant and child, *J Am Diet Assoc* 85:837, 1985.

83. Jacobs C, Dwyer JT: Vegetarian children: appropriate and inappropriate diets, *Am J Clin Nutr* 48:811, 1988.

84. Dwyer JT: Nutritional consequences of vegetarianism, *Annu Rev Nutr* 11:61, 1991.

85. Melina V, Davis B, Harrison V: *Becoming vegetarian,* Canada, 1994, Macmillan.

86. Robertson L, Flinders C, Ruppenthal B: *The new Laurel's kitchen,* Berkeley, Calif, 1986, Ten Speed Press.

87. Brody J: *Jane Brody's good food book,* New York, 1985, WW Norton.

88. Healthy People 2000: nutrition objectives, *J Am Diet Assoc* 91:1515, 1991.

10

Dietary Intervention to Prevent Chronic Disease

Peggy L. Pipes
Betty Lucas

+‡

Objectives

After studying this chapter, the student should:

✔ *Be aware of nutritional approaches to the prevention of chronic disease by changes in current dietary intake during childhood.*

✔ *Recognize factors that must be considered in controlling children's weight.*

✔ *Recognize the diversity of opinions regarding the screening of children for cardiovascular heart disease.*

✔ *Be aware of the studies about the effect of salt on the development of hypertension.*

✔ *Be aware of acceptable blood pressure levels during childhood.*

A significant number of longitudinal and other studies have indicated that the prevention of chronic disease should begin in childhood. As a result researchers and experts recommend dietary changes in the current diet consumed in childhood and adolescence, and they believe that such changes could extend the years of a healthy life for many. They recommend that obesity in childhood be prevented or corrected, that the current diet children consume be modified to decrease intakes of total fat, saturated fats, and salt, and to increase intakes of fiber. They also recommend the identification of and tracking and intervention for children at high risk for chronic disease.

OBESITY

Obesity is a frequent concern in clinics that serve adolescents. The lack of success in achieving sustained weight reduction of obese adolescents has focused on identifying children at risk and motivating families to alter lifestyles, environmental factors, and psychosocial factors that contribute to the development of this condition.

Obesity is a major health hazard predisposing affected adults to a greater risk of hypertension, cardiovascular disease, diabetes, gallbladder disease, and degenerative joint disorders than persons of normal weight. Even in children as young as 5 to 6 years of age a relationship has been found between fitness, fatness, and blood pressure.[1] In addition to these health risks, obese individuals are often subjected to sociocultural prejudices. Young children in elementary school have been shown to discriminate against the overweight peer.[2] Overweight and obesity in adolescence is discussed in chapter 14.

Incidence

Obesity in childhood is a growing problem. Data from the NHANES III survey conducted between 1988 and 1991 indicate a continuing increase in overweight and obesity in children and adolescents. Using body mass index (BMI), the prevalence of overweight was 10.9% based on the 95th percentile cutoff, and 22% based on the 85th percentile cutoff.[3] There are differences between age groups, races, and sexes. Among girls, both school-aged and adolescents, non-Hispanic blacks had the highest prevalence of overweight and non-Hispanic whites had the lowest prevalence (16.9% for black girls and 9.8% for white girls, 6 to 11 years, 95th percentile). For boys 6 to 11 years old, non-Hispanic whites had the lowest prevalence (10.4%), but for 12- to 17-year-olds, non-Hispanic blacks had the lowest prevalence (9.3%).[3] This data continues to document the increasing overweight among U.S. youth since the mid-1960s.

Prognosis of Obesity

Many obese children become obese adolescents and adults. It has been estimated that 40% of obese children at 7 years of age and 70% of obese adolescents are obese as adults.[4] Data from the Fels Longitudinal Study showed that BMI at age 35 years was highly predicted by BMI at age 18, but less so at younger ages, especially the BMI of children less than 13 years.[5] Tracking efforts find that overweight in adolescence and extreme overweight in youth tend to persist into adulthood. Obesity during the preschool and school-age years does increase the risk of obesity in later life—a channeling tendency that increases with age. Early-onset obesity is more severe and resistant to treatment than is obesity acquired later in life.

Definition

Obesity is defined as an excessive deposition of adipose tissue. It differs from **overweight,** which implies only weight in excess of the average for height. Overweight can result from increased lean body mass, adipose tissue, or both. Forbes[6] has suggested that there may be two types of obesity in childhood and adolescence: one type characterized by increased lean body mass in addition to fat, a tendency for tallness, advanced bone age, and a history of overweight since infancy; and another type with no increase in lean body mass, normal bone age and height, and weight gain in the midchildhood or late childhood years.

Weight greater than 20% of normal for height is one criterion that has been used to define obesity. Such standards, although they show trends for populations, are not applicable to individual children. The use of weight standards tends to underestimate fatness in children less than 6 or 7 years of age and frequently overestimates adiposity in adolescents. Diagnosis of grossly obese children is easily made by visual inspection. Differentiating between less severely obese children and those who are overweight because of increased muscle mass requires measurements that give indications of body composition. Identification of children who are overfat and are settled into patterns of growth indicative of future obesity also requires that measurements of body composition be included in health examinations, just as other measurements of growth are obtained. As described in chapter 1, standards for triceps fatfold measures with calipers have been published for all age groups. Standardized percentile curves of BMI (weight/height^2) have been developed for children and adolescents, and can be used to monitor obesity develop-ment as well as changes related to interven-tions.[7] Use of these measurements to define greater than normal increases in adipose tissue of children and adolescents as they grow older helps identify children for whom preventive measures should be applied.

Etiological Factors

Studies of rats and other animals have defini-tively shown that, in animals, genes carrying obese traits are transmitted to offspring. In humans, the heterogeneous etiology of obesity suggests that no single genetic locus is likely to explain all cases of obesity. However, genes asso-ciated with basal metabolism, dietary thermo-genesis, appetite, satiety, lipid metabolism, and fat storage are possible mechanisms for the inheritability of obesity in families.[8]

Definition of human genetic obesities has been more difficult because of the mixed racial heritage of most individuals and the many envi-ronmental factors known to contribute to obe-sity that cannot be controlled in studies. The high incidence of obesity among parents of obese children and the fact that early onset obe-sity appears to be almost intractable lead one to believe that hereditary factors are important. A study of Danish adoptees found that an individ-ual's relative weight strongly correlated with the body masses of his or her biological parents. There was no relation between the body masses of the individuals studied and their adoptive par-ents.[9] Another report of the BMI of adult twins reared apart found that there was strong evi-dence of the influence of heredity, but less impact of the environment on BMI.[10]

Dietz describes three critical periods for the development of obesity in childhood: prenatal, the adiposity rebound period (5 to 7 years of age), and adolescence.[11] The adiposity rebound is the natural increase in BMI following a dip in the preschool years. Its timing appears to be a predictor of fatness in adolescence and adult-hood. Children whose rebound occurs before age 5½ years have greater BMIs and subscapular skinfolds when they are older, compared with children with rebounds closer to age 7. These critical periods of adiposity development can be the focus of preventive efforts and intervention for the pediatric population.

Another study investigated whether parental obesity influenced **resting metabolic rate (RMR)** in children 3 to 5 years of age and 12 years later. These researchers found that parental obesity predicted a more rapid growth and an earlier decline in resting metabolic rate in males but did not predict adiposity. Also, childhood energy intake per kilogram of body weight in earlier years was not predictive of obesity in ado-lescent males. Among females they noted the opposite. Energy intake per kilogram of body weight in the early years was predictive of obesity 12 years later, even more than parental obesity. The RMRs of daughters of obese parents did not differ significantly from that of their peers who had higher energy intakes in childhood. The researchers felt that the differences between the sexes resulted from differences in the rates of maturation. They propose that children who are preobese have a faster rate of growth and decline of RMRs per kilogram, leading to earlier adoles-cence. They predict that children of obese par-ents will become obese themselves. They also think that sons who become obese as adults will have metabolic rates per kilogram similar to those of their nonobese peers.[12]

Inactivity is another cause of obesity. Obese adolescents and school-age children are less active than are those of normal weight. Most become obese despite ingesting kcalorie intakes equivalent to or less than their peers. This is also true in infancy. A longitudinal study of 31 infants at 6, 9, and 12 months of age found that the percentage of body fat was inversely related to activity level, but not related to energy intake.[13] Activity patterns are acquired in child-hood. Children learn to enjoy those activities in which their families and peers engage. Parents who enjoy hiking, swimming, and sports often teach their children to engage in and enjoy these physical activities. Parents who spend their hours at home urging their children to be still so that they can watch television or read reinforce inactivity and sedentary living.

Television viewing also contributes to obesity. Dietz and Gortmaker[14] found a dose-response effect: the more television viewed, the greater the

FIG. 10-1   Overweight infant became a lean, well-proportioned 12-year-old and a muscular 16-year-old boy.

risk of obesity. In addition to the inactivity while watching television, children are reported to eat more of the foods advertised on television as well as larger quantities of food during the programs than children not watching television. Another study, of prepubertal girls, found that they had a significantly lower resting energy expenditure while watching television than during rest, with an even larger decrease with the obese girls.[15]

Birth weight is not a good predictor of adult obesity. One report found that infants who were extremely obese at birth tended toward normal weight at 4 and 7 years of age, but an unusually high percentage retained their stocky physiques (fig. 10-1).[16] The children who were obese at 4 and 7 years of age tended to have stocky physiques at birth. By 7 years of age, however, they were joined in their obese and overweight statuses by children who had normal physiques at birth.

There has been speculation in the past that formula-feeding and the early introduction of semisolid foods might be one cause of excessive intakes of energy and obesity in infancy, and that obese infants often become obese adults. However, a number of studies have shown that breast-feeding, bottle-feeding, and the age of introduction of semisolid foods do not cause obesity in infancy or later childhood.[17,18] Obesity in infancy has not been found to be predictive of obesity in later life.[19] Fomon and others[18] found measures of fatness at 8 years of age no greater in children who had been bottle-fed compared with those who had been breast-fed. A longitudinal study of children found that obese infants at 6 months and one year of age become progressively thinner as they grow older. Weight gain in infancy was not found to be predictive of obesity at 9 years of age.[19]

Psychosocial factors and early parent-child interactions are important contributors to obesity in childhood. Johnson and Birch studied 3- to 5-year-olds' ability to self-regulate their energy intake at meals offered after consuming a caloric or noncaloric drink. Anthropometric data for children and parents, and mothers' child feeding practices were also collected.[20] The results found that the children with greater body fat stores were less able to regulate their energy intake accurately. Also, the children who had more difficulty regulating their energy intake had mothers who used more control over their children's food intake.

These children are often given food and material objects instead of love and the opportunity to have experiences that lead to the development of coping skills.[21] Anxious and insecure parents may overfeed children as expressions of their concern and love.

Psychological trauma has been observed to be another factor associated with the onset of obesity. Bruch[22] noted that fear of hospitalization was associated with the onset of obesity in some children. A 10-year follow-up study of Danish schoolchildren found that those who experienced parental neglect (little or no parent support and poor hygiene) had a significantly higher risk of obesity as young adults.[23] It has been noted in clinical practice that some superobese children come from families that include sexual or physical abuse or significant dysfunction.

Differences have been noted in the incidence of obesity among children from the lower and higher socioeconomic groups. Analysis of data compiled during the Ten-State Nutrition Survey of 1968–1970 and the Preschool Nutrition Survey found that after the first few years of life and into adolescence, the children of the poorest groups were leaner and the children of the affluent groups were fatter.[24]

Trends and surveys over the past 25 years, however, have suggested a reversal in leanness in some populations of low-income children. A compounding factor in comparing socioeconomic groups is the higher proportion of African American and Hispanics among low-income families. Children of African-American ethnicity tend to have advanced skeletal age, are taller, weigh more, and mature earlier than white peers. The recent NHANES III survey found that the highest percentage of overweight in 6- to 11-year-old children was among black and Mexican-American boys and girls.[3] Among teenagers, black boys had the lowest prevalence of overweight; black girls had the highest prevalence. A recent survey of 1,670 low-income school-age children from Harlem compared their growth with NCHS standards.[25] Nearly 90% of the students were black. Their height for age and weight for age was skewed to the higher percentiles, but so was their weight for height, suggesting that as many as a quarter of these children could be considered obese. Other causative factors of overweight in this population besides early maturation could include limited physical activity (due to lifestyle and safety issues), parental obesity, and diet.

Prevention

Regardless of its cause, obesity results when energy intakes exceed energy needs for growth, maintenance, and activity. Its manifestation is usually the result of small excesses of kcalorie intakes over expenditure for a period of weeks, months, or years. Monitoring rates of growth and deposition of adipose tissue helps to identify children who are accumulating more fat than would be anticipated, and measures to increase activity or decrease caloric intakes can be effected.

FIG. 10-2   Previously obese child and her mother exercise as part of a program to control the child's weight.

Due to long-term health and psychosocial consequences of obesity in childhood, prevention is an important public policy goal. Of particular importance in addressing obesity prevention is the lack of evidence showing increasing energy intakes in U.S. children. In fact, national surveys have shown stable or declining energy intakes over the past 20 years.[26] This suggests that decreased physical activity has been a significant contributor to higher levels of overweight. Therefore, dietary energy restriction may not be an automatic intervention approach.

Parents control the food available to younger children, create the environment that influences their acceptance of food, and can influence energy expenditure by the opportunities they create for physical activity for their children. It may be important to explore first with parents any reasons for allowing children to consume amounts of food that result in rapid weight gain. Some parents may not recognize that their expectations for the quantity of food they encourage their children to consume are excessive.

Parents may need help in developing appropriate parenting skills. They may need to learn how to respond to hunger and other needs of their infants or how to interact with their children. This includes avoiding verbal prompts and encouragement to get young children to eat, not using food for nonnutritious purposes (i.e., rewards, pacifiers), and allowing children to self-regulate their intake within developmentally appropriate limits.[27]

The activity pattern of both the child and the family should be explored; it may be important to help parents find ways of increasing their child's level of activity (fig. 10-2). Parents who live in apartments often reinforce sedentary activities to reduce the noise level and complaints from neighbors. Those who live in one-family dwellings may have limited space for activities for children. City park departments, preschools, and schools frequently have programs that offer opportunities to increase children's activity, such as swimming and team sports. Children of parents who bike, ski, and hike will also likely enjoy these activities, all of which can be continued throughout life.

TABLE 10-1　*Approximate Energy Value of Common Snack Foods Offered Young Children*

Food	Portion Size	kcal	Food	Portion Size	kcal
Cheese cubes	¼ oz	25	Homogenized milk	3 oz	60
Hard-boiled egg	½ medium	36	Chocolate milk	3 oz	80
Frankfurter, 5″ by ¾″	1	133	Cauliflower buds	2 small	2
Pretzel, 3″ by ½″	1	20	Green pepper strips	2	2
Potato chips	10	114	Cucumber slices	3 large	2
Popcorn with oil and salt	1 c	41	Cherry tomato	1	3
Bread stick, 4½″	1	38	Raw turnip slices	2	5
Saltines	1	12	Dill pickle, large	⅓	5
Graham cracker	2 squares	55	Apple wedges	¼ medium apple	20
Animal cracker	1	11	Banana	½ small	40
Brownie, 3″ by 1″ by ⅞″	1	97	Orange wedges	¼ medium orange	18
Chocolate cupcake	1	51	Orange juice	3 oz	35
Vanilla wafer	1	18	Grape juice	3 oz	60
Yogurt, plain	¼ c	40	Lemonade	3 oz	40

From Adams CF: *Nutritive value of American foods in common units,* Agriculture Handbook No 456, Washington, DC, 1975, US Department of Agriculture.

The range of appropriate energy intakes at any given age is large. Overweight children and children with familial trends to obesity may need fewer kcalories than their peers. Griffith and Payne[28] found that normal weight 4- to 5-year-old children of obese parents expended 1174 kcal/day as compared with 1508 kcal/day expended by children of the same size and age of normal weight parents. Children of normal weight parents expended twice as much energy in physical activity as did those of obese parents. Families of children with a familial tendency to obesity may need help in identifying the kinds and amount of food that provide energy intakes that support normal growth and weight gain.

Nutrition counseling should be family oriented and based on normal nutrition, using the Food Pyramid Guide, emphasizing foods that provide a balance of nutrients and appropriate kcalorie intakes. Families need to realize that efforts are directed at reduction in rates of weight gain and are not intended to effect weight loss. They must recognize that the food available and the models set for their child determine the child's response to efforts to control weight gain. Family meals may need to be modified to include fewer fried foods, less gravy, and fewer rich desserts. Parents and siblings may have to modify their own eating practices to set appropriate examples. Teachers, baby sitters and day-care workers should be alerted to and included in programs designed to control weight. Food experiences at school may need to be modified to exclude corn dripping with butter and chocolate cupcakes that are so frequently provided for special occasions. Low-kcalorie snacks such as raw fruits and vegetables can be provided instead of cookies, candy, and hot dogs. The use of food as reinforcers can be modified. Comparative energy values of snack foods are shown in table 10-1.

Care should be taken in approaches to prevention of obesity because overzealous preventive methods can have harmful results. For example, Pugliese and others[29] describe 14 normal children with growth failure and delayed maturation because of an inadequate intake because of fear of obesity.

If the child is grossly obese, a very slow rate of weight reduction may be attempted, however, linear growth should be frequently monitored.

Epstein and others[30] found that behaviorally family-based treatment procedures did not compromise the linear growth of obese children when height was adjusted for parental height. Clinical experience has indicated that in grossly obese preschool- and school-age children with developmental disabilities a weight reduction of 2 lbs/mo did not affect linear growth. Others, however, have reported that restricted kcalorie intakes did modify linear growth. Wolff and Lloyd[31] noted that children who had lost 2% or more of their weight per month grew in length at a less than expected rate. Children who (1) lost less than 2% of their body weight, (2) did not lose any weight, or (3) gained weight all grew at a rate faster than expected when energy intakes were increased to match energy expenditure.

Treatment programs for overweight and obese preadolescents are not commonly available despite the increasing prevalence of the problem. Any intervention for children should include the family as well as the child and provide nutrition/diet guidance, support of physical activity, and behavior therapy. Epstein and others recently reported a 10-year follow-up study of 158 children who had been participants in group treatment programs (weekly meetings for 8 to 12 weeks, with monthly follow-ups for 6 to 12 months).[32] They found that 10 years after treatment, 30% were not obese and 34% had decreased their percentage of overweight by 20% or more. The programs that were more family-based and included an exercise component had better outcomes after the 10 years. These long-term results are better than for similar programs for adults.

The many factors in the etiology of childhood obesity indicate that a multidisciplinary approach may be necessary. The team might consist of a psychologist or behaviorist, a physician, and a dietitian-nutritionist.

Parents and their children need continuing support as they implement programs to prevent obesity and face unwitting responses from other members of society. Well-meaning merchants and bankers who provide sweets for children should be encouraged to provide nonfood items as alternatives. Neighbors, relatives, and other children's parents should support weight control programs.

As children grow older, they must learn to make their own decisions regarding foods that result in a positive energy balance. The children should receive positive reinforcement for control of weight gain. They need continuing support, education, and understanding as they get older. An 8-year-old boy who has been on a weight control program for 6 years, since obesity was reversed at 27 months of age, expressed the difficulties encountered on such a program. He stated during a recent clinic visit, "It's really hard to control my weight. I'm often hungry. I can't eat as much as the other boys, and my food is different from that of the other children in my class. I don't want to get fat, but I don't like being different." He, however, understands his program and knows he will receive the guidance and support he desires from his family as he assumes control of his own food selection and management of weight control.

DIETARY FATS

It is generally believed that intakes of cholesterol and saturated fatty acids and food habits established in childhood are important factors in the development of coronary artery disease in later life. The Academy of Pediatrics[33] and the Expert Panel on Blood Cholesterol Levels in Children and Adolescents sponsored by the National Institutes of Health[34] recommend a reduction in dietary fat to 30% of total energy intake, 10% or less from saturated fat, 10% from monounsaturated fat, and less than 10% from polyunsaturated fat for all individuals over 2 years of age. They also recommend reducing cholesterol intakes to 250 to 300 mg/day or less.

The Expert Panel on Cholesterol Levels in Children and Adolescents recommends two approaches to the reduction of cardiovascular disease: (1) a population approach focusing on changes in the current diet of all children and adolescents over 2 years of age as described above, and (2) an individualized screening (determining cholesterol levels, and low-density lipoprotein cholesterol if indicated) for children and adolescents who are "at risk" (those with a family history of hyperlipidemia or early cardio-vascular events). Even though population screening identifies a number of false positives (children with elevated lipoprotein levels that will not remain elevated in adulthood), some researchers feel that screening of only "high-risk" individuals will miss 50% of children with elevated lipid levels, and that all children should be screened.[34]

Hyperlipidemia

Both cholesterol and triglycerides in the plasma are derived from two sources, dietary intake and endogenous synthesis in the liver and intestines. Dietary cholesterol is absorbed in proportion to the amount consumed. Increases in intakes reduce endogenous synthesis only partially. Endogenous triglycerides are synthesized from carbohydrate, fatty acids, and a variety of two-carbon fragments.

All plasma lipids, cholesterol, triglycerides, and phospholipids are transported in the blood bound to protein, which solubilizes them. Four macromolecule families of plasma lipoproteins are found in the blood. **Chylomicrons** transport the major portion of dietary triglyceride. **Very low-density lipoproteins** (pre-beta-lipoproteins) transport endogenous triglyceride. **Low-density lipoproteins** (beta-lipoproteins) transport one-half to two-thirds of the total plasma cholesterol. **High-density lipoproteins** transport cholesterol and phospholipids. Low-density lipoprotein cholesterol is transported primarily to peripheral tissue and the smooth muscle of the arterial intima. High-density lipoprotein cholesterol travels through the capillary bed of peripheral tissue and acquires redundant-free cholesterol. It is ultimately carried to the liver where it is released and excreted. Low-density lipoproteins appear to damage the arteries, whereas high-density lipoproteins are beneficial. The ratio of low-density lipoprotein cholesterol to high-density lipoprotein cholesterol has been found to be a good predictor for coronary heart disease.

Cholesterol concentrations are lower in cord blood than in maternal blood and rise after newborns are fed. At 6 months of age infants fed human milk or cow's milk have higher serum cholesterol concentrations than those fed formulas containing soy or corn oil. These differences are modified when other foods are added to the diet. At 1 year of age, differences in serum cholesterol levels between infants fed cow's milk or formula with unsaturated fatty acids and a variety of other food disappear. Total protein, total fat, and cholesterol intakes correlate with total serum lipoprotein cholesterol and serum low-density lipoprotein cholesterol at 1 year of age.[35] After weaning, serum cholesterol concentrations are unaffected by the method of feeding in early infancy.

Serum cholesterol levels vary at different age groups and into adulthood (table 10-2). There are significant changes between birth and 2 years of age and during sexual maturation. Researchers in Louisiana noted dramatic rises in the first 2 years of life. Low-density lipoproteins account for the major increase during the first year. However, a slow but progressive rise in high-density lipoproteins occurs.[36]

No dramatic changes occur in lipid or lipoprotein levels in school-age children. During adolescence, race- and sex-specific changes in cholesterol levels occur. There is a decrease in high-density lipoprotein serum cholesterol levels accompanied by an increase in low-density lipoprotein serum cholesterol levels in white males between 10 and 16 years of age. High-density lipoprotein cholesterol levels decline in black males of the same age, although not as dramatically. Black males also experience a slight drop in low-density lipoprotein cholesterol levels. Declines occur in high-density lipoprotein cholesterol levels with almost no change in low-density lipoprotein cholesterol levels in both black and white females between 9 and 14 years of age. The ratio of mean serum levels of low-density lipoprotein cholesterol to levels of high-density lipoprotein cholesterol rises dramatically in white boys beginning at 11 years of age, but it remains unchanged in black adolescent males and black and white adolescent females.[36] After 24 years of age, a progressive rise in total cholesterol for the next 30 years occurs.

The Louisiana study found that cholesterol levels in the first year were the most predictive factors studied of subsequent cholesterol levels. Of the children at the 90th and 10th percentiles

TABLE 10-2   *Serum Lipids and Lipoprotein Levels for Infants, Children,*
and Young Adults (Bogalusa Heart Study)

Age (Years)	Total Cholesterol		Triglycerides (mg/dl)	
	Median	(90th P)	Median	(90th P)
Birth	68	94	34	67
6 months	132	173	81	141
1–2	147	179	64	120
3–4	157	191	56	95
5–6	158	194	51	88
7–8	163	196	53	92
9–10	165	203	57	106
11–12	161	200	61	115
13–14	155	192	61	109
15–16	151	189	61	109
17–18	155	200	63	106
19–20	160	210	76	136
21–22	165	215	78	156
23–24	170	219	81	164
25–26	177	221	85	186

Cholesterol Fractions (mg/dl)

Age (Years)	HDL-C		LDL-C		VLDL-C	
	(10th P)	Median	Median	(90th P)	Median	(90th P)
Birth	18	35	29	43	2	9
6 months	27	51	73	99	9	22
1–2	33	55	85	113	6	16
3–4	36	59	92	122	4	13
5–6	43	67	86	117	4	13
7–8	43	66	91	123	4	14
9–10	40	67	91	127	5	17
11–12	38	62	90	123	7	19
13–14	37	61	84	117	7	19
15–16	35	58	82	118	8	19
17–18	35	57	89	128	8	19
19–20	24	51	101	143	9	22
21–22	23	50	102	155	10	27
23–24	23	52	106	155	10	29
25–26	23	52	116	156	12	34

From Berensen GS and others: Prevention of adult heart disease beginning in the pediatric age. In Frohoick ED (editor): *Preventive aspects of coronary disease,* and Brest AN: Cardiovascular Clinics, Philadelphia, 1990, FA Davis.

in the first year, 45% persisted at their respective levels in the second year. Children of parents with high serum cholesterol levels are 2.57 times more likely to have serum cholesterol levels greater than the 95th percentile.[37] Another longitudinal study in Iowa found that of those children with cholesterol levels above the 75th percentile 75% of boys and 56% of girls would not qualify for intervention as adults. Of the children with cholesterol levels above the 95th percentile, 57% of girls and 37% of boys would not qualify for intervention as adults.[38]

Studies have suggested that 5% of the children in the United States have serum cholesterol levels greater than 200 to 220 mg/100 ml. It appears that these individuals will maintain their elevated levels throughout childhood and into adulthood; they are considered at risk of developing coronary artery disease.[37] As they grow older, they will be joined by others who enter the ranks of the "at risk" population.

Etiological Factors in Atherosclerosis

Cardiovascular disease is responsible for more deaths in the United States than all other causes. **Atherosclerosis** is responsible for more than 50% of the deaths resulting from cardiovascular disease.

Atherosclerosis is a major specific type of **arteriosclerosis** and involves primarily the large elastic and medium-sized arteries. Lipids similar to those circulating in the blood accumulate on the intima of the arteries, to which an accumulation of connective tissue and various blood products are added, and plaques result. Several complications such as hemorrhage, thrombosis, or ulceration can occur in the atherosclerotic lesion and can transform plaques into rough, complicated lesions. The plaques narrow the lumen of the arteries and may produce a deficiency of blood flow to some degree. They set the stage for complete occlusion.

Fatty flecks and streaks are present by 3 to 5 months of age in the aortas of all children of all populations. As children age, the number and size of the streaks increase. Studies of animals have suggested that dietary intakes of cholesterol and fatty acids determine whether the fatty deposits are reabsorbed, remain, or develop into atherosclerotic plaques.[39,40]

The average extent of intimal involvement is small in the first 10 years of life. After the first decade the extent of the intimal surface involved by fatty streaks increases rapidly. The lipid in the juvenile fatty streak is predominantly intracellular with minimal connective tissue. Black children have more extensive fatty streaks than do children of other ethnic groups. Females have more extensive streaking than do males. This is true in all populations studied, regardless of the incidence of atherosclerosis. After 25 to 29 years of age, differences appear. Fatty streaks progress through continued lipid accumulation and lead to plaque formation. These fatty streaks contain much of their lipid in the form of extracellular accumulations in areas where intact cells are scanty. An increase in extracellular components of connective tissue also becomes apparent. Fibrous plaques then appear in a significant number of cases.

Autopsies of male soldiers in their early twenties who died in the wars in Korea and Vietnam revealed a striking incidence of atherosclerotic plaques. Of the males killed in Korea, 77% were found to have evidence of atherosclerosis, ranging from minimal thickening to complete occlusion of one or more of the main artery branches.[41] Autopsies of soldiers killed in Vietnam revealed a lesser but significant incidence of atherosclerosis. Of the casualties on whom autopsies were performed during this war, 45% were found to have atherosclerosis, but only 5% had gross evidence of coronary artery involvement.[42]

Autopsy studies of children from the Bogalusa Heart Study found an adverse effect of elevated risk factor levels including serum cholesterol and lipoprotein levels in accelerating the development of fatty streaks and fibrous plaques in adolescence.[43]

Risk Factors Associated with Atherosclerosis

Two hundred and forty-six risk factors have been identified for cardiovascular disease. However, the major risk factors include elevated serum levels of low-density lipoprotein cholesterol, cigarette smoking, hypertension, obesity, sedentary lifestyle, and a family history of heart disease. There is also some evidence that there is a relationship between watching television and cholesterol levels.[44] Children who watched the most television had the highest cholesterol levels, probably because they had less exercise. All risk factors have been found to be independent and continuous variables. No arbitrary serum cholesterol level exists at which the risk of developing cardiovascular heart disease is increased. As the serum cholesterol level increases, the risk for atherosclerosis increases. Also, the risk of developing atherosclerosis increases as the number of risk factors increases. Two or three risk factors increase the risk for atherosclerosis in an exponential manner. For example, the obese individual with a moderately elevated serum cholesterol level who has hypertension and smokes cigarettes has a higher risk of developing atherosclerosis than the person who has a more elevated serum cholesterol level but is lean, active, and does not smoke.

Elevated serum low-density lipoprotein cholesterol and low serum high-density lipoprotein cholesterol concentrations are clearly risk factors in the etiology of coronary artery disease. Populations that consume diets rich in cholesterol and saturated fats have higher serum cholesterol concentrations and higher incidences of and mortality rates from premature coronary heart disease than populations that consume diets low in cholesterol and saturated fats. The risk of developing premature atherosclerotic heart disease increases in any population group as the serum cholesterol concentration, especially LDL cholesterol, rises.[45]

Effect of Dietary Intervention

It has been proved that dietary alterations can reduce serum lipids. In adults who decrease total fat, saturated fat, and cholesterol, there is a reduction in serum lipids. Recommending similar diets in children, especially as a broad public health measure, has raised safety concerns, particularly during the peak growing years. These concerns have centered on the possibility of decreased growth, as well as inadequate nutrient intake and negative psychological effects.

The Dietary Intervention Study in Children (DISC) was a multicenter trial of 8- to 10-year-old children for three years. Those in the intervention group (receiving 28% of energy from fat) had lower levels of LDL cholesterol than those in the control group. There were no differences in height, weight, body mass index, or nutritional adequacy between the two groups, indicating that the diet was safe.[46] In another study of preschool children 3 to 4 years of age, a diet containing 27% of energy from fat did not compromise growth over a two-year period.[47]

Dietary factors other than fats have been shown to influence cholesterol levels. For example, fiber, especially pectin, has a **hypocholesterolemic** effect.

Recommendations

An effort to prevent cardiovascular heart disease has been recommended and is currently being implemented in most areas of the United States. Two efforts are directed toward children and adolescents; a change in the diet for all children limiting intakes of total fat, saturated fatty acids, and cholesterol, and the identification of the child "at high risk" because of a family history of cardiovascular heart disease. In addition, efforts need to be made to reduce the other risk factors such as smoking, stress, and obesity.

The Expert Panel from the National Institutes of Health (NIH) recommends a pattern of food intake for children over 2 years of age that includes foods low in saturated fatty acids, total fat, and cholesterol and that provides sufficient energy to support normal growth and development.[34] Specifically, they recommend a diet that includes (1) less than 10% of kcalories as saturated fatty acids, (2) no more than 30% of kcalories from total fat, and (3) less than 300 mg cholesterol per day.

Dietary Changes

It is probable that a reduction in total fat intake will aid in the prevention of obesity, since fat is a more concentrated source of energy than other nutrients. However, it is important that energy intake be maintained to support normal growth. This means that intakes of carbohydrate will be increased. The panel recommends an intake of 55% of energy using mostly complex carbohydrates. They recommend increasing intakes of pastas, breads and cereals, legumes, and fruits and vegetables. Most of these foods will also provide fiber.

The recommendation that children consume no more than 300 mg cholesterol per day will not be hard to achieve. Most children consume less than this. It has been suggested that a cholesterol intake based on energy intake might be more appropriate.

Lowering total fat in the current diet will mean that children will need to consume more low-fat dairy products, more low-fat cuts of meat, and few baked products made with fat. It will be important that the diets of children continue to be monitored for adequate energy intakes as children and adolescents implement the suggested changes. A diet that reduces total fat to the suggested level may include a number of high-fiber foods. The young child with a finicky appetite may soon be satiated.

Since most children consume a considerable percentage of food away from home, implementation of the recommendations will involve not only nutrition education for the children and their parents but changes in the menu patterns of many day-care and school feeding programs. The contents of school vending machines, snack bars, and student stores will need to include "heart healthy" foods. The food industry also has an important role to play in the implementation of the suggested changes by providing appropriate low-fat foods for children and labeling foods so that parents and children can identify the fat content of the products in the grocery store.

Dietary changes should be implemented by all of the health and educational professionals who interact with the child and family. Nutrition education at school can focus on teaching young children to make appropriate food choices at snack time and during meals; models have been developed for a "heart healthy" diet and lifestyle.[48] Physicians, dietitians, and nurses should include an assessment of the child's fat intake in their health surveillance programs and help the children and their parents implement a diet that provides no more than 30% of the kcalories as fat, no more than 10% of the kcalories as saturated fat, and no more than 300 mg cholesterol per day.

Selective Screening

The second approach recommended by the NIH panel is selective screening; that is, identification by physician and nurse practitioners of children "at high risk" for developing cardiovascular heart disease during health surveillance. Those at risk include children with a family history of hypercholesterolemia or cardiovascular disease, children who smoke, have high blood pressure, or whose diets include excessive amounts of cholesterol and saturated fatty acids. The screening protocol will vary with the reason for the high-risk designation. If one parent has high cholesterol levels, a determination of total cholesterol will be made. If the cholesterol level is borderline (table 10-3), a second measurement will be made.[34] If the total cholesterol is high, a lipoprotein analysis will be obtained. If the child is being tested because of a family history of premature cardiovascular disease, a lipoprotein analysis will be the first test performed. Acceptable ranges are shown in table 10-3.

If children have borderline or high low-density lipoprotein cholesterol levels, implementation of the diet previously described for the entire population is recommended. If the low-density lipoprotein cholesterol level is high and the diet does not sufficiently lower the lipid levels, a diet providing less than 200 mg cholesterol and 7% of total kcalories as saturated fatty acids is recommended. If diet fails to lower the lipid levels sufficiently, the use of cholesterol-lowering drugs should be considered.[34]

The recommendation for selective screening is based on the fact that population screening is costly and identifies a significant number of children with high cholesterol levels who will not be hypercholesterolemic as adults.[38] However, researchers are concerned that selective screening will miss a significant number of children with hypercholesterolemia. Steiner, Neinstein, and Pennbridge[49] found that one-third to one-half of teenagers with hypercholesterolemia will have been missed with selective screening. It is likely that one will find individual and mass screening in health care agencies and among individual practitioners.

TABLE 10-3   *Classification of Total and LDL Cholesterol Levels in Children and Adolescents from Families with Hypercholesterolemia or Premature Cardiovascular Disease*

Category	Total Cholesterol (mg/dL)*	LDL Cholesterol (mg/dL)*
Acceptable	<170	<110
Borderline	170–199	110–129
High	≥200	≥130

From Expert Panel on Blood Cholesterol Levels in Children and Adolescents: *Report of the health panel on blood cholesterol levels in children and adolescents,* Public Health Service, National Institutes of Health, Pub No 91-2732, Washington, DC, 1991, US Department of Health and Human Services.
*To convert cholesterol values in mg/dL to millimoles per liter (mmol/L), multiply by 0.02586.

SALT INTAKE

Essential hypertension, another risk factor in cardiovascular heart disease, as well as stroke and renal disease, is also a major health problem affecting over half of adults over 60 years of age. Epidemiological studies have suggested that as with hyperlipidemia, genetic and environmental factors interact to determine an individual's susceptibility to hypertension. Salt has been implicated as one factor that may cause this disorder.

Success in reducing blood pressure in hypertensive patients with the low-sodium rice diet designed by Kempner caused some researchers to hypothesize that excessive salt intakes could cause hypertension. Dahl[50] became so convinced that salt intakes were important in the development of hypertension that he devoted his life to this research. He studied the effect of salt intakes on thousands of rats, the effect of reduced sodium intake on hypertensive patients, and the relationship of sodium intakes to the incidence of hypertension in populations.

Evidence from Animal Studies

Meneely and others[51] induced hypertension in rats by mixing salt with their food and allowing them to consume as much water and food as they wished. They studied six groups of rats, each of which was fed an increasing amount of salt, and found that as sodium chloride intakes increased, elevations in blood pressures increased. Hypertension developed early in those animals who consumed the highest salt intakes, although individual variations within groups were noted.

Dahl and others[52] found that in unselected rats, blood pressure increases in response to high salt intakes ranged from none to gradually increasing blood pressures, including the malignant phase. Some rats died from hypertension within a few months. One-fourth of the animals showed no increase in blood pressure. The other animals developed increases in blood pressure that were associated with increasing morbidity and mortality.

In successive generations, rats were inbred and a strain of rats genetically susceptible to salt was developed. It was found that increased salt intakes of these animals during the first 12 to 13 months after weaning produced hypertension that was sustained regardless of later reductions in sodium intakes. Control rats fed low-sodium mixtures developed no hypertension.[53] Dahl, Heine, and Tassinari[54] concluded that salt intakes in infancy and early childhood may be more critical than those in later life to persons genetically determined to be responsive to salt intakes. In 1963 they fed commercially prepared salted infant foods to those rats bred to be genetically sensitive to salt. Five of seven rats developed hypertension, whereas none of the seven control rats who were fed low-sodium diets developed the disorder. At that time they suggested that there may be groups of human infants with similar genetic potentials who are at risk of induced hypertension from salt intakes in early life. They advocated reductions in salt intakes in infancy.

Srinivasan and others[55] found that systolic and diastolic blood pressure levels increased in spider monkeys that were fed salt and salt-sucrose diets as compared with the levels of monkeys fed a control diet. A greater rise was noted in blood pressure of those fed the salt-sucrose diet. They suggested a potentiating effect of sucrose on sodium-induced hypertension.

Studies of Populations

Dahl[50] studied five population groups whose lifetime salt intakes varied from 4 to 26 gm/day and found that as average salt intakes increased, the incidence of hypertension increased.

Gleibermann[56] reviewed studies of 27 populations. Sodium intakes had been estimated by urinary excretion of sodium for 24 hours in some and by estimated salt intakes in others. Her statistical analysis of these studies suggested a direct relationship between salt intakes and blood pressure across population lines.

The Intersalt Cooperative Research Group[57] studied the relationship between 24-hour urinary electrolytes and blood pressure in 10,079 men and women, 20 to 59 years of age, in 52 centers around the world. It was only in centers in which very low sodium excretion was found that a population was identified with low blood pressure and in which there was little or no increase in blood pressure with age. In the other centers sodium excretion was related to the slope of blood pressure with age but not to the prevalence of hypertension nor median blood pressure of the subjects. Within centers sodium excretion was related to blood pressure in individuals. The sodium to potassium excretion ratio and blood pressure in individuals had a pattern similar to sodium alone but was stronger and more consistent. Body mass index and alcohol consumption were positively associated with blood pressure in individuals.

Studies in children have not conclusively established a relationship between salt intakes and blood pressure. Whitten and Stewart[58] studied two groups of black males starting at 3 months of age: one fed a low level of salt; the other fed a high level of salt. They found no difference in blood pressure levels of the two groups at 8 months or 8 years of age.

Siervogelm and others[59] found a strong relationship between urinary sodium and systolic blood pressure in 8- to 18-year-old white children. However, the relationship was not significant when body size, obesity, and age were considered.

Falkner, Oresti, and Angelakos[60] found that adolescents with normal blood pressure from families with a history of hypertension who were fed a high-salt diet for 2 weeks and then stressed with difficult mathematical problems had a greater heart rate and blood pressure than did a control group. No differences were noted in children fed the high-salt diet and then stressed if their families had no history of hypertension.

The relationship of salt intakes of individuals to blood pressure has not been established, and high salt intakes do not necessarily guarantee the development of hypertension. However, some individuals are believed to be salt-sensitive, with significant response in their blood pressure after salt restriction or salt repletion.[61] At the present time there are no good methods for identifying salt-sensitive adults or children.[62]

Blood Pressure During Childhood

Blood pressure in adults is correlated with childhood blood pressure and body size. Children with higher blood pressure are more likely to become adult hypertensives, especially if they are obese and have a family history of hypertension.[63] Some individuals who are likely to be hypertensive adults can be identified in childhood and preventive intervention can be suggested. Goals during childhood are (1) surveillance, (2) possible prevention, and (3) identification and treatment of children who are already hypertensive. However, no mass screening is recommended.[62] Ideally, blood pressure measurements

TABLE 10-4   *Classification of Hypertension by Age Group*

Age Group	Significant Hypertension (mm Hg)	Severe Hypertension (mm Hg)
Newborn		
7 d	Systolic BP ≥96	Systolic BP ≥106
8–30 d	Systolic BP ≥104	Systolic BP ≥110
Infant (<2 yr)	Systolic BP ≥112	Systolic BP ≥118
	Diastolic BP ≥74	Diastolic BP ≥82
Children (3–5 yr)	Systolic BP ≥116	Systolic BP ≥124
	Diastolic BP ≥76	Diastolic BP ≥84
Children (6–9 yr)	Systolic BP ≥122	Systolic BP ≥130
	Diastolic BP ≥78	Diastolic BP ≥86
Children (10–12 yr)	Systolic BP ≥126	Systolic BP ≥134
	Diastolic BP ≥82	Diastolic BP ≥90
Adolescents (13–15 yr)	Systolic BP ≥136	Systolic BP ≥144
	Diastolic BP ≥86	Diastolic BP ≥92
Adolescents (16–18 yr)	Systolic BP ≥142	Systolic BP ≥150
	Diastolic BP ≥92	Diastolic BP ≥98

From Task Force on Blood Pressure Control in Children, American Academy of Pediatrics: *Pediatrics* 79:1, 1987.

are included during well-child and subsequent medical visits and at-risk children can be identified over time. Strong and colleagues have suggested using blood pressure and overweight status as criteria to identify, monitor, and treat hypertensive children.[64] Prevention in high-risk children includes avoiding overweight, consuming a moderate salt intake, and maintaining an active lifestyle.

Blood pressure readings increase from 3 months of age through adolescence. The definition of hypertension during childhood is age specific (table 10-4).

Sodium Intakes

Sodium intake of infants is relatively low when human milk and commercially prepared infant foods are consumed and relatively high when cow's milk and table foods are eaten. As the transition is made to table foods, salt intakes will reflect family food habits and cultural patterns. The use of convenience foods and the popularity of fast-food establishments

for feeding children past infancy have given the food industry a major role in determining salt intakes of children.

Commercially prepared infant foods have no salt added during preparation. Many parents prefer to make their own infant foods from a variety of foods prepared and seasoned for the family. Those who serve the highest sodium intakes to their infants have less education, feed salty snacks, and heavily salt their own food.[65] Salt intakes in the United States average 7 to 10 gm/day; intakes of 10 to 20 gm/day are common.

Need for Sodium

Sodium is an essential nutrient. It functions in the maintenance of water and acid-base balance and the regulation of blood volume. It regulates cell membrane and capillary permeability and is a constituent of tissues. It is estimated that total body sodium increases from 240 mEq in the 3.3-kg newborn to 3100 mEq in a 70-kg adult. Requirements are determined by the individual's needs for growth and by losses from the skin and in the urine and stools.[66] Needs for growth are estimated to be 0.5 mEq/kg/day during the first 3 months, 0.2 mEq/kg/day from 3 to 6 months, 0.1 mEq/kg/day from 6 to 12 months, and less than 0.1 mEq/kg/day after the first year. Skin losses depend on the ambient temperature. Sodium losses from stools are independent of intake, averaging 5% to 10% in the first year. Because of the variability of losses, Fomon[67] suggests an advisable intake of 80 mg of sodium per day during the first year of life. This is more than the estimated requirement, but less than the "minimum requirements" specified by the Food and Nutrition Board.[68] Humans adapt to a wide range of sodium intake by varying excretion in relation to intake and nonrenal losses. Safe limits for normal children appear to be between 8 and 100 mEq/day.

The Task Force on Blood Pressure Control in Children[62] recommends limiting sodium intake to 5 to 6 gm (85 to 100 mEq)/day if a child is hypertensive. It is also important to increase potassium-rich foods in the diet when intakes of salt are limited.

It is important to remember that iodized salt is a major source of iodine in the United States. Intakes by children who consume low-sodium diets should be carefully monitored for iodine. A palpable goiter has been noted in two adolescent females whose family had adopted a low-sodium dietary intake because of diagnosed hypertension in the father.

Summary

Obesity, hypertension, and hyperlipoproteinemia are all risk factors for adult cardiovascular disease and other disorders. A number of studies have indicated that the atherosclerotic process begins in childhood and that total cholesterol, low-density lipoprotein cholesterol, very low-density lipoprotein cholesterol levels, and high-density lipoprotein levels are correlated with the extent of the atherosclerotic lesions in adolescents and young adults.

It has been demonstrated that the lipid levels in the blood can be reduced by altering the present diet. Efforts have been directed to reduce intakes of fats and saturated fatty acids in the current diet of children and adolescents in hopes that reducing the risk factors of individuals will reduce the incidence of and the morbidity and mortality from cardiovascular heart disease. Recommendations have also been made to prevent obesity and moderate salt intakes.

REVIEW QUESTIONS

1. Define obesity and superobesity in childhood.
2. When should a weight reduction diet be planned for an obese child?
3. Why are there differences of opinion regarding individual and population screening for hyperlipidemia?
4. What dietary changes are recommended for children in the United States to reduce the incidence of cardiovascular heart disease?
5. What level of sodium restriction is recommended for children who are hypertensive?

SUGGESTED LEARNING ACTIVITIES

1. Plan a week's menu for a 5-year-old girl who weighs 21 kg and is 109 cm tall. The diet should maintain her weight.
2. Investigate and report on physical activities that are developmentally appropriate to increase energy expenditure for 2- and 8-year-old girls.
3. Describe how you would counsel the parents of an obese 8-month-old boy.
4. Describe children at risk of hyperlipoproteinemia. How would one counsel parents of these children?
5. Investigate the salt content of fast-food menu items.

REFERENCES

1. Gutin B and others: Blood pressure, fitness, and fatness in 5- and 6-year-old children, *JAMA* 264:1123, 1990.
2. Hill AJ, Silver EK: Fat, friendless, and unhealthy: 9-year-old children's perception of body shape stereotypes, *Int J Obes Relat Metab Disord* 19:423, 1995.
3. Troiano RP and others: Overweight prevalence and trends for children and adolescents. The National Health and Nutrition Examination Surveys, 1963–1991, *Arch Pediatr Adolesc Med* 149:1085, 1995.
4. Kalata G: Obese children: a growing problem, *Science* 232:20, 1986.
5. Guo SS and others: The predictive value of childhood body mass index values for overweight at age 35, *Am J Clin Nutr* 59:810, 1994.

❖ ❖ ❖

CASE STUDY

Weight Management for Obese Preschool Child

At the request of her local pediatrician, the 2½-year-old daughter of a single parent was seen at the Child Development and Mental Retardation Center at the University of Washington. She needed evaluation and therapy from several professionals. The child was visibly obese. Her weight plotted above the 95th percentile, her length was between the 25th and 50th percentiles, and her weight-for-height was over the 95th percentile.

During the nutrition interview it was reported that she was obviously overfat at 4 months of age. By 14 months of age her mother and grandmother became concerned. When she was 2 years of age she was often upset because she was "fat." Her mother tried offering her low-kcalorie foods. She, however, often gorged and sneaked food. The child, according to her diet history, was consuming 1500 to 1700 kcal/day, 75 to 85 kcal/kg, 16 to 18 kcal/cm of height. A diet supplying 850 kcal (9 cal/cm) was prescribed.

The mother and child lived with the mother's male friend and his father. The child was often cared for by her grandmother, and there was no coordination of efforts to control her food or energy intake.

The mother's friend, a rehabilitated drug addict, frequently told the child she was a "fatty" and ugly and then gave her food to keep her quiet. The child's mother did not want to move to her parents' home and doubted that she could "make it" on her own.

In the following 3 months the child lost 2 kg. Her linear growth proceeded in channel. Often when she came to the clinic she was very reluctant to be weighed, stating "I not a fatty; I not ugly." Play therapy for the child and therapy sessions for the mother as well as nutrition counseling were incorporated into the monthly visits.

The child's mother applied for and received a scholarship to a junior college, which carried a monthly stipend, and she was able to move to her own apartment and enroll the child in a preschool program that included a variety of daily physical activities. When she had lost 3 kg, her weight-for-height plotted below the 95th percentile, and her suggested energy intake was increased to 10.5 kcal/cm/day (950 to 1000 kcal/day) with a goal of weight maintenance. However, she began to gain weight.

It soon became apparent that each episode of weight gain was associated with psychosocial problems of the mother and that only the continuing counseling and play therapy made implementation of the plan for maintaining a normal weight possible. Even today, as a school-age child, her diet and weight gains must be carefully monitored. She is, however, no longer classified as obese. Continuing support has been necessary to maintain the gains toward prevention of future obesity (fig. 10-3).

Continued.

6. Forbes GB: Lean body mass and fat in obese children, *Pediatrics* 34:308, 1964.
7. Hammer LD and others: Standardized percentile curves of body mass index for children and adolescents, *Am J Dis Child* 145:259, 1991.
8. Burns TL, Moll PP, Lauer RM: Genetic models of human obesity—family studies, *Crit Rev Food Sci Nutr* 33:339, 1993.
9. Stunkard AJ and others: An adoption study of human obesity, *N Engl J Med* 314:193, 1986.
10. Stunkard AJ and others: The body-mass index of twins who have been reared apart, *N Eng J Med* 322:1483, 1990.
11. Deitz WH: Critical periods in childhood for the development of obesity, *Am J Clin Nutr* 59:955, 1994.
12. Griffiths M and others: Metabolic rate and physical development in children at risk of obesity, *Lancet* 336:76, 1990.
13. Ruowei L and others: Relation of activity levels to body fat in infants 6 to 12 months of age, *J Pediatr* 126:353, 1995.
14. Dietz WH, Gortmaker SL: Do we fatten our children at the television set? Obesity and television viewing in children and adolescents, *Pediatrics* 75:807, 1985.

❖ ❖ ❖

CASE STUDY

Weight Management for Obese Preschool Child—cont'd

FIG. 10-3   Weight/height grid of obese preschooler during and after nutrition counseling and psychosocial intervention.

15. Klesges RC, Shelton ML, Klesges LM: Effects of television on metabolic rate: potential implications for childhood obesity, *Pediatrics* 91:281, 1993.

16. Fisch RO, Bilek MK, Ulstrom R: Obesity and leanness at birth and their relationship to body habits in later childhood, *Pediatrics* 56:521, 1975.

17. Yeung DL and others: Infant fatness and feeding practices: a longitudinal assessment, *J Am Diet Assoc* 79:531, 1981.

18. Fomon SJ and others: Indices of fatness and serum cholesterol at age eight years in relation to feeding and growth during early infancy, *Pediatr Res* 18:1233, 1984.

19. Shapiro LR and others: Obesity prognosis: a longitudinal study of children from the age of 6 months to 9 years, *Am J Public Health* 74:968, 1984.

20. Johnson SL, Birch LL: Parents' and children's adiposity and eating style, *Pediatrics* 94:653, 1994.

21. Hertzler AA: Obesity-impact of the family, *J Am Diet Assoc* 79:525, 1981.

22. Bruch H: Obesity in childhood. III. Physiologic and psychologic aspects of food intake of obese children, *Am J Dis Child* 59:739, 1940.

23. Lissau I, Sorenson TIA: Parental neglect during childhood and increased risk of obesity in young adulthood, *Lancet* 343:324, 1994.

24. Garn SM, Clark DC, Guire KE: *Growth, body composition and development of obese and lean children*. In Winick M, editor: *Childhood obesity*, New York, 1975, John Wiley & Sons.

25. Okamoto E, Davidson LL, Conner DR: High prevalence of overweight in inner-city school children, *Am J Dis Child* 147:155, 1993.

26. Kennedy E, Goldberg J: What are American children eating? Implications for public policy, *Nutr Rev* 53:111, 1995.

27. Ray JW, Klesges RC: *Influence on the eating behavior of children*. In Williams CL, Kimm SYS, editors: Prevention and treatment of childhood obesity, *Ann NY Acad Sci* 699:57, 1993.

28. Griffith M, Payne PR: Energy expenditure in small children of obese and nonobese parents, *Nature* 260:698, 1976.

29. Pugliese MT and others: Fear of obesity: a cause of short stature and delayed puberty, *N Engl J Med* 301:513, 1983.

30. Epstein L and others: Growth in obese children treated for obesity, *Am J Dis Child* 144:1360, 1990.

31. Wolff OH, Lloyd JK: Obesity in childhood, *Proc Nutr Soc* 32:195, 1973.

32. Epstein LH and others: Ten-year outcomes of behavioral family-based treatment for childhood obesity, *Health Psych* 13:373, 1994.

33. American Academy of Pediatrics Committee on Nutrition: Statement on cholesterol, *Pediatrics* 90:469, 1992.

34. Expert Panel on Blood Cholesterol Levels in Children and Adolescents: *Report of the expert panel on blood cholesterol levels in children and adolescents*, Public Health Service, National Institutes of Health, Pub No (NIH) 91-2732, Washington, DC, 1991, US Department of Health and Human Services.

35. Farris RP and others: Influence of milk source on serum lipids and lipoproteins during the first year of life, *Am J Clin Nutr* 38:42, 1982.

36. Berenson GS and others: *Prevention of adult heart disease beginning in the pediatric age*. In Frohoick ED, editor: *Preventive aspect of coronary disease*, and Brest AN: *Cardiovascular clinics*, Philadelphia, 1990, FA Davis.

37. Berenson GS and others: Serum high-density lipoprotein and its relationship to cardiovascular disease risk factor variables in children—the Bogalusa Heart Study, *Lipids* 14:91, 1979.

38. Lauer RM, Clarke WR: Use of cholesterol measurements in childhood for the prediction of adult hypercholesterolemia: the Muscatine study, *JAMA* 264:3034, 1990.

39. Armstrong ML, Warner ED, Connor WE: Regression of coronary atheromatosis in rhesus monkeys, *Circ Res* 27:59, 1970.

40. Wissler RW and others: Atherogenesis in the cebus monkey, *Arch Pathol* 74:312, 1962.

41. Enos WF, Holmes RH, Beyer JC: Coronary disease among United States soldiers killed in action in Korea, *JAMA* 152:1090, 1952.

42. McNamara JJ and others: Coronary artery disease in combat casualties in Vietnam, *JAMA* 216:1185, 1971.

43. Cresanta JL and others: Prevention of atherosclerosis in childhood, *Pediatr Clin North Am* 33:835, 1986.

44. Wong ND and others: Television viewing and pediatric hypercholesterolemia, *Pediatrics* 90:75, 1992.

45. National Cholesterol Education Program: *Second report of the expert panel on detection, evaluation, and treatment of high blood cholesterol in adults* (ATP-11). NIH Pub. No. 93-3095, 1993.

46. DISC Collaborative Research Group: Efficacy and safety of lowering dietary intake of fat and cholesterol in children with elevated low-density lipoprotein cholesterol, *JAMA* 273:1429, 1995.

47. Shea S and others: Is there a relationship between dietary fat and stature or growth in children three to five years of age? *Pediatrics* 92:579, 1993.

48. Berenson GS and others: Cardiovascular health promotion for elementary school children. The Heart Smart Program. In Williams CL, Wynder EL: Hyperlipidemia in childhood and the development of atherosclerosis, *Ann NY Acad Sci* 623:299, 1991.

49. Steiner NJ, Neinstein LS, Pennbridge J: Hypercholesterolemia in adolescents: effectiveness of screening strategies based on selected risk factors, *Pediatrics* 88:269, 1991.

50. Dahl LK: Salt and hypertension, *Am J Clin Nutr* 25:231, 1972.

51. Meneely GR and others: Chronic sodium chloride toxicity in the albino rat. II. Occurrence of hypertension and a syndrome of edema and renal failure, *J Exp Med* 98:71, 1953.

52. Dahl LK and others: Effects of chronic excess salt ingestion: modifications of experimental hypertension in the rat by variations in the diet, *Circ Res* 22:11, 1968.

53. Dahl LK: Effect of chronic excess salt feeding induction of self-sustaining hypertension in rats, *J Exp Med* 114:231, 1961.

54. Dahl LK, Heine M, Tassinari L: High salt content of Western infants' diet: possible relationship to hypertension in the adult, *Nature* 198:1204, 1963.

55. Srinivasan SR and others: Effects of dietary sodium and sucrose on the induction of hypertension in spider monkeys, *Am J Clin Nutr* 33:561, 1980.

56. Gleibermann L: Blood pressure and dietary salt in human populations, *Ecol Food Nutr* 2:143, 1973.

57. Intersalt Cooperative Research Group: Intersalt: an international study of electrolyte excretion and blood pressure: results for 24 hour urinary sodium and potassium excretion, *Br Med J* 297:319, 1988.

58. Whitten CF, Stewart RA: The effect of dietary sodium in infancy on blood pressure and related factors, *Acta Paediatr Scand Suppl* 279, 1980.

59. Siervogelm RM and others: Blood pressure, electrolytes, and body size: their relationships in young relatives of men with essential hypertension, *Hypertension* 2(part II):183, 1980.

60. Falkner B, Oresti G, Angelakos D: Effect of salt loading on the cardiovascular response to stress in adolescents, *Hypertension* 3(part III):195, 1981.

61. Kotchen T: Evaluation of publicly available scientific evidence regarding certain nutrient-disease relationships: Sodium and hypertension, Life Sciences Research Office, *Federation of American Societies for Experimental Biology*, Bethesda, MD, 1991.

62. Task Force on Blood Pressure Control in Children, American Academy of Pediatrics: Report of the second task force on blood pressure control in children—1987, *Pediatrics* 79:1, 1987.

63. Mahoney LT and others: Childhood predictors of high blood pressure, *Am J Hypertension* 4:608S, 1991.

64. Strong WB and others: Integrated cardiovascular health promotion in childhood. A statement for health professionals from the subcommittee on atherosclerosis and hypertension in childhood of the Council on Cardiovascular Disease in the Young, *Circulation* 85:1638, 1992.

65. Schaefer LJ, Kumanyika SK: Maternal variables related to potentially high infant-feeding practices, *J Am Diet Assoc* 85:433, 1985.

66. Sperotto G: *Sodium chloride in pediatrics*. In Moses C, editor: *Sodium in medicine and health*, Baltimore, Md, 1980, Reese Press.

67. Fomon SJ: *Nutrition of normal infants*, St. Louis, 1993, Mosby-Year Book.

68. Food and Nutrition Board: *Recommended dietary allowances*, ed. 10, National Research Council, Washington, DC, 1989, National Academy Press.

11

Nutrition for Preschool-Age Children

Cristine M. Trahms
Peggy L. Pipes

✦✦

Objectives

After studying this chapter, the student should:

✔ *Be aware of nutrition concerns for preschool-age children.*

✔ *Understand that both physical and psychosocial development affects food choices in young children.*

✔ *Recognize that changes in growth rates, e.g., slowed and erratic, during the preschool-age period are reflected in food intake.*

✔ *Recognize cultural, community, and economic factors that affect food availability and choices for young children.*

✔ *Recognize factors that influence parents' provision of food for young children.*

✔ *Be aware of the value of snacks to a young child's daily total nutrient intake.*

✔ *Be aware of common concerns about food intake encountered by parents of preschool-age children.*

✔ *Have knowledge of feeding programs designed to improve the nutritional status of young children.*

The preschool-age period is considered to be 1 to 6 years of age. During this period, changes occur in children's rates of growth and continuing maturation of fine and gross motor skills. Personality development influences not only the amounts of food young children consume but also the foods that are acceptable to them. Food habits, likes, and dislikes begin to be established, some of which are transient and many of which form the base for a lifetime of food and nutrient intake. Environmental influences and parental behavior reinforce or extinguish food-related behavior.

There are common patterns of food and nutrient intake among preschool-age children. Feeding programs at day care and preschool contribute significantly to young children's total nutrient intake.

NUTRITION OF PRESCHOOL-AGE CHILDREN

Although overt clinical signs of malnutrition are rarely found in children in the United States, data indicate that children receive diets that are inadequate in quantity or quality. Iron, calcium, and zinc are the nutrients most frequently of concern for a lower-than-acceptable intake. Many surveys, comprehensive cross-sectional populations studies, and evaluations of small groups have been collected since 1936 to evaluate dietary intake and, less frequently, biochemical status of young children.

Regardless of population group, geographical location, or ethnic origin, some sociocultural factors appear to affect the nutrient intake of young children. A discussion of some of this information with a longer perspective will aid in understanding factors that have changed the pattern of nutrient intake of young children. Supplemental food programs, for example, have had a positive impact on iron intake of low-income children.

The data presented may appear to be contradictory, for example, preschool children are poorly nourished and poorly grown,[1] children have achieved acceptable height and weight attainment, and being overweight is more of a concern than being underweight.[2] These apparent contradictions result from circumstances affecting family economics, cultural influences, and food availability. They reflect the differences in groups of young children and point to areas of nutritional concern. Most of the reports of the dietary intakes of preschool children appropriately focus on those children believed to be at highest risk for deficient intakes—poor children. Younger children are more likely to be poor than older children or adults; one in four children under 6 years of age lives below the official **poverty line** (annual income of $15,600 for a family of four in 1996).[3]

Not all of the surveys evaluated the same nutritional components; for example, zinc, copper, and manganese have only recently emerged as nutrients of concern. Many surveys provide information on nutrient intake or consumption of food groups. Few studies report biochemical parameters of nutritional status.

Nutrient intakes of young children tend to be higher in families with incomes above poverty level. Intake data suggest that family income affects the energy intake of young children. Children whose families have incomes less than 131% of the poverty guidelines had energy intakes of about 1430 kcal/day, and those children in families with incomes greater than 300% of the poverty guidelines had energy intakes of about 1480 kcal/day.[4]

Race is often used as a substitute for income and is described as a factor that negatively affects nutrient intake. The adequacy of intake among three groups of young children (African-American, Mexican-American, and Caucasian) observed at day-care centers[5] was similar as was family socioeconomic status. Poverty or family income is often a better discriminator of nutrient intake than other factors.

The National Nutrition Status Study of preschool children conducted by Owen and others[6] found that cereal grains were the major contributors of iron. Vitamin C intakes were unrelated to energy intakes, and children of parents who had more money to spend for food consumed greater amounts of ascorbic acid.

Data from large surveys of dietary intake are often reported as a percentage of the RDA. This appears to be an appropriate use of the RDA if

TABLE 11-1 *Energy Intake for Young Children*

Age	NHANES I 1971–74	NHANES II 1976–80	NHANES III 1988–91
1–2 years	1350 kcal	1290 kcal	1290 kcal
3–5 years	1675 kcal	1570 kcal	1590 kcal

Adapted from Kennedy, *Nutr Rev*, 1995[8]

TABLE 11-2 *Fat and Carbohydrate Intakes of Preschool Children (NHANES II)*

Component	Reported Intake— All Children (% of total energy)	Recommended Dietary Guidelines (% of total energy)
Total fat	33%–36%	30%
Carbohydrate	49%–51%	55%
Protein	15%–16%	15%
Saturated fat	13%	10%
Polyunsaturated/ saturated fat intake ratio	0:4	1:1

Modified from Kimm SYS and others: *Prev Med*, 19:432, 1990.

the data are used as a reference, and not for interpretation of the status of an individual. Reporting mean levels of nutrient intakes can often "cover" large differences in actual consumption of a nutrient or nutrients. Acquiring nutrient intake data from groups of children can also be problematic because of difficulties children may have in remembering and reporting foods consumed. Preschool-age children as a group (2 to 5 years of age)—regardless of income (above or below poverty level), race (black or white), or gender—received intakes in excess of the recommendations for energy, protein, calcium, vitamins A and C, thiamin, and riboflavin. Intakes of iron varied with age. Iron is the nutrient of most significant concern.[7] Documentation of the nutrient intakes of young children includes the National Health and Nutrition Examination Surveys (NHANES), conducted from 1971 to 1974, 1976 to 1980, and 1988 to 1991. As shown in table 11-1, reported energy intakes of young children decreased from 1971 to 1976 but remained relatively stable over the next survey period.

The children enrolled in the Bogalusa Heart Study reported higher fat and carbohydrate intakes and lower protein intakes than the children surveyed for NHANES II.[9] The intake data of children enrolled in NHANES II are reported in table 11-2. These children as a group had fat intakes that were higher than those recommended for fat and cholesterol intakes[10] in objective 2.5 of the Healthy People 2000: Nutrition Objectives (table 11-3) and Dietary Guidelines for Americans (table 11-4).[11]

Black children generally had higher total fat and cholesterol intakes, and white children had higher energy intakes as complex carbohydrates. The reported protein intakes were similar for both groups.[12] Nicklas reported that mean cholesterol intake of children reaches adolescent levels by age 2 years; that is, about 300 mg/day. The composition of dietary intakes for children remains relatively constant at 13% of total energy as protein, 49% as carbohydrate, and 38% as fat regardless of age or gender.[13]

Preliminary reports from the 1988 to 1991 NHANES III noted that the range of reported intakes for energy, protein, and macronutrients, calcium and iron, is broad. Young children as a group appear to have energy intakes below recommendations (only about 40% of boys and 20% of girls under age 5 met the recommendation), adequate protein intakes (more than 90% of all children met the recommendation), and iron and calcium intakes that are relatively low as shown in table 11-5. However, the mean intakes of these nutritional components suggest that many children ingest excessive quantities of protein and appropriate energy, iron, and calcium (table 11-6). The pattern of low iron and calcium intakes does not consistently vary with family income. Iron intake has been increasing

TABLE 11-3 *Healthy People 2000 Objectives for Young Children*

Objective 2.4

Reduce growth retardation (height-for-age below the 5th percentile of NCHS reference data) among low-income children aged 5 years and younger to less than 10%.

In 1988, baseline estimates, depending on race and ethnicity, ranged from 13% to 16%.

In the 1992 baseline review, baseline estimates were revised to reflect improvement and were 8% to 15%, depending on race and ethnicity.

Objective 2.5

Reduce dietary fat intake to an average of 30% of energy or less and average saturated fat intake to less than 10% of energy among people aged 2 years and older.

In 1988, baseline estimates of total energy from fat was 36% and from saturated fat, 13%.

In the 1992 review, improvement was reflected as reported total energy from fat was 34% and from saturated fat, 12%.

Objective 2.10

Reduce iron deficiency to less than 3% among children aged 1 to 4 years.

Using the 1976 to 1980 NHANES II as baseline, prevalence of iron deficiency in low-income children ranged from 10% to 21% and in all children 4% to 5%.

No additional data were provided in the 1992 review.

Objective 2.17

Increase to at least 90% the proportion of school lunch and breakfast services with menus consistent with nutrition principles in the Dietary Guidelines for Americans.

The revised 1988 baseline data suggests that only 1% of school lunches met the goal.

No additional data were provided the 1992 review.

Objective 2.19

Increase to at least 75% the proportion of the nation's schools that provide nutrition education from preschool through grade 12, preferably as part of quality school health education.

The revised 1988 baseline data suggest that 60% met this goal.

No additional data were provided in the 1992 review.

Adapted from: *National Center for Health Statistics, Healthy People 2000 Review,* 1994. Hyattsville, MD, Public Health Service, 1995.

TABLE 11-4 *1995 Dietary Guidelines for Americans*

Balance the food you eat with physical activity—maintain or improve your weight.

Choose a diet with plenty of grain products, vegetables, and fruits.

Choose a diet low in fat, saturated fat, and cholesterol.

Eat a variety of foods.

Choose a diet moderate in salt and sodium.

Choose a diet moderate in sugars.

Adapted from: *J Am Diet Assoc,* 1996.[16]

TABLE 11-5 *Percentage of Young Children Meeting Recommended Intake for Age*

	Boys, 0–5 years old (%)	Girls, 0–5 years old (%)
Energy*	38	21
Protein#	95	92
Iron#	60	86
Calcium#	74	61

*100% of RDA for age, #75% of RDA for age
Adapted from Kennedy, *Nutr Rev,* 1995.[8]

TABLE 11-6　*Mean Average Three-Day Dietary Intakes of Young Children*

Mean Percentage of RDA for Age		
	Boys, 0–5 years (%)	Girls, 0–5 years (%)
Energy	>90	>80
Protein	>270	>240
Iron	>100	>100
Calcium	>100	>90

Adapted from Kennedy, *Nutr Rev*, 1995.[8]

TABLE 11-7　*Family Status of Children under 6 Years of Age*

	1960 (%)	1990 (%)
Living with two parents	90	70
Experienced divorce	<1	~50
Married women in workforce	~20	60

Adapted from Kennedy, *Nutr Rev*, 1995.[8]

in the past 20 years. The 1985 CSFII reported that 14% to 20% of young children under 5 years of age received less than 50% RDA for iron.[13] When vitamin and mineral intake were adjusted per 1000 kcals of energy, younger children (aged 6 mo. to 2 years) had a more nutrient dense diet than older children (aged 3–17 years). Preliminary reports from the 1988 to 1991 NHANES III noted that for children aged 3 and above the average sodium intake is more than 2400 mg/day.

A high percentage of children in all studies were receiving multiple vitamin and mineral supplements. In general, supplements are more often used by children from families with a head who is better educated. Fewer children are noted to take iron supplements than vitamin supplements. Supplemental iron is consumed most often as part of a multiple vitamin supplement.[14]

Nutrition Concerns of Children

A nutritional status study of low-income preschool children between 1977 and 1983 indicated that, although improvement in the nutritional status of children had been effected, 9% to 18% of the children studied had low or deficient serum levels of vitamins A and C, thiamin, riboflavin, or hemoglobin. Also, income level had dropped further and a greater number of the children were categorized as thin.[15]

Much has changed for families with young children in the past 30 years; see table 11-7. In 1990, only 70% of young children lived with

both parents; 50% had experienced the divorce of parents; and 60% of women with young children were working outside the home. It is clear that in the United States the lives of children have changed because of the profound changes in family constellations and lifestyles. The impact of these changes needs to be explored from a nutritional anthropology point of view.

Homelessness

Unfortunately, homelessness affects many young children. It is estimated that more than 100,000 children are homeless every night and about half of these children are under 6 years of age.[17]

When homeless children were compared with children living in homes, but of similar ages and income levels, homeless children showed a growth pattern compatible with moderate, chronic nutritional deprivation, for example, stunting without wasting. It was believed that the diets of these young children, 2 to 6 years of age, were not deficient in total energy but rather were inadequate in content of some nutrients and contained excessive amounts of less expensive, carbohydrate-rich foods.[18] Calculated intakes of nutrients indicated iron intakes at 40% of the RDA, and folic acid at 30% of the RDA. All other nutrients were ingested at amounts greater than or equal to 60% of the RDA. However, the overall dietary adequacy score was low at 9.8 (NORM = 16).[19]

Homeless children in Baltimore met the RDAs for all nutrients except calcium and zinc. Nutrient-fortified ready-to-eat cereals were a major contributor to the nutritional adequacy of food intakes. Sweetened beverages were consumed at meals. Fresh fruits and vegetables and dairy products were not available to these children. Foods high in sugar and sodium were often purchased by families because these foods are nonperishable.[17]

Foster Care

The numbers of young children in foster care are also increasing. Although little is known of the nutritional intake of this group, these children are vulnerable to nutritional deficiency and negative eating behavior because of the crises in their lives and the high incidence of health problems.[20]

WIC

Availability of specific nutrients has a positive impact on the diets of young children. Children of ages 1 to 5 years from low-income households were more likely to have low intakes of energy, vitamin C, and iron than children from high-income households. Children participating in the Supplemental Nutrition Program for Women, Infants, and Children (WIC) were less likely to have low-iron intakes than low-income children who were not enrolled in WIC. Vitamin A and calcium intake did not vary with WIC participation or by household income level.[21,22]

Iron. Some groups of children living in poverty have shown both clinical and biochemical evidence of malnutrition. All preschool children are at risk for iron-deficiency anemia, which appears to be a greater problem in children of low-income families than in children of other groups. For young children in Massachusetts overall iron deficiency was 9%. The highest rate was in the 0 to 12 month age group at 15%; the lowest rate was in the 37 to 59 month age group at about 5%. Low socioeconomic status is a predictor of community rates of iron deficiency.[23]

Iron-deficiency anemia causes long-term developmental effects. Costa Rican children whose iron status was documented in infancy were evaluated again at 5 years of age. All of the children had appropriate growth and iron status at age 5. However, those children who had moderately severe iron-deficiency anemia in infancy (hemoglobin levels less than 100 g/L)

TABLE 11-8   *Size Parameters of Massachusetts Head Start Children*

Size Parameter	Short Stature (height: <5th percentile)	Wasting (weight/ height: <5th percentile)	Overweight (weight/ height: >95th percentile)
% of children	7–9%	1–3%	9–13%

Adapted from Wiecha, *Public Health Reports,* 1994.[27]

had lower scores of mental and motor functioning at entrance into school.[24]

Iron intake appears to be a problem even for those children whose families have an annual income of more than $35,000 and who are in day care. Since 93% had height and weight measures within normal achievement, the apparently low energy intakes (mean = 70% of the RDA) were adequate to support growth. All nutrients met 75% of the RDA (1989) except for iron and folic acid (50% of the RDA). These children also had low biochemical indexes for iron status.[25] Healthy People 2000, Nutrition Objective 2.10 addresses the prevalence of iron deficiency anemia in this country (table 11-3). There has been a shift in public health from an emphasis on problems of underconsumption and nutritional deficiencies to those of overconsumption and imbalances in nutrient intake. Healthy People 2000, Nutrition Objective 2.4 data document the decrease in the prevalence of growth retardation among low-income children aged 5 years and under (table 11-3).[26]

The annual serial cross-sectional screening data from Head Start children in Massachusetts for four years were compared with the NCHS population data for children 36 to 59 months of age (table 11-8). The prevalence of children with short stature, wasting, and overweight was tabulated for each year. Children older than 48 months were more likely than younger children to be overweight.[27]

There is a great concern about the degree of overweight in preschool children. Because assessment techniques and interpretive guidelines have changed over time, there is no standard definition for obesity for children. Therefore, for this group it is difficult to state previous and current prevalence of overweight and obesity. However, concerns exist that the prevalence of obesity is increasing in this group of children. Potential reasons for the increasing prevalence of overweight include: nutrient intake trends, diminished physical activity, increased TV viewing, and genetics. Violent neighborhoods lead to children being "locked indoors" to protect them; often, even playgrounds are unsafe for children. Reports indicate that although energy intake of young children has remained fairly constant over the last decade; activity has decreased.[28] The concern about obesity in childhood is based on obesity to chronic disease relationships and child obesity to adult obesity relationships.

A group of children were followed from preschool to early school years. Children at the extremes of consumption tended to stay there; if at age 3 to 4 years children were in the highest quartile for foods/nutrients consumed, roughly half of them were still in the highest quartiles at age 5 to 6, and again at age 7 to 8. This would support the belief that food habits are developed early in life and persist. Food components with the strongest correlation to intake over time were carbohydrate and fat; components with the weakest correlation were cholesterol, sodium, and polyunsaturated fat.[29]

Other Concerns

Lead. Lead poisoning in young children can cause permanent stunting of growth, cognitive deficits, and other neurological problems. Children under 6 years old are at significant risk for lead toxicity because of their higher rate of lead absorption in the intestines, rapidly developing nervous system, and frequent exposure to lead (e.g., mouthing objects). Poor dietary intakes of energy, calcium, phosphorus, iron, and zinc increase susceptibility to lead effects (e.g., increased absorption and toxicity).[30] Improving intake and nutritional status of vulnerable groups offers some protection against toxicity.

Moderate concentrations of lead in children's blood (0.14 to 1.92 μmol/L) are associated with growth delay (e.g., short stature).[31] The FDA goal is to reach lead intakes of less than 100 μg/day from all food sources for children 1 to 5 years of age.[32]

A statement by the Centers for Disease Control offers these guidelines:[33] (1) offer regular meals to children, since more lead is absorbed on an empty stomach; and (2) include plenty of iron and calcium in the child's diet.

Dental caries. The prevention of baby bottle caries needs attention. In recent surveys 25% of 12- to 48-month-olds[34] and 35% of 9- to 36-month-olds[35] were put to bed with a baby bottle. Dental caries, as a result of excessive intakes of sweet foods, poor dental hygiene, and lack of dental care, is common among all groups of preschool-age children.

TV viewing. Children aged 2 to 5 years watch approximately 27 hours of television each week. In a recent survey more than half of the commercials on children's Saturday morning television were for food. It was estimated that a child viewed a food commercial every 5 minutes. Slightly less than half of the food commercials were for foods in the fats, oils, and sweets group; about 40% were for foods in the bread and cereals (sugared) group. The explicit message from the advertisements was "taste, fun, and free toys"; the implicit message was "healthful and nutritious." It is not possible to prove that food advertisements aimed at small children cause poor eating habits. However, since dietary patterns of children mirror adults, marketing of low overall nutritional value foods can be viewed as manipulative because young children cannot evaluate the advertising. It is believed that the effect of television food advertisements on children's diets and attitudes toward health are important public health issues.[36] There is an ongoing debate concerning the relationship among time spent watching television, physical activity, and body composition of children. Children who watched more television during the day and who watched television during longer periods of time were less likely to engage in physical activity.[37] The converse is also true; children whose circumstances prevented them from engaging in physical activity watched more TV.

Foods as Nutrient Sources

Food Consumption Survey data (table 11-2) indicate reported food intakes for young children. Most young children consume milk and meat, poultry, or fish as sources of protein. The percentage of young children consuming milk remains constant over the years while the proportion consuming low-fat or nonfat milk increases. About one-third of the vegetables reported to be consumed are white potatoes and over two-thirds of the fruits consumed are noncitrus fruits. Young Mexican-American children are reported to consume vegetables less often than other groups of children; for example, 25% of the Mexican-American children did not consume vegetables daily.[38]

Compared with Anglo-American children, Mexican-American children had diets with a greater density of micronutrients for energy intake. In spite of this, when the criterion of 66% of the RDA was used as a benchmark for adequacy, these children had deficient intakes of iron, zinc, vitamin D, vitamin C, and niacin. Low calcium intakes were of concern for Mexican-American girls.[39]

Food choices of young children shed light on the nutrients they ingest from foods. In a recent survey in New York State, about 40% of second graders did not eat vegetables except for potatoes and tomato sauce; 20% consumed no fruit; and about 60% of the children consumed no fruit other than juice.[40]

Snacking patterns of young children are of increasing concern; about 40% of children ate at least four different types of snack foods each day. After-school snack foods were generally cookies, soda, fruit drinks, chips, candy, milk, or juice. A child-prepared or a caretaker-prepared snack was less likely to include milk than a mother-prepared snack.[40]

GUIDELINES FOR FEEDING YOUNG CHILDREN

There are many statements about the appropriate guidelines for the diets of young children. Public health services in the United States are currently guided by the Healthy People 2000 Objectives. Of these objectives several focus directly on the nutritional state of preschool children. Table 11-3 lists the nutrition-related objectives and the current baseline data and steps toward achievement of each.

The Dietary Guidelines for Americans represent the best advice for persons 2 years of age and older about what to eat to stay healthy. Dietary Guidelines for Americans shown in table 11-4 relate to preschool-age children. The guideline for moderate use of alcohol, of course, does not apply to children who should avoid alcohol, and is not listed. These guidelines serve as the focal point for federal nutrition policy and education program planning.

FAMILY RESPONSIBILITY AND CHILDREN'S FOOD INTAKES

Preschool-age children depend on their parents or other care providers for the selection of food they consume (fig. 11-1). Since the preschool period is important in the formation of attitudes toward food, it is essential that foods that supply a variety of nutrients be available to young children. Parents also need to understand and support children in their food-related behaviors so that food habits are formed that are conducive to an adequate nutrient intake. Young children need some experience selecting food, yet parents and care providers need to set limits so that children eat foods that provide adequate amounts of nutrients.

The research data base for nutrition knowledge of parents and child care providers is limited. The data available have focused on nutrition knowledge and practices of mothers classified by income level rather than family constellation, for example, single-parent households and blended families. Recently, the role of day-care providers in the nutritional well-being of young children has been appreciated and evaluated.

The educational level and nutrition knowledge of the mother influence the nutritional quality of the diet. It has been noted that as the nutrition knowledge of the mother increased, preschool children's intakes of calcium, iron,

FIG. 11-1 Children consume food successfully in a comfortable setting free from stress.

riboflavin, and ascorbic acid increased. Nutrition knowledge was significantly related to positive attitudes toward meal planning and food preparation.[41,42] Also, the more positive mothers felt about meal planning, the importance of good nutrition for their children, and their roles as homemakers, the more likely were the children to receive good-quality meals; the more unhappy the mothers were with their roles as homemakers, the lower was the dietary quality of the children's food intakes.[43]

Although preschool children whose mothers were employed outside the home ate more meals at day-care centers, maternal employment did not negatively affect the dietary quality of these children.[44] This may also be related to other factors such as higher household incomes and fewer siblings in homes in which the mother was employed part time or full time outside the home. However, young children with mothers employed outside the home had less diverse diets than those with mothers at home.[40] It is not known how these data reflect the status of children in single-parent households.

Parents often need both help in interpreting the nutrition information to which they have been exposed and direction to valid sources of information. Sources of nutrition information vary among groups of parents. Low-income families and teenage parents reportedly receive their nutrition information from relatives and friends. Other families rely heavily on lay sources such as magazines, newspapers, books, radio, and television. Some of the information presented in these sources lacks validity, and conflicting information is often presented in any two sources. In addition, advertising and merchandising play on parents' emotional responses to suggestion and imply a false need for certain foods or supplements.

Preschool children often accompany their mothers to the grocery store and request specific foods. In this situation, 68% of mothers have reported that they sometimes buy foods that are requested and 18% stated that they always purchase the items. Sugar-coated cereal is the food most frequently requested.[45]

Young children have a significant impact on how families spend their food dollars. Child-prompted purchases comprised about 14% of the family food budget. The range was wide, as expected, varying from 1% to 44%. It is noteworthy that over half of the child-prompted food items were energy dense.[46] Mothers also reported a sense of guilt because they realized that their families, including young children, ate foods they preferred rather than foods the mothers felt to be nutritious.[47]

The ordinal position of the preschool child affected food choices and availability of foods, especially presweetened cereal. Preschool-aged children who were the oldest or the only child in their family received more foods than they specifically requested.[48]

Convenience is another factor many mothers consider when they select food for their families. Working mothers may rely heavily on convenience food and fast-food establishments. They have been known to leave the decision to the child as to what he or she would like to eat. Parents may need help selecting convenience foods and combinations of other foods that, when served together, provide a balanced nutrient intake. Parents may also need to learn how to plan other meals so that the daily intake is adequate when fast foods are consumed frequently.

Nearly half of young children receive foods away from home, and these meals comprise about 20% of their daily total energy intake.

Snacks comprise about the same percentage of the total energy intake as meals consumed away from home.

Low-income families have less money for food than more affluent families. If the purchasing power is reduced significantly, foods that provide essential nutrients may be partially or completely eliminated from the diet. However, not all children from low-income families are at risk for undernutrition. Undernourished, low-income children had parents who prepared fewer regular meals, and these children were less likely to eat vegetables and fruit and milk than adequately nourished children from homes with similar incomes. More convenience foods and fewer foods requiring preparation were served to undernourished children than to well-nourished children.[49]

Day Care

It is estimated that mothers of 15 million preschool children work outside the home. Of these 15 million children, 26% are enrolled in child-care centers (facility of 12 or more children); 22% are enrolled in family day-care (6–12 children in the caregiver's home); and 52% receive alternate care (with a relative).[50] Many children are in care centers or homes 8 to 10 hours/day, which means child care centers are responsible for two thirds of the child's total nutritional intake. Many children receive one or two meals a day at school or child care. Approximately three-fourths of young children in child care receive morning and afternoon snacks, and about 90% receive lunch at the child-care facility. The meals provided are a reflection of the hours of operation of the center and the schedules of the parents of the children (table 11-9).

It is clear that out-of-home child care has an impact on the foods and nutrients provided to young children. Although nutrition standards for day-care programs have been enacted,[52–56] the question still remains whether day-care programs provide adequate nourishment for young children.

Menus at child-care centers are primarily planned by either the center director or the cook. Both reported having received some training and viewed foods served at the center as an important part of the growth and health of the

TABLE 11-9   *Frequency of Meals Provided at Child-Care Centers*

Meal	Percentage of Centers Providing the Meal
Complete breakfast	57
Partial breakfast	38
Morning snack	71
Lunch	91
Afternoon snack	74
Late afternoon snack	87

Adapted from Pond-Smith, *J Am Diet Assoc*, 1993.[51]

young child.[57] There is concern that foods provided at child-care centers are those usually accepted by young children (hamburgers, fried potatoes, applesauce, cookies, milk) but not in large enough quantities to meet energy and iron needs of these children.[58] Poor combinations of foods provided less than 67% of the 1989 RDA for energy, iron, thiamin, and niacin even when foods were served at the recommended portion sizes.[59,60] The menus at family day-care homes had similar shortcomings.[61]

The goal of Healthy People 2000 Objective 2.17 (table 11-3) is to increase to 50% the number of child-care food services that provide foods consistent with the Dietary Guidelines for Americans.[10]

As family lifestyles have grown increasingly complex, and more children live in single-parent households, children at younger ages are increasingly independent in acquisition and preparation of food for themselves. Survey results show that children ages 5 to 8 years are frequently allowed to operate a microwave oven without supervision.[62] So it is no surprise that marketing for microwaveable frozen dinners is aimed at young children.

FACTORS AFFECTING FOOD INTAKE

Provision of appropriate amounts and kinds of food does not ensure that preschool-age children will consume foods that support an

FIG. 11-2 Parents provide role models for food choices and eating styles.

appropriate nutrient intake. Children imitate the models of food acceptance set for them. They learn to control concerned parents by the food they accept or reject.

Emotional factors influence food acceptance and intake. Parents and siblings provide a model of food acceptance and feeding behaviors that children imitate (fig. 11-2).

Attitudes of parents toward childrearing influence food intake. Permissiveness of parents in relation to eating was found to be negatively related to the nutritive value of food consumed by the children, adversely affecting all dietary components except fat. Less permissive mothers regulated the child's food intake to some degree, and as a result children consumed greater amounts of protein, vitamins, and minerals.[63] Children of more affluent, nonauthoritarian mothers had higher intakes of calcium and ascorbic acid, whereas children of parents with authoritarian attitudes toward child rearing had higher intakes of energy, carbohydrates, iron, and thiamin.[64] Parental monitoring (or threat of parental monitoring) decreased the number of nonnutritious foods chosen and thus the total energy content of a meal.[65]

The emotional environment at mealtime may influence food and nutrient intake. The dinner table is not the place for family battles or punitive action toward children. For eating to be successful, it should occur at a time and in a setting that is comfortable and free from stress and unreasonable demands.

THE PRESCHOOL CHILD'S DEVELOPMENTAL PROGRESS

During the preschool years, rates of growth decrease, and as a result appetites decrease. Children learn to understand language and how to talk and ask for food. Development of gross motor skills permits them to learn to walk and seek food for themselves. Development of fine motor skills allows them to learn to feed themselves and to prepare simple foods such as cereal with milk and sandwiches. They learn about food and the way it feels, tastes, and smells. Preschool children learn to eat a wider variety of textures and kinds of food, give up the bottle, and drink from a cup. They demand independence and refuse help in many tasks in which they are not skillful, such as self-feeding. As they grow older, they become less interested in food and more interested in their environment. They test and learn limits of behavior that are acceptable.

Self-Feeding

Children learn to feed themselves independently during the second year of life. Spilling and messiness are marked during the first half of the year. Handedness is established after 1 year of age. The 15-month-old child will have difficulty scooping food into the spoon and bringing food to the mouth without turning the spoon upside down and spilling its contents because of lack of wrist control. By 16 to 17 months of age a well-defined ulnar deviation of the wrist occurs and the contents of a spoon may be transferred more steadily to the mouth. By 18 months of age the child lifts the elbow as the spoon is raised and flexes the wrist as the spoon reaches the mouth so that only moderate spilling occurs, in contrast to earlier stages of self-feeding. By 2 years of age spilling seldom occurs (fig. 11-3).

FIG. 11-3   Preschool children refine their self-feeding skills as they grow older.

FIG. 11-4   Preschool children enjoy learning to feed themselves.

Younger preschool children are interested in how food feels and often prefer finger-feeding and feeding themselves. Foods that provide opportunities for finger-feeding should be provided at every meal. Children frequently will place food in the spoon with their fingers and may finger-feed foods commonly spoon-fed, such as vegetables and pudding (fig. 11-4).

By 15 months of age children can manage the cup, although not expertly. They have difficulty in lifting and tilting a cup and in lowering it to a tray after drinking. The cup is tilted, using the

TABLE 11-10   *Guidelines for Feeding Safety—Preschool Children*

Insist that children eat sitting down. It lets them concentrate on chewing and swallowing.

An adult should supervise children while they eat.

Food on which preschoolers often choke, such as hot dogs, nuts and crunchy peanut butter, hard pieces of fruit, and vegetables, should be avoided for children under 3 years of age.

Well-cooked foods, modified so that the child can chew and swallow without difficulty, should be offered.

Eating in the car should be avoided. If the child starts choking, it is hard to get to the side of the road safely.

Rub-on teething medications can cause problems with chewing and swallowing because the muscles in the throat may also become numb. Children who receive such medications should be carefully observed during feeding.

palm, and often is tilted too rapidly. By 18 to 24 months of age the cup is tilted by manipulation of the fingers.

Rotary chewing movements are refined in the second year and are well established by 2 years of age.

As the young child matures, self-help skills become more sophisticated. In general, a 2-year-old child uses arm muscles for tasks, a 3-year-old child uses hand muscles, and a 4-year-old child uses finger muscles.[66] This maturation enables the child to wipe, scrub, pour, mix, and peel foods for consumption.

Risk of Choking

Young children, especially preschoolers, are at risk of choking on food. Death from **food asphyxiation** has been described mostly in younger preschool children less than 2 years of age. Foods most often responsible for the deaths include hot dogs, candy, nuts, and grapes.

Actually children can choke on almost any food but are most likely to have trouble with foods that are hard, slippery, or just the right size to plug up the throat (e.g., hard candy, grapes, and popcorn). If the food becomes stuck, the plug prevents the child from coughing and bringing it back up. Other foods that may cause problems are thick, sticky foods such as peanut butter. These foods can line the back of the throat and build up so the children cannot clear their throats. Some types of cookies may crumble in the child's mouth and block airways.

Prevention is the most reasonable approach to childhood choking. Educating parents about developmentally appropriate foods is important. Guidelines for preventing choking are given in table 11-10.

Patterns of Food Intake

Few children pass through the preschool years without creating concern about their food intakes (fig. 11-5). Between 9 and 18 months of age a disinterest in food becomes apparent; this lasts from a few months to a few years.[67] Idiosyncratic food choices are common. Likes and dislikes may change from day to day and week to week. For example, a child may demand only a specific kind of cereal for snacks for a week and completely reject it for the next 6 months. Rituals become a part of food preparation and service. Some children, for example, accept sandwiches only when they are cut in half, and when parents quarter the sandwiches the children may throw tantrums. Others demand that foods have a particular arrangement on the plate or that their dishes be placed only in certain locations on the table.

Appetites are usually erratic and unpredictable during this period. The child may eat hungrily at one meal and refuse the next. The evening meal is generally the least well received and is of the most concern to the majority of parents. It is possible that a child who has consumed two meals and several snacks has met the energy and nutrient needs before dinnertime; in this instance consumption of limited amounts of

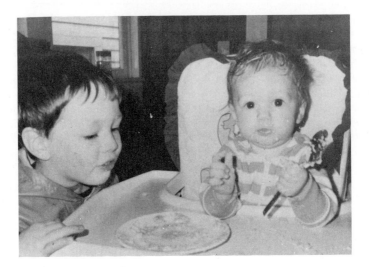

FIG. 11-5   Children want to eat the same food as their siblings, even if it means regressing to baby food.

food may be appropriate. It is also important to recognize that important social interaction occurs during the evening meal. This may be overwhelming for the preschooler who is learning not only to eat and interact at the same time but also to master the use of utensils and to eat harder-to-masticate foods.

A high percentage of parental dissatisfaction with children's appetites and interest in food between 2 and 4 years of age has been reported.[63,67] Concerns most frequently expressed are selection of a limited variety of foods, dawdling, limited consumption of fruits and vegetables, and consumption of too many sweets and too little meat.

More recently, mothers have described feeding problems among 2- to 7-year-old children that are very similar (table 11-11).[68] It is apparent that such problems are those of the parents' lack of insight into normal child development and, if properly managed, need not compromise a child's nutrient intake. Anticipatory guidance about children's food behavior is important for all parents, and intervention is imperative when battles are waged between parents and children about what is to be eaten.

Frequency of eating. Nearly 60% of 3- to 5-year-old children eat more than 3 times a day. Young children consume food an average of 5 to

TABLE 11-11   *"Problem" Food Behaviors of Children 2 to 7 Years of Age*

Consumes a restricted range of foods.
Eating habits are poor.
Eats insufficient quantity of food.
Is not interested in eating.
Dislikes new foods.
Likes "junk foods."

Adapted from Pelchat ML, Pliner D: *J Nutr Ed* 18:23, 1986.

7 times a day, although ranges of 3 to 14 times a day have been noted.[69] The frequency of food intakes was unrelated to nutrient intakes except when children consumed food less than 4 or more than 6 times a day.[70] Children who consumed food less than 4 times a day consumed less energy and calcium, protein, ascorbic acid, and iron than average intakes of other children their age. Those who consumed food more than 6 times a day consumed more energy, calcium, and ascorbic acid than average intakes of children their age. Snacks have been noted to provide one-fourth to one-third of the total energy, over one-third of the total sucrose, one-fifth of

the total calcium and ascorbic acid, and one-fifth of the protein ingested by children.

Food preferences. Parents report that preschool children enjoy meat, cereal grains, baked products, fruits, and sweets. They frequently ask for dairy products, cereals, and snack items such as cookies, crackers, and dry beverage mixes. Preschoolers seem to prefer the carbohydrate-rich foods that are easier to masticate. Cereals, breads, and crackers are often selected in preference to meat and other protein-rich foods. Dry fortified cereals are used as a primary source of many nutrients. Yogurt and cheese are popular among young children and provide calcium and protein.

Concerns of Parents

A concern of parents of many children between 1 and 3 years of age is that their children do not like meat and will not eat it. In the description of their dissatisfaction, it may become apparent that the children do eat and enjoy chicken and hamburger but refuse the more fibrous and harder-to-chew steaks and roasts. Foods have not yet been classified in relation to the pressure that must be applied to chew them well. Empirical observations, however, indicate that fibrous meats require the greatest pressure of any food consumed and may be difficult for the preschooler to eat. It may be important to focus parents' attention on the many softer, easier-to-chew meats and protein-rich foods that their children are consuming.

Food dislikes in childhood consistently include cooked vegetables and mixed dishes. Children accept raw vegetables more readily than they do cooked ones but often accept only a limited number. Acceptance of new foods appears to be age related. Only 6% of the youngest preschoolers but 18% of the oldest in their study would flatly refuse a new food.[5] Since familiarity with food is believed to influence its acceptance, new foods should be offered frequently, even though they have been previously refused.

Milk intakes are erratic and change with age. A reduction in milk intake begins at approximately 6 months of age.[67] Milk may be completely refused at times. Intakes of milk between ages 1 and 4 years approximate 1 to 2½ cups/day. After this age, the total volume of milk consumed increases.

Nutrient Intake Patterns

Both longitudinal and cross-sectional studies of nutrient and energy intakes of children have shown large differences in intakes between individual children of the same age and gender; some children consume two to three times as much energy as others.[45,71] Children are capable of regulating energy intake over a complete day, even though meal by meal, intake appears to be sporadic.[72,73,74] After a rapid rise in intake of all nutrients during the first 9 months of life, reductions can be expected in the intakes of some nutrients as increases occur in intakes of others.

Gender differences in intakes of energy and nutrients have been noted by several researchers. In all studies males consumed greater quantities of food and thus greater amounts of nutrients and energy.

During the preschool years a decrease occurs in intakes of calcium, phosphorus, riboflavin, iron, and vitamin A because of the omission of iron-fortified infant cereals in the diets of children, the reduction in milk intake, and the disinterest in vegetables. During this period children increase their intakes of carbohydrates and fats. Protein intakes may plateau or increase only slightly.[71] Between 3 and 8 years of age a slow, steady, and relatively consistent increase occurs in intake of all nutrients. Since intakes of vitamins A and C are unrelated to energy intakes, greater ranges of intakes of these nutrients have been noted.

Selection of a Nutritionally Appropriate Diet

Some clinicians mistakenly believe that if children are given a wide variety of food choices, they will instinctively select an adequate diet. These opinions are the results of studies designed to prove that infants and young children could tolerate and should receive a variety of foods in the first years of life. The studies, conducted in the 1920s and early 1930s, involved 6-month-old to 4½-year-old foundlings in a Chicago hospital.[75] The children under investigation were presented with 10 different fresh, unprocessed foods. They could eat as much or as many of the foods presented as they wished. At the completion of this study, the children were described as in good health, judged by physical growth, appearance, and vigor. It is important to note that the foods offered included only nutrient-dense, unsweetened items. There were no environmental factors that influenced food selection during the studies.

These studies indicate the kinds of food from which young children can select nutritionally adequate diets. They show that when natural, unmixed, unprocessed foods are presented in a neutral environment, children are likely to consume quantities to support normal growth and development. They do not prove that children in the free-living population and exposed to the number of combined and convenience foods available today will innately consume an appropriate nutrient and energy intake.[72,76]

Feeding Preschool Children

In spite of the reduction in appetite and erratic consumption of food, preschool children do enjoy food and gradually increase their average daily energy intakes. If simply prepared foods that provide a balance of nutrients are presented in a relaxed setting, children will consume an appropriate nutrient intake. Understanding and supportive help from parents and others who offer food to children lay the groundwork for the development of nutritionally sound and satisfying eating practices. Meals and snacks should be timed to foster appetite. Intervals necessary between meals and snacks may vary from one child to another; rarely can the clock be depended on to let one know appropriate intervals and times when it may be important for a child to eat.

Appetites may be satiated when energy needs are met regardless of a child's need for nutrients; thus a variety of food should be provided to ensure adequate nutrients and energy. The food should be presented without comment and the child permitted to consume amounts desired without any conversation focused on what or how much is being eaten. Portions served should be scaled to the child's appetite. When the meal is over, food should be removed and the child should be permitted to leave the table.

It is not unusual for a child to be "full" from foods offered at the meal; and still "have room" for dessert. This is often not manipulation on the part of the child but sensory specific satiety to the foods already offered.

Intervention for nutrition and feeding difficulties. Occasionally, anxious or concerned parents need help replacing food sources of nutrients usually supplied by food refused, or in establishing limits to preschoolers' food intakes and feeding behavior. Of the commonly expressed concerns, limited intakes of milk, refusal of vegetables and meat, consumption of too many sweets, and limited intakes of food appear to cause the most problems. It is important to recognize that 1 oz of milk supplies about 35 mg of calcium, and many children receive 6 to 8 oz of milk on dry cereal daily. Although they consume only 1 to 2 oz at a time, their calcium intakes may be acceptable when they consume milk with meals and snacks. When abundant amounts of fruit juice or sweetened beverages are available, children may simply prefer to drink them rather than milk. Other dairy products can be offered when milk is rejected. Cheese and yogurt are usually accepted. Powdered milk can be used in recipes for soups, vegetables, and mixed dishes.

Parents' perceptions of children's dislike of meat may need to be clarified. If preschoolers do consistently refuse all food sources of heme iron, their dietary intakes of iron should be carefully monitored. Parents concerned about children's excessive intakes of sweets may need help in setting limits on amounts of sweet foods they make available to their children. It may also be important to help parents convey their concern and the need to set limits on the availability of these foods to other family members, day-care providers, and preschool teachers.

When vegetables are consistently refused, wars between parents and children should not be permitted to erupt. Small portions (1 to 2 teaspoons) should continue to be served without comment and should be discarded if the child does not consume them. Preschool behavior modification programs that included token rewards when children consumed vegetables and another that provided education about specific vegetables served at mealtime have been found to increase children's acceptance and intake of them.[77]

If children's food intakes are so limited that their intakes of energy and nutrients are compromised, parents may need help in establishing guidelines so that the children develop appetites. Children who drink juice throughout the day may drink enough juice to take an "edge" off their appetite so they are never truly hungry and ready for a meal. Parents should offer food sufficiently often that children do not get so hungry that they lose their appetite, yet not so often that they are always satiated. Intervals of 3 to 4 hours are often successful. Very small portions of food should be offered, and second portions should be permitted when children consume the foods already served. Attention should always be focused on children when they eat and never when food is refused.

Group Feeding

As increasing numbers of children eat some of their meals outside the home, the role of child-care providers and preschools becomes more important in providing food, nourishment, and education in eating well. Day-care facilities and preschools offer snacks and meals, and food experiences are often included as part of the learning exercises provided for children.

Day-care centers are licensed by state agencies that mandate the meal pattern and types of snacks to be provided for the children and the percentage of the RDAs that must be included in the menus. Licensed centers may receive financial assistance by entering into an agreement with the Food and Nutrition Service of the Department of Agriculture. Rates of reimbursement are variable based on family size, income, and number of children in the program. Meal requirements for children 1 to 6 years of age are based on USDA guidelines (see tables 12-1 and 12-2).[78]

The Head Start Performance Standards are shown in table 11-12. Children who participate in part-day programs should receive one-third of their daily nutritional needs. Those children in full-day programs should receive one-half to two-thirds of their daily needs depending on the length of the program day.[54]

In day-care centers or schools, breakfast needs to be provided for children who receive none at home. Snacks should be planned to complement the daily food intakes. Small portions of food should be served, and children should be permitted second servings of those foods they enjoy. Disliked or unfamiliar foods may be offered by the teaspoon, and the child's acceptance or rejection should be accepted without comment. Children who eat slowly need to be served first and should be permitted to complete their meals without being rushed to other activities. Teachers should eat with the children without imposing their attitudes about food on them.

A new setting provides an opportunity for children to have exposure to many new foods. Day-care centers, kindergartens, and preschools can provide an important educational setting for both children and their parents (table 11-13). Children learn how to prepare food, how food grows, how foods smell, and what nutrients foods contain. Parents learn through participation, observation, and conversations with the staff. An organized approach to feeding children must include parents, teachers, and others who offer food to young children. Teachers and day-care workers can provide parents with important information about how children successfully consume food, the nutrients children need, and the foods that provide these nutrients. Parents offer important information to the centers about their children's food acceptance and needs. Parents and professionals need to positively reinforce each other to successfully provide food for children.

A study of 48 day-care and Head Start programs found that all participating children consumed appropriate intakes of nutrients. Total daily energy intakes were similar for all children regardless of whether one meal and one snack or two meals and two snacks were provided. In fact, when children consumed one meal and one snack in this setting, 82% of their energy intake was provided, but when they consumed two meals and two snacks, 84% of their energy intake was provided.[78]

The American Dietetic Association's recommendations for child nutrition services are shown in table 11-14. These guidelines address issues of food safety, nourishment, and development of healthy attitudes toward food. Table 11-15 lists resources that provide guidelines on the provision of nourishment to young children.

TABLE 11-12   Head Start Performance Standards: Nutrition Objectives

The objectives of the nutrition part of the health services component of the Head Start Program are to:

Help provide food that will meet the child's daily nutritional needs in the child's home or in another clean and pleasant environment, recognizing individual differences and cultural patterns, and thereby promote sound physical, social, and emotional growth and development.

Provide an environment for nutritional services that will support and promote the use of the feeding situation as an opportunity for learning.

Help staff, child, and family to understand the relationship of nutrition to health, factors that influence food practices, variety of ways to provide for nutritional needs and to apply this knowledge in the development of sound food habits even after leaving the Head Start program.

Demonstrate the interrelationships of nutrition to other activities of the Head Start program and its contribution to the overall child development goals.

Involve all staff, parents, and other community agencies as appropriate in meeting the child's nutritional needs so that nutritional care provided by Head Start complements and supports that of the home and community.

Adapted from Proposed Head Start Performance Standards, 1996.

TABLE 11-13   Nutrition Education Goals for Preschool Children

Nutrition education goals for young children should include developing:
1. An awareness of the physical and sensory characteristics of food.
2. The ability to distinguish the sources of different foods.
3. Knowledge that food is important for life and that a healthy body needs a number of different foods daily.
4. The ability to distinguish between many healthful and nonnutritious foods.
5. The realization of the negative consequences of consuming large amounts of sugar, salt, and fat.
6. The ability to select and enjoy nutritious foods for snacks and meals.
7. An attitude that demands verification of what is said and shown about food on television.
8. Knowledge that people of varied cultures, upbringing, and geographic locations have different eating patterns.
9. A willingness to taste a wide variety of foods, particularly fresh vegetables and fruits.
10. Skills and attitudes that facilitate consumption of a nutritious diet; tasting, sitting at the table, chewing food well, eating in a slow and relaxed manner, enjoying and valuing mealtime.
11. Skills to prepare and serve food, such as scrubbing, mixing, tearing, and pouring.
12. An acceptance of rules and limits about eating and cooking, and consideration of self and others.

TABLE 11-14   Recommendations for Child Nutrition Services

The American Dietetic Association recommends that these basic child nutrition services be available to all children, regardless of economic status, race, special needs, or national origin:

Access for all children to optimal amounts of health promoting foods.

Food programs that provide nutritious, appealing, wholesome foods that reflect the U.S. Dietary Guidelines for Americans, served in an environment that encourages its acceptance.

Meals that serve as a laboratory to apply critical thinking skills to food selection.

Nutrition education for parents and their children, and professional education and in-service training for teachers and others involved in the care of children.

Nutrition screening to identify children at nutritional risk.

Dietary assessment and counseling to meet special health needs.

Referral to food assistance programs and services.

Adapted from *J Am Diet Assoc*, 1993.[79]

TABLE 11-15 *Resource Materials for Child-Care Providers and Preschool Programs*

A Planning Guide for Food Service in Child Care Centers, USDA, Food and Nutrition Service, Jan, 1985.
  Meal patterns, menus, food preparation, sanitation and nutrition education guidelines for young children in child care centers

Head Start Program Performance Standards, US Department of Health and Human Services, Office of Human Development Services, Administration for Children, Youth, and Families, Head Start Bureau, 1996.
  Performance standards for menus, nutritional requirements and meal service that support developmental milestones for young children

Caring for Our Children—National Health and Safety Performance Standards: Guidelines for Out-of-home Child Care Programs: Joint Project of American Public Health Association and American Academy of Pediatrics, 1992.

Nutrition and your Health: Dietary Guidelines for Americans, ed 4, Home and Garden Bulletin No 232, USDA, US Department of Health and Human Services, US Government Printing Office, Washington, DC 1995.
  Provides guidelines for appropriate intakes of foods to support good health

Nutrition Standards in Day-care Programs for Children: Technical Support Paper, J Am Diet Assoc 87:504, 1987.
  Provides support for appropriate nutrient intake, emotional climate of food service, and nutrition education for young children

Meal Pattern Requirements and Offer Versus Serve Manual, USDA, Food and Nutrition Service, FNS-265, Aug, 1990.
  Provides USDA guidelines for foods to be served to young children at breakfast, lunch, or supper and snacks

Building the Future: Nutrition Guidance for the Child Nutrition Programs. US Department of Agriculture, Food and Nutrition Service, FNS-279, 1992.
  Based on Dietary Guidelines for Americans, promotes healthy eating for children and teens

Green, M (ed.): *Bright Futures: Guidelines for Health Supervision of Infants, Children, and Adolescents,* Arlington, VA, National Center for Maternal and Child Health, 1994.
  Guidelines for family-centered health supervision, anticipatory guidance, and developmental surveillance for all stages-infancy to adolescence

Healthy children 2000: *National Health Promotion and Disease Prevention Objectives Related to Mothers, Infants, Children, Adolescents, and Youth.* US Department of Health and Human Services, Public Health Service, Health Resources Services Administration, Maternal and Child Health Bureau, 1992.
  Proposes achievable goals for improved health and nutritional status for Americans

Lynch EW and Hanson MJ: *Developing Cross-Cultural Competence: A Guide for Working with Young Children and Their Families.* Paul H Brookes Pub Co. Baltimore, MD, 1992.
  Provides an awareness of cultural richness and differences in the United States and offers guidelines for appreciation of cultures and appropriate interactions for health care providers

Fenichel ES and Eggbeer L: *Preparing Practitioners to Work with Infants, Toddlers, and Their Families: Issues and Recommendations for the Professions.* National Center for Clinical Infant Programs, Arlington, VA, 1990.

Satter, Ellyn: *How to Get Your Child to Eat . . . But Not Too Much.* Palo Alto, CA, 1987, Bull Publishing Co.
  Provides guidelines to parents and health care providers as they work with children to develop a healthy relationship with food

Summary

Children between 1 and 6 years of age develop at a steady rate. They acquire many new skills, learn a great deal about the environment in which they live, and test the limits of behavior that the environment will accept. All of these factors influence their food and therefore nutrient intake. Parents need to provide appropriate foods and supportive guidance so that food patterns that support an appropriate nutrient intake are developed. Nutrition knowledge of the parents positively influences children's nutrient intake. Advertising and television programs also affect children's requests for and acceptance of food.

Although most young children are well nourished, groups exist within our population with both clinical and biochemical evidence of malnutrition. Nutrients most often consumed in inappropriately limited amounts are iron, calcium, and vitamins B_6 and C. Because changes in families affect the lives and nourishment of young children, programs for young children as well as schools, child-care facilities, and other community services must include both the child and the family.

REVIEW QUESTIONS

1. Which nutrients are most likely to be consumed at low levels in the preschool-age period?
2. What influence does rate of growth have on energy intake?
3. Which physical and developmental factors most influence the foods that young children are willing and capable of consuming?
4. How do family food habits most significantly effect the foods that are consumed by young children?
5. In what ways do cultural and community factors effect the foods that are available to young children?
6. What are the most common concerns of parents about the food intake of young children?

SUGGESTED LEARNING ACTIVITIES

1. Observe a preschool feeding program and describe the feeding environment.
2. Describe factors that influence food acceptability in the preschool child.
3. Describe appropriate snacks for preschool-age children.
4. Describe factors that influence foods acceptable to preschool-age children.
5. Plan a nutrition lesson for a Head Start Program class.

❖ ❖ ❖

CASE STUDY

Nourishment of a Preschool-Age Child

Kim is 3 years old and will start preschool/ day care this fall. She has previously received her care from a relative at home. Kim's mother is required to be at her work by 7:30 A.M. and will be able to pick up Kim at school by 5:30 P.M. Kim is a healthy child who has grown at the 10th percentile for length, weight, and weight for length since infancy. Kim's mother is concerned about Kim's growth and how it may be affected at preschool because of Kim's preference for a limited variety of foods and her "slow" style of eating, which has required encouragement at home. Currently Kim's favorite foods are ready-to-eat breakfast cereal, macaroni and cheese, applesauce, bananas, rice, french fries, and milk. Because of her mother's work schedule Kim will receive her breakfast, morning snack, lunch, and afternoon snack at preschool. The preschool provides foods in a family-style meal service with an adult at each table with the children.

1. Would you be concerned about Kim's growth?
2. Kim's mother wonders if she should provide foods from home for Kim because of her limited choices of foods? What would you suggest?
3. As a preschool director and teacher, describe the strategies that your preschool might have in place to encourage Kim to try a wider variety of foods.

6. Plan brown bag lunches for a preschool-age child for one week that provide variety and are nutritionally appropriate.

REFERENCES

1. Jones DY, Nesheim MD, Habicht JP: Influences in child growth associated with poverty in the 1970s: an examination of HANES I and HANES II, cross-sectional US national surveys, *Am J Clin Nutr* 42:714, 1985.

2. Kumanyika SK and others: Stature and weight status of children in an urban kindergarten population, *Pediatrics* 85:783, 1990

3. Nutrition Week, *Community Nutrition Institute* 26:8, 1996.

4. Nationwide food consumption survey: CSFII—continuing survey of food intake by individuals—1986: Nutrition Monitoring Division, Human Nutrition Information Service, *Nutr Today* Sept/Oct:36, 1987.

5. Friedman BJ: Differences in dietary intake of young Caucasian, Mexican-American, and African-American children, *J Am Diet Assoc* 91:A–77, 1991.

6. Owen GM and others: A study of nutritional status of preschool children in the United States, 1968–1970, *Pediatrics* 53:597, 1974.

7. Caloric and selected nutrient values for persons 1–74 years of age: First Health and Nutrition Examination Survey, US, 1971–1974. US Department of Health, Education and Welfare, Public Health Service, Office of Health Research, Statistics, and Technology. National Center for Health Statistics, DHEW Pub No (PHS) 79-1657, 1979.

8. Kennedy E, Goldberg J: What are children eating? Implications for public policy, *Nutr Rev* 53:111, 1995.

9. Nicklas TA and others: Cardiovascular risk factors from birth to 7 years of age: the Bogalusa Heart Study—dietary intake, *Pediatrics* 80(suppl 5): 797, 1987.

10. Healthy People 2000: *National health promotion and disease prevention objectives,* US Dept HHS, PHS, HRSA, MCHB, 1992.

11. *Nutrition and your health: dietary guidelines for Americans,* ed 4, Home and Garden Bulletin No 232, USDA, US Department of Health and Human Services, Washington, DC, 1995, US Government Printing Office.

12. Kimm SYS and others: Dietary patterns of US children: implications for disease prevention, *Prev Med* 19:432, 1990.

13. Nicklas TA: Dietary studies of children: the Bogalusa heart study experience, *J Am Diet Assoc* 95:1127, 1995.

14. Terry RD, Oakland MJ: Parents' reasons for giving vitamin and mineral supplements to their preschoolers, *Top Clin Nutr* 5:67, 1990.

15. Zee P and others: Nutritional improvement of poor urban preschool children: a 1983–1977 comparison, *JAMA* 253:3269, 1985.

16. Kennedy E, Meyers L, Layden W: The 1995 dietary guidelines for Americans: an overview, *J Am Diet Assoc* 96:234, 1996.

17. Taylor M, Koblinsky SA: Dietary intake and growth status of young homeless children, *J Amer Diet Assoc* 93:464, 1993.

18. Fierman AH and others: Growth delay in homeless children, *Pediatrics* 88:918, 1991.

19. Drake MA: Dietary adequacy of children residing in temporary shelters, *J Am Diet Assoc* 91:A-77, 1991.

20. DuRousseau PC and others: Children in foster care: are they at nutritional risk? *J Am Diet Assoc* 91:83, 1991.

21. Brown E, Tieman P: Effect of income and WIC on the dietary intake of preschoolers: results of a preliminary study, *J Am Diet Assoc* 86:1189, 1986.

22. Smith AL and others: Effectiveness of a nutrition program for mothers and their anemic children under 5 years of age, *J Am Diet Assoc* 86:1039, 1986.

23. Sargent JD, Stukel TA, Dalton MA, Freeman JL, Brown MJ: Iron deficiency in Massachusetts communities: socioeconomic and demographic risk factors among children. *Am J Public Health* 86:544, 1996.

24. Lozoff B and others: Long-term developmental outcome of infants with iron deficiency, *N Engl J Med* 325:687, 1991.

25. Drake MA: Anthropometry, biochemical iron indexes, and energy and nutrient intake of preschool children: comparison of intake at day care center and at home, *J Am Diet Assoc* 91:1587, 1991.

26. National Center for Health Statistics, *Healthy people 2000 review, 1994,* Hyattsville, Maryland, Public Health Service, 1995.

27. Wiecha JL, Casey VA: High prevalence of overweight and short stature among Head Start children in Massachusetts, *Public Health Reports* 109:767, 1994.

28. Schlicker SA, Borra ST, Regan C: The weight and fitness status of United States children, *Nutr Rev* 52:11, 1994.

29. Singer MR, Moore LL, Garrahie EJ, Ellision RC: The tracking of nutrient intake in young children: the Framingham children's study, *Am J Public Health* 85:1673, 1995.

30. Mahaffey KR: Environmental lead toxicity: nutrition as a component of intervention, *Environ Health Perspect* 89:75, 1990.

31. Frisancho AR, Ryan AS: Decreased stature associated with moderate blood lead concentrations in Mexican-American children, *Am J Clin Nutr* 54:516, 1991.

32. Mushak P, Crocetti AF: Methods for reducing lead exposure in young children and other risk groups: an integrated summary of a report to the US Congress on childhood lead poisoning, *Environ Health Perspect* 89:125, 1990.

33. Preventing lead poisoning in young children: a statement by the Centers for Disease Control, US Department of Health and Human Services, Public Health Service, Centers for Disease Control, Oct, 1991.

34. Faine MP, Oberg D: Snacking and oral health habits of Washington state WIC children and their caregivers, *ASDC J Dent Child* 61:350, 1994.

35. Brenard-Bonnin AC, Petit N, and others: Cariogenic feeding habits and fluoride supplementation during infancy and early childhood, *Canadian J Public Health* 84:90, 1993.

36. Kotz K, Story M: Food advertisements during children's Saturday morning television programming: Are they consistent with dietary recommendations?, *J Am Diet Assoc* 94:1296, 1994.

37. DuRant RH, Baranowski T, Johnson M, Thompson WO: The relationship among television watching, physical activity, and body composition of young children, *Pediatrics* 94:449, 1994.

38. Murphy SP and others: An evaluation of food group intakes by Mexican-American children, *J Am Diet Assoc* 90:388, 1990.

39. Zive MM, Taras HL, Broyles SL, Spoher F, Nader PR: Vitamin and mineral intakes of Anglo-American and Mexican-American preschoolers, *J Am Diet Assoc* 95:329, 1995.

40. Wolfe WS, Campbell CC: Food pattern, diet quality, and related characteristics of schoolchildren in New York state, *J Amer Diet Assoc* 93:1280, 1993.

41. Eppright ES and others: Nutrition of infants and preschool children in the North Central region of the United States of America, *World Rev Nutr Diet* 14:269, 1972.

42. Eppright ES and others: The North Central Regional study of diets of preschool children. II.

Nutrition knowledge and attitudes of mothers, *J Home Econ* 62:327, 1970.

43. Caliendo MA and others: Nutritional status of preschool children, *J Am Diet Assoc* 71:20, 1977.

44. Johnson RK and others: Effect of maternal employment on the quality of young children's diets—NFCS 1987–1988, *J Am Diet Assoc* 91:A–67, 1991.

45. Crawford PB, Hankin JH, Huenemann RL: Environmental factors associated with preschool obesity, *J Am Diet Assoc* 72:589, 1978.

46. DeWalt KM: The use of itemized register tapes for analysis of household food acquisition patterns prompted by children, *J Am Diet Assoc* 90:559, 1990.

47. Kirk MC, Gillespie AH: Factors affecting food choices of working mothers with young families, *J Nutr Educ* 22:161, 1990.

48. Phillips DE and others: Use of food and nutrition knowledge by mothers of preschool children, *J Nutr Educ* 10:73, 1978.

49. Karp R and others: Parental behavior and the availability of foods among undernourished inner-city children, *J Fam Pract* 18:731, 1984.

50. Dietitians teach value of good nutrition in food-service for young children, *ADA Courier* 31:1, 1992.

51. Pond-Smith D, Richarz SH, Gonzalez NL: A survey of foodservice operations in child care centers in Washington state. *J Amer Diet Assoc* 92:483, 1992.

52. Nutrition standards in day-care programs for children: technical support paper, *J Am Diet Assoc* 87:504, 1987.

53. *A planning guide for food service in child care centers,* Food and Nutrition Services, USDA, Washington, DC, 1985.

54. *Head Start Program Performance Standards,* US Department of Health and Human Services, Office of Human Development Services, Administration for Children, Youth, and Families, Head Start Bureau, 1984.

55. *Caring for our children: national health and safety performance standards: guidelines for out-of-home child care programs:* joint project of American Public Health Association and American Academy of Pediatrics, 1992.

56. Position paper on nutrition in child care settings, *J Nutr Educ* 23:49, 1991.

57. Briley ME and others: Who plans the menu at the child care center? *J Am Diet Assoc* 91:A-75, 1991.

58. Briley ME and others: What is on the menu at the child care center? *J Am Diet Assoc* 89:771, 1989.

59. Briley ME: Nutrition of young children in child care programs, *Food and Nutr News* 62(4):21, 1990.

60. Albertson AM, Tobelman RA, Engstrom A, Asp EH: Nutrient intakes of 2- to 10-year-old American children: 10 year trends. *J Am Diet Assoc* 92:1492, 1992.

61. Briley ME and others: Nutrition knowledge and attitudes and menu planning skills of family day-home providers, *J Am Diet Assoc* 89:694, 1989.

62. Microwave meals attract children, *J Am Diet Assoc* 91:720, 1991.

63. Eppright ES and others: Eating behavior of preschool children, *J Nutr Educ* 1:16, 1969.

64. Sims LS, Morris PM: Nutritional status of preschoolers, *J Am Diet Assoc* 64:492, 1974.

65. Klesges RC and others: Parental influence on food selection in young children and its relationship to childhood obesity, *Am J Clin Nutr* 53:859, 1991.

66. Hertzler AA: Preschoolers' food handling skills—motor development, *J Nutr Educ* 21:100B, 1989.

67. Beal VA: On the acceptance of solid foods and other food patterns of infants and children, *Pediatrics* 20:448, 1957.

68. Pelchat ML, Pliner P: Antecedents and correlates of feeding problems in young children, *J Nutr Educ* 18:23, 1986.

69. Huenemann RL: Environmental factors associated with preschool obesity. II. Obesity and food practices of children at successive age levels, *J Am Diet Assoc* 64:489, 1974.

70. Eppright ES and others: The North Central Regional study of diets of preschool children. III. Frequency of eating, *J Home Econ* 62:407, 1970.

71. Beal VA: Dietary intake of individuals followed through infancy and childhood, *Am J Public Health* 51:1107, 1961.

72. Birch LL and others: The variability of young children's energy intake, *N Engl J Med* 324(4):232, 1991.

73. Sanjur D and others: Dietary patterns and nutrient intakes of toddlers from low-income families in Denver, Colorado, *J Am Diet Assoc* 90:823, 1990.

74. Stanek K and others: Diet quality and the eating environment of preschool children, *J Am Diet Assoc* 90:582, 1990.

75. Davis CM: The self-selection of diet experiment: its significance for feeding in the home, *Ohio State Med J* 34:862, 1938.

76. Story M, Brown JE: Do young children instinctively know what to eat? The studies of Clara Davis revisited, *N Engl J Med* 316:103, 1987.

77. Ireton CL, Guthrie HA: Modification of vegetable-eating behavior in preschool children, *J Nutr Educ* 4:100, 1972.

78. *Meal pattern requirements and offer versus serve manual,* USDA, Food and Nutrition Service, FNS-265, Aug, 1990.

79. Position of the American Dietetic Association: Child Nutrition Services. *J Amer Diet Assoc* 93:334, 1993.

12

Nutrition for School-Age Children

Betty Lucas

✦✦✦

Objectives

After studying this chapter, the student should:

✔ *Be aware of nutrition concerns of school-age children.*

✔ *Recognize factors that influence food choices and attitudes of children and their families.*

✔ *Be aware of the value of snacks to a child's daily total nutrient intake.*

✔ *Have knowledge of feeding and educational programs designed to improve the nutritional status of children.*

✔ *Understand nutrition and food intake approaches to the control of dental caries.*

✔ *Understand the primary nutritional considerations for children participating in sports.*

✔ *Recognize the effects of diet on learning and school performance.*

✔ *Be familiar with the various dietary treatments for hyperactivity and the studies of their effectiveness.*

✔ *Understand the natural course and dietary management of lactose intolerance.*

The school-age years, generally considered to be 6 to 12 years of age, are marked by more quiet, stable changes compared with the extremes of growth and development seen in infancy and adolescence. Children in this age group show a consistent but slow rate of physical growth, continuing maturation of fine and gross motor skills, and gains in cognitive and social-emotional growth. By the end of this period, girls are typically well into puberty, and boys will soon follow.

There are common patterns of food and nutrient intake among school-age children. Food habits, likes, and dislikes are established, many of which form the base for a lifetime of food and nutrition intake. Food choices are influenced more by factors from outside and less by parents and family. Feeding programs at daycare and school continue to contribute significantly to children's total nutrient intake.

NUTRITIONAL STATUS OF SCHOOL-AGE CHILDREN

Although clinical signs of malnutrition are rarely found in children in North America, there are children who receive diets inadequate in quantity or quality. Nutrients most likely to be low or deficient are calcium, iron, vitamins B_6 and A, and zinc.[1,2] Conversely, national survey data indicate that children continue to consume more total fat, saturated fat, and sodium than recommended by the Dietary Guidelines.[2]

Children living in poverty or those chronically hungry are likely to have diets low in energy, vitamins A, C, E, B_6, folate, iron, zinc, thiamin, and magnesium.[3] The more limited the diet is in energy, the more likelihood for low or deficient nutrient intakes.

Vitamin and Mineral Supplements

The use of multiple vitamin and mineral supplements decreases after infancy to about 23% of school-age children.[4] Supplements are generally used by families who are better educated and in less need of them. Most children take iron supplements as part of a multiple vitamin supplement.

Except for fluoride supplementation in unfluoridated areas, the American Academy of Pediatrics does not support routine supplementation for healthy children. Four groups of children at nutritional risk, however, are identified as potentially benefiting from supplements. These include: (1) children from deprived families, especially those abused or neglected; (2) children with anorexia, poor appetites, and poor eating habits; (3) children consuming vegetarian diets without dairy products; and (4) pregnant adolescents.[5]

Children needing supplements can be determined by a nutritional assessment, and in addition to the above, might include those with food allergies, limited food acceptances, or frequent or chronic illness. There is no risk if parents wish to give their children a standard pediatric multivitamin but **megadose** levels (greater than 10 times the RDA) should be discouraged.

FACTORS AFFECTING FOOD INTAKE

Several influences determine the food habits and intake of children. Major factors include family, peers, and the media.

Family

Eating habits and food likes or dislikes are formed in the early years and continue into adulthood. Parents and siblings provide a model of food acceptance and feeding behavior that children imitate. In a study of parents and 6- to 19-year-old children, there was a positive correlation between parent and child intakes of kcalories, carbohydrates, saturated fats, and polyunsaturated fats.[6] The correlation was greater for black children than for white children.

The emotional environment at mealtime may influence food and nutrient intake. The dinner table is not the place for family battles or punitive action toward children. For eating to be successful, it should occur at a time and in a setting that is comfortable and free from stress and unreasonable demands.

Almost 75% of mothers of school-aged children in two-parent families are employed outside the home. These children receive more meals at school and day care, but there is no evidence that they eat more often in restaurants.[7] Although working mothers have less time available for food preparation, studies have not found negative effects of employment on the dietary intakes of their children.[7] More specific research is needed, however.

One out of every five children lives in a family with income below the poverty line, increasing the risk of poor health.[8] Low-income families have less money for food than more affluent families. The large percentage of single-parent families headed by women often means a reduced purchasing power. Foods that provide essential nutrients may be partially or completely eliminated from the diet. However, not all children from low-income families are at risk for undernutrition. One study found that undernourished children from low-income families had parents who prepared fewer regular meals and who were less likely to eat vegetables and milk than parents of adequately nourished children from homes with similar incomes. More **convenience foods** and fewer foods requiring preparation were available to undernourished children than to the well-nourished children.[9]

An emerging trend in the United States is the increased responsibility for family shopping and cooking by children not yet in their teenage years. Some of these children frequently prepare their own breakfasts, lunches, snacks, and even evening meals.[10] They also shop for food on a regular basis and have a significant influence on family food purchases. Factors contributing to this trend include working parents, increased use of microwave ovens, more money available to spend on convenience and prepared foods, and less emphasis on family meals. Along with this trend there is increasingly sophisticated advertising aimed at these children.[10] Although children need experience selecting food, parents need to provide guidance so that children select foods that provide adequate amounts of nutrients.

Peers

As children move into the wide world, their food choices are influenced by those outside the immediate family. Day care, the homes of friends, and school provide broad food experiences, with both positive and negative impacts on nutritional status. The credibility of parents is often questioned in the face of advice from teachers, peers, or peers' parents. The school-age child has more access to money, to grocery stores, and therefore to foods with questionable nutrient value.

Participation in the school lunch program may be determined as much by friends as by the menu. Being part of the group can be a problem for a child who has a chronic illness or disorder that requires diet modification such as diabetes, food allergies, or phenylketonuria (PKU). These children need education regarding diet rationale appropriate to their developmental level and methods of problem-solving food choices when in a group of peers.

Media

Television is the primary media influence on children of all ages. The typical school-age child watches nearly 3½ hours of television per day.[11] One-half of all commercials advertise food during children's programs.[11] Foods most frequently advertised are those high in fat, sugar, and salt (e.g., sweetened cereals, soft drinks, fast foods, snack foods, and candy). The message from these food commercials has a primary emotional and psychological appeal, with little basis on sound nutrition. Although school-age children are better at cognitive discrimination between the program and commercial messages than younger children, they are still very responsive to these commercials.

FEEDING THE SCHOOL-AGE CHILD

The school-age period is one of relatively steady growth and few apparent feeding problems. School schedules provide a more ordered routine. Children attempt to master physical skills, and they expend energy in organized sports and games. A natural increase in appetite is responsible for normal increases in food intake. Differences in intake between males and females increase gradually up to 12 years of age and then become marked. Boys consume greater quantities of energy and nutrients than do girls.

School-age children are not without food and nutrition concerns. Unresolved conflicts from the preschool years may persist. Children in their early school years may continue to refuse a food that touches another on the plate or to demand a special arrangement of dishes and utensils on the table. Likes and dislikes, although established, are not necessarily permanent, but they may become so if parents do not offer the food or if the food dislike is such a frequent focus that children become fully patterned into their **food idiosyncrasies.**

Undernutrition may have serious consequences for the school-age child; for example, the child may become easily fatigued, unable to sustain prolonged physical effort, or unable to participate fully in learning experiences. Because the risk of infection is greater in undernourished children, a child with limited nutrient reserves may have frequent absences from school.

Food Intake Patterns

School-age children eat less frequently than younger children, about four to five times per day on school days. They almost always want snacks after school, which they often prepare themselves. It has been reported that their snacks contribute about one-third of their total energy intake.[12] Although some children increase the variety of foods they accept, many continue to reject vegetables, mixed dishes, and some meats, or to accept a limited range of foods.

Breakfast is an important meal. Children have to rise early to eat an unhurried and balanced meal and may have to prepare it themselves. Most children consume breakfasts that contribute at least one-fourth of the RDA.[13] A larger percentage of children in the lower grades eat breakfast than of those in the middle and upper grades. Children who skip breakfast have lower intakes of energy (200 to 500 fewer calories) and other nutrients than those who eat breakfast.[14,15]

Regular family meals may be less frequent as participation in organized sports, music lessons, and other activities increases. Even when eating at the same time, some family meals have been moved from the dining room to trays in front of the television. In addition to limiting the social interaction of family meals, it has been observed that some children become so engrossed in the shows that they lose interest in their food.

Snacking between meals and while watching television is an important factor in the school-age child's nutrient intake and food habits. Not only does television viewing encourage snacking, but it is a **sedentary** activity and has been linked to the development of obesity in childhood.[16] Parents can help by planning regular snack times and providing appropriate foods (see chapter 10 for a thorough discussion of obesity and its management).

SCHOOL MEALS

Feeding and nutrition education programs in schools, when adequately implemented, provide not only important nutrients for children but also an opportunity for them to learn to make responsible choices regarding dietary intake. Since its inception in 1946, the **National School Lunch Program (NSLP)** has been administered by the US Department of Agriculture (USDA), which provides cash reimbursement and supplemental foods to feeding programs that comply with federal regulations. These regulations require that school meals be sold at reduced prices or be given free to children whose families cannot afford to buy them.

Begun as a pilot project in 1966, the **School Breakfast Program (SBP)** is also administered by USDA. Supported by consumer groups and low-income advocates, the program has slowly expanded in the past 25 years. Some states have passed legislation requiring breakfast programs in schools where there is a high percentage of children receiving free or reduced price lunches. In 1994, breakfasts were provided in almost 70% of the schools participating in the lunch program.[17]

Menus must be planned to meet the guidelines established for the NSLP. Lunch provides about one-third of the RDA for the particular age group. Tables 12-1 and 12-2 show minimum quantities of food required for the lunch and breakfast patterns for the various age groups.

Historically, problems with the NSLP program have included **plate waste,** poor menu

TABLE 12-1   *School Lunch Pattern—National School Lunch Program*

Meal Component	Minimum Quantities Required				Option
	Ages 1–2	Preschool	Grades K–6	Grades 7–12	K–Grade 3
Milk (as a beverage)	6 ounces	6 ounces	8 ounces	8 ounces	8 ounces
Meat or meat alternate (quantity of the edible portion as served)					
Lean meat, poultry, or fish	1 oz	1½ oz	2 oz	2 oz	1½ oz
Cheese	1 oz	1½ oz	2 oz	2 oz	1½ oz
Large egg	½	¾	1	1	¾
Cooked dry beans or peas	¼ cup	⅜ cup	½ cup	½ cup	⅜ cup
Peanut butter or other nut or seed butters	2 tbsp	3 tbsp	4 tbsp	4 tbsp	3 tbsp
The following may be used to meet no more than 50% of the requirement and must be used in combination with any of the above: Peanuts, soynuts, tree nuts, or seeds, as listed in program guidance, or an equivalent quantity of any combination of the above meat/meat alternate (1 oz of nuts/seeds = 1 oz of cooked lean meat, poultry or fish).	½ oz = 50%	¾ oz = 50%	1 oz = 50%	1 oz = 50%	¾ oz = 50%
Vegetables/Fruits (2 or more servings of vegetables or fruits or both)	½ cup	½ cup	¾ cup plus extra ½ cup over a week[1]	1 cup	¾ cup
Grains/Breads—must be enriched or whole grain. A serving is a slice of bread or an equivalent serving of biscuits, rolls, etc., or ½ cup of cooked rice, macaroni, noodles, other pasta products or cereal grains.	5 servings per week— minimum of ½ per day[1]	8 servings per week— minimum of 1 per day[1]	12 servings per week— minimum of 1 per day[1,2]	15 servings per week— minimum of 1 per day[1,2]	10 servings per week— minimum of 1 per day[1,2]

[1]For the purposes of this chart, a week equals five days.
[2]Up to one grains/breads serving per day may be a dessert.

From Food and Consumer Service, U.S. Department of Agriculture: *Child Nutrition Programs: School Meal Initiatives for Healthy Children*, Federal Register, 7 CFR, Part 210, June 13, 1995.

TABLE 12-2   School Breakfast Pattern—School Breakfast Program

Meal Component	Minimum Quantities Required			Option
	Ages 1–2	Preschool	Grades K–12	Grades 7–12
Milk (Fluid) (As a beverage, on cereal or both)	½ cup	¾ cup	8 oz	8 oz
Juice/Fruit/Vegetable: Fruit and/or vegetable; or full-strength fruit juice or vegetable juice	¼ cup	½ cup	½ cup	½ cup
Select One Serving from Each of the Following Components or Two from One Component:				
Grains/Breads—One of the following or an equivalent combination:				
Whole-grain or enriched bread	½ slice	½ slice	1 slice	1 slice
Whole-grain or enriched biscuit, roll, muffin, etc.	½ serving	½ serving	1 serving	1 serving
Whole-grain, enriched, or fortified cereal	¼ cup or ⅓ oz	⅓ cup or ½ oz	¾ cup or 1 oz	¾ cup or 1 oz Plus an additional serving of one of the grains/breads above
Meat or Meat Alternates:				
Meat/poultry or fish	½ oz	½ oz	1 oz	1 oz
Cheese	½ oz	½ oz	1 oz	1 oz
Egg (large)	½	½	½	½
Peanut butter or other nut or seed butters	1 tablespoon	1 tablespoon	2 tablespoons	2 tablespoons
Cooked dry beans and peas	2 tablespoons	2 tablespoons	4 tablespoons	4 tablespoons
Nut and/or seeds (as listed in program guidance)[1]	½ oz	½ oz	1 oz	1 oz

[1]No more than 1 oz of nuts and/or seeds may be served in any one meal.
From Food and Consumer Service, U.S. Department of Agriculture: *Child Nutrition Programs: School Meal Initiatives for Healthy Children,* Federal Register, 7 CFR, Part 220, June 13, 1995.

acceptance by students, and concerns regarding excessive amounts of fat, sugar, and salt. Factors believed to be responsible for food waste include unpalatability of the food, limited menu choice, off-site food preparation, children's low preference for vegetables, and the availability of sweets and sodas in vending machines. **Family-style service** has been shown to result in less waste than cafeteria-style service.[18] Other factors believed to compromise children's food intakes include short lunch periods, long cafeteria lines, and a hurried, unsupervised atmosphere.

Efforts have addressed these problems by including students in menu planning, improving the eating environment, program promotion, and related activities. Programs have offered popular foods that comply with the NSLP (e.g., pizza, hamburger, tacos, salad bars, and fruits). To provide variety and to increase participation and consumption, schools are encouraged to provide a selection of foods. Students may be permitted to decline one or two items, depending on age and local discretion.

School meals have not always accommodated the needs of a child on a weight management program, and more recent concerns about preventing cardiovascular disease have focused on the levels of fat, sugar, and salt in the menus. School lunch may provide as much as 40% of calories from fat.[13,19] Current guidance from USDA, the School Meal Initiatives for Healthy Children, has encouraged the development of menus that will strive to meet the U.S. Dietary Guidelines, including reducing the fat content of recipes, offering fewer baked desserts and more fresh fruits and vegetables, and incorporating more whole-grain products.

Vending machines and school stores used as fund-raisers for school activities have been a concern to many interested in dental health, prevention of obesity, and the development of sound food habits for all children. Although common items offered are candy, soda pop, and chips, some school districts have made efforts to provide more fruit, juice, milk, nuts, and seeds. These more healthy options have met with partial success, since they may not sell as well and the profit margin is slimmer than with the candy and soda.

Federal legislation stipulates that foods sold in competition with school lunch in snack bars or vending machines must provide at least 5% of the RDA for one or more of the following nutrients: protein, vitamin A, ascorbic acid, niacin, riboflavin, thiamin, calcium, and iron. The original legislation was amended to restrict this competition to the food service area during the lunch period. Other items not meeting this criteria (e.g., soda pop, chewing gum, some candies) can be sold anytime outside the restricted area. Thus, these competitive foods continue to be daily choices for schoolchildren.

Children who do not participate in the school lunch program generally bring a packed lunch from home. Studies have indicated that, compared with the school lunch, sack lunches provide significantly fewer nutrients, but they are also lower in saturated fats.[19] Little variety is seen in the packed lunches because favorite foods tend to be consistently packed and lack of refrigeration limits the food choices.

Although elementary school children are making more decisions regarding food selection, some supervision and supportive guidance may be necessary at lunchtime. Children may give priority to activities other than eating, often rushing through their meals. They may prefer to do without meals rather than reveal the fact that they must receive reduced price or free lunches. Some may refuse to eat many foods on the menu. In addition, disposable trays and plastic utensils are not always easy for children to use.

Some children and their families may need assistance in making school meals meet the child's needs. Overweight and obese children will need more fresh fruit desserts and fewer sauces and gravies as well as a low-fat milk. As more children with special health care needs participate in school meals, some may need to have their meals modified in some manner. These children are eligible for special meals, but written documentation by a health care provider is needed, as well as planning with school staff and families.[20]

NUTRITION EDUCATION

As children grow older, have money to spend, attend school, and interact with larger numbers of individuals, selection of food increasingly becomes their own responsibility. Nutrition education during the school years is an important method of developing a nutritionally informed population. This occurs formally in school classrooms and clubs such as 4-H, but also informally from the media, advertising, written materials, family, and peers.

A 1995 Gallup survey of 9- to 15-year-old children showed positive attitudes and awareness about healthy eating and physical activity.[21] At the same time, there were misconceptions about low-fat diets and "good" versus "bad" foods. Unfortunately nutrition is frequently a low priority in the curriculum and few teachers have had basic nutrition information during their teacher training. Many have considered it a boring subject and difficult to integrate into an already crowded curriculum. Other reasons cited for ineffective nutrition education programs include lack of adequate research, resource materials, and specific curriculum guidelines that would be interdisciplinary and sequential. Nutrition education activities have been a part of some private sector programs, primarily the Dairy Council, American Heart Association, and American Cancer Society, and of some governmental agencies.

Children's developmental level should be taken into consideration when teaching nutrition concepts. **Piaget's theory of learning** through the growing years is the basis of many educational programs.[22] Table 12-3 correlates Piaget's learning theory with progress in feeding and nutrition. School-age children will do best with a hands-on food experience that relates to them personally, not written or verbal nutrition concepts. Based on Piaget's theory, the play approach is suggested as a method to teach school-aged children about nutrition and fitness.[23] In addition, a recent review of nutrition education for school-aged children addresses the theoretical frameworks used, the effectiveness of interventions, and the implications for nutrition education policy and research.[24]

Nutrition Education Training Program

Because of concern that lack of adequate nutrition information was contributing to unwise food choices and to food waste in the school lunch programs, Congress enacted the **Nutrition Education Training Program (NETP)** in 1977. Administered by the USDA, the program offered states grants to develop and implement a state nutrition education plan.

During the program's most active phase, states provided nutrition education for school lunch employees and teachers. Curriculum guidelines and materials for children in schools and child-care settings were also developed. Classroom activities that involved the cafeteria were initiated in some schools.

When the effect of these programs was evaluated, they were found to have a strong positive impact on nutrition-related knowledge. There was an increase in the number of children willing to select and taste new foods and in reported food preferences and food-related attitudes. However, the behavioral and attitudinal effects were neither as strong nor as consistent across grade levels as were the effects on knowledge.[25]

During the 1980s, the NETP budget was drastically reduced with little program impact noted at the local level. Recent years have seen a small but relatively stable funding level. Current efforts are directed toward school food service employee training, coordination of curriculum and food service activities, and integration of nutrition into health education and other curriculums.

As children prepare to enter adolescence, attitudes toward food will be well established. The nutrition knowledge and attitudes acquired during this period become a basis for the future when decisions of food selection become their own. It is important that we learn new methods of nutrition education that may have a greater impact on behavioral change in school-age children.

SPORTS AND FITNESS

Interest in sports and physical fitness has increased dramatically among children and adolescents. No longer are athletic competition and training restricted to boys in varsity team sports. Much enthusiasm has developed among girls, and individual sports have gained in popularity among girls and boys of all ages.

On the other hand, overweight and obesity has increased substantially in the school-age and adolescent population compared with children of the same age groups in the 1970s.[26] It has been reported that American youth are becoming less fit. A decline in physical activity throughout childhood is observed and accepted, although results of national fitness tests are not necessarily linked to health outcomes.[27]

Some factors believed to be at blame for a sedentary lifestyle include an increase in time spent watching television and playing computer

TABLE 12-3 *Piaget's Theory of Cognitive Development in Relation to Feeding and Nutrition*

Developmental Period	Cognitive Characteristics	Relationships to Feeding and Nutrition
Sensorimotor (Birth–2 years)	Progression from newborn with automatic reflexes to intentional interaction with the environment and the beginning use of symbols	Progression is made from sucking and rooting reflexes to the acquisition of self-feeding skills Food is used primarily to satisfy hunger, as a medium to explore the environment, and to practice fine motor skills
Preoperations (2–7 years)	Thought processes become internalized; they are unsystematic and intuitive Use of symbols increases Reasoning is based on appearances and happenstance Approach to classification is functional and unsystematic Child's world is viewed egocentrically	Eating becomes less the center of attention than social, language, and cognitive growth Food is described by color, shape, and quantity but there is limited ability to classify food into "groups" Foods tend to be classed as "like" and "don't like" Foods can be identified as "good for you" but reasons are unknown or mistaken
Concrete operations (7–11 years)	Child can focus on several aspects of a situation simultaneously Cause/effect reasoning becomes more rational and systematic Ability to classify, reclassify, and generalize emerges Decrease in egocentricism permits child to take another's view	Beginning of realization that nutritious food has a positive effect on growth and health, but limited understanding of how or why this occurs Mealtimes take on a social significance The expanding environment increases the opportunities for, and influences on, food selection (peer influence rises)
Formal operations (11 years and older)	Hypothetical and abstract thought expand Understanding of scientific and theoretical processes deepens	The concept of nutrients from food functioning at physiological and biochemical levels can be understood Conflicts in making food choices may be realized (knowledge of nutritious food vs. preferences and nonnutritive influences)

From Mahan LK, Arlin MT: *Krause's food, nutrition, and diet therapy,* ed 8, Philadelphia, 1992, WB Saunders.

and video games and less physical education in the school curriculum. With two working parents there is less free or spontaneous play and more organized sports, dance classes, swimming lessons, and gymnastics classes. Budget cuts can eliminate extramural school sports or recreational activities in community centers. In addition, safety issues, especially in urban areas, frequently mean that children are restricted to their homes.

Interest in athletic performance is beneficial to the health of our youth, provided that the intensity of involvement is not excessive. Activities that focus on winning rather than skill development and pleasure can have negative physical and emotional consequences. Positive

❖

THE YOUNG ATHLETES' BILL OF RIGHTS

1. The right to have the opportunity to participate in sports regardless of one's ability level.
2. The right to participate at a level commensurate with the child's developmental level.
3. The right to have qualified adult leadership.
4. The right to participate in a safe and healthy environment.
5. The right of each child to share leadership and decision making.
6. The right to play as a child and not as an adult.
7. The right to proper preparation for participation in sports.
8. The right to equal opportunity to strive for success.
9. The right to be treated with dignity by all involved.
10. The right to have fun through sports.

From Strong WB: *Am J Dis Child* 142:143, 1988.

TABLE 12-4 *Activities of Different Energy Expenditures**

Energy Output	Activities
Low (<4 kcal/min; up to 240 kcal/hr)	Baseball, cycling (up to 9 mi/hr), walking, gymnastics, table tennis, moderate football
Moderate (4–7 kcal/min; 240–420 kcal/hr)	Basketball, cycling (10–13 mi/hr), roller skating, ice skating (9 mi/hr), running (more than 12 min/mi), touch football, hiking with a pack (3 mi/hr)
High (>7 kcal/min; ≥420 kcal/hr)	Cycling (more than 14 mi/hr), running (more than 6 mi/hr), judo, karate, vigorous calisthenics (e.g., some aerobic dance)

Modified from Peterson M, Peterson K: *Eat to compete*, St Louis, 1988, Mosby–Year Book.
*Based on a reference child weighing 100 lbs.

goals for children in sports are listed in the box above. Sensible health practices for growing athletes are multifaceted, including attention to appropriate diet, fluid, sleep, and training and an accepting, supportive home environment.

Few studies have been done on the nutritional needs of growing athletes. Most published research has been taken from adolescents who agreed to be studied while training for specific sports.

Adequate energy and water are the key nutrients to be considered in the typical school-age athlete. Besides being needed for basal metabolism and physical activity, energy is required to support normal growth. Growing athletes therefore demand more kcalories per kilogram of body weight than adults performing the same activity. During adolescence when the growth rate is extremely rapid (especially for boys), the energy needs may be great.

The amount of energy needed will depend on the intensity, duration, and frequency of the activity (table 12-4 gives examples of activities with different levels of energy expenditure). The average 10-year-old boy may expend between 2000 and 2800 kcal/day, but those who are running long distances or exerting themselves in other physical activities may need an additional 300 to 700 kcal/day. The energy needs of preadolescent girls are similar to those of boys for moderate and heavy exercise, but may be greater at ages 11 to 12 as they go into puberty.

Fluids are especially critical in hot, humid weather or when participating in endurance activities. Dehydration not only decreases performance but also can result in serious health consequences such as increased body temperature, muscle cramps, and heatstroke. Children are more at risk for these disorders than adults, so diligent attention to fluids is needed during children's physical activities.[28] Although thirst is a normal cue to drink, children frequently do not instinctively drink enough fluid to replenish losses during prolonged exercise. They should be encouraged to drink plenty of fluids before, during, and after exercise. A rule of thumb is to drink every 15 minutes during

❖

> ### AMERICAN MEDICAL ASSOCIATION'S GUIDELINES FOR WEIGHT MANAGEMENT IN YOUNG WRESTLERS
>
> 1. The amount of body fat desirable for the wrestler is 7% to 10%.
> 2. The wrestler should participate in a 6-week intensive training and conditioning program with no regard for his weight.
> 3. Weight at the end of this period is to be his minimum effective weight for competition and certification.
> 4. Any effort to maintain a weight below this would be a hardship to the body.

FIG. 12-1   Biking is a physical activity that can be enjoyed throughout life.

practice. Electrolytes lost from sweat can be replenished easily by eating food after the physical exertion, and the use of special supplements will not be necessary.

A group particularly at health risk are competitive wrestlers who may restrict food and fluids to "make weight" in their weight class. Studies of college wrestlers have shown that they are unable to fully rehydrate themselves by competition time and may enter a match in a state of dehydration, with compromised performance as a result.[29] The American Medical Association's guidelines for weight management in young wrestlers should be used as the foundation for practice by coaches and trainers in this sport (see the box above).

Diet and sports is unfortunately filled with superstition and myth about "optimum practices." Special diets or foods are sometimes promoted, and supplements are frequently recommended. These diets and supplements often have no scientific proof to support their use; however, the enthusiasm of the coach or trainer may influence the child to follow these practices. Carbohydrate-loading is inappropriate for children, extra protein will not increase performance, and various supplements will not energize the body.[30]

Common sense is much needed in assessing the nutritional needs of the growing athlete. Sufficient kcalories must be consumed to support growth and activity. For the young athlete with a busy schedule, frequent, portable snacks are essential in addition to regular meals. Fluid and electrolytes lost during practice or competition must be replaced to avoid the consequences of dehydration and electrolyte imbalance. Weight management efforts should be approached sensibly without trying to achieve minimal weight through promotion of fluid loss. Eating before competition should be scheduled to allow enough time to avoid retention of undigested food material in the gut at the time of the event. Foods that are easy to digest should be selected, avoiding unnecessary fat, fiber, and gas-forming fruits and vegetables. No special diets or supplements are recognized to be the answer to greater performance or success. However, if eating a particular food provides a psychological edge, choosing it might be considered potentially advantageous.

Many children do not participate in organized sports because of lack of interest, finances, or family support. However, all children should be encouraged and supported in physical fitness through individual activities of their interest, unorganized group play, or other recreational activities (e.g., camping, hiking, nature exploration). The optimal physical activities or sports are those that the child can continue to perform into and throughout adulthood (fig. 12-1).

Parents and other family members are significant models and should provide opportunities for family activities such as biking, walking the dog, or exploring a local park or beach. Families may also consider limiting the time children spend watching television or playing computer games. Beyond the family, the fitness of youngsters will be boosted by local support for community recreational programs and the availability of physical education in the school curriculum.

HEALTH PROMOTION

Increased interest in health and concern about heart disease, cancer, and obesity have caused Americans to change their eating habits in recent years. Various recommendations from the government and nonprofit organizations, such as the Dietary Guidelines, are promoting healthy eating to the public.

The **National Cholesterol Education Program (NCEP)** recommends that everyone over 2 years of age consume a diet of no more than 30% of kcalories from fat (10% or less from saturated fat, up to 10% from unsaturated fat, 10% to 15% from monounsaturated fat) and no more than 300 mg cholesterol per day.[31] Cholesterol screening is also recommended for children at risk for cardiovascular disease. Secular trends over the past 15 years have been reported by the Bogalusa Heart Study, including significant decreases in total fat intake, saturated fat intake, and percent of kcalories from fat (from 38% in 1973 to 1974 to 36% in 1987 to 1988).[32] These dietary trends, however, did not alter serum lipid and lipoprotein levels and do not meet the NCEP guidelines. Although there remains controversy about the appropriateness of the dietary and screening recommendations for children, school-age children and adolescents apparently are able to consume low-fat diets (less than 30% of kcalories from fat and less than 300 mg cholesterol) without negatively influencing the level of micronutrients.[33] See Chapter 10 for further discussion.

Prevention of **osteoporosis** in later years is critically dependent on calcium retention during adolescence and young adulthood. Calcium needs in childhood are usually met by the inclusion of typical amounts of dairy products in the diet. By ages 10 to 12 years in females, however, the needs increase significantly to match pubertal growth. Balance studies suggest that young adolescent girls may need to consume more than the RDA level of 1200 mg/day to achieve maximum calcium intake and balance.[34] This may also be true of school-aged children. In a three-year, double-blind study of prepubertal twins, those supplemented up to 1600 mg of calcium per day had significantly greater increases in bone mineral density.[35] The National Institutes of Health Consensus Development Conference Statement recommends an optimal calcium intake of 800 to 1200 mg daily for children 6 to 10 years of age.[36] Therefore the preteen years are critical for establishment of dietary habits that include optimal calcium sources to carry them through the next decades.

Although there has been emphasis on dietary fiber in the American diet for some time, little information has been available on the dietary fiber intake of children. Recent data suggest that school-aged children consume about 12 gm of dietary fiber per day, which may not be adequate for health promotion and disease prevention.[37,38] A new recommendation, endorsed by several national organizations concerned with child health, suggests that children over age 2 should consume a minimum dietary fiber of age plus 5 gm per day, with a safe intake up to age plus 10 gm per day.[39]

Common sense and moderation are probably the best policy in promoting a healthy diet in school-age children. Beneficial food habits consolidated in these years will likely be maintained into adulthood. The use of low-fat dairy products, lean animal protein, and fewer high-fat foods is appropriate for healthy, growing children. Restricting the intake of fermentable carbohydrate in the diet will improve dental health and nutrient density. Increasing children's intake of fruits, vegetables, whole grains, and legumes above usual reported levels has several benefits including (1) increasing the fiber content, (2) reducing the percentage of dietary fat, (3) increasing the amount of beta-carotene and other dietary factors that may help in cancer prevention, and (4) providing a diet that is more nutrient dense.

NUTRITION CONCERNS

Diet and Behavior

Does sugar make a child "hyper"? Does skipping breakfast really make any difference in school performance? Are food additives or allergies a cause of behavioral problems in children? These and similar questions are often asked by parents, teachers, and health care workers. A good deal of information on diet and behavior is available, but some of it is myth, some of it is controversial, and some of it is based on sound scientific research.

Nutrition and learning. Dozens of studies over the last few decades have documented the negative effect of malnourishment on children's intellectual development (see chapter 1 for a thorough discussion). A more gray area of any diet-cognitive connection is whether "marginal" malnutrition or skipping meals affects behavior or school performance. A recent literature review of the effects of breakfast on school performance and cognition supports the findings that omitting breakfast has a negative impact on children's academic performance, especially in those at nutritional risk.[40]

Studies of healthy school-age children in a laboratory setting have measured cognitive abilities, such as problem solving, memory, and attentiveness, after the children had eaten or not eaten breakfast. The children who had fasted generally made more errors in their performance.[41] Another report using similar methodology compared healthy children with those stunted, those experiencing severe malnutrition in early life, and those currently wasted (low weight for height). Although variation occurred among the groups in their response to the cognitive tests, all of the malnourished and undernourished children were adversely affected in their performance when they missed breakfast.[42]

In a community-based study, the academic performance of children in six schools in a low-income area was compared before and after the schools began the SBP. The children participating in the breakfast program showed improved performance as measured by standardized achievement tests compared with children qualifying for the breakfast program but not participating.[43] These results support the expansion of nutrition education and feeding programs so that children at risk might be successful in school.

Iron deficiency, a common nutrient deficiency in children, has long been implicated in negative changes in behavior and performance. Iron is involved in the functioning of many molecules in the brain and nervous system, and these systems are sensitive to lowered iron levels long before overt anemia is diagnosed. Compared with control subjects, iron-deficient infants and preschool children (with and without anemia) tend to score lower on standard scales of mental development and are less likely to pay attention to relevant cues in problem-solving situations.[44,45] A recent report suggests that iron deficiency's negative impact on cognitive performance can have long-term consequences on children into the school years.[46] This information has clinical implications in terms of assessing the overall nutrient quality of the diet of a "behavior problem" child, as well as implications for public policy in addressing the nutrition needs of low-income, high-risk children.

A relatively new research focus has been on the relationships between nutrition and behavior and the brain. Studies have addressed the influence of dietary components on the synthesis of brain neurotransmitters that affect behaviors such as appetite, mood, and depression. Tryptophan and choline intake can stimulate the increased release of the neurotransmitters serotonin and acetylcholine.[47] Studies in adults suggest that mental alertness is lower and lethargy and drowsiness are greater after a high-carbohydrate rather than a high-protein meal.[47] Although there seems to be a general relationship between diet, brain chemistry, and behavior, further research will be needed to reveal the significance of individual variability and to discern clinical implications for children.

Attention deficit hyperactivity disorder. Frequently referred to as **hyperactivity, attention deficit hyperactivity disorder (ADHD)** is most commonly seen among school-age children in the United States. ADHD is a clinical diagnosis requiring the following specific criteria: inattention, impulsivity, and hyperactivity; onset before 7 years of age and duration of at least 6 months; and absence of schizophrenia, affective disorder, or mental retardation.[48]

An estimated 3% to 5% of schoolchildren are believed to be affected by ADHD with boys affected six to nine times more often than girls.[48] Although a true diagnosis is a result of assessment by medical or educational specialists, many children are labeled hyperactive by less formal measures of behavior in the school or home. Regardless of the looseness of the diagnosis, the main focus of those involved with the child becomes treatment and management.

Various causes of ADHD have been proposed over the years, yet the etiology remains relatively unknown. Perinatal complications such as anoxia, toxemia, prematurity, and infection have long been suggested as causes, as have insults during the early years including head injuries, seizures, toxic agents, or infections. Greater incidence of a family history of hyperactivity and learning disabilities in the identified children suggests a genetic component. Some studies have suggested a biochemical basis for ADHD, and environmental factors such as exposure to fluorescent lights and heavy metals (e.g., lead) have also been suggested. Dietary factors, including food additives, sugar, and allergies, have also been implicated as causes of hyperactivity.

Stimulant medication. The most widely used and accepted forms of treatment for ADHD are stimulant medications, behavioral management, and special education. Methylphenidate (Ritalin) is the most common medication, with dextroamphetamine (Dexedrine) and pemoline (Cylert) used less frequently. Although the exact mechanism of these medications is not fully understood, children with ADHD respond to them with reduction in such undesirable behaviors as motor restlessness, short attention span, and irritability. Many people assume that when the child is calmed down and paying more attention, academic performance improves. Some evidence, however, suggests that stimulant medications do not necessarily improve school learning and that long-term outcomes are no different from those of children who have no medication.[49]

One of the appeals of stimulant medication is its immediate results with few toxic side effects. Anorexia is frequently noted and can eventually result in growth suppression.[50] There appears to be a direct relationship between the dosage and the degree of suppressed appetite.[51] Although more tolerance to the medication's negative effect on growth is expected over time, the response is very individual. Children discontinuing the medication during vacations and summers usually have a growth rebound, but this is unlikely to compensate completely for the growth suppression incurred during the school year. However, evidence suggests that adult height of boys treated with Ritalin for up to five years was no different from control boys, suggesting a compensatory growth rebound after discontinuation of the medication.[52]

Although the mechanisms by which stimulant medication may inhibit growth is unclear, decreased energy intake is a factor. Children receiving stimulant medication present a variety of feeding problems, including being picky about foods eaten, dawdling at mealtime, refusing school lunches, and being disinterested in food. Some children have been observed to consume large amounts of sweets and other low-nutrient foods because parents are concerned that the child will refuse to eat something. Because of poor appetites and slow growth, families frequently resort to bribery, indulgence, and threats to induce their children to eat. It is easy to understand how a preoccupation with food and eating can lead to frustration for parents and children, resulting in inappropriate behaviors and interactions at mealtimes. When the children discontinue medication during vacations, their parents often note dramatic increases in appetite and food consumption.

Since stimulant medications can result in growth suppression, frequent measurement of weight and height is essential to monitor longitudinal changes in growth. The efficacy of the medication should be assessed periodically using standard double-blind procedures. For practical dietary management, it is important to know the type, dosage, and administration time of the medication. Since it takes about 30 minutes for the medication's effect to be clinically manifested, the medication should be given before or with meals to take advantage of optimal appetite. The medication's effect is usually minimal or absent after 4 to 6 hours, and foods of high energy and nutrient density should be offered then. Each child should be evaluated with regard to medication administration, meal and snack routine, and appetite response. Some families may benefit from counseling regarding specific feeding problems.

Food additives. Of the various proposed dietary causes of ADHD, artificial colorings and flavorings in food is one of the most common. This theory, supposedly supported by parallel increases of food additives in the food supply and the prevalence of ADHD, was proposed by Feingold and became popular in the 1970s. Although most concerns regarding additives center on safety issues and potential carcinogenicity, adverse physical reactions are reported with monosodium glutamate, which precipitates the Chinese restaurant syndrome, and tartrazine, which causes an allergic response in persons who are also sensitive to aspirin.[47]

Treatment by the Feingold diet consisted of removing these additives, natural salicylates (found mostly in fruits), and some preservatives (BHA, BHT) from the child's diet. Initial reports, mostly open trial and subjective, were positive and caused the diet to become popular with the public at a time when medication use and overuse were being questioned. Subsequent challenge and diet replacement studies using controlled double-blind procedures have not supported the Feingold diet as an effective therapy for ADHD.[53,47] It is accepted, however, that as many as 5% to 10% of children may benefit from a trial of the diet, and preschool children appear to be more sensitive to these substances than older children.[47] One diet replacement study in preschool hyperactive boys used the Feingold diet plus elimination of any other foods to which the child seemed to react (e.g., chocolate, sugar, or caffeine). Using accepted rating scales, results showed some behavioral improvement in almost one-half of the boys.[54]

For families using the Feingold diet, nutritional evaluation of the modified version (including the natural fruits and vegetables) has shown that it compares favorably with the RDA and thus poses little nutritional risk for the child.[55] It is certainly understandable that a family with a child with ADHD might expect a positive outcome from a diet that is relatively simple and without side effects. In addition to the possibility of a placebo effect, the diet may create a positive focus for the family rather than the negative attention to problem behaviors. Children using the diet should receive nutritional assessment, and families should be counseled not to disregard the potential help provided by special education, behavioral management, and other therapies that can combine appropriately with the diet.

Sugar. Sugar (sucrose) has been implicated, mainly in popular books and anecdotal reports, as a causative factor in a multitude of diseases and disorders. Some of these include diabetes, obesity, heart disease, and hypoglycemia, as well as mental and behavioral disorders such as ADHD, depression, and psychoses. Some parents, teachers, and school nurses report dramatic negative changes in some children after receiving a load of sugar. Anecdotal stories describe children "climbing the walls" the day after Halloween. All of these reports, however, are subjective and are not based on controlled studies.

An early report suggested that there was a positive correlation between sugar consumption and destructive-aggressive behavior in 4- to 7-year-old hyperactive children.[56] Correlation, however, does not imply a cause-effect role for sugar in behavior problems of children. Other factors such as a permissive home environment or a child who demands foods high in sucrose may be involved.

Sucrose double-blind challenge studies have not detected significant negative behavioral effects of sucrose. Contrary to popular belief, one study found that the children who consumed sugar were less active and quieter after a challenge than those given the placebo.[57] These results may support the theory that a high carbohydrate intake facilitates production of serotonin, or the results may derive from other unknown factors.

Wolraich, Wilson, and White recently reported a meta-analysis of sugar's effect on behavior and cognition in children.[58] Sixteen studies met the criteria of using sugar and placebo challenges, being double blind, and reporting statistical results based on observational data and standardized measurements. The results of this analysis found that sugar has no effect on behavior or cognition in children.

At this time the only direct cause-effect relationship between sugar and disease is the role of sugar in dental caries, but this does not preclude the possibility that an individual child might be responsive to a large sucrose load.

Americans consume approximately 125 pounds of sweeteners per year, of which sucrose represents about 65 pounds.[47] Many foodstuffs that are high in sugar are low in nutrients, and thus they dilute the nutrient quality of the diet. Reducing or eliminating sugar in the diet serves to improve the overall nutritional and dental health of both child and family. These positive changes in families' diets have been observed in personal clinical experience. The professional can reinforce the dietary changes while stressing the lack of data supporting a sugar-behavior association.

Megavitamin therapy. The use of large doses of certain vitamins to treat ADHD frequently originates from lay groups, the popular press, and some professionals. The basis of megavitamin therapy is that children with ADHD or learning problems have biochemical imbalances and that these disturbances can be eliminated by this therapy.

Megavitamin therapy, using nicotinic acid, was first used to treat schizophrenia. Suspecting vitamin deficiency as a cause of mental and behavioral problems is a result of existing nutritional knowledge on deficiency states. Classic examples are the neurological and mental changes noted in persons with niacin deficiency (pellagra) and thiamin deficiency (beriberi).

Most commonly, megavitamin therapy includes niacin, ascorbic acid, pyridoxine, and calcium pantothenate. On the other hand, personal clinical experience has indicated that children receiving megavitamin therapy may be taking a wide assortment of vitamin or mineral supplements with or without professional guidance.

A few studies have tested megavitamin therapy using double-blind controlled studies. Arnold and others[59] reported on 31 children with minimal brain dysfunction who received either placebos or megavitamins during a 2-week trial. Parent and teacher behavior ratings taken before and after the trial showed no significant difference in the two groups. Only two children responded so well that stimulant medication was not considered necessary; they were both in the placebo group.

Other studies have had similar results. In one, children with learning disabilities were put on a low-carbohydrate, high-protein diet and then given either megavitamins or placebos for 6 months.[60] Evaluations before and after this period with a combination of intellectual, school achievement, perceptual, and behavioral measures showed no difference between the two groups. In another report, behavioral and classroom performance of children with ADHD actually worsened following megavitamin therapy, while the behavior of those receiving a placebo improved.[61]

Studies have been unable to support the theories advocated by proponents of megavitamin therapy, and established medical professionals have not supported the treatment. In addition, potential dangers exist from consuming large doses of vitamins. Toxicity can result from excessive intake of fat-soluble vitamins A and D. These vitamins are not included in the standard megavitamin treatment, yet clinical experience reveals that some practitioners commonly recommend vitamins A and D, or that families on their own initiative may include them in their regimen. Other complications that have been reported from megadoses of water-soluble vitamins are **hyperbilirubinemia** and liver damage from large doses of nicotinic acid, and sensory neuropathy from large doses of vitamin B_6.[47] Megavitamin therapy as an unfounded treatment for mental retardation is discussed in chapter 15.

It is easy to understand why a family would respond to the appeal of megavitamin therapy, but too often it plays on the false hopes and guilt of the parents or provides a focus for blame. Some families can spend considerable money on vitamins and yet not deal with the basic problem related to the child's behavior. Although there are no sound data to support the use of megavitamins with hyperactive children, it is possible that some individuals may have increased needs for certain nutrients. The nutritional status of each child should be assessed and appropriate dietary intervention should be planned. In working with parents who choose to use megavitamins for their child, one needs to help them recognize the practice as helpful, neutral, or harmful and to provide accurate information. At times counseling may be indicated to help families recognize and consider other treatment options.

Dental Health

Dental caries, one of the most common nutritional diseases, affects children at all ages and income levels. Recent national data show an average of 2.5 decayed, missing, and filled tooth surfaces (DMFS) in children ages 5 to 17 years.[62] The rate increases with age, from 0.9 DMFS in school-aged children to 4.4 DMFS in adolescents. The same report found that 74% of children 5 to 11 years were caries-free, but this decreased to 33% by the teen years.[62]

Once the tooth has erupted, the composition of the diet, the presence of acid-producing bacteria, and the buffering capacity of the saliva interact and result in the control or development of dental caries. Some children appear to be more susceptible to dental caries than others, suggesting a hereditary influence. Calcified dental tissues, unlike the long bones, which are subject to constant remodeling and repair, do not have the ability to repair themselves. Tooth destruction by decay is permanent.

The development of dental caries requires fermentable carbohydrate, bacteria, and a susceptible tooth. The decay process starts with the interaction of bacteria *(Streptococcus mutans)* and a carbohydrate on the surface of the tooth. The bacteria, within the sticky, gelatinous dental plaque, metabolize the carbohydrate, producing organic acids. When the pH is decreased to 5.5 or less, degradation and demineralization of the tooth enamel begin.[63] The saliva, with a pH of 6.5 to 7.0, acts as a buffer and provides mechanical cleansing of the teeth.

Although any fermentable sugar is cariogenic, sucrose is considered the most cariogenic because it is the most common in the diet. The three major food sources of sucrose in the diets of children and adolescents are beverages, candies, and desserts. Starch is considered to be less cariogenic than sugars, but it is readily broken down to fermentable carbohydrate by salivary amylase. In addition, many high-starch foods also contain sucrose, which could make them more cariogenic than sugar alone because starch is retained longer in the mouth.[63]

The presence of sugar, or even the total amount of carbohydrates in the diet, may not be the determining factor in the incidence of dental caries. Other important factors are the frequency of eating and the retentiveness of the food to the teeth. These elements as a whole influence the length of time that the teeth are exposed to an acidic environment, which leads to tooth decay.

Protein foods such as hard cheeses, nuts, eggs, and meats do not reduce plaque pH and thus are believed to be protective against caries.[64] The exact mechanism involved is unknown, but these foods have a relatively high protein content with basic amino acids, a moderate fat content, a strong buffering capacity, a high mineral content including calcium and phosphorus, and a pH greater than 6.0. They also stimulate saliva flow.

Prevention and control of caries. Fluoride is the single most effective factor in caries prevention. It reduces the incidence of dental caries by suppressing sugar metabolism by bacteria, making enamel more resistant to acid, and stimulating remineralization of the teeth. A fluoridated water supply is a critical part of prevention. In areas without fluoridation, a supplement is recommended through the growing years.

Dietary management continues to be a most important and effective approach to the control of dental caries. Three factors are interdependent in determining the cariogenicity of a particular food: (1) sucrose content; (2) physical properties; and (3) consumption patterns. For example, sweets and desserts eaten with meals will be less cariogenic than when eaten alone; dried fruits are less retentive when in cereal, baked goods, or salads; and sweetened beverages may be less damaging than starchy foods containing sugar.[63]

Snacks for children should emphasize foods that are low in sucrose, are not retentive, and

NUTRITIONAL SNACKS FOR DENTAL HEALTH

*Protein foods**
Natural cheese (cheddar, jack, string)
Milk
Cooked turkey, chicken, beef, ham
Plain yogurt
Peanut butter
Cottage cheese
Unsalted nuts and seeds
Tuna
Hard-cooked egg
Breads and cereals†
Whole-grain breads
Whole-grain cereals
Whole-grain, low-fat crackers
Tortillas
English muffins
Rice crackers
Pita bread
Popcorn
Bagels

Fruits†
Apples
Bananas
Pears
Berries
Oranges, other citrus fruits
Melon
Grapes
Unsweetened canned fruit
Unsweetened fruit juices
Vegetables
Carrots
Celery
Green pepper
Radishes
Cucumbers
Cabbage
Cauliflower
Broccoli
Tomatoes
Jicama
Vegetable juices

Examples: Apple wedges with peanut butter; egg salad sandwich; raw vegetables with yogurt or cottage cheese dip; plain yogurt with unsweetened applesauce and cinnamon; tortilla with melted cheese; pita bread with tuna; popcorn with parmesan cheese; frozen banana rolled in plain yogurt and chopped nuts; rice cracker with peanut butter or cheese.

*These foods may be protective against lowering plaque pH when eaten with foods that contain fermentable carbohydrate.
†Fruits, juices, and most cereal/bread products contain fermentable carbohydrate; limit to 1 serving in a snack.

stimulate saliva flow (the box above lists some examples). Eating cheese, nuts, and meats at the same time as higher sugar foods will help prevent a decrease in plaque pH. Chewing sugarless gum after eating fermentable carbohydrate may also be beneficial in controlling acidity.[65]

Good dental health will be most likely when families purchase few cariogenic foods, provide routine eating schedules, encourage daily oral hygiene, and schedule routine dental examinations. In addition, group feeding at schools, day-care facilities, camps, and other programs should practice positive dental nutrition, and dental health education should be a part of the school health curriculum.

Lactose Intolerance

Many adults throughout the world experience lactose malabsorption or intolerance. The exceptions include Northern Europeans, the Fulani and Tussi tribes of Africa, the Punjali of India, Finns, Hungarians, and probably Mongols. An estimated 70% of black American adults and 100% of homogenous Native Americans have limited ability to hydrolyze lactose.[66] The onset of reduced lactase levels occurs in childhood and adolescence, but rarely before 3 years of age. In some countries (e.g., Greece and Israel) there is a linear progression in the prevalence of lactose malabsorption throughout the school-age years, but in other countries (e.g.,

China, Jamaica, Peru, and Bangladesh) this transition occurs more quickly between 3 and 5 years of age.[67] In the United States, clinical symptoms are usually not manifested until after 5 to 7 years of age.

Unaffected individuals hydrolyze and absorb ingested lactose in the small intestine. If lactase activity is low, only a portion of the sugar will be hydrolyzed to glucose and galactose. Undigested lactose remains in the lumen of the intestine and has a hyperosmolar effect, drawing large amounts of fluid into the gut. As the sugar is transported to the ileocecal region and the first part of the colon, it is fermented by bacterial flora. This causes production of carbon dioxide, hydrogen, and low molecular weight acids that interfere with the reabsorption of fluids and electrolytes. The increased fluid load and products of bacterial fermentation cause the symptoms of bloating, flatulence, abdominal cramping, and diarrhea.

The response of individuals with lactase deficiency to the ingestion of milk varies. Some manifest no symptoms, and others experience symptoms shortly after milk is ingested. The amount of milk that must be consumed at one time to produce symptoms ranges from less than 240 ml to 1000 ml. Many persons with lactase deficiency are not intolerant to lactose or to milk. Adults and older children with low lactase levels have usually consumed milk in infancy and early childhood without symptoms.

There are two common tests for lactose intolerance.[66] A lactose tolerance test measures change in blood glucose for 2 to 3 hours after a load of lactose is given. A flat glucose curve suggests lactose intolerance but is not diagnostic for lactose malabsorption. The lactose breath-hydrogen test, which more directly indicates lactose maldigestion, measures expired breath hydrogen.

Milk is an important source of protein, calcium, riboflavin, and vitamins D and A. Children in racial groups known to have a high incidence of lactose intolerance should not be limited in their milk intake unless they manifest symptoms. Those with symptoms should be encouraged to consume dairy products in which lactose has been fermented (e.g., yogurt, buttermilk, and aged cheese). Heating or pasteurizing yogurt loses its effectiveness because the bacteria are killed; thus products with active cultures are most beneficial.[68] Ice-cold milk and milk consumed alone seem to cause greater discomfort than milk consumed with food or at room temperature. Many children can tolerate up to one cup of milk at a time when consumed with meals.

Lactose-free milks or milk treated with lactase are commercially available for children whose symptoms are severe. These products provide a 70% to 100% reduction of the lactose.[68] Commercial preparations are also available either as drops to add to milks or formulas, or as tablets to take orally at the same time as a lactose-containing meal. Since lactose is added to many prepared foods, parents of children with lactose intolerance should read labels carefully so that additional loads of lactose can be avoided. Lactose is found in whey powder, casein, casein hydrolysate, sodium caseinate, and lactalbumin.[68]

Diets of all children who limit their intakes of milk should be carefully monitored for vitamin D and calcium levels. Supplements should be prescribed when appropriate. In healthy subjects the percentage of calcium absorbed from carbonate, acetate, gluconate, and citrate salts is similar to the percentage absorbed from whole milk.[69]

The previous discussion applies to primary lactase deficiency acquired after the weaning years. Primary lactase deficiency can occur in infancy as a result of a congenital condition or inborn error of metabolism, but this is rare.[68] Secondary lactase deficiency may result from infectious diarrhea, medications that alter the intestinal mucosa, and gastrointestinal diseases. These periods are usually temporary, and normal levels of lactase activity usually return when the disease is controlled. Despite long-standing therapy to omit the offending sugars in these cases, current practice suggests continuing to offer the dairy products after an initial 24-hour glucose-electrolyte solution.[68]

Summary

School-age children grow at a steady rate and acquire many physical and cognitive skills. Their food and nutrient intake is influenced by many factors, including family, peers, and media. As children prepare to enter adolescence, their attitudes toward food will be well established. Parents need to provide appropriate foods and supportive guidance so that positive food patterns are developed. School feeding programs and educational curricula provide an opportunity for nutrition education that can improve nutrition knowledge and behavior.

Although most school-age children clinically appear to be well nourished, some groups are at risk for malnutrition because of socioeconomic factors, limited food resources, lack of education, or health conditions. Others are at risk for obesity and poor physical condition as a result of poor food selection and poor lifestyle habits.

REVIEW QUESTIONS

1. Discuss the major problems and criticisms of the NSLP. What factors are responsible for these problems?
2. List the NCEP dietary guidelines for children.
3. Discuss the various dietary treatments for ADHD and critique the rationale for each.
4. List three practical, but reasonable, dietary recommendations that would decrease the risk of dental caries in children.
5. Describe major societal trends in the United States over the last two decades that have influenced the dietary intake and health status of school-age children.
6. List the four groups of at-risk children who might benefit from routine vitamin-mineral supplements.

❖ ❖ ❖

CASE STUDY

Stimulant Medication and Diet

J. H. is an 8-year-old boy with attention deficit hyperactivity disorder (ADHD) who was put on a trial of Ritalin (a stimulant medication) because of increasing difficulties in school performance and behavior, and outbursts at home. After a month there were positive improvements documented by the school and family, so J. H. was continued with a regimen of 10 mg in the morning and 10 mg at noon. However, his parents noticed that he wasn't eating very much breakfast now, and they tried offering him other foods (including sweets) to get him to eat. His teacher also reported that J. H. frequently ate less than half of his school lunch, even though he had enough time. When his parents became more concerned about his poor eating as well as a recent 2-pound weight loss, they were referred to a nutritionist.

The nutrition evaluation determined that J. H. had decreased his energy intake significantly since starting the Ritalin, primarily at the morning and noon meals. During the interview, parents reported a medication schedule of giving the Ritalin about 30 to 40 minutes before meals, which explained its dramatic effect on appetite and intake. The nutritionist provided information regarding the appetite-suppressing effect of Ritalin, including the likelihood that J. H. would develop a tolerance to it over time. She and the family discussed various intervention options, with the family agreeing on the following: (1) J. H. would get the morning dose at breakfast rather than before, and parents would request the school staff to do the same at lunch, (2) the parents would communicate with J. H.'s day-care provider to request an energy-dense after-school snack, (3) the parents would offer him a bedtime snack, and (4) the parents would obtain weight measures monthly until growth shows slow but stable progress. Parents were also encouraged to offer a variety of nutritious foods at meals and snacks, and to avoid using nagging or rewards to get their son to eat.

SUGGESTED LEARNING ACTIVITIES

1. Assess the nutrient intake of a school-age child.
2. Review a daily activity log of an elementary school child and categorize according to levels of energy expenditure.
3. Describe factors that influence food choices in the school-age child.
4. Assess the nutritional status of a child who has been on long-term stimulant medication. What is the growth pattern? The appetite?
5. Eat a school lunch with children and assess the menu, palatability, cafeteria atmosphere, amount of time to eat, and children's interaction.
6. Plan a nutrition lesson emphasizing dental nutrition for an elementary school class.
7. Plan brown bag lunches for a school-age child for one week that provide variety and are nutritionally appropriate.

REFERENCES

1. Alaimo K, McDowell MA, Briefel RR and others: *Dietary intake of vitamins, minerals, and fiber of persons ages 2 months and over in the United States: third national health and nutrition examination survey, phase I, 1988–91,* Advance Data from Vital Statistics; No. 258, (PHS) 95-1250 Hyattsville, MD, National Center for Health Statistics, 1994.
2. Kennedy E, Goldberg J: What are American children eating? implications for public policy, *Nutr Rev* 53:111, 1995.
3. Cook JT, Martin LS: *Differences in nutrient adequacy among poor and non-poor children,* Medford, MA, May, 1995, Tufts University School of Nutrition Center on Hunger, Poverty and Nutrition Policy.
4. Bowering J, Clancy KL: Nutritional status of children and teenagers in relation to vitamin and mineral use, *J Am Diet Assoc* 86:1033, 1986.
5. Committee on Nutrition, American Academy of Pediatrics: Vitamin and mineral supplementation needs in normal children in the United States, *Pediatrics* 66:1015, 1980.
6. Laskarzewski P and others: Parent-child nutrient intake interrelationships in school children ages 6 to 19: The Princeton School District Study, *Am J Clin Nutr* 33:2350, 1980.
7. Johnson RK, Crouter AC, Smiciklas-Wright H: Effects of maternal employment on family food consumption and children's diets, *J Nutr Educ* 25:130, 1993.
8. Wright JD: Homeless children. Two years later, *Am J Dis Child* 147:518, 1993.
9. Karp R and others: Parental behavior and the availability of foods among undernourished inner-city children, *J Fam Pract* 18:731, 1984.
10. Guber S: Marketing to kids: it's elementary, *Prepared Foods* 158:48, 1989.
11. Kotz K, Story M: Food advertisements during children's Saturday morning television programming: Are they consistent with dietary recommendations? *J Am Diet Assoc* 94:1296, 1994.
12. Nicklas TA and others: Nutritional studies in children and implications for change: the Bogalusa Heart Study, *J Adv Med* 2:451, 1989.
13. Nicklas TA: Dietary studies of children: The Bogalusa Heart Study experience, *J Am Diet Assoc* 95:1127, 1995.
14. Nicklas TA, Bao W, Webber LS and others: Breakfast consumption affects adequacy of total daily intake in children, *J Am Diet Assoc* 93:886, 1993.
15. Sampson AE, Dixit S, Meyers AF and others: The nutritional impact of breakfast consumption on the diets of inner-city African-American elementary school children, *J Natl Med Assoc* 87:195, 1995.
16. Klesges RC, Shelton ML, Klesges LM: Effects of television on metabolic rate: Potential implications for childhood obesity, *Pediatrics* 91:281, 1993.
17. Community Nutrition Institute, vol 25, no 41; Oct 27, 1995.
18. Lind BA and others: Effect of family versus cafeteria style service on students' attitudes, food intake, and food waste, *Sch Food Serv Res Rev* 10:18, 1986.
19. Ho CS and others: Evaluation of the nutrient content of school, sack and vending lunch of junior high students, *Sch Food Serv Res Rev* 15:85, 1991.
20. Horseley JW, Allen ER, White PA: *Nutrition management of school age children with special needs: a resource manual for school personnel, families and health professionals,* 2nd ed., 1996. Virginia Department of Health and Virginia Department of Education, Richmond, VA.
21. Borra ST, Schwartz NE, Spain CG and others: Food, physical activity, and fun: inspiring America's kids to more healthy lifestyles, *J Am Diet Assoc* 95:816, 1995.
22. Brainerd CJ: *Piaget's theory of intelligence,* Englewood Cliffs, NJ, 1978, Prentice-Hall.
23. Rickard KA and others: The play approach to learning in the context of families and schools: an alternative paradigm for nutrition and fitness education in the 21st century, *J Am Diet Assoc* 95:1121, 1995.

24. Contento I, Balch GI, Bronner YL and others: The effectiveness of nutrition education and implications for nutrition education and policy, programs, and research: a review of research, *J Nutr Educ* 27:298, 1995.

25. St. Pierre RG, Rezmovic V: An overview of the national nutrition education and training program evaluation, *J Nutr Educ* 14:61, 1982.

26. Troiano RP, Flegal, KM, Kuczmarski RJ and others: Overweight prevalence and trends for children and adolescents. The national health and nutrition examination surveys, 1963–1991, *Arch Pediatr Adolesc Med* 149:1085, 1995.

27. Rowland TW: *Exercise and children's health,* Champaign, Ill, 1990, Human Kinetics Books.

28. American Academy of Pediatrics: Clinical heat stress and the exercising child, *Phys Sports Med* 11:155, 1983.

29. Vaccaro P, Zauner CW, Cade JR: Changes in body weight, hematocrit and plasma protein concentration due to dehydration and rehydration in wrestlers, *J Sports Med Phys Fitness* 16:45, 1976.

30. Jennings DS, Steen SN: *Sports nutrition for the child athlete,* Chicago, 1993, The American Dietetic Association.

31. National Cholesterol Education Program: *Report of the expert panel on blood cholesterol levels in children and adolescents,* NIH Pub No 91-2732, National Heart, Lung, and Blood Institute, NIH, Public Health Service, Bethesda, Md, 1991, US Department of Health and Human Services.

32. Nicklas TA and others: Secular trends in dietary intakes and cardiovascular risk factors of 10-year-old children: the Bogalusa Heart Study (1973–1988), *Am J Clin Nutr* in press.

33. McPerson RS and others: Intake and food sources of dietary fat among schoolchildren in The Woodlands, Tex, *Pediatrics* 86:510, 1990.

34. Matkovic V, Heany RP: Calcium balance during human growth: evidence for E threshold behavior, *Am J Clin Nutr* 55:992, 1992.

35. Johnston CC, Miller JZ, Slemenda CW and others: Calcium supplementation and increases in bone mineral density in children, *N Engl J Med* 327:82, 1992.

36. National Consensus Conference: Optimal calcium intake, *JAMA* 272:1942, 1994.

37. Williams CL: Importance of dietary fiber in childhood, *J Am Diet Assoc* 95:1140, 1995.

38. Nicklas TA, Myers L, Berenson GS: Dietary fiber intake of children: the Bogalusa heart study, *Pediatrics* 96(suppl):988, 1995.

39. Williams CL, Bollella M, Wynder EL: A new recommendation for dietary fiber in childhood, *Pediatrics* 96(suppl):985, 1995.

40. Pollitt E: Does breakfast make a difference in school? *J Am Diet Assoc* 95:1134, 1995.

41. Pollitt E, Leibel RL, Greenfield D: Brief fasting, stress, and cognition in children, *Am J Clin Nutr* 34:1526, 1981.

42. Simeon DT, Grantham-McGregor S: Effects of missing breakfast on the cognitive functions of school children of differing nutritional status, *Am J Clin Nutr* 49:646, 1989.

43. Meyers AF and others: School breakfast program and school performance, *Am J Dis Child* 143:1234, 1989.

44. Pollitt E and others: Iron deficiency and behavioral development in infants and preschool children, *Am J Clin Nutr* 43:555, 1986.

45. Walter T and others: Iron deficiency anemia: adverse effects on infant psychomotor development, *Pediatrics* 84:7, 1989.

46. Lozoff B, Jimenez E, Wolf AU: Long-term development outcome of infants with iron deficiency, *N Engl J Med* 325:687, 1991.

47. Kanarek RB, Marks-Kaufman R: *Nutrition and behavior: new perspectives,* New York, 1991, Van Nostrand Reinhold.

48. American Psychiatric Association: *Diagnostic and statistical manual of mental disorders,* ed 3 (rev), Washington, DC, 1987, The Association.

49. Varley CK: Attention deficit disorder (the hyperactivity syndrome): a review of selected issues, *Dev Behav Pediatr* 5:254, 1984.

50. Mattes JA, Gittelman R: Growth of hyperactive children on maintenance regimen of methylphenidate, *Arch Gen Psychiatry* 40:317, 1983.

51. Lucas B, Sells CJ: Nutrient intake and stimulant drugs in hyperactive children, *J Am Diet Assoc* 70:373, 1977.

52. Klein RG and others: Hyperactive boys almost grown up. III. Methylphenidate effect on ultimate height, *Arch Gen Psychiatry* 45:1131, 1988.

53. Lipton MA, Mayo JP: Diet and hyperkinesis—an update, *J Am Diet Assoc* 83:132, 1983.

54. Kaplan BJ and others: Dietary replacement in preschool-aged hyperactive boys, *Pediatrics* 83:7, 1989.

55. Harper PH, Goyette CH, Conners CK: Nutrient intakes of children on the hyperkinesis diet, *J Am Diet Assoc* 73:515, 1978.

56. Prinz RJ, Roberts WA, Hantman E: Dietary correlates of hyperactive behavior in children, *J Consult Clin Psychol* 58:760, 1980.

57. Behar D and others: Sugar challenge testing with children considered behaviorally "sugar reactive," *Nutr Behav* 1:277, 1984.

58. Wolraich ML, Wilson DB, White JW: The effect of sugar on behavior or cognition in children: a meta-analysis, *JAMA* 274:1617, 1995.

59. Arnold LE and others: Megavitamins for minimal brain dysfunction: a placebo-controlled study, *JAMA* 240:2642, 1978.

60. Kershner J, Hawke W: Megavitamins and learning disorders: a controlled double-blind experiment, *J Nutr* 109:819, 1979.

61. Haslam RHA, Dalby JT, Rademaker AW: Effects of megavitamin therapy on children with attention deficit disorders, *Pediatrics* 74:103, 1984.

62. Kaste LM, Selwitz RJ, Oldakowski JA and others: Coronal caries in the primary and permanent dentition of children and adolescents 1–17 years of age: United States, 1988–1991, *J Dent Res* 75:631, 1996.

63. White-Graves MV, Schiller MR: History of foods in the caries process, *J Am Diet Assoc* 86:241, 1986.

64. Navia JM: Carbohydrates and dental health, *Am J Clin Nutr* 59(suppl):719S, 1994.

65. Jensen ME: Responses of interproximal plaque pH to snack foods and effect of chewing sorbitol-containing gum, *J Am Dent Assoc* 113:262, 1986.

66. Committee on Nutrition, American Academy of Pediatrics: The practical significance of lactose intolerance in children, *Pediatrics* 86(suppl):643, 1990.

67. Ladas SD, Katsiyiannaki-Latoufi E, Raptis SA: Lactose maldigestion and milk intolerance in healthy Greek schoolchildren, *Am J Clin Nutr* 53:676, 1991.

68. Sinden AA, Sutphen JL: Dietary treatment of lactose intolerance in infants and children, *J Am Diet Assoc* 91:1567, 1991.

69. Sheikh MS, and others: Gastrointestinal absorption of calcium from milk and calcium salts, *N Engl J Med* 317:532, 1987.

13

Nutrition for Adolescents

Jane Mitchell Rees
Peggy L. Pipes

++

Objectives

After studying this chapter, the student should:

✔ *Be able to define and contrast the terms* adolescence *and* puberty.

✔ *Know the milestones of adolescent physical development.*

✔ *Be able to describe the emotional and intellectual components of adolescent psychological development.*

✔ *Be able to list influences on adolescent eating habits.*

✔ *Know the elements of nutritional assessment of males and females during puberty.*

Adolescence is a dynamic phase of life. The normal human develops a mature body in the 5 to 7 years during puberty. The mind also develops, advancing to adult thought patterns and emotions. To understand nutritional issues of this stage of the life cycle, one needs to learn about growth and development processes that determine what teenagers need nutritionally and how they eat. Learning about adolescence is an exciting challenge and a valuable lesson because it provides a basis for understanding much about human life and the principles of nutrition that support it.

ADOLESCENT GROWTH AND DEVELOPMENT
Physiological Growth

Puberty. During late childhood growth begins to accelerate with the initiation of **puberty** until linear growth (in centimeters per year) during the teen years compares with that of the second year of life (fig. 13-1). About 20% of adult height and 50% of adult weight are acquired during pubertal growth. Most body organs double in size. The body develops sexual organs, larger hips and thighs, and breasts

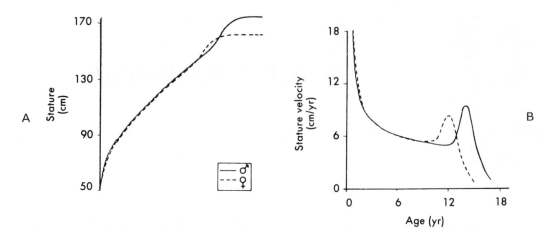

FIG. 13-1 **A,** Growth in stature of typical boy (*solid line*) and girl (*interrupted line*). **B,** Growth velocities at different ages of typical boy (*solid line*) and girl (*interrupted line*). (From Marshall WA: *Clin Endocrinol Metab* 4:4, 1975.)

(in females) called the **secondary sexual characteristics.**

Initiation of puberty. The exact factor, or combination of factors, that triggers the upsurge in hormonal activity to initiate puberty is still unknown. A sequence of hormonal changes culminating in feedback mechanisms that allow increased production of estrogen, testosterone, and progesterone with the onset of puberty has been described.[1] An association between **menarche** and the attainment of a critical body weight in North American and most European females has also been noted.[2] They theorize that the achievement of the critical body weight of 47.8 kg (105 lb) or body fatness of 17% causes a change in metabolic rate, which triggers menarche. Most researchers acknowledge an association between change in body composition and the onset of menarche, but they do not view it as triggering puberty.[2]

Physical Growth and Development

Stage. Each characteristic of sexual maturity and growth occurs gradually but at any one time can be described as being at a certain stage (or phase). The stages of sexual development are listed in table 13-1.

Sequence. Maturation takes place in a predictable sequence. For example, genital development always occurs before the period of most rapid growth in height. The sequence of sexual maturity and growth in height is shown in figure 13-2.

Timing. The "tempo" (or timing) of initiation and moving from one stage to another during physical maturation is different from one individual to another (see fig. 13-2). The years of age at which sexual maturation may begin or end are shown with each characteristic listed. The menarche typically occurs between 10.5 and 15.5 years of age, for example. Males of the same chronological age may be very different in size as shown in figure 13-3 because they are at different stages of development.

Sexual development. Sexual maturity begins with enlargement of genitalia in males and breast development in females (figs. 13-4 and 13-5). Pubic hair distribution is first sparse and becomes thicker and covers a large area. Completion of genital growth in males corresponds

TABLE 13-1   Stages of Sexual Maturation (Sexual Maturity Ratings)

Boys	Pubic Hair	Genitalia
Stage 1	None	No change from childhood
Stage 2	Small amount at outer edges of pubis; slight darkening	Beginning penile enlargement; testes enlarged to 5 ml volume; scrotum reddened and changed in texture
Stage 3	Covers pubis	Longer penis; testes 8–10 ml; scrotum further enlarged
Stage 4	Adult type; does not extend to thighs	Larger, wider, and longer penis; testes 12 ml; scrotal skin darker
Stage 5	Adult type; now spread to thighs	Adult penis; testes 15 ml

Girls	Pubic Hair	Breasts
Stage 1	None	No change from childhood
Stage 2	Small amount; downy on labia majora	Breast bud
Stage 3	Increased; darker and curly	Larger; no separation of nipple and areola
Stage 4	More abundant; coarse texture	Increased size; areola and nipple form secondary mound
Stage 5	Adult type; now spread to thighs	Adult distribution of breast tissue; continuous outline

Modified from Tanner JM: *Growth at adolescence,* ed 2, Oxford, 1962, Blackwell Scientific Publications. In Mahan LK, Rees JM: Seattle, Wash, 1989. Originally published in Mahan LK, Rees JM: *Nutrition in adolescence,* St Louis, 1984, Mosby–Year Book.

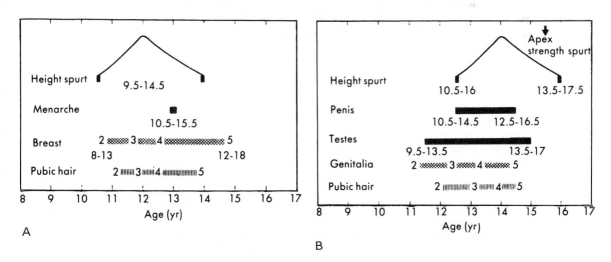

FIG. 13-2   Diagram of sequence of events at puberty in, **A,** girls and, **B,** boys.
(From Marshall WA, Tanner JM: *Arch Dis Child* 45:13, 1970.)

FIG. 13-3   Two boys of same chronological age in different stages of adolescent development.
(Copyright Mahan LK, Rees JM: Seattle, Wash, 1989. Originally published in Mahan LK, Rees JM: *Nutrition in adolescence,* St. Louis, 1984, Mosby–Year Book.)

with stage 5, or adult status of sexual maturity. In females menstrual cycles begin when breasts are nearly mature and height growth is nearly complete.

Existing data indicate that during the past century young women have gradually come to experience the menarche at a younger age. The so-called **secular trend** is probably due to improved nutrition, sanitation, and health care, allowing modern children to mature more rapidly. The current mean age of menarche is 12 years and 4 months compared with approximately 16 years in 1890. This theory is generally accepted, although records of menstrual age are scarce enough that it has been criticized. Total maturation probably occurs earlier for males as well. The mean age of onset of sperm emission **(spermarche)** currently is 13.4 years.

Height and weight. Throughout the approximately 5 to 7 years of pubertal development, rapid growth continues although a great percentage of height will be gained during the

FIG. 13-4 Female adolescents in all stages of adolescent development.

(Copyright Mahan LK, Rees JM: Seattle, Wash, 1989. Originally published in Mahan LK, Rees JM: *Nutrition in adolescence,* St Louis, 1984, Mosby–Year Book.)

FIG. 13-5   Male adolescents in all stages of adolescent development.
(From Farrow JA: *Semin Fam Med* 2[3]:146–153, 1981. By permission of Grune & Stratton, Inc.)

TABLE 13-2	Postmenarcheal Growth in Stature (N = 408)
Growth (in)	Percent of Sample
<1.00	6.0
1.00–1.99	21.0
2.00–2.99	34.0
3.00–3.99	22.0
4.00–4.99	9.0
5.00–5.99	4.0
6.00–6.99	1.5
7.00–7.99	1.5

Data from Fried RI, Smith E: *J Pediatr* 61:562, 1962.

TABLE 13-3   *Approximate Increments in Weight of Postmenarcheal Women*

Postmenarcheal Year	lbs	kg
1	10.12	4.6
2	6.16	2.8
3	2.42	1.1
4 and 5	1.76	0.8

Data from Frisch RE: *Hum Biol* 48:353, 1976. Copyright Mahan LK, Rees JM: Seattle, Wash, 1989. Originally published in Mahan LK, Rees JM: *Nutrition in adolescence*, St Louis, 1984, Mosby–Year Book.

"growth spurt." Like the initiation of puberty, the 18- to 24-month period of the peak growth velocity will occur at different ages for different individuals, fitting into the sequence of overall sexual development. Peak growth velocity occurs earlier for girls than for boys. Following the achievement of sexual maturity, linear growth and weight acquisition continue at a much lower rate and then cease, as shown by the downward slope of the height spurt curve (see fig. 13-2). For rare females it will continue into the late teens and for males into the twenties. Most females will gain no more than 2 to 3 inches (5.1 to 7.6 cm) after the onset of menses (table 13-2). Approximate weight gain following the menarche is shown in table 13-3.

Body composition. Body composition changes during maturation. The proportion of fat and muscle in prepubertal males and females tends to be similar, with body fat about 15% and 19%, respectively, and lean body mass is about equal for both sexes. During puberty females gain proportionately more fat. By age 18 body fat is normally about 27% in females and 16% in males.[3] Males, meanwhile, gain twice as much muscle as females do (fig. 13-6). This striking difference in adolescent growth between males and females influences nutritional needs. Since adolescent males experience greater gain in bone and lean tissue than females, they require more protein, iron, zinc, and calcium for development

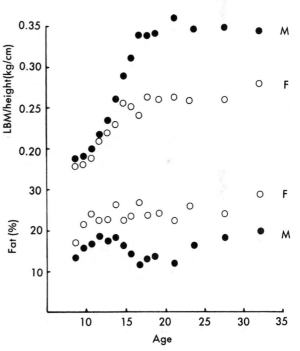

FIG. 13-6   Mean lean body mass/height ratio and percent body fat. *LBM,* Lean body mass.

(From Forbes GB: *Nutritional requirements in adolescence.* In Suskind RM, editor: *Textbook of pediatric nutrition,* New York, 1981, Raven Press.)

of these tissues. The male's larger requirements for these nutrients is also related to his greater *rate* of growth.

Monitoring growth. Knowing the relationship between the milestones of sexual development and physical growth will enable the clinician to assess growth in an adolescent at a particular time and indicate the extent of future growth. Thus pubertal development can be monitored clinically by using weight and height tables and sexual maturity ratings. Excessive or less-than-normal growth can be detected by plotting height changes on standard growth charts (see appendix). Height and weight changes should be plotted on gender-specific charts. The major cause of short stature during adolescence is genetically late initiation of puberty, although such conditions as chronic disease and skeletal or chromosomal abnormalities also account for certain children being shorter than expected. Cases of hormonal imbalances or malnutrition leading to abnormal growth rate are rare in the United States.

Weight can be plotted on a chart similar to the one for height to determine if an individual is either keeping pace with or exceeding the weight of peers at a particular year of age. Because of the wide variation in weights seen in sample individuals in the adolescent period, some of whom were obese, the frequency distribution represented by the charts cannot be used for evaluation of weight-for-height proportion as it is used for younger children. Evaluation of weight-for-height proportion in adolescents is described in the assessment section of this chapter.

Psychosocial Development

Tasks of adolescence. The term "adolescence" refers to the period when both mind and body are maturing and therefore applies to humans before and after, as well as during, puberty. Emotional, social, and intellectual development are rapid during adolescence. Milestones in psychological development of humans are shown in table 13-4. The ability to use abstract thinking that adolescents develop, as opposed to the concrete thought patterns of childhood, enables the individual to accomplish these tasks. Planning ahead and connecting facts into integrated ideas become possible. With the accomplishment of the developmental **tasks of adolescence** as shown in figure 13-7, the person is prepared for a role in adult society. An adolescent can plan to get the food he or she needs throughout the day, for example, while a younger child will need to have food provided by others.

Successfully accomplishing the tasks of adolescence can contribute to the nutritional health of the individual. For example, emotional maturity allows teenagers to develop their own value system. As a result they may choose foods that will enhance their health rather than responding to less healthful characteristics of foods as they may have done in childhood. They may go through a time of experimentation while they are learning to make choices.

Body image. Developing an image of the physical self that includes an adult body is an intellectual and emotional task intertwined with nutritional issues. Adolescents often feel uncomfortable with their rapidly changing bodies. At the same time, being much affected by influences outside themselves, they want to be like their most perfect peers and the idols of their culture. Stereotypes in the mass media reinforce such images. Teenagers may wish that certain body parts were larger and that other parts were smaller. They may want to grow faster or slower. Many are dissatisfied with their body weight. These feelings can lead them to try to change their bodies by manipulating their diets.

Young women who have not developed a mature **body image** may restrict food to reduce the size of hips and thighs they have developed during puberty. Young men are tempted to use nutritional supplements, steroids, or growth hormones to speed up their muscular development.[4,5,6]

REQUIREMENTS FOR NOURISHMENT
Nutritional Requirements Related to Growth

Limitations of the Recommended Dietary Allowance. Studies of the nutritional requirements of adolescents take age as well as stage of physical maturity into account. The research

TABLE 13-4 *Erikson's and Piaget's Models for Emotional and Cognitive Development*

Age (Years)	Erikson (Emotional)	Piaget (Cognitive)
0–2	**Phase I** Basic trust versus mistrust	**Sensorimotor period** Learning through senses and manipulation
2–4	**Phase II** Autonomy versus shame and doubt	**Preconceptual period** Classification by a single feature (e.g., size); no concern for contradictions
4–8	**Phase III** Initiative versus guilt	**Initiative thought period** Intuitive classification (e.g., awareness of conservation of mass concept)
8–12	**Phase IV** Industry versus inferiority	**Concrete operations period** Logical thought development; learning to organize
12–20	**Phase V** Ego identity versus role confusion	**Formal operations period** Comprehension of abstract concepts; formation of "ideals"
20 and older	**Phase VI** Intimacy versus isolation	—
Middle adulthood	**Phase VII** Generativity versus stagnation	—
Late adulthood	**Phase VIII** Integrity versus despair	—

Developed by LL Eggert, University of Washington. Copyright Mahan LK, Rees JM: Seattle, Wash, 1989. Originally published in Mahan LK, Rees JM: *Nutrition in adolescence,* St Louis, 1984, Mosby–Year Book.

base on which recommendations are made is limited because appropriate studies are not generally available. The Recommended Dietary Allowance (RDA)[7] for three adolescent age groups is stated, but is not related to stages of maturity. The highest levels of nutrients are recommended for the group assumed to be growing at the most rapid rate. Adolescents at the peak of their growth velocity have been shown to incorporate twice the amount of cal-cium, iron, zinc, magnesium, and nitrogen into their bodies during the years of the growth spurt as compared with that of other years (table 13-5).

Calculation of individual needs. Dividing the RDA total of a nutrient by the reference individual's height in centimeters provides a quantity of the nutrient in units per centimeter that can be applied to any size teenager.[8] For example, the RDA for protein for the male 11 to

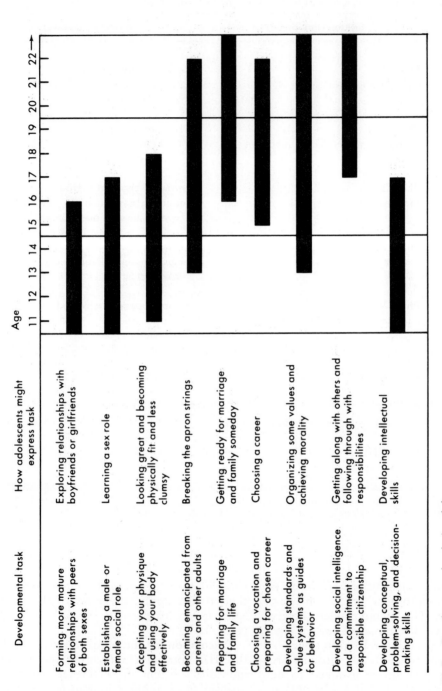

FIG. 13-7   Developmental tasks in adolescence.

Developed by LL Eggert, University of Washington. Modified from Thornburg H: *Contemporary adolescence: readings*, ed 2, Monterey, Calif, 1975, Brooks/Cole Publishing. Copyright Mahan LK, Rees JM: Seattle, Wash, 1989. Originally published in Mahan LK, Rees JM: *Nutrition in adolescence*, St Louis, 1984, Mosby–Year Book.

TABLE 13-5 Daily Increments in Body Content Due to Growth

	Average for Period 10–20 yr (mg)	At Peak of Growth Spurt (mg)
Calcium		
Male	210	400
Female	110	240
Iron		
Male	0.57	1.1
Female	0.23	0.9
Nitrogen*		
Male	320	610 (3.8 g protein)
Female	160	360 (2.2 g protein)
Zinc		
Male	0.27	0.50
Female	0.18	0.31
Magnesium		
Male	4.4	8.4
Female	2.3	5.0

From Forbes GB: *Nutritional requirements in adolescence.* In Suskind MR, editor: *Textbook of pediatric nutrition,* New York, 1981, Raven Press.
*Maintenance needs (2 mg/basal calorie) at age 18 are 3500 mg and 2700 mg for males and females, respectively.

TABLE 13-6 Recommended Dietary Allowances for Energy for Adolescents (Kcalories per Day)

Age (Years)	Allowance	Reference Height (cm)	Energy (kcal) per cm Height
Children			
7–10	2000	132	15.2
Males			
11–14	2500	157	15.9
15–18	3000	176	17.0
Females			
11–14	2200	157	14.0
15–18	2200	163	13.5

Data from Food and Nutrition Board, National Research Council: *Recommended Dietary Allowances,* ed 10, Washington, DC, 1989, National Academy of Sciences.

14 years old is 45 gm/day. The reference height is 157 cm. Thus 0.29 gm/cm would be recommended. Then the total protein need would be 39 gm for the 135-cm male and 54 gm for the 185-cm male. This example of variation in size during the teenage years is quite realistic, since persons experience the growth spurt at different ages. Nutrient recommendations will come closest to meeting needs when the largest quantity of nutrient per centimeter is suggested for those experiencing the most rapid growth, even if the age does not coincide with the age at which the highest RDA is made.

Recommendations for Specific Nutrients

Energy. The recommended energy intake in the RDA for adolescents as shown in table 13-6 reflects average needs of teenagers. To determine the needs of the individual, level of exercise and growth rate will need to be considered.

Protein. Less is known about the protein requirements of adolescents than of other age groups. The current recommendation is that protein intake should provide 15% to 20% of the total energy consumed.[9] Gender, age, nutritional status, and quality of the protein must be considered in estimating the amount an individual will need. The range of total protein need, about 39 to 56 gm, usually is obtained in the typical diet. Usually it need not be emphasized during nutrition counseling. Protein stores of adolescents should be carefully monitored and supported in situations in which nutritional depletion may occur so that physical development will not be impaired.

Calcium. An optimal intake of calcium in adolescence provides levels of intake that permit maximization of peak adult bone mass. There are indications that this intake may be one important factor in the prevention of osteoporosis.

During the adolescent growth spurt, 37% of total bone mass is accumulated. The calcium accumulation, between 140 to 165 mg/day in earlier childhood, increases to as high as 400 to 500 mg/day. There is an intake threshold below

TABLE 13-7   *Calculated Iron Requirements for Males and Females at the 3rd, 25th, 75th, and 97th Percentile for Body Weight (From 10 to 16 Years of Age)*

| | Calculated Iron Requirements (mg) | | | | | |
| | Daily Dietary Need* | | Peak Daily Dietary Need* | | Cumulative Need† | |
Percentile Rating	Male	Female	Male	Female	Male	Female
3rd	6.6	5.1	13.2	10.3	966	751
25th	9.3	5.2	18.6	10.4	1360	772
75th	11.0	5.5	21.9	11.0	1610	794
97th	12.9	5.7	25.8	11.9	1885	836

From McKigney JI, Munro HN, editors: Nutrient requirements in adolescence, Cambridge, Mass, 1978, The MIT Press.
*Period of adolescent growth spurt.
†Total body iron increment represented by muscle tissue increase during 10 to 16 year interval.

which adolescents will not reach genetically predetermined peak bone mass. This threshold is highly variable and depends on body size as well as stage of development. The threshold during adolescence appears to be 1400 mg/day with a retention of 396 mg/day. It is important that a positive calcium balance be maintained during adolescence. Many believe that the current 1200 mg/day recommendation for calcium intake is not high enough and that new recommendations for calcium intake during growth may be indicated.[10]

Iron. Males and females have high requirements for iron during adolescence as shown in table 13-7. Males require more iron because the buildup of muscle mass is accompanied by greater blood volume. Adolescent females require more than children because they lose iron monthly during menstruation.

Zinc. Zinc is known to be essential for growth and sexual maturation and is therefore of great importance in adolescence. The retention of zinc increases, especially during the growth spurt, leading to more efficient use of dietary sources of the nutrient.

Other minerals. The roles of other minerals in the nutrition of adolescents have not been extensively studied. Magnesium, iodine, and phosphorus as well as copper, chromium, cobalt, and fluoride, however, are known to be important. The possibility that these nutrients interact cannot be overlooked. The recommendations for safe levels should be followed so that imbalances will not develop.

Vitamins. Adolescents require large amounts of thiamin, riboflavin, and niacin because of their high energy requirements. Vitamin D is necessary for rapid skeletal growth. Recommended amounts of vitamins A, E, C, and B_6 and folic acid are the same as those for adults. Often the quantity of vitamins recommended for adolescents has been interpolated from studies in adults and children.

PHYSICAL FITNESS

All teenagers should be encouraged to fit exercise into their lives as part of balanced nourishment. Adolescents who participate in sports should adopt personal fitness programs between seasons.

Lack of Fitness

As the energy requirements of modern life are decreasing, adolescents are less fit than in earlier decades.[11] Only about 50% of young people today are regularly involved in vigorous exercise. When tested, 30% of males and more than 50% of females ages 6 to 17 years could not do one pull-up.[12]

FIG. 13-8   Adolescents can maintain fitness with daily activity.

Benefits of Physical Fitness

Physical activity can benefit individuals because it:

1. Helps maintain optimal body composition
2. Facilitates weight loss (when necessary)
3. Increases the efficiency of energy use by muscle fibers
4. Increases the efficacy of hormones (insulin, lipoprotein lipase, epinephrine) in the regulation of energy metabolism
5. Decreases the production of lactic acid, which interferes with energy production
6. Strengthens the heart, lungs, and circulatory system
7. Increases levels of HDL over LDL and decreases some triglycerides
8. Raises rates of basal metabolism
9. Helps control appetite

Elements of Fitness

Each teenager should participate in activities that maintain the elements of fitness, which are (1) cardiorespiratory function, (2) body composition, and (3) muscular strength, endurance, and flexibility (fig. 13-8).

Maintaining Fitness

The principles of maintaining fitness are incorporated into the testing and improvement protocol (fig. 13-9). Raising the heart rate to at least 50% but not more than 75% of the maximum heart rate for 15 minutes with 5 minutes warm-up and cool-down at least 3 days a week will maintain cardiorespiratory fitness. The maximum heart rate of adolescents is about 200. This number can be used until age 20, when the usual calculation for adults, subtracting the age from 220 to determine the maximum heart rate, can begin. Stressful exercise is ineffective, but continuous gradual improvement and maintenance is effective. A few well-chosen calisthenics will maintain muscular strength, flexibility, and endurance.

EATING HABITS
Nutrient Consumption

Surveys of nutrient intake have shown adolescents likely to be obtaining less vitamin A, thiamin, iron, and calcium than recommended.[13,14] They also ingest more fat, sugar, protein, and sodium than is thought to be optimal.[13,14,15]

Snacks

Concern is often expressed about snacking patterns of adolescents because many popular and highly available snacks are high in sugar and/or fat. However, teenagers can obtain substantial nourishment from foods outside traditional meals. The choice of foods they make is of greater importance than the time or place adolescents eat. Emphasis should be placed on fresh vegetables, fruits, low-fat milk products, and whole-grain products to complement the foods high in energy value and protein that they commonly choose.

FITNESS: TESTING AND PLANNING IMPROVEMENT PROGRAMS

1. a. Have client sit quietly and relax for 3 to 5 minutes.
   b. Take pulse for 10 seconds.*
   c. Record resting heart rate (RHR):_____.
2. a. Find intensity of exercise required to reach training heart rate (THR)†immediately after exercise (THR for teens: 20 to 22 beats/10 seconds).
      Stop with the exercise that achieves 20 to 22 beats/10 seconds. This is the exercise to use initially in the improvement program.

	Run for 5 minutes
	Jog for 5 minutes
Intensity increases	Jog for 2 minutes—walk for 2 minutes—jog for 2 minutes
	Walk uphill or upstairs for 2 to 3 minutes
	Walk for 5 minutes at a more rapid pace
START	Walk for 5 minutes at a moderate pace

   b. Monitor pulse return toward RHR after each exercise level—it should be below 16 beats/10 seconds

   Immediate → _____   1 minute → _____   2 minutes → _____   3 minutes → _____   5 minutes → _____

3. Improvement program: To maintain THR for 15 minutes 4 to 5 days/week:
   a. Work with client to design an individualized program that is comfortable for him/her.
   b. Plan 5-minute warmup—move at level below the level that maintains THR.
   c. Exercise at intensity that maintains THR.
   d. 5-Minute cool down—back to warmup speed—client should not sit or lie down immediately.
   e. Use a combination of exercise levels and types, if necessary.
   f. If the client is ill, he/she should begin after illness at lower intensity and return slowly to intensity achieved before illness.
4. a. Retest every 3 to 4 weeks.
   b. Increase intensity of exercise to maintain THR.
   c. Client can increase time spent doing the exercise by 5-minute increments, up to 30 minutes.
   d. When client has reached jogging level and maintained it for 6 to 8 weeks, increase THR to 22 to 25 beats/10 seconds.
   e. Client can use any aerobic activities (e.g., jogging, bicycling, skating, or dancing) or combinations that the client prefers.

FIG. 13-9   Testing and improvement protocol.

(Developed by Scott B, Rees J: Adolescent Program, University of Washington, Seattle.)

*10-second time segment is easiest to measure and use.

†*Maximum heart rate* (MHR): ≈200 beats/minute for persons under 20 years of age (Cumming GR, Everatt D, Hastman L: Bruce treadmill test in children: normal values in a clinic population, *Am J Cardiol* 41:69, 1978). THR is 60% of MHR for persons with poor initial fitness, 75% of MHR for persons who are fit (e.g., 60% of 200 = 120 beats/minute = 20 beats/10 seconds [20 to 22 beats/10 seconds for normal variation]).

Note: Contraindications for testing and initiating fitness program are revealed by routine medical history and physical examination.

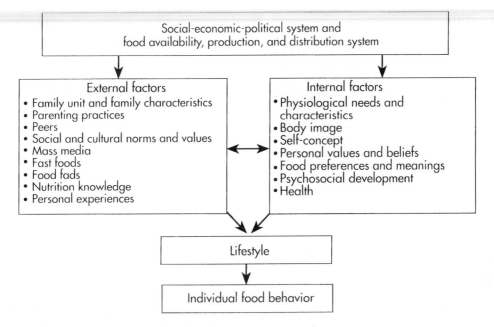

FIG. 13-10   Schematic diagram of factors influencing adolescent food behavior.

(Developed by M Story, University of Minnesota. Copyright Mahan LK, Rees JM: Seattle, Wash, 1989. Originally published in Mahan LK, Rees JM: *Nutrition in adolescence,* St Louis, 1984, Mosby–Year Book.)

Meals

The number of meals teenagers miss and eat away from home increases from early adolescence to late adolescence, reflecting the growing need for independence and time away from home. The evening meal appears to be the most regularly eaten meal of the day. Females skip meals more often than males.

Breakfast is frequently neglected and is omitted more often by teenagers than other age groups. A likely explanation for why females are more likely to miss breakfast than are males is the pursuit of thinness and frequent attempts at restricting food intake. Many teenage girls believe that they can control their weight by omitting breakfast or lunch. Young women who are attempting to manage their weight should be counseled that this approach is likely to accomplish just the opposite. By midmorning or lunchtime they may be so hungry that they eat more than if they had eaten at least simple foods in the early morning.

Racial differences have been noted in specific foods chosen. The Bogalusa Heart Study noted that white adolescents reported more servings of beef, cheese, and vegetables with meat than did their black peers. More servings of eggs, luncheon meat, pork, poultry, and total protein were reported by black than white adolescents. The total protein intake of adolescent boys was greater than that of girls.[16]

Influences on Eating Habits

By the time a person reaches adolescence, the influences on eating habits are numerous. Formation of those habits is extremely complex (fig. 13-10). Adolescents' growing independence, increased participation in social life, and generally busy schedule of activities have a decided impact on what they eat. They are beginning to buy and prepare more food for themselves, and they often eat rapidly and away from home.

Advertising

Although families provide the basic foundation for eating habits, many influences on eating behavior originate outside the home. Teenagers are vulnerable to advertising messages. Television food commercials and the eating habits portrayed in program content have influenced people for more than a decade by the time they become adolescents.[17] The average teenager will have watched more than a million food commercials, the majority of which are for products with a high energy concentration from sugar and fat.

Ready-to-Eat Foods

The ease of obtaining food that is ready to eat also influences the eating habits of teenagers. In vending machines and at movies, sporting events, fast-food outlets, and convenience groceries, food is available at numerous times throughout the day. During the time of their peak growth velocity, adolescents may need to eat often and in large amounts and are able to use foods with a high concentration of energy. However, they will usually need to eat more carefully when growth has slowed.

Nutritional Limitations of Fast Food

The following factors appear to be the major nutritional limitations of **fast-food** meals:[18]

1. *Calcium, riboflavin, and vitamin A.* These essential nutrients are low unless milk or a milkshake is ordered. In addition, extensive consumption of soft drinks contributes to low intakes of magnesium and vitamin C.
2. *Folic acid and fiber.* There are few fast-food sources of these key factors.
3. *Fat.* The percentage of energy from fat is high in many meal combinations.
4. *Sodium.* The sodium content of fast-food meals is high.
5. *Energy.* Common meal combinations contain excessive energy when compared with the amounts of other nutrients provided.

Although fast foods can contribute nutrients to the diet, they cannot completely meet the nutritional needs of teenagers. Both adolescents and health professionals should be aware that fast foods are acceptable nutritionally when they are consumed judiciously and as *part* of a well-balanced diet. If they become the mainstay of the diet, there is cause for concern. Food sources of nutrients not consumed in fast foods should be included in nutrition education plans.

SUBSTANCE USE AND ABUSE
Adolescent Experience

Substance use and abuse among adolescents are of major concern.[19] Tobacco, smokeless tobacco, alcohol, marijuana, and cocaine are the substances most widely abused. Over 90% of high school seniors have consumed alcohol, and in one study one in seven seniors admitted they had been inebriated once a week. The use of marijuana has been declining in recent years while there was a steady increase in cocaine use throughout the 1980s. Although rates of tobacco use have remained stable since the early 1980s, the rate among females has increased and the age of beginning use has declined for all teenagers. Smokeless tobacco is typically used by 7% to 25% of male adolescents in rural areas and young white male athletes in populations studied. It is responsible for significant oral damage, including cancer.

Overall, about 10% to 15% of teenagers have had no experience with drugs and alcohol, 70% to 80% have experimented, 10% to 15% have definable problems, and less than 1% are chemically dependent. Cognitive, emotional, and social development is likely to be retarded in the last group.[19]

Impact on Nutritional Status

In studies of nutritional status of drug and alcohol abusing teenagers, one study of a racially mixed and the other of a Native American population, deficient nutrient levels were not found in blood samples from either group.[20,21] Neither reported consuming less of the nutrients studied than they needed or than nonusing peers. However, abusers acquired nutrients from a different group of foods than nonabusers. They consumed more snack foods and meat products while fruits, vegetables, and

TABLE 13-8 *Drug Use Indications*

Rash	Dyspnea on exertion
Muscle weakness	Faintness
Vomiting	Hangover
Diarrhea	Blackouts
Stomach pain	Nervousness
Nausea	Depression
Indigestion	Tiredness
Bleeding gums	Insomnia
Sore tongue	Somnolence
Taste loss	Headache
Appetite loss	Seizures
Memory loss	

milk were left out of their dietary patterns.[20] The long-term effects of alcohol abuse coupled with an imbalance of nutrients probably account for development of nutritional disorders as they reach adulthood. Overall, the effect of substance abuse on nutritional status of any individual depends on the substance, the amount, duration and frequency of use, prior health and nutritional status, stage of physical growth, and nutritional adequacy of the diet consumed.

Identification and Rehabilitation

All health professionals need to be aware of the indicators of drug use (see table 13-8) so that they can refer adolescents with a definable problem for treatment before they reach a more advanced stage of chemical dependency. Nutritional assessment, intervention, and support are included in rehabilitative programs for adolescent substance abusers.

Role of Parents in Supporting Healthful Habits

To encourage adolescents to form reasonably healthy eating habits, parents should give their children increased responsibility and choice of nourishing foods as they are growing up. By the time they are teenagers, they will need some freedom to use the kitchen; this is true for young men as well as for young women.

NUTRITIONAL ENVIRONMENT

Because adolescent life is increasingly complex, the health professional will need to know a great deal about a teenager to assess his or her nutritional status. Intelligence, emotional status, social functioning, and physical status are relevant factors. General medical history, socioeconomic status, medications, alcohol or tobacco use, family attitudes, and peer group food practices are part of the nutritional environment of an adolescent and influence food choices. Table 13-9 summarizes the significance of each of these influences. A probing interview by a nutritionist who has had experience communicating with adolescents about these topics will reveal how an individual teenager feels about and manages food.

Evaluating Nutritional Status

To fully assess the nutritional status of adolescents, the health professional will evaluate the progress of physical development (see the following list), the usual laboratory tests, and the measures of dietary intake.
Weight/age
Height/age
Weight/height/age
Body mass index
Mid (upper) arm circumference/age/sex*
Triceps skinfold/age/sex*
Subscapular/skinfold/age/sex*
Arm fat area/age/sex*
Arm muscle circumference/age/sex*
Arm muscle area/age/sex*
Percentage body fat/age/sex
Sexual maturity rating of males and females
Females
    Age (or absence) of menarche
    Timing of menses

Anthropometry

Weight, height, weight-for-height proportion, skinfold measurement, and muscle mass are evaluated by comparing the measurements of an individual with measurements of subjects

---

*Measurements for African-American adolescents available.[3]

TABLE 13-9   *Nutrition Environment Evaluation Guide*

Influences	Key Issues	Significance
Likes and dislikes	Does patient dislike any particular food that is a major source of a specific nutrient (for example, milk is a major source of calcium; citrus fruits of vitamin C; meat of high-quality protein)?	Points out need to explore alternative ways to supply nutrients (for example, substitute cheese and yogurt for milk; broccoli and green peppers for citrus fruit; proper combinations of plant foods for meat)
Environment and attitudes		
Individual	Does patient express interest in his or her diet?	Gives clues to attitude toward role of nutrition in health care
	Are there any behavioral problems that influence patient's food choices?	May indicate need to work with other health team members to resolve problem that temporarily precludes nutrition intervention
	Has patient ever followed a special diet? If so, who prescribed it, what type of diet was it, and when was it prescribed? What instructions did patient receive?	Self-prescribed diet may signal inappropriate or unreliable approach toward control of health by diet; points out medical and educational considerations needed in design of care plan
	Does patient think he or she has been following the diet? Is there evidence to substantiate this?	If discrepancy exists, indicates lack of understanding of diet by patient or unwillingness or inability of patient to make dietary changes
	What difficulties if any does patient see in making dietary changes?	Focuses on issues that need consideration in design of individualized care plan
Family	Who purchases and prepares food in home (that is, partially controls patient's food supply)?	Sets scene for type of action plan suitable to patient and family
	Does patient have adequate cooking facilities and equipment or access to other resources?	May indicate need to provide basic nutrition guidelines, including personalized menu plan
	Are there any cultural, regional, or religious factors that affect patient's food choices?	Requires consideration to tailor care plan to individual needs
Peers	How often does patient eat away from home? Where and with whom does patient eat? Are there specific food intake patterns related to peer influences?	Indicates potential influences of peers on food choices; points out potential efficacy of patient- versus family-oriented care plan

Developed by R Rosebrough, University of Maryland. Copyright Mahan LK, Rees JM: Seattle, Wash, 1989. Originally published in Mahan LK, Rees JM: *Nutrition in adolescence,* St Louis, 1984, Mosby–Year Book.

TABLE 13-9 *Nutrition Environment Evaluation Guide—cont'd*

Influences	Key Issues	Significance
Environment and attitudes—cont'd		
Schools	Does patient eat at school? Does patient participate in school feeding programs?	School feeding programs with their standardized composition assure minimal nutrient availability and provide reference for accuracy of reported information
	Is there anything about school schedule or cafeteria environment that may discourage appropriate nutrient intake?	"Too little time for lunch" or "no one to eat with" may necessitate consultation with other team members or school to resolve lifestyle problems
	Is patient in appropriate grade in school? Has patient received food and nutrition information in school courses?	Gives clues to current knowledge of nutrition and level of intellectual functioning; allows practical planning for educational aspects of care plan
Limited food funds	Is patient or family eligible for food stamps; Women, Infants, and Children program (WIC), reduced-price, or free school lunch? Do they participate in programs? Does patient or family receive other social assistance?	Indicates family has limited income and may need assistance with food buying and preparation to assure nutritionally adequate diet; points out need to consider referral to appropriate food program or nutrition education resource
Health-related concerns	Does patient have any food allergies or intolerances (as distinguished from dislikes)?	Excludes foods from diet; indicates need to plan and assure adequacy with alternative food choices
	Are there any physical conditions affecting ability to consume adequate nutrients (for example, mouth sores, swallowing problems, taste abnormalities)?	Indicates need to consider flavor, consistency, and temperature of food in care plan
	Are there any problems in digestion, absorption, or metabolism that will interfere with nutrient utilization? Will any other therapy (drugs, exercise, radiation) affect nutrient needs?	Indicates need to address these problems in diet preparation

of the same age and sex in large studies. Measurements are also available for African-American adolescents. It is not possible to use the growth charts to determine ideal body weight of adolescents as is the practice for younger children because weight-for-height charts were not constructed for adolescents.

Body Mass Index

Body mass index as described in chapter 1 should be used routinely to define excess body mass. The index is easily determined: weight/height^2 (kg/m^2), or it may be charted from available tables (table 13-10). When plotted on BMI nomograms, the BMI will identify the current status; over time the BMI will identify changes in percentile of body mass status (fig. 13-11). An index between the 5th and 85th percentile indicates a healthy weight. Adolescents who have a BMI greater than the 95th percentile for age are considered overweight and need to be screened further. An investigation of blood pressure, family history of cardiovascular death and risk factors, and indications from the adolescent of weight concerns need to be explored.[22]

Increments in BMI over previous recordings may indicate an excessive rate of weight gain. This may indicate the need to institute measures to prevent obesity.

In addition, a skinfold evaluation will yield a more precise assessment of the proportion of fat to muscle and therefore weight to height. For example, a low value for triceps skinfold measurement in an individual above the 75th percentile for weight and height indicates that the adolescent is overweight but not overfat. An assessment of midarm circumference and arm muscle area will confirm the muscular body composition.

Sexual Maturity Rating

The evaluation of **sexual maturity** is an essential factor in making a valid nutrition assessment of an adolescent in a normal clinical setting. By knowing the stage of sexual maturity of the adolescent (see fig. 13-2) it is possible to determine if the full height has been reached or if growth can still occur. Also it is possible to determine whether the proportion of fat to lean body mass measured in a person at a given time

TABLE 13-10 *Recommended Cutoff Values for Body Mass Index (BMI, in kg/m^2) for Adolescents Who Are Overweight or at Risk of Overweight during Adolescence*

Age (y)	At Risk of Overweight		Overweight	
	Males	Females	Males	Females
10	20	20	23	23
11	20	21	24	25
12	21	22	25	26
13	22	23	26	27
14	23	24	27	28
15	24	24	28	29
16	24	25	29	29
17	25	25	29	30
18	26	26	30	30
19	26	26	30	30
20–24	27	26	30	30

From: Himes JH, Dietz WH: Guidelines for overweight in adolescent preventive services: recommendations from an expert committee, *Amer J Clin Nutr* 59:307, 1994.

is likely to change because maturation is incomplete. Thus if a young woman at stage 1 of sexual maturity is at the 90th percentile of weight-for-height, she will continue to grow in height and has a greater potential to achieve more normal body composition by maintaining a stable weight as she grows than has a female of the same age, the same weight-for-height, but who has experienced menarche and is at stage 4 of sexual maturity. The young woman described last would not grow taller and would have to lose weight to improve the proportion of weight-to-height.

Prevention of Hyperlipidemia and Hypertension

Excessive intakes of fat, energy, and sodium should be discouraged to reduce risk factors for cardiovascular disease. In the case of hyperlipidemia, fat and total energy intake should be controlled. The risks of particular levels of blood lipids for ages 2 to 19 years are listed in

OVERWEIGHT IN ADOLESCENCE

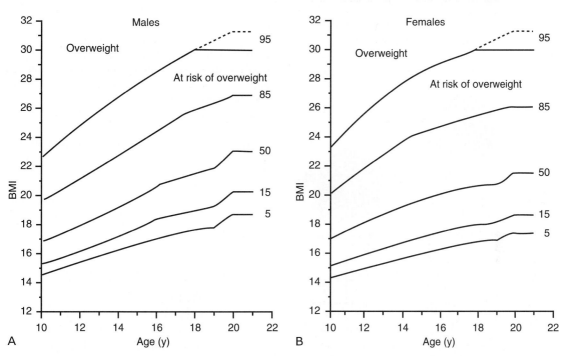

FIG. 13-11 **A,** Recommended percentiles of BMI (in kg/m²) for males from Must et al (64), modified so that the limit separating at risk of overweight from overweight does not exceed 30. The broken line from 18 y onward is the 95th percentile as originally published. **B,** Recommended percentiles of BMI (in kg/m²) for females from Must et al (64), modified so that the limit separating at risk of overweight from overweight does not exceed 30. The broken line from 17 y onward is the 95th percentile as originally published.

(From Himes JH and Dietz WH: Guidelines for overweight in adolescent preventive services: recommendations from an expert committee, *Am J Clin Nutr* 59:307, 1994.)

figure 13-12. If an adolescent is hypertensive or has a strong family history of hypertension, a diet controlled in sodium and total energy is part of long-term nutritional care.

Dental Caries and Periodontal Disease

The cause of dental caries is a complex process involving the interaction of several factors. The minerals of the tooth enamel are in constant equilibrium with the oral environment. It is necessary therefore to consider not only the presence of fermentable carbohydrate but also such factors as food solubility, mineral composition, and the buffering capacity of the oral environment. Adolescents' propensity to snack on refined carbohydrates is conducive to tooth decay. Since 80% of the average person's total incidence of dental lesions occurs in the teenage years, this is the time to encourage habits built on choosing alternatives to sugar-containing foods.

Gingivitis increases in prevalence during the teenage years, and periodontal disease often follows. Little is known about nutrition's role in periodontal disease, although deficiency in ascorbic acid has received a great deal of attention as an important cause. Vitamin A deficiency has also been implicated because it is

High risk > 95th percentile

Moderate risk 75th–95th percentile

Low risk < 75th percentile

Mg/dL

300
275
225
200
175
150
125
100
75
50

Male Female
Total
cholesterol
age 2-19 years

Male Female
Low density
lipoprotein
cholesterol
age 2-19 years

FIG. 13-12   Cholesterol and low density lipoprotein cholesterol (LDL-C) reference ranges for risk assessment.

(Developed by MS Jacobson, Director, Center for Atherosclerosis Prevention, Schneider Children's Hospital, New Hyde Park, NY.)

common in underdeveloped countries with high incidences of periodontal disease. Inadequate intake of these nutrients in the teen years can have an adverse effect on the health of the gums in later life.

Acne

About 85% of all adolescents have acne caused by action of high levels of hormones on the sebaceous glands. Severity in individual teenagers varies. Stress and phase of the menstrual cycle are two of the factors that determine severity. Traditionally, dietary factors have been blamed for the appearance of acne, but studies have shown no correlation between ingestion of foods and the appearance or degree of this condition.

Education about the cause of acne helps teenagers learn to control it. Antibiotics given orally and benzoyl peroxide and tretinoin to apply on skin surfaces are usually effective, as are special cleansing agents.

Medicinal levels of vitamin A derivatives are useful in treating acne. Because they are linked to deformities in fetal development, they should not be used by young women who may become pregnant. In general, while no research is available to confirm the effect, it would seem that the optimally nourished body will be best able to cope with the development of acne as with many conditions.

NUTRITION EDUCATION
Potential Application

Well-developed nutrition education has components devoted to (1) communicating facts, (2) influencing attitudes, and (3) changing behavior.[23] Print media are usually the most successful in communicating information, while audio, visual, combined audiovisual, and hands-on experience communication techniques effectively influence attitudes and model healthful behavior.

Because teens normally begin to look outside the family for information, it is logical to expect that they can be educated about nutrition by institutions with which they interact in the community at large (fig. 13-13). Coordinated efforts could educate them in schools, malls, libraries, grocery stores and convenience stores, fast-food outlets, detention facilities, and mass media (magazines, television, radio, newspapers, and books).

Current Status

At present, nutrition education of adolescents is not well designed or financed so they are generally influenced more by advertising, sensationalized material in magazine and newspaper stories, and peer-generated information than by health educators. Health education is usually confined to print techniques, brief units in the health curriculum, and occasional encounters

FIG. 13-13 Adolescents are interested in the composition of foods and influenced by marketing.

with health professionals. As a result, typical teenagers know something about healthy use of foods but do not put most of that knowledge into practice. It is obviously a challenge, but health educators and health policymakers will have to build coalitions to develop strategies for funding and carrying out programs for teenagers to improve the health of the adults of the future.[24]

Summary

Physical and psychosocial developments are rapid and all encompassing in the adolescent period of human life. The nature of physical growth is the basis for determining nutritional needs. Nutrition efforts should include a focus on prevention of chronic disease in later life. Eating behavior is influenced to a great extent at this time by the developing body image and, as a result of breaking ties with the family, by the total culture. Emphasis must be placed on physical fitness to help all adolescents balance energy intake and output. The multitude of factors influencing teenagers at a time of so much change makes it an ideal time to provide nutrition education. Messages relayed in a style that they find appealing can help them sort out the conflicting information they get from family, peers, mentors, and media.

REVIEW QUESTIONS

1. What are the main characteristics of adolescent eating behavior patterns?
2. Why might two 16-year-old males be of different heights?
3. Discuss the current age of menarche as compared with 1900 and the reasons for the difference.
4. What is the relationship between puberty and adolescence?
5. What elements of a nutritional assessment are unique to adolescents?
6. How do the thinking patterns of older teenagers compare with those of younger children?
7. Describe the sequence of events in adolescent maturity for males. For females.

SUGGESTED LEARNING ACTIVITIES

1. Seek out a fast-food restaurant that provides information to customers about nutrient content of its foods. Pick out a menu that contains the major nutrients and appropriate energy for an adolescent female whose statural growth is complete.
2. Assess 3-day food records kept by an adolescent male and an adolescent female who are still growing. How do their intakes and eating patterns compare with published reports?
3. Assess the material in a magazine popular among teenagers. Are the weight management methods safe? Is the nutrition information sound? Do the human images portray healthy weights and varied body types?
4. Interview an adolescent to obtain the types of information needed to assess that person's nutritional environment.
5. Prepare a talk describing physical growth and development during puberty and the interaction with nutrition for a Girl Scout group.

REFERENCES

1. Neinstein LS: *Adolescent health care: a practical guide,* ed 2, Baltimore, 1991, Urban & Schwarzenberg.
2. Trussel J, Frisch RE: Menarche and fatness: reexamination of the critical body composition hypothesis, *Science Zoo* 1506, 1978.

❖ ❖ ❖

CASE STUDY

Obesity Prevention for an Adolescent

M. L., a 13-year-old, is concerned that she is gaining too much weight. She has kept a record of her food intake for three days and now asks for help to define an appropriate weight for herself, and to know how she can change her diet so that she does not gain weight so fast.

1. See the growth chart in figure 13-14. Based on her body mass index, is M. L. at risk for becoming obese?
2. Is her nutrient intake appropriate for a 13-year-old girl?
3. How would you suggest she modify her food intake to increase her intake of nutrients and to reduce her current energy intake?

Food Diary

Day 1

6:30	English muffin with butter and jelly
	Orange juice ½ cup
12:00	Bagel with cream cheese 1
	Banana 1
	Potato chips 1 oz
	Sugar cookie 2
	Dried apples ¼ cup
	Carbonated cola drink 12 oz
3:30	Candy 1 2-oz bar
6:00	Beef stew with veggies 1 cup
	English muffin with butter 1
	Raw peppers and cucumbers 5 pieces
	Lemon pie 1 slice
	Milk 8 oz

Day 2

6:30	Granola cereal with milk 1 cup
	Orange juice ½ cup
12:00	Peanut butter and jelly sandwich
	Corn chips 1 oz
	Apple 1 medium
	Candy bar 2 oz
	Carbonated cola beverage 12 oz
3:00	Popsicle 1
	Oatmeal cookies 3
6:00	Pizza 2 slices
	Pineapple 2 slices
	Root beer 12 oz
	Banana 1
8:00	Chocolate chip cookies 2
	Kool-Aid 6 oz

Day 3

6:30	Toast with butter and jelly 1 slice
	Orange juice ½ cup
12:00	Bagel with cream cheese 1
	Banana 1
	1% milk 8 oz
3:30	Peanut butter and jelly sandwich 1
	Milk 10 oz
7:00	Fish and chips 4 pieces fish
	½ cup french fries
	1% milk 8 oz
	Banana 1
9:00	Chocolate chip cookies 4

❖ ❖ ❖

Obesity Prevention for an Adolescent—cont'd

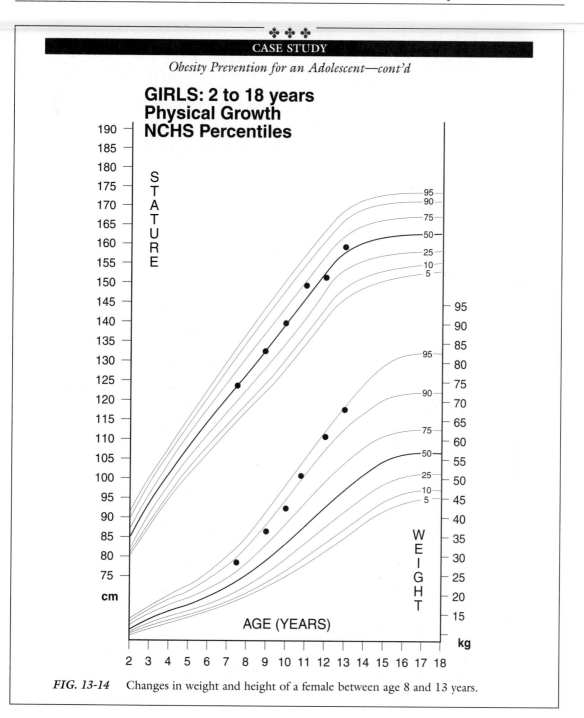

GIRLS: 2 to 18 years
Physical Growth
NCHS Percentiles

FIG. 13-14 Changes in weight and height of a female between age 8 and 13 years.

3. Report of a WHO Expert Committee. *Physical status: the use and interpretation of anthropometry.* WHO Technical Report Series 854, Geneva, Switzerland, 1995.

4. Moore DC: Body image and eating behavior in adolescent boys, *Am J Dis Child* 144:475, 1990.

5. Johnson, MD and others: Anabolic steroid use by male adolescents, *Pediatrics* 83:921, 1989.

6. Rickert VI and others: Human growth hormone: a new abused substance among adolescents? (Abstract), *J Adolesc Health Care* 13:47, 1992.

7. Food and Nutrition Board, National Research Council: *Recommended Dietary Allowances,* ed 10, Washington, DC, 1989, National Academy of Sciences.

8. Mahan LK, Rosebrough RH: *Nutrition requirements and nutritional status assessment in adolescence.* In Mahan LK, Rees JM: *Nutrition in adolescence,* St Louis, 1984, Mosby–Year Book.

9. National Cholesterol Expert Panel on Blood Cholesterol in Children and Adolescents, NIH Publication No. 91-2732, National Heart, Lung and Blood Institute, Public Health Service, September, 1991.

10. Matkovic V, Ilich JZ: Calcium Requirements for growth: are current recommendations adequate? *Nutr Rev* 51:171, 1993.

11. Raunikar RA, Strong WB: The status of adolescent physical fitness, *Adolesc Med: State of Art Rev* 2:65, 1991.

12. American Medical Association and American Dietetic Association: *Targets for adolescent health: adolescent nutrition and physical fitness,* Chicago, 1991, American Medical Association.

13. Farthing MC: Current eating patterns of adolescents in the United States, *Nutr Today* 26:35, 1991.

14. Pennington JAT and others: Mineral content of foods and total diets: the selected minerals in foods survey, 1982 to 1984, *J Am Diet Assoc* 86:876, 1986.

15. Chan G: Dietary calcium and bone mineral status of children and adolescents, *Am J Dis Child* 145:631, 1991.

16. Frank GC, Nicklas TA, Webber LS and others: A food frequency questionnaire for adolescents: defining eating patterns, *J Amer Diet Assoc* 92:313, 1992.

17. Morton HN: A survey of the television viewing habits, food behaviors and perception of food advertisements among South Australian year 8 high school students, *J Home Econ Assoc Aust* 22:34, 1990.

18. Franz MJ: Fast food facts: *Nutritive and exchange values for fast-food restaurants,* Wayzata, Minn, 1990, Diabetes Center Inc.

19. Farrow JA: Adolescent chemical dependency. In Farrow JA editor: Adolescent medicine, *Med Clin North Am* 74:1265, 1990.

20. Farrow JA, Rees JM, Worthington-Roberts BS: Health, development and nutritional status of adolescent alcohol abusers, *Pediatrics* 79:218, 1987.

21. Story M, Van Zyl York P: Nutritional status of Native American adolescent substance users, *J Am Diet Assoc* 87:1680, 1987.

22. Himes JH, Dietz WH: Guidelines for overweight in adolescent preventive services: recommendations from an expert committee, *Amer J Clin Nutr* 59:307, 1994.

23. Rees JM, Dixon-Docter A, Worthington-Roberts BS: *Nutrition education: a support for reproduction.* In Worthington-Roberts B, Williams SR: *Nutrition in pregnancy and lactation,* ed 5, St Louis, 1983, Mosby–Year Book.

24. Panzarine S, editor: *Promoting the health of adolescents: proceedings from the 1990 state adolescent health coordinators conference,* Washington, DC, 1991, National Center for Education in Maternal and Child Health.

14

Adolescent Nutrition in Special Situations

Jane Mitchell Rees
Cristine M. Trahms

✛✛✛

Objectives

After studying this chapter, the student should:

✔ *Be able to describe the major eating disorders.*

✔ *Know the psychological and physiological factors fostering obesity.*

✔ *Be able to describe dietary issues for adolescents who are athletes.*

✔ *Understand how the growth of the fetus influences the growth of the adolescent during pregnancy.*

✔ *Be aware of the main principles of counseling adolescents.*

Nutritional support for growth and development in such diverse circumstances as eating disorders, competitive sports, and pregnancy follows specific principles. Modifications may be required to ensure that physical development is normal and continuous in the face of wide swings in nutritional requirements based on the characteristics of an adolescent's life. The nature of psychological development requires that the most sophisticated counseling techniques available today be applied in helping teenagers change long-standing food-related behaviors that impair their nutritional health.

✛ Eating Disorders in Adolescence

The number of overweight adolescents has increased dramatically in the past decade. Using NHANES II data, more than 20% of youth, ages 12 to 17 years, in the United States are overweight.[1] Further, one-half to three-quarters of all adolescent females report a history of dieting. There appear to be differences between adolescents who diet and those who do not. Adolescents who diet are more likely to have poor body image and to indulge in fasting,

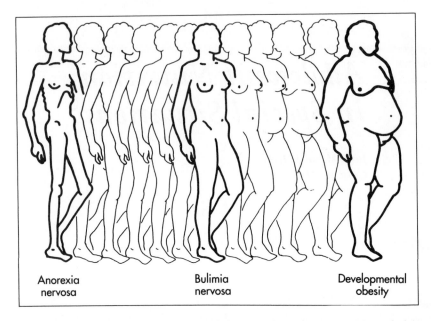

FIG. 14-1 Spectrum of eating disorders. Although physical conditions vary, underlying psychological characteristics are held in common across the spectrum.

(From Rees JM: *Eating disorders.* Copyright Mahan LK, Rees JM: Seattle, Wash, 1989. Originally published in Mahan LK, Rees JM: *Nutrition in adolescence,* St Louis, 1984, Mosby–Year Book.)

vomiting, taking diet pills, and binge eating.[2] It is believed there may be a spectrum of abnormal eating attitudes and behaviors that are not actual physiopathology but may place adolescents at risk for adopting potentially unhealthy eating practices or even for development of eating disorders under the right emotional or environmental circumstances.[2] It is now realized that unhealthy weight control behaviors are not confined to upper socioeconomic status females. About 15% to 20% of all adolescent females have used vomiting as a weight control measure; 25% to 35% reported binge eating, and 10% to 15% reported out-of-control eating. Some of these unhealthy weight control behaviors are more frequent in ethnic/racial subgroups than whites, regardless of socioeconomic status (SES) or BMI.[3] The number of adolescents with diagnosed **anorexia nervosa** or **bulimia nervosa** is growing. Because these disorders are so common among adolescents, health professionals interested in adolescent nutrition must understand them. Eating disorders provide effective models for study of other adolescent nutrition problems and their treatment. Therefore this chapter will explore these disorders in depth.

✣ Eating Disorder Spectrum

Characteristics

The physical symptoms of eating disorders can be viewed as a spectrum, with **developmental obesity** at one end and anorexia nervosa at the other (fig. 14-1). In the middle of this spectrum are persons at normal and abnormal weights. Along the spectrum these persons have in common basic underlying psychological problems that interfere to varying degrees with normal functioning.

A "psychology of dieting" appears to exist among adolescents that involves cognitive self-regulation processes.[4] The desire to "diet" regardless of body weight may interfere with the development of appropriate responses to hunger, appetite, and food. In developing responses to life, affected persons often use food inappropriately. Food-related behaviors and the resulting deviation in weight, the two most obvious aspects of these disorders, are usually the main focus of attention of the person affected, the public, and often the health professional. The underlying neurophysical and psychodevelopmental mechanisms, however, are the essential features of knowledge needed by nutritionists.

Adolescent Growth and Body Image Development

Because of rapid physical growth and body image development in adolescence, eating disorders are of special concern at this stage of life. These changes intensify associated **self-esteem** problems. Anorexia nervosa, for example, is a disorder so tied to **body image distortion** that it is most commonly seen in adolescence, the period when a person is struggling with self-identity and is most vulnerable to body image problems. Progress in adopting a normal adult body image will be interrupted for the teenager with an eating disorder. Bruch[5] has provided classic descriptions of distorted body images in both anorexic and obese adolescents.

Psychosocial Developmental Tasks

Teenagers with severe eating disorders fail in varying degrees to accomplish the developmental tasks of adolescence. The developmental problems of these persons are summarized in table 14-1. The most striking of their problems is failure to develop autonomy.

FAMILY INTERACTION

In recent years, studies of factors contributing to the origin of these problems have turned to the structure and interaction of the adolescent's family. Although obese teenagers are a much less homogeneous group than anorectic persons, the family patterns have much in common. Minuchin and others[6] have described families of persons with anorexia as being psychosomatic. They are enmeshed, rigid, and overprotective and have a low tolerance for conflict.

TABLE 14-1 *Developmental Problems Associated with Eating Disorders in Adolescence*

Difficulty in accomplishing the normal tasks of adolescence
Failure to develop autonomy
Inability to develop and use formal operational thought processes, especially in reference to themselves
Inability to experience bodily sensations originating within themselves as "normal" and "valid"
Unrealistic expectations for themselves
Unrealistic perceptions of body size
Preoccupation with weight and food, reflecting dependence on social opinion and judgment
Failure to normalize eating and exercise patterns

From Rees JM: *Eating disorders.* Copyright Mahan LK, Rees JM: Seattle, Wash, 1989. Originally published in Mahan LK, Rees JM: *Nutrition in adolescence,* St Louis, 1984, Mosby–Year Book.

Biopsychosocial Etiology

Eating disorders are very complex and may have developed throughout life or appear in adolescence. Individual and familial, biological, and psychological characteristics influenced by the modern social milieu contribute to their origin.

ANOREXIA NERVOSA
Symptoms

The term *anorexia nervosa* is actually a misnomer.[6] The implication that affected persons have a lack of appetite has been shown to be invalid. Superficially, the motivation to be thin keeps the person with anorexia nervosa from eating. In over 100 years of description in the literature, however, a combination of symptoms has come to be recognized as characteristic of the disorder. Although certain of these symptoms may be seen in other disorders, the combination is unique in anorexia nervosa. This unique combination of symptoms has been defined by the American Psychiatric Association.[7]

The criteria are as follows:

- The individual maintains a body weight that is below a minimally typical level for age and height, that is, less than 85% of the weight that is considered typical for that person's age and height or BMI ≤17.5.
- The individual, although underweight, intensely fears gaining weight or becoming fat.
- The individual has distorted experience and perception of body weight and shape.
- The postmenarcheal female has amenorrhea.

The principal psychological features of anorexia nervosa are "a relentless pursuit of thinness" and "a misuse of the eating function in efforts to solve or camouflage problems that otherwise would appear insolvable," that is, problems resulting from arrested normal development.[5]

Incidence

The majority of persons with anorexia nervosa are females in late adolescence and early adulthood. About 1% of young women present with the full criteria for anorexia nervosa; individuals with subthreshold criteria for the disorder are more commonly identified. The disorder has not been commonly seen in males, but 5% to 10% of anorectic teenagers are male. Males who develop the disorder appear to experience anorexia nervosa in essentially the same form as females.[8] Because of the predominance of females in the population seen with anorexia nervosa, the feminine pronoun will be used in this discussion.

Anorexia nervosa occurs predominantly in affluent classes and nations and is supported by a **cultural paradox** in which food is abundant and used lavishly for purposes other than survival on the one hand, and slimness is highly valued on the other. These cultural values are strong internal messages that have great impact on a young adolescent who has not developed autonomy. The lack of a similar value on slimness in males probably accounts for the small number of males seen with the disorder, although the influence of rock stars and other celebrities with excessively thin bodies is beginning to affect the ideals of young males.

Etiology

Theories about the etiology of anorexia nervosa have evolved from the initial psychoanalytic idea that the disease stemmed from an inability to deal with innate sexual drives, through periods when it was ascribed to endocrine deficits, and then disturbed patterns of family interaction, to the present when a combination of these biological, psychological, and social factors is thought to contribute to the development of the disorders.[10]

Effect of adolescence. As adolescence approaches, the body develops and life requires decisions and performance in many areas. The teenager panics at her lack of ability to cope independently. She develops rituals related to eating in an effort to be thin and "good." To gain her "independence," the teenager regresses to the period when independence ordinarily begins. In this early stage the principal manner to demonstrate growing independence open to the child is eating behavior.

Family system. Minuchin and others[6] describe how interrelationships within the family system foster anorexia nervosa. If family members are enmeshed in a system that does not allow development of appropriate roles, the system can produce a variety of psychosomatic problems. The particular direction toward anorexia nervosa may be determined when the main themes of family interaction are related to food, fitness, and appearance.

Biochemical processes. The possibility that a biochemical process may be responsible for development of anorexia nervosa continues to be investigated. Although various mechanisms have been proposed, so far none have been shown to be primary or causative. These mechanisms appear to result from psychological stress, malnutrition, and starvation. The fact that patients and their families fit such characteristic and complex patterns would raise doubt that a single primary physiological cause exists in most cases. However, it may be found that biochemical factors contribute to the development of the disorder.

Psychological State

The physical manifestations of anorexia nervosa may be sudden, although unrecognized underlying characteristics may have been previously present. Intervention strategies must address both the psychological and physiological states of the patient.

Progressive development. From the family's point of view, the anorectic teenager is usually a "model child" until she begins to develop a compulsive attitude about her weight. She has fit into the family unit and met their high expectations. She has worked extremely hard at school, being satisfied with nothing less than excellent grades.

Suddenly the whole family erupts in conflict over her eating behavior. The teenager herself has become troubled about her role in life. She is unable to sustain peer friendships and she is very anxious about relationships with males. She is confused by the need to establish more adult behavior patterns and clings to the rigid standards of childhood. She isolates herself. Life appears to be out of her control. She has conflicting feelings about living as her parents direct her to live, and she is hurt by their critical comments and begins to realize that she must assert herself. She takes a stand and will not compromise on her eating and exercise habits. She feels that she is too fat and must be slim to prove that she is a worthy person. She is increasingly preoccupied with her rituals and is angry when her family interferes. She denies her illness.

Distorted perceptions. A wide range of distorted perceptions has been noted, related specifically to body size, sex, hunger, rest, satiety, body temperature, pleasure, control, and "feeling states" in general. The anorectic teenager has often been described as wishing to stave off adulthood. But the question remains as to whether she wishes to avoid maturation or whether maturation eludes her.

Family problems. Although most families with anorectic teenagers would describe themselves as normal and without problems until the manifestations of anorexia nervosa arise, these families often have a multitude of problems. The parents may have been dominating and intrusive. They may have overlooked the *actual* (including nutritional) needs and emotions of their children, even in times when the children have been ill. By adopting a "helpless" stance, the affected children may be thoroughly manipulative and involved in their parents' conflicts. Both parents and children become locked into a system in which problems go unresolved and responses are stereotyped.[6]

Physiological State

In the initial stage of anorexia nervosa, physical symptoms are related to weight, diet, exercise, menses, and nutritional status.

Weight. In some cases the anorectic teenager is overweight when the disorder begins. The anorectic young woman is typically hypersensitive to developing breasts and hips. These young patients often recall a chance statement about their needing to lose weight by a relative or close friend, or a weight reduction plan suggested by a health professional, as the trigger for their initial weight loss behavior.

Diet. The anorectic adolescent usually develops a personal philosophy about her diet, limiting herself by eating food only from certain categories and in certain ways. She may manipulate the fluid or sodium content of her intake. In addition, she may force herself to vomit and misuse laxatives or diuretics to rid herself of food energy and weight. Vomiting may follow episodes of gorging.

Exercise. The practice of exercise rituals is equally varied. Anorectic teenagers include excessive calisthenics and other strenuous activities in their schedules. They may limit rest and use stimulants. They are so frequently involved in junior and senior high school athletics and dancing that coaches and teachers should be educated about the disorder. Good coaches should recognize which of their students may be exercising to their detriment by compulsively training beyond reasonable endurance while losing weight at a rapid rate.

Menses. Although a young woman in a state of starvation would be expected to become **amenorrheic,** indications are that cessation of menses occurs in most patients with anorexia nervosa before they have lost sufficient weight and body fat to cause an interruption of the cycle and lasts beyond the time they have regained weight and body fat.[9,11] Psychological factors probably contribute to the problem as well as true hormonal disturbance since stressful states are known to interfere with the endocrine system regulating the menstrual cycle.

Nutritional status. During the initial phase of an anorectic teenager's energy restriction, the body does not exhibit the effects of malnutrition to a measurable degree other than a decrease in weight. Infections are not generally seen. Deficiencies in specific nutrients have not been reported, but they may exist subclinically depending on the food habits of the individual. If weight loss continues unchecked, however,

TABLE 14-2   *Issues to Address in a Clinical Assessment of Eating Disorders*

Motivation
Appropriateness of weight goals
Desire to change unhealthful habits
Insight into problem

Emotional/psychological status
Depression
Locus of control
Body image
Self-esteem
Oral expression
Coping skills
Compulsivity
Perfectionism
Independence

Mental function
Intellectual ability
School performance
Attitude toward school
Ability to articulate

Family characteristics
Eating disorders
Other diseases
Natural or other parent
Intrusiveness
Enmeshment
Rigidity
Conflict resolution
Role of food
Exercise patterns
Perceptions of problem
Attempts to intervene
Willingness to participate in therapy

Social relationships
Friends
Social habits
Social skills
Attitude of peers

Eating behavior
Knowledge/acknowledgment of nutritional needs
Meal pattern
Bizarre eating habits
Personal philosophy toward eating
Nutritional adequacy
Control over food supply

Physical status
Signs of bulimia
Signs of starvation
Terminal signs of starvation
Thyroid status (obesity)
Resting heart rate
Exercise to reach 60% maximum heart rate

Growth and adiposity
Weight/height/age percentile
Triceps skinfold/age percentile
Arm muscle area/age percentile
Weight/height history
Growth velocity
Maturational stage
Age

Physical activity
Exercise patterns
Hobbies/interests
Personal feelings about exercise

From Rees JM: *Eating disorders.* Copyright Mahan LK, Rees JM: Seattle, Wash, 1989. Originally published in Mahan LK, Rees JM: *Nutrition in adolescence,* St Louis, 1984, Mosby–Year Book.

the symptoms of severe starvation may become apparent and additional nutritional problems begin to undermine basic health. This state indicates the onset of a crisis.

Intervention Strategies

Early recognition of symptoms. A recognition of the developing symptoms is the most important early intervention strategy. A protocol for assessing anorexia nervosa and bulimia nervosa is provided in table 14-2. Friends, school personnel, family, and health professionals are among those who observe the growing problems and can take steps to initiate treatment.

Psychotherapy. Individual and family psychotherapy by experienced therapists will enable both the affected adolescent and her family to adopt more appropriate roles. It will also help the anorectic teenager to complete the psychological developmental processes that have been arrested.

Nutritional therapy. Other than general monitoring of height and weight, it may not be necessary to treat the patient physically at this stage. Refocusing her attention on the primary emotional and interactional problems rather than the power struggle over food and exercise patterns will often enable the patient to abandon her compulsive striving for thinness. The patient should have access to a professional who can answer her questions about nutrition and make sure that she has the information she needs to begin to regulate her eating patterns to meet her physical needs. Information should be given in the context of the adolescent's desire to change rather than imposed as a rigid system of dietary planning by a professional. The overall disorder should not be defined as solely a nutritional problem, although nutrition counseling is an important component of therapy.

Crisis Stage: Psychological State

Overall, a lack of progress toward positive family interaction patterns during the initial therapy or continuing avoidance of intervention will often lead to physical and mental deterioration. When the crisis stage of anorexia nervosa develops, severe psychological and physiological symptoms appear and intervention must be directed toward the deteriorating condition.

Psychological effects of starvation. The anorectic teenager in crisis can cause panic among family, friends, and professionals. The family generally sees the adolescent's bizarre eating behavior as the problem and fails to understand the extent of developmental and interactional patterns. As a result, they often seek treatment that does not demand their involvement with the patient in therapy. As she becomes truly cachectic, the psychological changes inherent in starvation described by Keys and others[9] in his classic studies become evident:

1. Cognitive processes center around food. Thoughts of food intrude constantly; the major part of the waking hours are spent in contemplating it.
2. Behavior around food includes toying with it and hoarding, especially during **renourishment.**

3. Coherent creative thinking is impaired.
4. Mental function is characterized by apathy, dullness, exhaustion, and depression.
5. Interest in sexual function is lacking.

These effects of starvation are superimposed on the anorectic teenager's already disturbed psychological state. The behavior pattern, distorted perceptions, and weight phobia become more pronounced.

Behavior pattern. Many patients resist what they see as intrusions by professionals. They are secretive and hide the fact that they are carrying out their rituals. Their behavior may otherwise reflect the apathy typically seen in starving people. In obsessional preoccupation, they plan menus, read recipes, cook and serve food to others, cut or manipulate food before eating it, and record all that they eat. They usually have a detailed knowledge of "calorie content," but not of the energy value of foods. They may pretend to eat and then hide and dispose of the food. The disturbed adolescent's fear of gaining weight becomes increasingly evident as her weight phobia intensifies.

Crisis Stage: Physiological State

In the crisis stage of anorexia nervosa, the physiological state deteriorates with physical signs of starvation, endocrine abnormalities, and undeniable signs of approaching terminal starvation.[12]

Physical signs of starvation. As the crisis stage develops, the individual is unable to take care of herself. The physical state of starvation is now superimposed on the other problems inherent in the disorder. These physical signs of starvation include:

Fat store depletion
Muscle wasting
Amenorrhea
Cheilosis
Desquamation
Dry skin
Hirsutism
Thin, dry, brittle hair
Alopecia
Degradation of fingernails
Acrocyanosis
Postural hypotension
Inability to regulate body temperature

Additional nutritional problems. In addition to the clinical signs, recent research has focused on zinc nutriture, bone demineralization, growth failure, and structural changes in the brain, which result from severe long-term malnutrition in anorectic patients.[13,14] The possibility that bone demineralization, growth retardation, and brain structural abnormalities may prove irreversible to some degree is especially troublesome and warrants further examination.[15-17] The relationship of depressive symptoms, sex role, and body image distortion to lowered body weight, and the suggestion that fewer than the expected number of children are born to patients formerly diagnosed with anorexia nervosa are equally disturbing long-term effects of chronic malnutrition with implications for dancers, gymnasts, and other athletes who keep themselves in a state of starvation as well as for anorectics.[18-20]

Endocrine abnormalities. The endocrine abnormalities in women with anorexia nervosa are such that the body essentially reverts to a prepubertal hormonal state. As a result of hypothalamic change, the anorectic adolescent is amenorrheic, is unable to adapt to heat and cold, suffers sleep disturbances, and is unable to conserve body water. There is no interest in sex.

Terminal starvation signs. During the crisis, professionals must monitor the physical state of the patient and take remedial action when signs of starvation approach a terminal state. The most outstanding of these signs include:

Fluid and electrolyte imbalance indicating inability of the body to maintain homeostasis (dehydration and edema)

Severe cardiac abnormalities in the absence of electrolyte imbalances, indicating a wasted myocardium

Absence of ketone bodies in the urine, indicating a lack of fat stores for metabolic fuel

Concurrent infection, indicating increasing nutritional needs

Crisis Intervention Strategies

When the anorectic adolescent's condition reaches the crisis stage, hospitalization is necessary to provide comprehensive care involving nutritional therapy.

Hospitalization. For some clinicians, the decision to hospitalize an anorectic patient depends on her reaching a life-threatening physical state. However, if the goal is to renourish the individual so that she will be able to benefit from psychotherapy without semistarvation neurosis, as many authoritative therapists recommend, the anorectic patient must be hospitalized before a critical stage has been reached. The patient can be released from the hospital when she has been nutritionally rehabilitated, usually confirmed by reaching a particular weight-for-height goal.

Comprehensive treatment. Nutritional components of therapeutic regimens for anorexia nervosa patients in the crisis stage are intertwined with the psychological aspects of the treatment. Team care is essential. Certain principles can be observed that will apply regardless of the treatment modality. Renourishment obviously will begin with a gradual increase in energy intake.

Diet therapy. In some programs the patient will be allowed to choose anything available on the hospital menu. Other programs impose rules, make additions to what is ordered, or serve a set menu. If a diet is prescribed following the principles established for renourishing malnourished individuals, it should have adequate protein to meet basic needs with additional energy made up of complex carbohydrates and a small amount of fat.

Nutritional supplements. If a patient refuses food, a nutritional supplement, which is prescribed and dispensed as a medicine, may be used. If a life-threatening state is reached at any time with the patient refusing oral feeding, nourishment by nasogastric tube or parenteral methods may be necessary. These methods will be presented as life-saving procedures and not as punishment for refusing to eat. Nourishment by mouth is the preferred route and is possible in most cases.

Renourishment edema and body image. Edema generally appears with renourishment and can be a problem because of the anorectic patient's phobia of weight gain. The edema is seen by her as proof that she will "expand" as she feared. Some anticipatory guidance can help her accept such a development. Assurance that professionals will aid her in gaining appropriate weight, which will be strengthening for her but will not form excess fat, can help desensitize the issue.

Role of the clinical nutritionist. The clinical nutritionist/dietitian on the therapeutic team provides nutritional care while maintaining the psychotherapeutic goal of redirecting the focus of the patient's concern. The nutritionist's knowledge of energy balance as it applies to the individual is needed in determining appropriate weight goals throughout therapy, especially as related to the patient's release from the hospital.

Long-Term Therapy

Psychological state. The anorectic teenager who has recovered from a starvation crisis by gaining a certain amount of weight to improve her physical state will still have to deal with the developmental arrest that brought her to the crisis, a process that usually requires several years. There will continue to be problems concerning vocational choices and preparation, economic stability, relationships with peers and especially with the opposite sex, weight management, and body image.

Physiological state. The anorectic young woman will often experience wide swings in weight from extreme thinness to obesity before she will be able to bring her anorexia into control. She may see herself as somewhat detached from her body and experiment with various food habits before putting food into a more normal perspective. She may keep herself sufficiently thin that she may not resume her menses. She may feel bloated and have bouts of edema, physical responses to starvation and refeeding, and **carotenemia,** a symptom of anorexia.

Intervention strategies. In the recovery period the psychotherapeutic goal will be to facilitate normal development in the anorectic teenager, to prepare her for a full adult role in society, and to enable her to function without depending on bizarre eating and exercise habits. She will need information and retraining about food and the physical aspects of life. Many of the techniques described in the section on obesity will be useful. Issues such as the state of nourishment necessary to maintain the menstrual

cycle will resurface from time to time as development proceeds. Returning to such issues will enable her to deal more capably with them as time goes on. Guided food experiences in cafeterias, grocery stores, cooking, and entertaining help ready the person for managing food in her environment. The objective is to help the individual put food into a reasonable perspective and give up overfocusing on food out of ignorance. A team consisting of medical, psychological, and nutrition specialists may provide care, or the care may be left to a single therapist who will be responsible for all aspects of therapy with consultation from others.

Outcome. Common features of anorexia nervosa are the strong resistance to treatment and the high incidence of relapse and partial recovery. Some patients will manifest varying degrees of the anorectic symptoms in adulthood. Although outcome criteria have been inconsistently used by researchers, results reported to date indicate that although weight-for-height proportion improved in about 75% of the patients, menstrual cycles were often unsatisfactorily maintained, ideas about food and weight were disturbed, and psychosocial maladjustment was common.[21]

BULIMIA NERVOSA

First called bulimarexia, *bulimia nervosa* is the most recently recognized eating disorder and is characterized by gorging followed by self-induced vomiting or diarrhea. Although these symptoms may be a part of anorexia nervosa, they also constitute a separate syndrome.

Symptoms

The person suffering from bulimia nervosa generally maintains close-to-normal weight (fig. 14-1) while gorging, bingeing, eating abnormally large amounts of food, and vomiting or purging (forcing bowels to empty) on a regular basis. The bulimic teenager may have somewhat less severe distortions in body image and less restrictive weight goals than the adolescent with anorexia nervosa. She is often older at age of onset.

American Psychiatric Association criteria. The diagnostic criteria for bulimia nervosa has been established by the American Psychiatric Association (APA).[7]

The criteria are as follows:

- The individual demonstrates recurrent episodes of binge eating that are characterized by (1) eating a larger amount of food in a period of time than most people would under similar circumstances, and (2) a sense of lack of control over eating.
- The individual repeatedly uses inappropriate methods to prevent weight gain (vomiting, laxatives, and diuretics).
- The individual demonstrates binge eating and inappropriate compensation twice a week for three months.
- The individual is overly concerned with body shape and weight.

Incidence

The syndrome of bulimia nervosa should be differentiated from the recent behavior of many normal adolescent females who occasionally use self-induced vomiting as a means of controlling weight.[22] As many as 20% of college age females may engage in bulimic behaviors with an estimated 1% to 3% of adolescent and young adult females meeting the criteria for diagnosis of bulimia nervosa.[7]

A serious condition will be uncontrollable, and the psychological features of the disorder will impair normal functioning. Bulimia nervosa sometimes develops after a serious bout with anorexia nervosa or obesity. The bulimic person is more likely to be fertile than the individual with anorexia nervosa. Therefore, certain young women will be bulimic during pregnancy.

Psychological State

Separation anxiety is one of the important issues for the bulimic teenager. Her self-esteem is extremely low and is tied to her feelings about her body. She demonstrates excessive need for control and approval. She thinks of herself as physically unattractive, although she is well groomed and has a normally attractive physique. She develops guilt over her habits and her secret feelings of inadequacy. Superficially, she may be responsible and keep a heavy social schedule. In reality she has few close friends and feels that no one really knows her. In contrast

to the more rigid anorectic adolescent, the young woman with bulimia nervosa often demonstrates poor impulse control, abuses substances, and becomes easily enraged. By all accounts, the gorging, vomiting, and purging serve to release tension for the sufferers. However, the residual guilt feelings bring renewed tension that perpetuates an uncontrolled cycle. Social isolation is also perpetuated because of the fear that the secret will be found out. If pregnant, the bulimic teenager may be committed to protecting the fetus but retain ideas that inhibit normal nourishment of herself, her fetus, and the child after birth.

Food behavior. The bulimic teenager periodically eats large amounts of food and then voluntarily vomits or purges. Each person with bulimia nervosa defines what a binge is for herself. Because of distortions in thinking about food, as little as one doughnut may be thought of as a binge by one person while as much as an entire package of doughnuts may constitute a binge for another. As the duration of the habits extends, it becomes easier for her to vomit. Eventually, the vomiting is a nearly automatic response. In addition, she may take laxatives to purge herself of the energy she has ingested or use diuretics to remove body fluid.

Physiological Symptoms

As a result of these behaviors, physiological symptoms of the bulimic adolescent will include:

Tooth damage

Throat irritation

Esophageal inflammation (all of the above symptoms are caused by exposure of unprotected tissues to acidic vomitus)

Swollen salivary glands (caused by acidic reflux or constant stimulation)

Broken blood vessels in face (from force of vomiting)

Cracked, damaged lips

Rectal bleeding (caused by overuse of laxatives)

Life-threatening situations are rarer in bulimics than in anorectics. They are:

Dehydration and electrolyte imbalance

Fistulas or ruptures in the upper gastrointestinal tract

Kidney damage

Concerns during pregnancy are the adverse biochemical environment for the mother and fetus, the mother's abnormal weight gain pattern (weight loss, lack of weight gain, inordinate gain), and the mother's unrealistic ideas about infant feeding.

Intervention Strategies

The techniques most frequently reported in treating bulimia nervosa patients are similar to those used during the long-term recovery period of anorexia nervosa patients. Psychotherapy, nutritional therapy, and care of any pregnancy that may occur must be included.

Psychotherapy. The emphasis of therapy is on freeing the person from guilt, facilitating gains in self-esteem, and helping her deal with anxiety as well as challenging distorted goal setting based on perfection. Ideally, the young woman's family or partner will be included in the therapy.

Nutritional therapy. While she deals with the psychological problem, the bulimic individual will still have an eating disorder and will need reeducation to nourish herself properly. Physical and nutritional education can fill gaps in knowledge these teenagers have about their body functions. Over time, myths about weight management can be dispelled and more normal eating habits developed. Because of distorted feelings about food, the bulimic person may feel guilty every time she eats, despite the fact that food is necessary for life. The family often reinforces the guilt by a misguided overfocus on food, thinness, and the physical aspects of life. The bulimic teenager usually restricts her food intake to match the ideal plan she conceives for herself. Binges may thus arise from the natural need for adequate food and the desire for additional gratification.[23]

Role of the clinical nutritionist. The clinical nutritionist on the professional team will help the young person with bulimia nervosa to see food in a more appropriate context and accept more realistic weight goals using the techniques described in the following section. Helping her understand the physiological processes of energy balance and nutrient functions as well as the effects of bingeing, vomiting, and purging as they affect her personally is especially useful.

This education, however, must be done gradually in a counseling mode, allowing time for alteration of her rigid system of beliefs. Family and individual psychotherapy will continue concurrently. It is necessary to deal with the underlying causes of the obsessional food behavior. Group therapy has also been used.

Pregnancy care. The bulimic teenager who is pregnant can be helped to accept the idea that the baby she wants must be nourished. She can then be supported in learning to retain those foods that the fetus needs even if she cannot give up bingeing and vomiting totally. She should also be helped in learning to recognize her baby's natural hunger signals.

OBESITY

At the other end of the physical spectrum of eating disorders is obesity. Unlike anorectic adolescents, persons who are abnormally heavy do not fit into a homogeneous group and may be carrying excessive weight for a variety of reasons. Factors leading to obesity can be broadly divided into those that are psychological and those that are physiological. In any individual a combination of these factors may operate in the development and maintenance of obesity. Because of the cultural response to obesity, the adolescent whose obesity may be physiologically based will generally be subject to many of the same problems as those whose obesity is more psychologically based.

Psychological Factors

Various psychological factors are associated with adolescent obesity, whether it develops during earlier childhood or is related to more severe psychiatric disorders.

Developmental obesity. Bruch[5] described a form of obesity that primarily results from psychological factors within the family. Thus it is termed *developmental obesity.* It is an eating disorder comparable to anorexia nervosa in that it originates in the early life of the child. The families of developmentally obese teenagers fit descriptions of the psychosomatic family. The family's attitudes and behavior thus stunt the child's psychological development and serve as primary causes of the obesity. The obesity itself further inhibits normal development, and this in turn leads to maintenance or increase of body weight. The affected children are made to feel pressure, inappropriate responsibility, and specialness to an abnormal degree in family interactions. They become rigid, isolated, and enmeshed. They develop misperceptions about their basic physical needs and rely on coping skills based on the abuse of food. Obese teenage girls rated their families low on cohesion, expressiveness, democratic family style, that is, a family style that did not provide adequate emotional support and viewed the girls as having lack of control.[24] As obese teenagers, these persons may not develop their full potential as competent, well-functioning adults, but they are less likely to experience the complete developmental arrest that the anorectic teenager does.

Body image. The teenager who is overweight is vulnerable to body image disturbances. The type and extent of the disturbance depend on the length of time the person has been heavy, the amount of excessive weight carried, the person's sex, and the life situation surrounding the individual's unique development. For example, teenagers who have been heavy from childhood may react differently from those who have gained weight only during later adolescence. Like anorectic teenagers, many tie thoughts of success or failure to their weight status.

Associated psychological disorders. In some teenagers, obesity may be associated with severe psychiatric disorders. In others, the overeating behavior may act as an emotionally stabilizing influence helping to maintain the person at a functioning level. Interference in such a situation without substantial support provided can cause the disintegration of the person's affect into an anxious or depressed state.

Cultural and Family Influences

The abundance of food and lack of necessity to expend energy in American society make it easy for children to gain unwanted weight. In families where food intake and exercise patterns are not appropriate for dealing with this situation, an overweight state can result without other specific psychological or physiological origins.

Behavior Patterns in Obese Teenagers

The usual overweight or obese teenager is passive in interactions with others and with the environment. This response further reinforces the weight problem and leads to social isolation, lack of exercise, and disturbed patterns of eating and family interaction.

Social isolation. The **passive response pattern** of the obese adolescent in contact with others creates social isolation and an increased dependence on the family for relationships, even though the family interaction patterns may be unpleasant and the parents may constantly exhibit intrusive and negative attitudes. Adolescents often react to the stigma of obesity by adopting a stereotyped lifestyle with a narrow range of activities.

Sedentary lifestyle. The eating and exercise functions in the lives of obese teenagers generally become distorted. They may never feel comfortable eating in social situations. Their isolation leads them to opt out of many activities that would expend energy. They fear being seen wearing gym clothes or swimsuits or doing physical activities because they feel they are the object of attention and even ridicule. Instead they spend an inordinate amount of time in passive pursuits such as watching television or reading. Both of these activities may be paired with eating. Commercial television, especially, fosters this behavior with frequent food-related cues.

Eating patterns. Although many studies of teenagers after they have become obese have shown that on the average they eat no more, and sometimes less, than their normal weight peers, they often have disturbed, unstructured patterns of eating. They may eat only in the latter part of the day, feeling nausea when eating earlier, and eat rapidly and indiscriminately.

Family patterns. Parents in some families may be locked into power struggles with their children, attempting in vain to control what they eat. Overanxiety regarding even slight overweight may actually contribute to growing obesity. In other families overeating may be the main theme, with most interactions revolving around food.

Physiological Factors

In certain individuals physiological factors are principally responsible for their obesity. These factors are summarized in table 14-3. Two of these underlying factors deserve note here.

TABLE 14-3   Processes Leading to and Sustaining Obesity: Therapeutic Implications

Process	Therapeutic Implications
Genetic predisposition Certain inherited biochemical, morphological, and histological features foster excess storage of energy as fat.	Teach to control energy intake and output to exert any possible control and need to be vigilant even if unable to avoid being greater than normal size.
Sodium pump activity Less activity in cells of obese decreases energy usage, making more available for storage.	No direct intervention; not known if process is reversible.
Body temperature differences Defect in regulation with failure to maintain normal core temperature by obese increases energy available for storage.	As above
Adipose tissue lipoprotein lipase activity Rate-limiting enzyme in triglyceride storage is more active in the obese, enhancing adipose tissue synthesis.	As above
Insulin resistance Obese bodies are less sensitive to insulin. Resulting hyperinsulinemia tends to maintain obese state.	Exercise improves sensitivity to insulin even without weight loss; also reversible with weight loss.
Thermogenesis Less energy is spent in obligatory (food processing) or facultative (response to sympathetic nervous system) thermogenesis in obese.	Complex carbohydrates increase obligatory thermogenesis in some individuals; timing exercise before or after meals increases facultative thermogenesis in some.
Adipocyte hypertrophy When energy is available for storage fat cells enlarge.	Decrease energy available by changing intake/output; cell size is reduced with energy deficit.
Adipocyte hyperplasia When fat cells are filled, new cells will be formed if energy continues to be available for storage.	Already obese can decrease energy available to prevent formation of even more cells; cell number does not decrease even with energy deficit.

Modified from Rees JM: *Eating disorders.* Copyright Mahan LK, Rees JM: Seattle, Wash, 1989. Originally published in Mahan LK, Rees JM: *Nutrition in adolescence,* St Louis, 1984, Mosby–Year Book.

Continued.

TABLE 14-3 *Processes Leading to and Sustaining Obesity: Therapeutic Implications—cont'd*

Process	Therapeutic Implications
Regional distribution of adipose tissue	
Typically, males have more central (abdominal) adipose tissue with higher waist/hip ratios than females who have more peripheral (femoral and gluteal) fat with lower waist/hip ratios. Male distribution associated with diabetes, hypertension, and cardiovascular disease; female distribution more difficult to change. Difference in cell size and lipoprotein lipase activity in various sites may be important.	Assessing waist/hip ratio helps determine difficulty of achieving weight loss and harm in remaining obese.
Set-point weight	
Bodies of certain individuals defend high body weights. Others defend low weights or no particular weight.	Decrease excess energy through exercise and substituting complex carbohydrates for fat, so as to reverse any processes that are reversible. If obese adolescents have control of energy intake and output, psychological support for physiologically sustainable weight is reasonable.

Set-point theory. One theory that cannot be overlooked is that certain individuals may be subject to a body weight **set point.** A certain body weight may be physiologically normal for each person, and body characteristics may be tuned to keep the body at that weight.

Lower basal energy needs. A decreased requirement of the amount of energy used in biochemical reactions may increase the amount of energy available in the systems of some people for storage as fat. Based on present theory, the longer the teenager has been obese and the greater the extent of the obesity, the greater the effect these factors will have. The adolescent whose obesity was originally caused by other factors such as social, psychological, or family influences will, as time passes, have added problems of physiological obesity. This pattern increases the complexity of the obese state.[25]

Intervention Strategies

An effective program in working with obese teenagers and their families will provide personalized care, giving attention to identifying individual needs and attitudes, setting realistic goals, developing related strategies within a comprehensive approach (see table 14-4), and evaluating outcome.

Assessment

The combination of psychological and physiological circumstances by which an individual teenager has become obese must be identified so that intervention can be directed toward specific aspects of the problem. The degree of overweightness must be considered.

Body mass index (BMI) should be routinely used to screen adolescents for overweight. BMI is significantly correlated with subcutaneous fat and total body fatness in adolescents and is highly specific for those with the greatest amount of body fat. BMI is useful because suitable reference data are available and BMI can be derived from stature and weight.[26] Overweight criteria that use BMI must be age specific. This is necessary because during growth and maturation, body proportions, bone mass, and ratio of lean to fat tissue change at different times and at different rates.[1] The WHO Expert Committee recommends the following criteria: (1) Adolescents whose BMI ≥ 85th percentile are considered to be at risk for overweight and

TABLE 14-4   *Components of a Comprehensive Weight Management Program with Applicable Treatment Modalities*

Food Management	Energy Time Management	Psychosocial Adjustment
Food use retraining	Fitness testing and improvement programs	Supportive counseling
Nutrition education	Relaxation training	Family counseling
Behavior modification	Movement and dance therapy	Social skills training
Diet prescription	Expanded interest stimulation	Assertion training
		Psychotherapy
		Group support

From Rees JM: *Eating disorders.* Copyright Mahan LK, Rees JM: Seattle, Wash, 1989. Originally published in Mahan LK, Rees JM: *Nutrition in adolescence,* St Louis, 1984, Mosby–Year Book.

(2) adolescents whose BMI ≥ 85th percentile BMI and triceps skinfold and subscapular skinfold thickness both ≥ 90th percentile are considered obese.[27] The Expert Committee on Clinical Guidelines for Overweight in Adolescent Preventive Services provides a slightly different criteria: (1) Adolescents whose BMI ≥ 95 percentile for age and sex, or >30, should be considered overweight, and (2) adolescents whose BMI ≥ 85th percentile but ≤ 95th percentile, or ≤ 30 should be considered at risk for overweight. Percentiles for BMI for male and female adolescents are shown in table 14-5. Triceps and subscapular skinfold percentiles are shown in the appendix.

Among all of these persons some will suffer from hidden eating disorders such as bulimia nervosa or anorexia nervosa (recovery stage). The information needed to assess adolescent obesity (fig. 14-2) may best be gathered by a team of professionals. Many of these aspects will need to be explored over time. The basic initial steps to assess physical status and personal attitude include:

1. Physical status. A physical examination will disclose the stage of puberty and rule out any endocrine abnormalities or complications of the obese state. Endocrine disorders are rarely found. Most physiological abnormalities associated with obesity indicated by clinical laboratory measures will respond to weight reduction.
2. Personal attitude. The most important aspect of initial evaluation is whether the

individual is committed to making changes. The teenager's feelings must be assessed initially and at each visit. It is of no value for other persons to have goals related to weight management if the teenager is not ready to change the status quo. The question needs to be, "Are you ready to make changes?" rather than, "Do you want to lose weight?" Many teenagers will answer yes to the second question but remain totally passive, the implication being that the process of weight management for them is a passive one in which the professional administers treatment.

Reasons for Not Starting a Weight Loss Program

A weight loss program should not be instituted if (1) the adolescent has not reached full height; (2) there is a lack of commitment; (3) it is likely to be another in a series of failures harmful to the individual's self-esteem; or (4) the individual is obviously predisposed to obesity by overwhelming physiological factors. If obese teenagers keep fit, maintain energy equilibrium, and are emotionally healthy, they will be candidates for weight loss only if they understand the physiological aspects of obesity and are determined to test these aspects in a healthful manner. Those adolescents who are still growing in height should not be encouraged to lose weight because the level of energy restriction required to do so is inadequate to support growth.

text continues on page 351

TABLE 14-5A   Percentiles of BMI-for-Age: Male Adolescents, 9–24 Years[a]

Age (years)	Percentiles				
	5th	15th	50th	85th	95th
9	14.03	14.71	16.17	18.85	21.47
10	14.42	15.15	16.72	19.60	22.60
11	14.83	15.59	17.28	20.35	23.73
12	15.24	16.06	17.87	21.12	24.89
13	15.73	16.62	18.53	21.93	25.93
14	16.18	17.20	19.22	22.77	26.93
15	16.59	17.76	19.92	23.63	27.76
16	17.01	18.32	20.63	24.45	28.53
17	17.31	18.68	21.12	25.28	29.32
18	17.54	18.89	21.45	25.92	30.02
19	17.80	19.20	21.86	26.36	30.66
20–24	18.66	20.21	23.07	26.87	31.26

[a]Reference data are based on the first National Health and Nutrition Examination Survey (NHANES I) in the United States of America (*2, 3*).

TABLE 14-5B   Percentiles of BMI-for-Age: Female Adolescents, 9–24 Years[a]

Age (years)	Percentiles				
	5th	15th	50th	85th	95th
9	13.87	14.66	16.33	19.19	21.78
10	14.23	15.09	17.00	20.19	23.20
11	14.60	15.53	17.67	21.18	24.59
12	14.98	15.98	18.35	22.17	25.95
13	15.36	16.43	18.95	23.08	27.07
14	15.67	16.79	19.32	23.88	27.97
15	16.01	17.16	19.69	24.29	28.51
16	16.37	17.54	20.09	24.74	29.10
17	16.59	17.81	20.36	25.23	29.72
18	16.71	17.99	20.57	25.56	30.22
19	16.87	18.20	20.80	25.85	30.72
20–24	17.38	18.64	21.46	26.14	31.20

[a]Reference data are based on the first National Health and Nutrition Examination Survey (NHANES I) in the United States of America (*2, 3*).

From Report of a WHO Expert Committee. *Physical status: the use and interpretation of anthropometry.* WHO Technical Report Series 854, Geneva, 1995.

Rate on a scale of 0 to 5 the contribution to weight management
0 = Minimum; 5 = Maximum

	0	1	2	3	4	5
NOURISHMENT						
Knowledge of:						
Meaning of "kcalories"						
Role of food in life						
Relationship of energy intake/output						
Major nutrients—physiological role						
energy value						
amount needed						
food sources.						
amount of food needed						
Choosing food in a variety of situations.						
Behavior modification techniques						
Appropriate wt/ht/age/genetic heritage						
Attitude						
Acceptance of responsibility for nourishing self.						
Commitment to health-promoting habits						
Obtaining appropriate foods						
Nutrition education						
Eating behavior						
Control of food supply.						
Fat content.						
Types of food						
Amounts of food						
Meal pattern.						
Between-meal eating						
Binges/night eating/other aberrations						
Uses behavior modification techniques						
Eats in social situations—						
with family.						
with peers						
Family						
Eating meal together.						
Place.						
Distractions (TV).						
Serving methods						
Support for weight control via use of						
Food						
Knowledge						
Autonomy allowed to choose food						

FIG. 14-2   Format for weight management assessment of adolescents. The initial rating in each category can be used to set short-term goals and subsequently can be used to monitor improvement between assessments.

Continued.

	0	1	2	3	4	5
ENERGY TIME MANAGEMENT						
Knowledge of:						
Exercise in energy balance						
Fitness—cardiorespiratory						
muscular						
Exercise—aerobic						
anaerobic						
Monitoring pulse						
Attitude						
Commitment to exercising regularly						
Without others, equipment, or money if necessary						
Interest in fitness education						
Pleasure in moving						
Behavior						
Fitness tested						
Program planned						
Program maintained						
Level of fitness						
Relaxation						
Rest/sleep						
Activities shared—with friends						
with family						
Consciously plans exercise/relaxation/rest						
Family						
Support of activities						
Family activities						
Understanding of exercise in weight management						
PSYCHOSOCIAL HEALTH						
Knowledge of:						
Emotional factors in weight management						
Cues to eat—internal						
external						
Impact on emotional health of:						
physical activity						
nourishment						
Responsibility for weight managment						
Need to seek guidance for insoluble problems						
Attitude						
Commitment to mental health						
Learning about weight control						
Solving problems						

FIG. 14-2, Cont'd.

	0	1	2	3	4	5
PSYCHOSOCIAL HEALTH—cont'd						
Behavior						
Pleasurable experiences						
Relationships—peers						
family						
teachers						
counselors						
School activities						
Social skills						
Intellect—insight						
communication						
problem solving						
school performance						
Goal setting—short term						
long term						
Self-rewards						
Emotional status						
Body image						
Self-efficacy						
Locus of control						
Depression vs. nondepression						
Sense of humor						
Oral gratification						
Coping skills						
Compulsivity						
Perfectionism						
Independence						
Parental support						
Perception of weight problem						
Support vs. intrusion—emotional						
financial						
Rigidity						
Conflict resolution						
Commitment to treatment						

FIG. 14-2, Cont'd.

OBJECTIVE INFORMATION:

Age _____ yr

	Infancy	Toddlerhood	Early childhood	Elementary school	Jr. high	Sr. high
Length of obesity Reduction attempts	Yo-yo Anorexia nervosa	Severe Bulimia nervosa	Diets	Exercise	None	Reasonable
Parents	Birth Anorexia nervosa	Adoptive Bulimia nervosa	Obesity	Overweight		
Grandparents	Birth Anorexia nervosa	Adoptive Bulimia nervosa	Obesity	Overweight		
Maturation stage	0	1	2	3	4	5
Menarche	0	+1 yr	+ 2yr	+3 yr	+4 yr	+5 yr
Thyroid screen Cholesterol	(mg/dL) _____		HDL (mg/dL) _____		LDL (mg/dL) _____	
Wt percentile*	>95	95	95–75	75	75–50	50
Ht percentile*	95	90	75	50	25	10
Wt/Ht percentile*	(100–50 lb) >95	(50–25 lb) >95	>95	95	95–75	75
BMI percentile†						
TSF percentile‡	>95	95	95–75	75	75–50	50
SSF percentile (male)‡	>95	95	95–75	75	75–50	50
MAC percentile‡	>95	95	95–75	75	75–50	50
AMA percentile‡	>95	95	95–75	75	75–50	50

Waist circumference _____ in
Hips circumference _____ in
Waist/hip ratio _____

FIG. 14-2, Cont'd.

*National Center for Health Statistics: *Height and weight of youths 12–17 years,* United States. In Vital and health statistics, series 11, no 124, Health Services and Mental Health Administration, Washington, DC, 1973, US Government Printing Office. From Mahan LK, Rees JM: *Nutrition in adolescence,* St Louis, 1984, Mosby–Year Book.
†Body Mass Index (kg/m²). Guidelines in Hammer LD and others: Standardized percentile curves of body-mass index for children and adolescents, *Am J Dis Child* 145:259, 1991.
‡TSF (triceps skinfold); SSF (subscapular skinfold); MAC (midarm circumference); AMA (arm muscle area). Guidelines in Frisancho AR: *Anthropometric standard for the assessment of growth and nutritional status,* Ann Arbor, 1990, University of Michigan Press. From Rees JM: Management of obesity in adolescents. In Farrow JA, editor: Adolescent medicine, *Med Clin North Am* 74:1275, 1990.

EXERCISE

HR to reach 120 beats/min	Slow walk	Moderate walk	Fast walk	Walk up hill	Walk/jog	Jog
Entry Date _____		+3 mo _____	+6 mo _____	+12 mo _____	+18 mo _____	+24 mo _____
Weight __ lb	+ 10 _____ + 5 _____ − 2.5 _____ − 5 _____ − 10 _____ − 15 _____					
%BF§ _____	+ 3 _____ + 2 _____ − 2 _____ − 5 _____					
RHR‖ _____ beats/min	+ 5 _____ + 3 _____ − 3 _____ − 5 _____					
Height _____ in	+ 3 _____ + 2 _____ + 1 _____					
AMA‡ _____ mm²	+500 _____ +200 _____ +100 _____ −100 _____ −200 _____					

FIG. 14-2, Cont'd.

§Percent body fat
‖Resting heart rate

Goals

Realistic planning of goals includes a series of short-term steps to achieve the long-term goal:

1. Short-term goals. These continuing short-term goals need to be based not on changes in weight but on positive changes in food intake and exercise-related attitudes and behaviors with appropriate rewards built in. It is especially necessary to build a program around short-term manageable goals related to behavioral change, since physiological factors may make actual weight loss a difficult, long-term achievement. The teenager should be made aware that over the long term,

deficit will eventually lead to weight loss, however slowly. Working toward improved knowledge, attitudes, or behaviors is a worthy short-term goal.

2. Weight goal. The initial weight goal in a **weight management** program is usually maintenance, that is, cessation of weight gain. In certain situations an even more basic change from *rapid gain* to *slow gain* is the more appropriate goal. Immature adolescents who have not completed linear growth can bring weight and, more specifically, percentage of body fat into better proportion with height by holding their weight stable or by reducing gains to a lower rate as height increases. This pattern eliminates nutritional risk to the individual from severe diet restrictions at a time of rapid growth and development. For teenagers who have stabilized their weight and are no longer gaining in height, the next step will be a slow, steady *loss* based on reeducation in the use of energy. A *loss* of 0.9 kg/wk (2 lb/wk) should not be exceeded. If this rate appears insignificant to the teenager, point out that it would add up to more than 45 kg (100 lb) loss over 1 year. Improvement in any of the physical measures of figure 14-2 constitutes achievement of a long-term goal.

Intervention Strategies: Physiological Factors

Strategies planned to deal with the physiological factors of obesity must be based on the laws of energy exchange and balance, address positive changes in personal food behaviors, avoid the dangers of "crash diets" and life-threatening situations, and increase physical activity and fitness.[25]

Basic individual energy balance. Whatever the reasons are for a teenager's being overweight, the method for intervention remains the same: decreasing the body's energy intake and increasing the energy output until the appropriate deficit state is established. There is no way of knowing the exact use of energy by a particular body except by testing it over time. To lose weight an energy deficit must be achieved at the cellular level. Because this state is not measurable under normal clinical circumstances, there is no set formula that ensures weight loss. It is an error to count kcalories of food energy being eaten and assume that this amount of energy will be available within the biochemical system. Thus a deficit of 3500 kcalories calculated at the point of intake does not necessarily lead to a loss of 1 lb of body weight. This does not imply that the second law of thermodynamics is inoperative, but simply that energy from food may be used in a variety of ways once it is in the body, as indicated previously (table 14-3). Thus both the physiological and the psychological aspects of weight management are unique to the individual.

Eating habits. Each individual teenager must be guided in learning the level of energy intake and output that produces weight gain, loss, and maintenance for that individual if the treatment is to be effective. An understanding of physiological factors must be incorporated. The teenager must be made aware that however bleak the physiological situation appears, the possibility of weight management has not been tested until the individual has control over energy intake and output. There is usually some potential for improvement in the diet that will help even those persons who are physiologically prone to obesity to become more fit and healthy and to stabilize and perhaps to reduce their weight in small amounts.

Dietary change. Strategies for dietary change must address the issues of (1) energy and nutrient content of the food intake; (2) circumstances of eating related to timing, place, accompanying social factors, and emotions; and (3) principles of nutrition regarding weight management.

Food use retraining. Specific diets have rarely achieved long-term changes in eating behavior. This result is especially true for teenagers, who tend to rebel against authoritarian techniques and hold a number of negative views about diets. Food use retraining, a series of habit changes planned jointly by the teenager and the therapist and instituted in succession over time, will be more acceptable to most adolescents and is a more realistic way to approach a complex problem.

Time factor. Because eating habits have been developed over a number of years, the teenager will need considerable time to make changes. A person cannot suddenly pick up a musical instrument and play it well but will need education, practice, and support to become proficient. Even so, most teenagers will not be able to learn a new food pattern or "diet" and perfect it immediately. Usually, intensive treatment will need to be continued for a year or more to accomplish major dietary changes. Breaking down the problem of food misuse into small components makes change more probable. What habit will be the initial focus, how change will be accomplished, what foods will be eaten, and what motivations and rewards will be effective are topics to be developed and clarified in counseling sessions between the therapist and the teenager.

Therapy objective. The nutritional therapist's objective is eventually to focus on each time of day and point of environment where teenagers meet with food and to help them to *retrain themselves* in the use of food. Most teenagers will have some reasonable habits that can be supported and used as a foundation for the emerging positive patterns.

Self-responsibility. Teenagers will need help at every stage to take responsibility for their actions. Coupled with psychological support, the process can lead to effective change. Even those who are unsuccessful in retraining themselves during the adolescent period will have a model for the future, when they may be able to take greater control. Education regarding the physiological factors of obesity will help teenagers avoid the harmful quick-loss plans to which they are so vulnerable.

Dangers of "crash" diets. An important component of programs in weight management education involves helping the teenager understand that rapid weight loss by either starvation or too low an energy intake is ineffective. Since the loss is in lean body mass and fluids, inevitably weight will be regained when usual eating is resumed and muscle (and the ability to use energy), not fat, will have been lost.[28] The deprivation in such a regimen often leads to even greater overeating. Thus the final result of a "crash" diet is often a net gain.[29] It is not difficult to convince those who have had the experience a few times that such practices are ineffective, but it is important to support their impressions by teaching them the physiological reasons. Teenagers who will not be convinced that such methods and "diet aids" are unhealthy will be deterred from using them by the knowledge that they will not lose fat.

Morbid obesity. There are certain life-threatening situations for very obese persons when drastic intervention will be necessary. The physical condition should be monitored to detect any rapid deterioration. The following conditions warrant hospitalization:

Sudden changes in cardiac or respiratory function

Inability to move, maintain balance, or travel

Rapid weight increase because of the above factors

Inability to fit into furniture and having to rest on the floor

Ulcerations at pressure points and friction areas

As with the anorectic teenager, a period of separation from the family may break up a pernicious cycle leading to physical deterioration.[30] Comprehensive treatment using a **modified fast** as the dietary component is at present the most practical therapy. Although it is still controversial whether lean body mass can be spared, such dietary methods appear less objectionable than other radical procedures.

Physical activity and fitness. One of the most important concepts of weight management is that energy output must be increased. Individualized exercise programs need to be developed with the obese teenager to achieve a gradual increase in physical activity. The fitness test shown in chapter 13 is designed to be a conservative tool that can safely be used with even an extremely obese person. It can be used with or without professional help. Increasing activity can be rewarding in itself, whereas denying oneself an accustomed food may seem more like punishment. Besides fitness testing and improvement, various strategies can be directed toward increasing energy output by increasing physical activity. Activities should be (1) built into everyday life; (2) something the person enjoys or finds useful; (3) independent of help from others or complex equipment; and (4) nonstressful by not causing embarrassing exposure of the body or awkwardness.

Intervention Strategies: Psychological Factors

Weight management for teenagers should be a total rehabilitation program. It demands a significant length of time and must be individualized. Like the physiological component, the psychological component of any weight management problem cannot be overlooked. Activities planned to meet these needs include motivational support, psychotherapy, and counseling.[31-33]

Motivation. In a short-term situation where the teenager has only a few pounds to lose, the problem is one of motivation. This support can be provided in school settings and in many other community settings.

Psychotherapy. With extreme developmental obesity, changes usually require extensive psychotherapeutic intervention. This includes the family when the teenager is living at home.[34]

Counseling. For teenagers falling between these two extremes, a variable degree of supportive counseling will be needed to increase self-acceptance, to decrease stress, to facilitate development, and to enable adolescents to carry out weight management strategies. Teenagers need help in learning to experience the body's signals related to hunger and satiety and to adopt nondestructive coping mechanisms to replace the misuse of food.

Comprehensive Approach

To provide a comprehensive approach to a weight management program for teenagers, attention must be given to additional resources available. These resources include group activities applied with professional guidance, parent education and counseling, and school and community support.

Group activities. Strategies such as camp settings, support groups, peer counseling, social skills and assertiveness training, body awareness experience, physical fitness training, and behavior modification can be used successfully with some individuals. Groups and preplanned programs will help those adolescents with mild, relatively simple problems. *Camps and other groups that provide for only short-term weight loss are detrimental and should be avoided.*

Professional guidance. No group setting provides a solution for all aspects of obesity. To be effective, weight management techniques must be applied within the context of ongoing supportive counseling by professionals who assess the specific problems of the individual over time and choose appropriate treatment methods. A team of professionals will be best able to carry out a comprehensive program as described here.

Parent education and counseling. Counseling will enable parents to support their teenagers in learning to manage weight. Education about the physiological factors involved and rational approaches to management will help dispel parents' myths. Helping them develop a nonintrusive attitude toward their teenagers is extremely important. The counselor can demonstrate this by stressing the need for the teenager, not the counselor or the parent, to establish his or her own goals.

School and community support. Although they are rarely in the position to carry out therapy because of the complexity of the problem, teachers, school counselors, nurses, coaches, and other community leaders have many opportunities to educate and support overweight teenagers. Curriculum materials such as those represented in figure 14-3 have been designed to help adolescents understand the complexity of weight management.

Outcome

Reviews of the outcome of weight management therapies for teenagers are uniformly gloomy. In general, such programs are designed as studies of *weight loss* when informed workers in the field of adolescent health have stressed the importance of focusing on the other benefits of *weight management* programs such as increased self-esteem. Added knowledge, increased readiness to work for change, and improved practices are important outcomes of weight management programs for adolescents.

SUMMARY: EATING DISORDERS

The spectrum of eating disorders affects adolescents physically, psychologically, personally, and socially. Intervention strategies must be directed toward both the nutritional and the developmental aspects of these disorders for them to be effective. Goals must be established

BE SIZEWISE
Don't Lose Your Balance.

Nourishment	Activities	Feelings
Be good to your body—give it what it needs	Do interesting things—quiet as well as energetic	Learn to know and like yourself
Don't starve or stuff yourself	Take time to relax every day	Have realistic goals for yourself
Know what's in the food you eat	Don't let eating be your only recreation	Don't substitute food for love and companionship
	Do some strenuous activity every day	Build satisfying relationships with your family and friends
	Share active and quiet time with friends	Get help for problems you can't cope with alone

FIG. 14-3 Be sizewise—materials for clinicians, educators, and teenagers. (From Rees JM and others: *Be size wise,* Seattle, 1979, American Heart Association of Washington.)

in relation to all aspects of eating disorders. Helping teenagers put food into reasonable perspective in their lives will be a principal goal of nutritional therapy. A recognition of the amount of time required for effective intervention is essential for a basic understanding of eating disorders.

♣Athletics
NUTRITIONAL SUPPORT FOR ADOLESCENT ATHLETES

Adolescent athletes require nutritional support to maintain normal growth and physiological maturation in spite of physical stress. Energy is the basic factor here. The additional energy needed depends on the intensity, duration, and type of exercise and the size and state of development of the adolescent.

Source of Energy

Energy is best utilized if it is supplied as carbohydrates. The need for carbohydrate as fuel instead of protein to build muscle even for a teenager who is still growing is one of the most misunderstood principles among adolescent athletes.

Protein requirement. An additional intake of 6 to 7 gm of protein/day is sufficient in a muscle-building phase (during initial training). Thereafter, intakes of 2 to 3 gm of protein/day above the recommended daily allowance (RDA) will support body maintenance in most athletes. Abnormally high levels of protein or amino acid supplements are counterproductive, leading to dehydration as the body rids itself of nitrogenous waste products.

Weight Management

Weight should be gained or lost following safe effective methods. To support normal growth successfully, weight should be maintained at an optimal level over the long term rather than be subjected to seasonal, or especially weekly, manipulation as is often urged by wrestling and crew coaches during competition.[35] The development pattern of skeletal growth and weight gain must be considered. Two problems in this area are common among teenage athletes who become too thin in trying to reduce the percentage of body fat:

(1) women interrupt their menses, and (2) men stunt their linear growth. **Anabolic steroids** taken by men to increase weight cause stunting of growth and disturbed development of secondary sex characteristics. Both males and females may increase the tendency to gain weight as fat if they repeatedly gain and lose weight rapidly through drastic dietary and related manipulation.[36,37]

Supplements

The increased dietary intake should provide sufficient amounts of vitamins and minerals, including the B vitamins essential in energy production.[38] Supplementation of nutrients in amounts above those recommended has not resulted in benefits during competition.

Iron Nutriture

Of the non-energy-producing nutrients, iron is particularly important to young athletes because "sports anemia" is associated with reduced oxygenation. There is some evidence that adolescents involved in athletics are more likely to become iron deficient than adolescents who are not athletes. The increased needs of both males and females during physical growth and development may impair their ability to maintain body stores when they engage in strenuous activity. Teenage athletes should be tested for iron deficiency before and during each season and treated for any problem found. Other than consuming foods with enough iron to meet the RDA and taking supplements at that level if dietary sources are inadequate, teenagers are not advised to use additional iron on a routine basis.[23,39]

Anabolic Steroids

An estimated 5% to 10% of adolescents are using anabolic steroids. Use is greater among male athletes who say they use them to increase muscle, size, strength and speed and to improve personal appearance and athletic performance. Young people are using these substances without appropriate knowledge of the profound effects they have been found to have throughout the bodies of adults.

Dietary Issues for Adolescents in Competition

The science of managing food and drink to keep athletes healthy and in condition for competing is constantly advancing.[40,41] All teenagers who are participating in athletics, as well as their coaches and parents, need to know the latest principles of dietary intake with the following issues in mind as they apply to younger athletes.

Adequate fluids and electrolytes. Younger people are at greater risk for dehydration and heat illness than adults. They have a lower output of water from the sweat glands and lower cardiac output, resulting in less blood being carried to the skin to lower the core body temperature. Adolescents are especially at risk when they start strenuous workouts at the beginning of a season in an unconditioned state and when humidity as well as temperature is high.[42]

Appropriate balance between complex and simple carbohydrates during competition and training. Because adolescents are vulnerable to advertising and mythology repeated by others, they may follow unsound practices instead of using glucose and starches effectively. Teenagers may not take the time or realize the need to appropriately nourish their bodies for grueling, long-term sporting events.

Teenagers also do not clearly understand the need for sufficient but not excess fuel for short-term sporting events. The subtleties of balancing the various sources of simple and complex carbohydrates are especially important during these often anaerobic events because sufficient oxygen cannot be provided by the cardiorespiratory system without adequate fuel.

Because young teenagers may lack experience in choosing foods, they may not choose a meal of reasonable composition before competition and thus may impair their performance. Foods that should be eliminated are those with excess roughage or fats and gas-forming foods.

Long-term adequacy. Food intake must be balanced with energy output, but also with sufficient energy and nutrients to support growth and development. Total energy and calcium are especially important for normal skeletal development and maintenance.[43]

Support from Adults

Maintaining appropriate weight for height as the adolescent grows is a good general guide to dietary adequacy as long as the foods eaten to attain that weight are nutrient rich. Obtaining sufficient food may prove difficult for teenage athletes whose days are filled from early morning to late evening with practices as well as normal activities including classes and study assignments. Parents, coaches and school officials need to support teenagers by helping them plan specifically to obtain adequate acceptable foods at times when rigorous schedules allow them to eat.

✣ Adolescent Pregnancy
DEVELOPMENTAL ISSUES

Teenage pregnancy must be studied in light of the highly dynamic nature of adolescence. Both the psychological and the physical status of the adolescent have implications for the course of any pregnancy. The many interactions of factors in adolescent development and reproduction have great clinical significance for all aspects of the pregnancy including nutrition.[44] Indeed, adolescents are changing so profoundly that pregnancy for the younger, less mature teenager will be different than for the older, more mature adolescent.

Less mature teenagers will be more dependent on others and less able to act and make decisions on their own. They will be more **narcissistic** and less able to comprehend the needs of others. These young women will be less realistic, engage in more fantasy and wishful thinking, and have less insight into their own behaviors and motives. In general, younger teenagers will have fewer intellectual and physical skills to be able to cope with any situation, especially a complex reproductive experience. Many of the difficulties related to pregnancy in adolescence stem from this immaturity. As development advances, a person is able to carry out reproduction and childrearing in a more normal, less problem-fraught way. As shown in figure 14-4, the time line of events in teenage pregnancy has great potential for affecting the nutritional well-being of the adolescent.

✣ Reproduction During Adolescence

The pregnant adolescent's nutritional needs are influenced by many factors. Primary influences are her growth and nutrient stores, her gynecological age, and her nutritional status at conception.

ADOLESCENT GROWTH AND NUTRIENT STORES

The assumption that pregnant adolescents need an additional supply of nutrients to support their own growth plus that of the growing fetus has been questioned. Because hormone levels are high in pregnancy, even the slower statural growth that usually follows menarche may not occur. Growth does continue to some degree during adolescent pregnancy.[45,46] Whether or not actual growth continues for an adolescent who becomes pregnant, she will have experienced rapid growth more recently than her adult counterparts. There will have been less opportunity for storage of nutrients. Thus there may be greater physiological risk to young women who conceive in the early years after the onset of menses.

GYNECOLOGICAL AGE

The number of years between the onset of menses and conception is calculated to determine gynecological age. Those adolescents who are more sexually mature, that is, of greater gynecological age, share a vulnerability to physiological stresses but appear to have no more physically based complications during pregnancy than adult women. It is the young women of lower gynecological age who carry more risk and need more nutritional support. Only a small number of adolescents become pregnant in the first 2 years following menarche because most of them will not be ovulating during that time, although they are menstruating. Those who do become pregnant, however, are of great concern to clinicians and researchers.

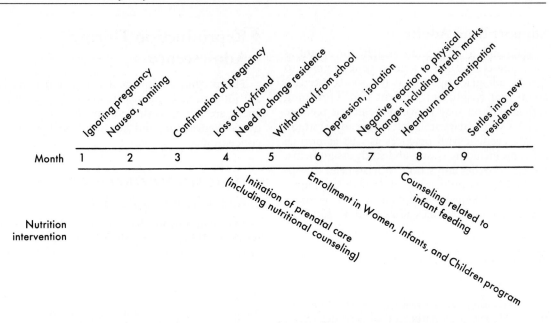

FIG. 14-4   Typical events in teen pregnancy that could affect intake or utilization of nutrients. (From Rees JM, Worthington-Roberts BS: *Adolescence, nutrition and pregnancy: interrelationships.* Copyright Mahan LK, Rees JM: Seattle, Wash, 1989. Originally published in Mahan LK, Rees JM: *Nutrition in adolescence,* St Louis, 1984, Mosby–Year Book.)

NUTRITIONAL STATUS AT CONCEPTION

Pregnant adolescents who are of young gynecological age and are malnourished at the time of conception are at double risk. They appear to have the greatest need for nutrients to support a pregnancy and maintain optimal health themselves.[46]

HAZARDS TO THE MOTHER

Given the complexity of pregnancy in the adolescent period, it is logical to question how these young women fare during pregnancy. They have more complications, a higher risk of maternal mortality, and more problems in personal psychological development and education that carry long-term implications for economic well-being.[47]

Complications

The variety of complications often described for the teenage mother during gestation includes:

First and third trimester bleeding
Anemia
Difficult labor and delivery
Cephalopelvic disproportion
Pregnancy-induced hypertensive disorders including preeclampsia and eclampsia
Infections

Of these complications, the most common physical problem is infection, while the most serious problem is preeclampsia, which usually manifests itself in the third trimester by increased weight gain, fluid retention, high blood pressure, and proteinuria and does not appear to run a different course in pregnant teenagers than in older women. Some researchers point out that it is a disease of first pregnancies. In addition, the harmful effects of preeclampsia, or the more serious state of eclampsia, may be greater in teenagers. Damage to the cardiovascular and renal systems initiated with a first pregnancy early in life and intensified by insults such as other pregnancies can increase the risk of developing renal and cardiovascular problems with increasing age.[48]

Maternal Mortality

The serious risk of maternal mortality is also a problem. The rate is 2.5 times greater for mothers under 15 years of age than for those 20 to 24 years of age.

Effect on Normal Developmental Steps

Apart from the physical sequelae, pregnancy often affects teenagers' psychological development, education, and ability to gain economic independence. Clearly these developmental steps are difficult to achieve in any case, and for many adolescents pregnancy is not a cause of failure but a coinciding event. The situations responsible for early pregnancy often remain unresolved, and many teenage mothers have additional pregnancies before the adolescent years are over.

HAZARDS TO THE INFANT

Infants born to teenage mothers suffer a higher incidence of morbidity and mortality in the perinatal period than do infants of older mothers. Problems seen more frequently include.[49]

Prematurity
Stillbirth
Low birth weight (LBW), the major hazard in adolescent pregnancy
Physical deformities

It is difficult to compare the likelihood of these problems occurring in infants born to teenage versus older mothers, or to younger versus older teenage mothers, but it is generally agreed that the problems do occur in a considerable number of teenage pregnancies. For example, the incidence of LBW is far greater when the mothers are adolescents.

TABLE 14-6 *Approximate 9-Month Increments in Weight of Postmenarcheal Women*

Postmenarcheal Year	Pounds	Kilograms
1	8	3.45
2	5	2.0
3	2	.90
4 and 5	1.32	.60

Modified from Frisch RE: *Hum Biol* 48:353, 1976. In Rees JM, Worthington-Roberts BS: *Adolescence, nutrition and pregnancy: interrelationships.* Copyright Mahan LK, Rees JM: Seattle, Wash, 1989. Originally published in Mahan LK, Rees JM: *Nutrition in adolescence,* St Louis, 1984, Mosby–Year Book.

WEIGHT GAIN
Specific Requirements

There is evidence that adolescents need to gain substantial weight during gestation to deliver optimal weight infants. Their infants will be somewhat smaller than the infants born to adults with the same gestational weight gain.[50,51] For example, when adolescents gain 26–35 lb, the incidence of LBW (under 2500 gm) is 6.3%, equivalent to the incidence for adult women who have gained 21 to 25 lb.[52] The incidences of fetal mortality and morbidity are thus linked to weight gain because they are linked to LBW.

The continuing growth and development of the adolescent may account for the extra weight that is needed.[53] Table 14-6 shows the amount of weight a young woman could be expected to gain in the 9-month period corresponding to her gynecological age if she were not pregnant. That amount plus the amount she would have to gain to be normal weight for her height and age if she is underweight probably constitute the extra amount she will gain in pregnancy.[54] Some authors refute this idea, theorizing (1) that teenagers may retain extra weight following delivery if they gain more than adults, and (2) that the teenagers' infants may be small in a natural adaptation to the less mature maternal biological state of the adolescent, and therefore not at risk simply because their birth weights are lower.[55,56] However, a critical factor in the outcome of adolescent pregnancy may be the maturity of the mother. Data have suggested that growing adolescents have infants that weigh less compared with nongrowing adolescents and mature controls.[57] Further, it has been shown that despite apparently sufficient weight gain and accumulation of stores during pregnancy, young, still growing women apparently did not mobilize fat stores late in pregnancy to enhance fetal growth.[58,59] This suggests that a larger weight gain during pregnancy is needed for adolescents.

Rate of Gain

Provisional recommendations in the 1990 Institute of Medicine Report are that women gain at the following rates in the last two trimesters of pregnancy, depending on their prepregnant weight status.[60]

.361 to .529 (.440 average) kg/wk if normal weight

.386 to .588 (.490 average) kg/wk if underweight

.218 to .386 (.300 average) kg/wk of overweight

Further, it was suggested that adolescents gain at the upper portion of these ranges. The report stated, however, that there was insufficient evidence to make separate recommendations for teenage mothers.

In the meantime, data show that the rate of gain by adolescents in the final trimesters of pregnancy is, on average, above .500 kg/wk. In one study a multiethnic group of adolescents who delivered term infants with a mean birth weight of 3258 gm (calculated from data given) gained at the rate of .505 to .531 kg/wk (50th percentile) during the last 18 weeks.[61] Weight gain at the rate of .692 to .893 kg/wk represents the 75th percentile. Of term infants delivered following relatively uncomplicated pregnancies, 5% weighed under 2500 gm, putting them in the category of high risk. To decrease the number of infants weighing less than optimal, the average rate would have to be greater.

In another study the mean rate of gain during the second and third trimesters of mothers delivering normal weight (3000 to 4000 gm), term infants was .588 kg/wk, while mothers of less than 3000 gm infants gained at the rate of .510 kg/wk in the same period (fig. 14-5).[62] The mean rate of gain for adolescents to bear infants weighing close to 3500 gm would appear to be about .588 kg/wk.

In summary, the evidence does not suggest restricting the natural weight gain of adolescents to levels recommended for adults. The upper and lower limits of optimal weight gain still need to be established to guide young women who find it difficult to gain at a reasonable rate.

MONITORING WEIGHT IN PRENATAL CARE

In both studies described above, the rates of gain were observed during prenatal care, rather than from the mother's report of what she weighed when she conceived. Keeping track of weekly weight gains is an effective way to evaluate the progress of adolescents during pregnancy.

In addition, measuring triceps skinfolds indicates adequacy of initial stored energy while changes have been related in later pregnancy to infant birth weight (fig. 14-6).[63]

ASSESSMENT AND MANAGEMENT OF NUTRITION
Risk Factors

So that nutrition services can be provided efficiently and effectively, pregnant teenage clients should be screened for those risk factors most closely linked to poor outcomes. Significant factors include:

Low gynecological age

Low prepregnancy weight for height or other significant evidence of malnutrition

Low pregnancy weight gain

Infections during pregnancy

Excessive pregnancy weight gain

Excessive weight for height at conception

Anemia

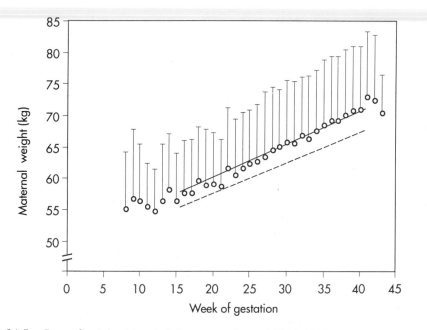

FIG. 14-5   Rate of weight gain of adolescent mothers of 3000-4000 gm (——) and <3000 gm (- - - -) infants described by regression statistics from 15 to 40 weeks' gestation (n of week 8 to 15 and after 40 too small to include in analysis). Means of weekly weight measures are shown for the total study population (o) and standard deviation (T). Symbols represent 6 to 313 measures at a given week.

(From Rees JM and others: *Am J Clin Nutr,* 56:868, 1992.)

FIG. 14-6   Monitoring body composition of adolescent during prenatal care.

TABLE 14-7   *Recommended Dietary Allowances for Pregnant Adolescent Females*

| | Age (Reference Height) | | | |
| | 11–14 Years (157 cm) | | 15–18 Years (163 cm) | |
Nutrient	Total RDA	RDA/cm†	Total RDA	RDA/cm†
Energy (kcal)*	2500	15.9	2500	15.3
Protein (gm)	56	0.38	54	0.36
Calcium (mg)	1200	7.6	1200	7.4
Phosphorus (mg)	1200	7.6	1200	7.4
Iron (mg)	30	0.19	30	0.18
Magnesium (mg)	300	2.0	320	2.1
Iodine (μg)	175	1.1	175	1.1
Zinc (mg)	15	0.09	15	0.09
Vitamin A (μg RE)	800	5.1	800	4.9
Vitamin D (μg)	10	0.06	10	0.06
Vitamin E (mg α-TE)	10	0.06	10	0.06
Ascorbic acid (mg)	60	0.38	70	0.43
Niacin (mg NE)	17	0.11	17	0.10
Riboflavin (mg)	1.6	0.01	1.6	0.01
Thiamin (mg)	1.5	0.01	1.5	0.01
Folate (μg)	400	2.3	400	2.5
Vitamin B_6 (mg)	2.0	0.01	2.1	0.01
Vitamin B_{12} (μg)	2.2	0.01	2.2	0.01

Data modified from Food and Nutrition Board, National Research Council: *Recommended dietary allowances,* ed. 10, Washington, DC, 1989, National Academy of Sciences.

Modified from Rees JM, Worthington-Roberts BS: *Adolescence, nutrition and pregnancy: interrelationships.* Copyright Mahan LK, Rees JM: Seattle, Wash, 1989. Originally published in Mahan LK, Rees JM: *Nutrition in adolescence,* St Louis, 1984, Mosby–Year Book.

*Second and third trimester.

†Dividing total allowances by reference height provides a suitable allowance/cm unit that can be used with adolescents who vary in height because of differing maturational ages.

Other risk factors gathered from history include:
Unhealthy lifestyle (including use of tobacco, drugs, and alcohol)
Unfavorable reproductive history
Chronic diseases or eating disorders
Overall assessment of nutritional status of the pregnant teenager follows more or less the general pattern for nutritional assessment of all pregnant women.

Nutrient Needs

A summary of recommended amounts of nutrients is provided in table 14-7. It combines the allowance for pregnancy in adult women with the amounts recommended for nonpregnant adolescents. A clinically practical way of ensuring nutrient adequacy is to encourage the pregnant adolescent to gain the recommended amount of weight by consuming nutrient-rich foods. Sources of protein, calcium, iron, micronutrients, and dietary fiber are also important. Table 14-8 translates these recommendations into food groups, which will assist the adolescent in evaluating food choices to meet nourishment goals. Many adolescents are willing to choose different foods while they are pregnant. When surveyed, pregnant adolescents reported including more dairy products, citrus fruits and juices, candy and

TABLE 14-8   *Daily Food Guide for Pregnancy*

	Minimum Daily Recommended Servings		
Food Group	Nonpregnant Adolescent	Pregnant Adolescent	Pregnant Adult
Dairy products—equivalents of 300 mg calcium and 8 gm protein	4	4–5	4
1 cup milk 1½ cup ice cream or pudding			
2 slices cheese 1 cup yogurt			
1¾″ cube cheese 2 cups cottage cheese			
¾ cup custard			
Meat and meat alternatives—equivalents of 14 gm protein/serving	2	3–4	3
2 oz meat, fish, poultry 2 oz cheese*			
1 cup dried beans, peas 4 slices bologna			
4 T peanut butter ½ cup cottage cheese*			
2 eggs 6 oz tofu			
Vegetables and fruits			
Vitamin A equivalents 1000 RE/serving	1	1	1
½ cup greens ½ cup green peppers			
½ cup spinach 1 cup broccoli			
½ cup carrots 1 cup apricots			
½ cup sweet potatoes 1 cup cantaloupe (¼ medium)			
Vitamin C equivalents 60 mg/serving	1	2	2
½ cup orange juice, grapefruit juice 1 orange			
1 grapefruit			
½ cup juices fortified with vitamin C 1 cup watermelon			
2 tomatoes			
¼ cantaloupe 1 cup cabbage (raw)			
⅔ cup strawberries 1½ cups tomato juice			
½ cup broccoli, brussel sprouts, green peppers			
Other fruit or vegetables	2	2	2
Breads and cereals—equivalents of 2 gm protein/serving	4	5–6	4
1 slice bread ½ cup cooked cereal, grits			
½ cup cooked rice ¾–1 cup dry cereal			
½ hot dog or 5 crackers			
hamburger bun 4″ pancake			
cornbread 1½″ × 2″ × 1½″ 1 biscuit, roll			
½ cup cooked macaroni ½ english muffin			
or spaghetti noodles ½ frozen waffle			
Fats and oils—provides 45 kcal/serving size	2	2	2
1 teaspoon margarine, ¾″ cube pork fat			
butter, oil, bacon fat 2 tablespoons sour cream			
1 tablespoon cream cheese 2 teaspoons salad dressing			
1 strip bacon or mayonnaise			

*Count cheese as a serving of milk or meat, not both simultaneously.

From Story M: Nutrient needs during adolescent pregnancy. In Story M (ed): *Nutrition management of the pregnant adolescent: a practical reference guide.* Washington, DC, MCH National Clearinghouse, 1990.

TABLE 14-9   *Warning Signs of Nutrition Problems in Pregnant Adolescents*

Medical/Obstetrical Factors	Nutrition/Dietary Factors	Psychosocial Factors
Adolescent with a gynecological age (chronological age minus age at menarche) of <3	Inadequate refrigeration or cooking facilities	Inadequate income
A previous pregnancy	Lack of transportation or accessibility to grocery store	Living alone or in an unstable family or other environment
History of poor obstetrical or fetal performance	Cultural or religious dietary restrictions	Little family or peer support
Chronic systemic disease	Frequent eating away from home	Denial or failure to accept the pregnancy
Past or present eating disorder: anorexia nervosa or bulimia nervosa	Frequent snacking	Significant emotional stress or depression
Underweight or overweight before pregnancy	Poor appetite	
Inadequate weight gain during pregnancy	Limited, monotonous, or highly processed diet	
Excessive weight gain during pregnancy	Irregular meal patterns (skipping meals)	
Persistent nausea or vomiting during pregnancy	History of frequent dieting	
Iron deficiency anemia or other nutritional deficiencies	Exclusion of a major food group(s)	
Infections during pregnancy	Binge eating episodes	
Heavy smoker	Eating of nonfood substances (pica)	
Alcohol or drug use	Nontraditional dietary pattern (e.g., vegetarianism)	
	Overuse of nutritional supplements	
	Heavy caffeine intake	

From Story M: *Nutrition assessment of pregnant adolescents.* In Story M, editor: *Nutrition management of the pregnant adolescent: a practical reference guide.* Washington, DC, MCH National Clearinghouse, 1990.

chocolate, and main dishes and less carbonated beverages and salty snacks.[64] Table 14-9 shows warning signs that a pregnant adolescent may demonstrate when having nutritional problems.

Contact with health professionals during prenatal care provides many important opportunities to teach adolescents about feeding themselves and their families. See table 14-10 for a clinical protocol for nutritional management of adolescent pregnancy.

Economic and Psychosocial Needs

The economic instability of pregnant adolescents makes it impossible to assume that they will have an adequate food supply. The impact of lifestyle, economics, and other stressful issues

on the nutritional well-being of young pregnant women is great and must be acknowledged in any program to improve their nutritional status.[65,66] A summary of these issues is provided in table 14-11. Above all, the stage of social and emotional development will determine the mother's ability to cope with all aspects of reproduction.

Involving the Baby's Father

When the partner of the young pregnant woman is available, he should be included in counseling sessions to build mutual nutritional support for the pregnancy. Specific outreach to the father of the baby can be beneficial.[67] If he is employed or in school, an effort should be made

TABLE 14-10   Protocol for Assessment and Management of Normal Teenage Pregnancy

Initial evaluation

Review intake material, social, and lifestyle history

Review clinical data

    Height and weight

    Gynecological age

    Physical signs of health

    Expected delivery date

Review laboratory data

    Hematocrit or hemoglobin

    Urinalysis

Begin to build relationship with the client (and partner if available)

Assess clients' perspective of nutrition issues

Assess attitude about, and acceptance of, prepregnancy with and feelings about weight gain during pregnancy

Assess intake patterns using dietary methodology best suited to client and professional

Make preliminary assessment of food resources and refer to supportive agencies if necessary

Check for nausea and vomiting and suggest possible remedy

Discuss supplemental vitamins and minerals

Make initial plan that sets priorities for issues

Come to agreement with patient about any initial changes and steps to take; have client state plan as she perceives it

Determine client understanding of relation between nutrition and health

Do initial anthropometrics, calculate reasonable weight gain

Second visit

Check on referrals to other agencies

Discuss results of initial evaluation and suggest any changes necessary in dietary patterns (use educational materials as appropriate)

Do any further investigations when necessary

Laboratory studies

    Specific diagnosis of anemia

    Protoporphyrin heme or serum ferritin

    Serum or red cell folate

    Serum vitamin B_{12}

    Further probing of dietary habits if necessary

Monitor weight gain; discuss projected weight gain for following visit and total for gestation

Assess and address issues affecting nutritional status in order of priority for the individual:

- Activity level
- Appetite changes
- Pica, food cravings, and aversions
- Allergies/food intolerances
- Supplementation practices (prescribed and self-selected)

Subsequent visits

Monitor and support appropriate weight gain: include discussion of fitness and encourage habitual safe exercise

Support upgrade in nutritional pattern in support of the woman and the developing infant; augment knowledge of principles of nutrition; continue to address issues affecting nutritional status

Check for heartburn, small food intake capacity, and elimination problems; suggest dietary interventions

Begin preliminary discussion and comparison of advantages/disadvantages of breast feeding and formula feeding

Final prenatal visit(s)

Discuss infant feeding if client will keep infant

If breast-feeding is chosen, provide preliminary guidance about breast-feeding practices

If formula-feeding is chosen, discuss product selection and preparation; define important details about feeding techniques

Postpartum visits

Help client understand safe methods of managing weight following delivery

Review infant feeding practices and infant growth; provide assistance when problems are identified

Modified from Rees JM, Worthington-Roberts BS: *Adolescence, nutrition and pregnancy: interrelationships.* Copyright Mahan LK, Rees JM: Seattle, Wash, 1989. Originally published in Mahan LK, Rees JM: *Nutrition in adolescence,* St Louis, 1984, Mosby–Year Book.

TABLE 14-11   *Issues in Adolescent Pregnancy That Influence Nutritional Well-Being*

Acceptance of the pregnancy
Desire to carry out successful pregnancy
Acceptance of responsibility (even if child is to be
    relinquished)
Clarification of identity as mother separate from her
    own mother
Realistic acceptance versus fantasy and idealization

Food resources
Family meals (timing, quantity, quality,
    responsibility)
Self-reliance
School lunch
Fast-food outlets
Socially related eating
Food assistance (WIC program and others)
Mobilization of all resources

Body image
Degree of acceptance of an adult body
Maturity in facing bodily changes throughout
    pregnancy

Living situation
Acceptance by living partners and extended family
Role expectations of living partners
Financial support
Facilities and resources
Ethnic group (religious, cultural, and social
    patterns)
Emancipation vs. dependency
Support system vs. isolation

Relationship with the child's father
Presence or absence of father
Quality of relationship
Influence on decision making
Contribution to resources
Influence on mother's nutritional habits and
    general lifestyle
Understanding of physiological processes
Tolerance of physical changes in pregnancy and
    physical needs of mother and child
Influence on child feeding

Peer relationships
Support from friends
Influence on nutritional knowledge and attitudes
Influence on general lifestyle

Nutritional state
Weight-for-height proportion
Maturational state
Tissue stores of nutrients
Reproductive and contraceptive history
Physical health
History of dietary patterns and nutritional status,
    including weight-losing schemes
Present eating habits
Complications of pregnancy (nausea and vomiting)
Substance use
Activity patterns
Need for intensive remediation

Prenatal care
Initiation of and compliance with prenatal care
Dependability of supporting resources
Identification of risk factors

Nutritional attitude and knowledge
Prior attitude toward nutrition
Understanding of role of nutrition in pregnancy
Knowledge of foods as sources of nutrients and of
    nutrients needed by the body
Desire to obtain adequate nutrition
Ability to obtain adequate nutrition and to control
    food supply

Preparation for child feeding
Knowledge of child-feeding practices
Attitude and decisions about child feeding
Responsibility for feeding
Understanding the importance of the bonding
    process
Support from family and friends

From Rees JM, Worthington-Roberts BS: *Adolescence, nutrition and pregnancy: interrelationships.* Copyright Mahan LK, Rees JM: Seattle, Wash, 1989. Originally published in Mahan LK, Rees JM: *Nutrition in adolescence,* St Louis, 1984, Mosby–Year Book.

by the counselor to see him at least occasionally. This effort will be especially important if for some reason he is interfering with the young woman's ability to nourish herself. Sharing what is known about the father's contribution to the outcome of pregnancy helps some adolescent males become more interested in maintaining healthy living habits.

Individualized Counseling

To be effective, the clinician must work within the context of an individualized counseling relationship with the young pregnant adolescent and her partner.[68] The counselor will not "prescribe" but will make practical suggestions and give support to help the teenager change her habits, usually in small increments throughout the pregnancy.

Benefits of Nutrition Counseling

The benefits of nutrition counseling will be seen more in the long term than in a particular pregnancy. Prenatal care is one of the best opportunities to teach a vulnerable group of teenagers sound nutritional information. Even if they seek care later in pregnancy and miss appointments, for most of them these contacts constitute the greatest input of health care during their adolescence.

Effective Counseling Strategies

Helping pregnant adolescents follow the suggested rate of gain can ensure sufficient energy intake to support the pregnancy and the mother's own developmental needs. Following the guidelines demonstrates dramatically in a few months the possibility of exerting personal control over eating, as well as the effect on both weight and nutritional status, in a way the teenager can understand. There is great appeal in discussing with adolescents the effects of various events on their bodies and on the growing fetus. Learning about the physiological needs of both her own body and her developing infant can be the teenager's impetus for upgrading the quality of her diet to keep pace with the increase in energy intake needed to support adequate weight gain. Repeated counseling sessions to review those needs may motivate the young mother to try new foods to obtain additional

sources of nutrients. Attention to nutritional health in the prenatal period can become a model for taking responsibility for feeding a family. The young woman can gain experience in the use of community resources to obtain food for herself and her family.

In summary, nutrition counseling in prenatal care for teenagers can accomplish the following goals:

1. Serve as a model for exerting control over what a person eats with visible results in terms of the optimal weight gain pattern and the quality of foods contributing to it.
2. Be an impetus for trying new foods.
3. Serve as a model for taking responsibility and using community resources to feed a family.

The nutrition counselor will be most effective when working within a clinical program designed especially for adolescents. Such programs have been shown to improve overall outcome in adolescent pregnancy.[49]

✣ Nutritional Counseling for Adolescents

FACILITATING CHANGE

Attempts to help adolescents improve their nutritional status must be approached with skill, especially because of their growing independence. Nutrition counselors must know adolescents' physical and psychological development, lifestyles, and habits as well as appropriate methods of communicating with the adolescents.[68]

Strategies for Change

Sophisticated strategies to add knowledge, alter attitudes, and change behavior must be used in any setting if the objective is to influence an adolescent's eating habits.[69] Providing knowledge or teaching can be done in a variety of settings from the classroom to the hospital bedside. Altering attitudes is much more difficult and usually demands an individualized experience. Facilitating the adoption of new behavior is even more difficult and requires a lengthy period of time. The adolescent will have to feel positive about any plan before it can succeed. In fact, much effort must be directed toward encouraging the person to want to change before introducing steps to bring about the change.

Personalized counseling. Besides changes in attitude, the counselor must impart knowledge in an especially meaningful and individualized manner. Finally, behavior change can be approached in increments that are sufficiently realistic to ensure personal success.[70]

Nutritional counseling, unlike nutrition education activities or specific dietary teaching techniques, is based on a continuing interactive relationship between counselor and client. The mutual goal for the relationship is improvement of the adolescent's nutritional well-being. This relationship has been characterized as one of mutual participation, as opposed to the activity-passivity relationship seen in acute care or the guidance-cooperation model, which usually is used with younger children.[71] The way in which a message is presented is as important as the message itself.

Nature of counseling process. The counseling process is a specialized conversation that has a specific purpose and takes place within a relationship.[72] The professional will be primarily responsible for guiding the process so that the mutual goals are met. It can never be a unilateral responsibility, however, but must be shared by the adolescent client. In fact, the professional will need to help clients feel a responsibility for contributing if they do not do so spontaneously. In these conversations the purposes will be to obtain information about the client, to provide information to the client, and to stimulate the client to take action.

Content vs. process. The exchanges in counseling can be divided into the content (the information exchanged) and the process (the way the exchange takes place).[73,74] The content that is brought forth for discussion by adolescents consists of what they want to talk about, what they are concerned about, and in some situations, irrelevant material used to avoid focusing on problems. It ultimately will be the responsibility of the counselor to guide them in presenting material that contributes to the overall goals of counseling. The counselor will also be responsible for bringing in content that is suited to the

client's needs in terms of quantity, type, and level of understanding.

The process on the adolescents' part is made up of their attitude toward the discussion, the way they express themselves, and their emotional response to the counseling session. The counselor's expression (beginning from the first meeting with the client in the waiting room or at the bedside), verbal and nonverbal reinforcement of the client's responses, and overall guidance of the session constitute the counselor's contributions to the process. Examples of the content of a nutritional counseling session would include information from the client about his or her eating habits and recommendations from the counselor about changes that need to be made. The process would include the way the client described his or her eating patterns and the kind of approach the counselor took in securing the information and in suggesting changes following an evaluation.

Both the content and process of counseling exchanges contribute to the results of a therapeutic relationship. When the approach of the clinician is overly authoritarian, a working relationship becomes impossible. The other extreme is the relationship that builds rapport on irrelevancies but fails to deal with difficult issues.

Obtaining and providing information are relatively common processes, and it is easy to conceive of how this is done in counseling. Stimulating a client to take action by means of a conversation, however, is a much more complex process to visualize and to accomplish than that of obtaining information. The following are descriptions of accomplishments in counseling that lead to change on the part of the client:

Increasing self-awareness
Realizing existence of alternatives
Problem solving
Experiencing positive communication style
Experiencing control over one's life
Building self-esteem

Building self-esteem. Adolescents must believe that they are worthy individuals so that they may find the energy to make changes in their lives. Table 14-12 describes some of the specific methods nutritionists use to foster self-esteem in encounters they have with adolescents.

TABLE 14-12 *Strategies for Fostering Client Dignity*

Address the client's presenting agenda.

Provide information so that a structure can be developed that will encourage and support an honest, mutual interaction.

Assess and respect the client's coping style (e.g., What is her behavior telling you? Is she withdrawn? Talkative? A caretaker? Childlike? Mature beyond her years?).

Allow the client choices whenever possible so that she can feel she is making her own decisions.

Normalize variations in feeling and mood so that the client does not fear or harshly judge the changes in her emotions since pregnancy.

Provide words for feelings.

Provide education about physical and emotional aspects of pregnancy so that the client has a simple base of knowledge from which to participate in her pregnancy.

Reinforce adult (not childlike) behaviors.

Focus on her positive attributes to foster self-esteem and positive coping.

Draw out positive coping by recognizing and complimenting coping behaviors that are obviously functional and healthy.

Focus away from pathology and avoid unhelpful commiseration so that you will represent a person who can remain a neutral mirror for her.

Proceed at a pace that is comfortable for the client.

From Reynolds S, Faulkner P: *Interviewing and counseling skills.* In Story M, editor: *Nutrition management of the pregnant adolescent: a practical reference guide,* Washington, DC, 1990, National Center Education Maternal Child Health.

Role of parents. Parents must be appropriately involved in the counseling process. They need help in being supportive, as opposed to being intrusive, as the adolescent makes changes. Both adolescents and their parents must be helped to see the importance of focusing on the process of making change rather than solely on the desired goal of self-care. An understanding of both the physical and social sciences, along with a liberal injection of art, is needed in nutrition counseling for adolescents and their parents. It is indeed a challenging field.

Common problems in counseling. Health care professionals must often overcome a lack of training in counseling techniques. Some of the common pitfalls that indicate a need for improved skills are listed below:

Setting inappropriate goals

Communicating in overly authoritarian style

Losing the adolescent's attention

Being deterred by the adolescent's defenses

Losing control and therefore losing credibility

Being confused over the direction counseling should take

Failing to treat the adolescent as an individual

Preparation for counseling. By constantly improving skills, a counselor will be more effective in a greater variety of settings. Resources for improving counseling skills are listed below:

Classes

Workshops

Experience

Observation of others

Working with other disciplines

Reading

Self-monitoring

    Video or audio

    Client surveys

Feedback from colleagues

Assessing clinical outcome

Self-assessment

Counseling environment. Adolescents will often need to be counseled in their own environment, whether that be in a school, a mall, or a community-based clinic.

TABLE 14-13   Adaptations to Counseling in Undesirable Settings

Verbally acknowledge and apologize for the inconvenience, reassuring the adolescent of your concern for him or her.

Reschedule the appointment if conditions might be better another day.

Acknowledge your own feeling of anger, frustration, anxiety, or tension elicited by the situation, and be aware that the adolescent may feel similarly.

Consider going for a walk or sitting outside to conduct the counseling session.

When time is inadequate, prepare in advance and prioritize needs:

- Review the chart and previous "progress notes" (if available) before the meeting.
- Have available at the meeting any materials that might be useful.
- If there are no immediate or obvious needs, allow the adolescent to use the time as she or he wants (e.g., ask if the teen has any particular questions or concerns to discuss).

If permissible, display in the lobby or examination room posters that might be appealing and informative to pregnant adolescents.

From Reynolds S, Faulkner P: *Interviewing and counseling skills.* In Story M, editor: *Nutrition management of the pregnant adolescent: a practical reference guide,* Washington, DC, 1990, National Center Education Maternal Child Health.

Table 14-13 provides suggestions for making adolescents feel comfortable in any setting.[69] Taking a walk with a teenager or inviting the teenager to share some other activity often puts him or her more at ease than sitting face to face with a counselor. An adolescent who has had little experience conversing with adults will often be more verbal when he or she can move freely.

✣ The Health Care Team

Adolescent health care is one of the most demanding of clinical problems. As such, it is best handled as a team effort. Any one professional will generally not possess the skills to meet all the client's needs. Table 14-14 lists types of issues that will arise throughout the course of teenage pregnancies with a suggested list of professionals to guide clients in managing these issues. This does not mean that certain problems are the responsibility of any one profession to the exclusion of others. Each professional team member can support the messages and guidance provided by other team members. Team conferences aid in coordination of care and team efficiency in meeting identified needs and noting the client's progress in solving various problems. Nutritionists and other professionals who are in positions to influence program planning can help develop clinical teams for care of adolescents.

Working with a team requires specialized skill. Team members bring their backgrounds, both professional and personal, with them. These characteristics determine how that professional will carry out a role on a team. The structure of the team, which may be any one of those in figure 14-7, will affect their work in a basic fashion. Structure determines communication patterns between professionals and between professionals and clients. Interrelationships between team members are complex and must be carefully developed by clinicians who are highly motivated to work together. The reward will be seen in improved comprehensive care for adolescents with complex problems.

Summary

In the context of rapid physical and psychological growth during adolescence, appropriate nourishment cannot be taken for granted.

TABLE 14-14 *Suggested Members of Health Care Team to Guide Adolescents in Issues Arising in Pregnancy*

Issues	Discipline					
	Obstetrician	Adolescent Medical Specialist	Nurse	Nutritionist	Social Worker	Psychologist
General health and planning of continuous care		X	X	X	X	
Complications of pregnancy	X	X	X	X		
Labor and delivery preparation	X	X	X			
School program					X	X
Economic resources			X		X	
Substance abuse (cessation and education)		X	X	X	X	X
Psychological adjustment and stress	X	X	X	X	X	X
Developmental delay			X		X	X
Infant-care education		X	X	X		
Relinquishment counseling			X		X	X
Nutritional care		X	X	X		
Education		X	X	X		
Resource coordination			X	X	X	
Family or marital conflict					X	X

From Rees JM: *Nutritional counseling in adolescence.* In Mahan LK, Rees JM: *Nutrition in adolescence,* St Louis, 1984, Mosby–Year Book.

Extrapolations cannot always be made from the known requirements of adults or children. There will be specific nutritional objectives in each of the special circumstances of adolescent life.

In dealing with a client with an eating disorder, the overall objective is to help the individual put the eating function into proper perspective. The athlete must obtain sufficient nourishment to support a growing body that is subjected to stress. If a pregnancy should occur, the adolescent will need support in nourishing herself and her developing infant during a chaotic time. Although a great deal is still unknown about nutritional needs of adolescents, the growing interest in this age group should stimulate the research necessary to close gaps in our knowledge.

Structure	Communication pathways	Best serves
Undisciplinary (Pt)◄──────►(A) (Case manager)	Direct from patient to professional	Uncomplicated problems in competence area of one discipline
Serial undisciplinary (Pt) ►(A) ►(B) ►(C) (Case manager)	Direct from patient to professional; lack of contact between disciplines; patient coordinates care	Complicated problems necessitating more than one discipline
Multidisciplinary (Pt)◄──►(A)►(B) ►(C) ►(D) (Case manager)	Direct from patient to professional who acts as case manager; other professionals consult with case manager but do not communicate with other disciplines or with patient apart from assessment	Multiple problems falling in purview of several disciplines; some disciplines may overlap
Interdisciplinary (A) (Pt) (B) (D) (C) (Case manager)	Direct among patient and all professionals; case manager coordinates care	As above

FIG. 14-7   Structure of health care teams. *Pt,* Patient; *A, B, C, D,* health care specialists of various disciplines.

(From Rees JM: *Nutritional counseling in adolescence.* In Mahan LK, Rees JM: *Nutrition in adolescence,* St Louis, 1984, Mosby–Year Book.)

❖ ❖ ❖

CASE STUDY

Nourishment of an Adolescent Athlete

Kevin is a 16½-year-old, 6-foot, 150-lb high school student who is a dedicated swimmer. His weekly workout schedule is:

 6:00–7:00 A.M. swim, 3 days/week
 5:00–6:30 P.M. swim, 5 days/week
 8:00–9:00 P.M. swim, 5 days/week
 Saturday: 8:30–10:00 A.M. swim
 Sunday: rest day

Swimming workouts often require 3 to 4 hours/day and include 11,000 to 12,000 yards of swimming.

Kevin goes directly from his morning workout to school. He takes a sack breakfast and lunch from home. After school he prepares and eats a dinner meal at 3–3:30 P.M. He consumes another meal after the afternoon workout at 7:00 and a snack after the evening workout at about 9:30 P.M.

Kevin is often hungry and must "work" at maintaining his weight. A one-day record of Kevin's intake is:

 7:30 Breakfast: 4 cups skim milk, 5 maple bars, 16-oz cran-grape juice
 11:30 Lunch: 1 8-oz blueberry yogurt, 1 candy bar (Starburst)

 3:30 Dinner 1: ½ 10-in. cheese pizza, 4 cups skim milk, 1 can soda
 7:30 Dinner 2: 4 cups skim milk, 1 maple bar
 9:30 Dinner 3: 1 bagel, 3 oz beef, mustard, 4 cups skim milk,
 Extras: 4½-oz package butterscotch hard candies

This pattern of food choices provides about: 4400 kcal energy, 200 gm protein, 65 gm fat, 15 mg iron, and 5600 mg calcium.

1. What would you recommend as a usual daily energy intake?
2. What protein intake would you recommend?
3. What calcium and iron intakes would you recommend?
4. Would you assess Kevin's current intake as adequate?
5. Would you recommend a vitamin/mineral supplement?
6. What changes would you recommend to optimize nutrient intake?

REVIEW QUESTIONS

1. Discuss the commonalities and differences of specifically recognized syndromes across the spectrum of eating disorders.
2. Describe how a comprehensive weight management program would be set up for teenagers in a community where none had previously existed.
3. It has been proposed that adolescents need to gain more weight during pregnancy than adult women. What aspects of adolescent growth and development lead to the idea that these larger gains are beneficial?
4. What are the most important dietary issues for adolescent athletes?
5. What are the characteristics of effective counseling for adolescents?

SUGGESTED LEARNING ACTIVITIES

1. Prepare a discussion about the specific dietary issues important to adolescent athletes for a high school track team.
2. Develop an explanation you can give to a 15-year-old pregnant teenager as to why she will be counseled to gain more weight than her mother did when she was pregnant with her daughter.
3. Explain to an obese teenage boy who has not experienced a growth spurt why he should not try to lose weight rapidly. Test his fitness (as described in chapter 13) and help him develop an improvement plan.
4. Speak with a teenager about lowering the fat content in his or her diet.
5. Develop a graph depicting all the factors that contribute to the development of eating disorders in adolescents.

REFERENCES

1. Troiano RP, Flegal KM, Kuczmarski RJ, Campbell SM, Johnson CL: Overweight prevalence and trends for children and adolescents: the National Health and Nutrition Examination Surveys, 1963–1991, *Arch Pediatr Adolesc Med* 149:1085, 1995.
2. Moore DC: Body image and eating behavior in adolescents, *J Am Coll Nutr* 12:505, 1993.
3. Story M, French SA, Resnick MD, Blum RW: Ethnic/racial and socioeconomic differences in dieting behaviors and body image perceptions in adolescents, *Int J Eating Disord* 18:173, 1995.
4. Contento SR, Michels JL, Williams SS: Adolescent food choice criteria: role of weight and dieting status, *Appetite* 25:51, 1995.
5. Bruch H: Developmental considerations of anorexia nervosa and obesity, *Can J Psychiatry* 26:212, 1981.
6. Minuchin S and others: *Psychosomatic families: anorexia nervosa in context,* Cambridge, Mass, 1978, Harvard University Press.
7. *Diagnostic and statistical manual of mental disorders,* ed 4, Washington, DC, 1994, American Psychiatric Association.
8. Farrow JA: The adolescent male with an eating disorder, *Pediatr Ann,* 1992.
9. Keys A and others: *The biology of human starvation,* vols I and II, Minneapolis, 1950, University of Minnesota Press.
10. Thompson JK, Covert MD, Richards, KJ, Johnson S, Cattarin, J: Development of body image, eating disturbance and general psychological functioning in female adolescents: covariance structure modeling and longitudinal investigations. *Int J Eating Disord* 18:221, 1995.
11. Meyer AE and others: Psychoendocrinology of remenorrhea in the late outcome of anorexia nervosa, *Psychother Psychosom* 45:174, 1986.
12. Commerci G: Medical complications of anorexia nervosa and bulimia nervosa. In Farrow JA, editor: Adolescent medicine, *Med Clin North Am* 74:1293, 1990.
13. Bachrach LK and others: Decreased bone density in adolescent girls with anorexia nervosa, *Pediatrics* 86:440, 1990.
14. Nussbaum M and others: Cerebral atrophy in anorexia nervosa, *J Pediatr* 96:867, 1980.
15. Rigotti NA and others: The clinical course of osteoporosis in anorexia nervosa: a longitudinal study of cortical bone mass, *JAMA* 265:1133, 1991.
16. Nussbaum MP and others: Blunted growth hormone responses to clonidine in adolescent girls with early anorexia nervosa: evidence for an early hypothalamic defect, *J Adol Med* 18:145, 1990.
17. Dolan RJ and others: Structural brain changes in patients with anorexia nervosa, *Psychol Med* 18:349, 1988.
18. Laessle RG and others: Depression as a correlate of starvation in patients with eating disorders, *Biol Psychiatry* 23:719, 1988.
19. Steiger H and others: Relationship of body-image distortion to sex-role identification, irrational cognitions, and body weight in eating-disoriented females, *J Clin Psychol* 45:61, 1989.
20. Brinch M and others: Anorexia nervosa and motherhood: reproduction pattern and mothering behavior of 50 women, *Acta Psychiatr Scand* 77:611, 1988.
21. Rock CL, and Curran-Celetano J: Nutritional disorder of anorexia nervosa: a review, *Int J Eating Disord* 15:187, 1994.
22. Polivy J, Herman CP: Diagnosis and treatment of normal eating, *J Consult Clin Psychol* 55:635, 1987.
23. Rowland TW and others: The effect of iron therapy on the exercise capacity of nonanemic iron-deficient adolescent runners, *Am J Dis Child,* 142:165, 1988.
24. Mendelson BK, White DR, Schliecker E: Adolescents' weight, sex and family functioning, *Int J Eating Disord* 17:73, 1995.
25. Rees JM: Management of obesity in adolescents. In Farrow JA, editor: Adolescent medicine, *Med Clin North Am* 74:1275, 1990.
26. Himes, JH and Dietz, WH: Guidelines for overweight in adolescent preventive services: recommendations from an expert committee, *Am J Clin Nutr* 59:307, 1994.
27. Report of a WHO Expert Committee: *Physical status: the use and interpretation of anthropometry,* WHO Technical Report Series 854, World Health Organization, 1995.
28. Pencharz PB and others: The effect of a weight-reducing diet on the nitrogen metabolism of obese adolescents, *Can J Physiol Pharmacol* 66:1469, 1988.
29. Bennett W: Dietary treatments of obesity, *Ann NY Acad Sci* 499:250, 1987.
30. Boxer G, Miller BD: Treatment of a 7-year-old boy with obesity hypoventilation (Pickwickian syndrome) on a psychosomatic inpatient unit, *J Am Acad Child Adolesc Psychiatry* 26:798, 1987.
31. Hoerr SLM, Nelson RA, Essex-Sorlie D: Treatment and follow-up of obesity in adolescent girls, *J Adolesc Health Care* 9:28, 1988.

32. Ikeda JP and others: Two approaches to adolescent weight reduction, *J Nutr Educ* 14:90, 1982.

33. Mellon LM, Slinkard LA, Irwin CE: Adolescent obesity intervention: validation of the SHAPE-DOWN program, *J Am Diet Assoc* 87:333, 1987.

34. Kinston W and others: Interaction in families with obese children, *J Psychosom Res* 32:513, 1988.

35. Marquardt LF, Koszewski W, Sobal J: Motivation, risks, and nutrition counseling for weight loss in athletes, *Top Clin Nutr* 10:48, 1994.

36. Steen SN, Oppliger RA, Brownell KD: Metabolic effects of repeated weight loss and regain in adolescent wrestlers, *JAMA* 260:47, 1988.

37. Woods ER, Wilson CD, Masland RP: Weight control methods in high school wrestlers, *J Adolesc Health Care* 9:394, 1988.

38. Buzina K and others: Vitamin C status and physical working capacity in adolescents, *Int J Vitam Nutr Res* 54:55, 1984.

39. Nickerson HJ and others: Causes of iron deficiency in adolescent athletes, *J Pediatr* 114:657, 1989.

40. Mahan LK, Escott-Stump S: *Krause's food, nutrition and diet therapy*, ed 9, Philadelphia, 1996. WB Saunders.

41. McArdle WD and others: *Exercise physiology: energy, nutrition, and human performance*, ed 2, Philadelphia, 1986, Lea & Febiger.

42. Squire DI: "Heat illness: fluid and electrolyte issues for pediatric and adolescent athletes," *Pediatr Clin North Am* 37:1085; 1990.

43. Drinkwater BL and others: Bone mineral density after resumption of menses in amenorrheic athletes, *JAMA* 256:380, 1986.

44. Story M, editor: *Nutrition management of the pregnant adolescent: a practical reference guide*, Washington, DC, 1990, MCH National Clearinghouse.

45. Scholl TO and others: Maternal growth during pregnancy and decreased infant birth weight, *Am J Clin Nutr* 51:790, 1990.

46. Harrison KA and others: Growth during pregnancy in Nigerian teenage primigravidae. In Harrison KA, editor: Child-bearing, health and social priorities: a survey of 22,774 consecutive hospital births in Zario, Northern Nigeria, *Br J Obstet Gynaecol* 55:32, 1985.

47. Story M, Alton I: Nutrition issues and adolescent pregnancy, *Nutr Today* 30:142, 1995.

48. Rees JM, Lederman SA: Nutrition for the pregnant adolescent, *Adol Med: State of the Art Reviews* 3:439, 1992.

49. Rees JM and others: Position of the American Dietetic Association: nutrition management of adolescent pregnancy, and technical support paper, *J Am Diet Assoc* 89:900, 1989.

50. Haiek L, Lederman SA: The relationship between maternal weight for height and term birth weight in teens and adult women, *J Adolesc Health Care* 10:16, 1988.

51. Frisancho AR and others: Developmental and nutritional determinants of pregnancy outcome among teenagers, *Am J Phys Anthropol* 66:247, 1985.

52. Taffel S: *National Center for Health Statistics: maternal weight gain and the outcome of pregnancy*, United States, 1980, Vital and Health Statistics, Series 21, No 44, DHHS Pub No (PHS) 86-1922, Washington, DC, June 1986, US Government Printing Office.

53. WHO Collaborative Study: Maternal anthropometry and pregnancy outcomes. *Bull WHO* 73:1, 1996.

54. Rosso P, Lederman SA: *Nutrition in the pregnant adolescent*. In Winick M, editor: *Adolescent nutrition*, New York, 1982, John Wiley & Sons.

55. Garn SM, Petzold AS: Characteristics of the mother and child in teenage pregnancy, *Am J Dis Child* 137:365, 1983.

56. Stevens-Simon C, McAnarney ER: Adolescent maternal weight gain and low birth weight: a multifactorial model, *Am J Clin Nutr* 47:948, 1988.

57. Scholl TO, Hediger ML: A review of the epidemiology of nutrition and adolescent pregnancy: maternal growth during pregnancy and its effect on the fetus, *J Amer Coll Nutr* 12:101, 1993.

58. Scholl TO, Hediger ML, Schall JI, Khoo CS, Fischer, RL: Maternal growth during pregnancy and the competition for nutrients, *Am J Clin Nutr* 60:183, 1994.

59. Scholl TO, Hediger ML: Weight gain, nutrition, and pregnancy outcome: findings from the Camden study of teenage and minority gravidas, *Semin Perinatol* 19:171, 1995.

60. Institute of Medicine, National Academy of Sciences: *Nutrition during pregnancy*, Washington, DC, 1990, National Academy Press.

61. Hediger ML and others: Rate and amount of weight gain during adolescent pregnancy: associations with maternal weight-for-height and birth weight, *Am J Clin Nutr* 52:793, 1990.

62. Rees JM and others: Weight gain in adolescents during pregnancy: rate related to birthweight outcome, *Am J Clin Nutr,* 56:868, 1992.

63. Maso MJ and others: Anthropometric predictors of low birth weight outcome in teenage pregnancy, *J Adolesc Health Care* 9:188, 1988.
64. Skinner JD, Carruth BR: Dietary quality of pregnant and nonpregnant adolescents, *J Am Diet Assoc* 91:718, 1991.
65. Farrow JA: *Homeless pregnant and parenting adolescents: service delivery strategies,* Maternal and Child Health Technical Information Bulletin, Public Health Service, USDHHS, Nov, 1991.
66. Ketterlinus RD, Henderson SH, Lamb, ME: Maternal age, sociodemographics, prenatal health and behavior: influences on neonatal risk status, *J Adolesc Health Care* 11:423, 1990.
67. Hardy J, Duggan AK: Teenage fathers and the fathers of infants of urban, teenage mothers, *Am J Public Health* 78:919, 1988.
68. Rees JM: *Nutritional counseling in adolescence.* In Mahan LK, Rees JM: *Nutrition in adolescence,* St Louis, 1984, Mosby–Year Book.
69. Reynolds S, Faulkner P: *Interviewing and counseling skills.* In Story M, editor: *Nutrition management of the pregnant adolescent: a practical reference guide,* Washington, DC, 1990, National Center Education Maternal Child Health.
70. Faulkner PL: *Strategies for dietary change.* In Story M, editor: *Nutrition management of the pregnant adolescent: a practical reference guide,* Washington, DC, 1990, National Center Education Maternal Child Health.
71. Silber TJ: Physician-adolescent patient relationship, *Clin Pediatr* 19:50, 1980.
72. Rogers CR: A counseling approach to human problems, *Am J Nurs* 56:994, 1956.
73. Hackney H, Cormier LS: *Counseling strategies and objectives,* Englewood Cliffs, NJ, 1979, Prentice-Hall.
74. Brill NI: *Teamwork: working together in the human services,* Philadelphia, 1976, JB Lippincott.

15

Nutrition and Special Health Care Needs

Peggy L. Pipes
Robin Pritkin Glass

+++

Objectives

After studying this chapter, the student should:

✔ *Be aware of the many physical and environmental factors that affect food and nutrient intake in children with special health care needs.*

✔ *Be able to identify children at risk for nutritional problems for whom preventive intervention is appropriate.*

✔ *Have knowledge of ways to secure anthropometric indices for children with contractures.*

✔ *Recognize factors that may modify the energy needs of children with special health care needs compared with those of average children.*

✔ *Be able to screen children with motor difficulties that affect eating and who need referral to a therapist.*

✔ *Have knowledge of the many factors that must be assessed to design an intervention program for any nutritional and feeding problems that may be found in developmentally delayed children.*

Between 10% and 15% of children in the United States have special health care needs that include chronic illnesses, motor difficulty and/or developmental disorders. Many of these children have more than one developmental or medical problem. A significant number have issues that result from maternal abuse of alcohol or drugs during pregnancy or from maltreatment and neglect. Children with **acquired immune deficiency syndrome (AIDS)** have unique problems that must be addressed.

Many children and families will require several disciplines or programs to control or resolve nutrition concerns. Currently the development of community-based interdisciplinary teams is encouraged. Since many of the children are at risk of difficulties in achieving an adequate nutrient intake, the inclusion of a dietitian/nutritionist on the team is essential. Services should be family centered and delivered in a culturally relevant manner.[1]

DEVELOPMENTAL DELAYS

Approximately 3% of all infants and children are developmentally delayed. Often these children also have medical conditions (such as heart disease or seizure disorders) that may increase or modify their nutrient and energy needs. In addition, psychosocial factors, developmental delays, or motor dysfunctions may create nutritional and feeding concerns.

Nutritional problems in this population range from severe undernutrition to gross obesity; activity patterns range from immobility to hyperactivity. Often a nutritional problem is caused by several etiological factors. For example, a child with failure to thrive and osteomalacia may be undernourished because of inadequate energy intake secondary to oral motor dysfunction and parent-child interactions; the osteomalacia may result from the metabolic interaction of drugs and nutrients.

Commonly reported parental and professional concerns relating to handicapped children's food and nutrient intakes include the following:

1. Slow growth in length and lack of appropriate weight gain
2. Excessive weight gain in relation to length gains
3. Obesity
4. Iron deficiency anemia
5. Refusal of the child to consume specific foods or groups of foods
6. Refusal of the child to progress in feeding behavior when developmentally ready
7. Pica
8. Bizarre feeding patterns
9. Lack of appetite
10. Excessive appetite
11. Gagging, vomiting, or rumination
12. Food allergies
13. Limited fluid intake
14. Constipation
15. Abnormal motor patterns that affect the child's ability to consume food
16. Inability or unwillingness of the child to finger feed or self-feed
17. Limited attention span at mealtime
18. Disruptive behavior at mealtime

Difficulties in weight control are often clustered in specific syndromes. Obesity is common in children with **Down syndrome, Prader-Willi syndrome, Carpenter syndrome, Cohen syndrome,** and **Laurence-Moon-Biedl syndrome.** Underweight is frequently noted in children with **Rett syndrome,** athetoid cerebral palsy, hyperactivity, and behavior problems.

Underweight children with limited energy intakes commonly have less than desirable intakes of several nutrients because of the limited volume of food they consume. Inadequate intakes of vitamins A, C, and D and folate are the most frequent problems.

Feeding problems and growth retardation appear to be issues most often in children with cerebral palsy, congenital heart disease, and who are deaf and blind. Children who have oral motor dysfunction and who require assisted feeding have lower nutrient and energy intakes and are shorter and leaner than children with normal oral patterns and who can feed themselves.[2,3]

NUTRITIONAL NEEDS OF CHILDREN WITH DEVELOPMENTAL DELAYS

Children with developmental delays require the same nutrients as any individual. However, no dietary recommendations exist that are applicable to groups of developmentally delayed children. Many of these children, although not all, are growth delayed because of a genetic or biological defect. Syndromes with which growth retardation is associated include Down syndrome, Prader-Willi syndrome, **trisomy 13 and 18 syndromes, Cornelia de Lange's syndrome, Hurler syndrome, Russell-Silver syndrome,**

FIG. 15-1   Arm span measured from tip of one middle finger to the other.

Williams syndrome, and many syndromes and conditions whose etiology remains unknown.

Early studies of the growth and nutrient intake of developmentally delayed children were conducted primarily in institutions on children with cerebral palsy. More recent studies have focused on children in the free-living population and on nutrition problems encountered in specific syndromes.

Measurements of Children with Physical Disabilities

Evaluating the adequacy of a child's nutrient and energy intake includes assessment of his or her physical growth. This means the child must be accurately weighed and measured and the data plotted on growth charts (see chapter 1). However, difficulties may be encountered in securing and interpreting the data for children who have developmental delays.

Accurate measurements of linear growth may be impossible to secure for children who have contractures or cannot stand. Crown-rump length or sitting height can be used to estimate height. The measurements, however, cannot be considered accurate when a child's trunk or torso is affected. Arm span can be used to estimate length in children so affected. For those

who have contractures of the arm, tibia length, though less accurate, can also be used with a formula to estimate length.

Arm span measurements are made with an anthropometer, a stainless steel detachable rod approximately 7 feet long with etched gradations to 0.1 cm and one movable sleeve. The arm span has been defined as the greatest distance between the outstretched fingers of the right and left hands with the arms and forearms extended horizontally sideways and the back pressed against a flat surface. To secure this measurement, the subject stands in the erect position with arms outstretched (fig. 15-1). The fixed end of the anthropometer is held by one individual at the tip of the individual's middle finger of one hand, while another individual positions the sleeve at the tip of the middle finger of the person's other hand. The person is then told to stretch his or her arms, and the movable sleeve is adjusted to the maximum arm span.

Estimation of linear length and height using tibia length had higher standard errors because of the dynamics of relative tibial length. Although less accurate than arm span, this measurement is believed to provide useful information for individuals who have contractures in the arms and have previously been mobile.

Tibia length is defined as the distance between the medial tibial epicondyle to the medial malleolus.[4] To measure tibia length, individuals are seated with their feet resting as flat on the floor as possible. The top of the right tibia is located by palpating downward from the medial condyle of the femur to the zone of articulation between the femur and the tibia. This point is marked at the closest approximation to the highest point of the medial condyle of the tibia, which is buried. The tip of the medial malleolus is easily identified and marked. The distance between these two points is measured with a sliding anthropometer (fig. 15-2). Height is estimated from the equation:

$$\text{Height (cm)} = 3.54 \times \text{tibial length} + 32.23$$

Although more data are needed on typical children to establish guidelines, arm span can be used to estimate linear height for children who cannot stand, and tibia length can be used for children with contractures in their arms.

Syndrome-specific growth expectations. Some classifications of handicapped children show expected growth, whereas others with **congenital** or metabolic disorders are associated with significant growth deviation. Researchers realize that the growth curves for typical children are not applicable for individuals with some handicapping conditions and that syndrome-specific reference data are needed. Anthropometric guidelines and growth curves have been developed for several syndromes and have been used successfully in managing patients.[5–10] These growth charts should be used for plotting measurements of these children. For other children who have developmental delays, monitoring the rates of gain in height and weight, weight for height percentiles, midarm circumference, and triceps skinfold measurements over time provides useful information. The professional interpreting this data should have knowledge of specific syndromes associated with growth retardation.

Energy Requirements

Early studies in institutions indicated that retarded children who are ambulatory have energy requirements similar to those of normal children, if height is used as a standard for energy needs. Because short stature was common in the

FIG. 15-2   Tibia length measurement.

population studied, the energy requirements were less than those of other children the same age. Only when motor dysfunction became severe enough to cause children to be nonambulatory did it reduce the energy requirement per centimeter of height significantly.[11] Another early study indicated that a group of emaciated institutionalized children had energy requirements in excess of those of typical children. Even though such children consumed energy intakes recommended for their ages, they remained emaciated. Other studies in the free-living population have indicated that some children with special health care needs have a reduced need for energy compared with the average.

Prepubescent children with Down syndrome have been found to have reduced resting metabolic rates compared with controls.[12] Children with the Prader-Willi syndrome have reduced energy requirements per centimeter of height compared with the average child of the same age. The mean energy requirements for some children with myelomeningocele is 11 kcal/cm of height compared with ~15 kcal/cm of height for the average child; an intake of 7 kcal results in only a slight weight loss.[13]

Children with **spasticity (hypertonia)** frequently become overweight for their heights consuming low-energy intakes for their age. One obese 16-year-old female quadriplegic with spasticity has been described who had a basal energy expenditure of a person half her body weight.[14] Children with athetosis (mixed pattern of too much and too little muscle tone) consume greater intakes of energy than do those with spasticity and are less likely to become obese because they are able to engage in greater amounts of activity. Some children with **athetosis** expend energy constantly in involuntary movements. Basal energy expenditures have been noted to be similar to average children while the energy cost of activity depends on the child's capacity for muscular work. As levels of activity reach limits, activity becomes costly and uneconomical.

Many children with developmental delays are less active than their peers because of low muscle tone, immobility, or general disinterest in their environments. This inactivity limits their energy expenditure and therefore their energy requirements. Children with cerebral palsy who have decreased levels of activity have been noted to need 10 kcal/cm of height, whereas those with normal or increased levels of activity need 15 kcal/cm of height.[14]

Recommendations for energy intakes of children with developmental delays must be individualized. Because physical activity of these children frequently deviates from the typical, kcalories of energy per centimeter (kcal/cm) may prove to be a more useful reference on which to base estimated energy needs than kcalories per kilogram of energy (kcal/kg) of body weight.

DRUG AND NUTRIENT INTERRELATIONSHIPS

Many drugs affect the gastrointestinal tract, appetite, absorption, and/or metabolism of nutrients. Those most often of concern to the nutritional well-being of children with special health care needs are the anticonvulsants. These drugs prescribed to control seizures increase children's need for vitamin D and alter their folate metabolism.

Evidence of vitamin D deficiency has been found in both institutionalized patients and outpatients treated with anticonvulsant drugs for longer than 6 months for control of seizures. Serum calcium levels may be normal or low; serum parathyroid hormone concentrations may be increased; serum phosphate levels may be low; and serum alkaline phosphatase levels may be elevated. Plasma 25-OHD levels have been found to be low. The degree of reduction of serum 25-OHD concentrations correlates with the relative decreases in serum calcium concentration, intestinal calcium absorption, and bone mass.[15] The result of these biochemical anomalies can be rickets and osteomalacia, most often when the drugs have been taken longer than 6 months. All drugs commonly used to control seizures have been implicated. The incidence of abnormalities increases with duration of therapy. Multiple drug regimens cause the most problems. The abnormalities may result from an increase in hepatic microsomal catabolism or a biliary excretion of vitamins. The drugs may also have an inhibitory effect on calcium transport and bone metabolism. In addition, some believe that anticonvulsant drugs may affect the metabolism of vitamins D_2 and D_3 differently.

Rickets and osteomalacia are most often diagnosed in nonambulatory individuals who have infrequent exposure to sunlight and receive a combination of anticonvulsant medications. Amounts of vitamin D necessary to prevent deficiency and rickets in children receiving anticonvulsant therapy appear to vary depending on the number and dosage of anticonvulsant drugs, the duration of therapy, the pattern of mobility, and the exposure to sunlight.

Folate. Drug-induced disturbances of folate metabolism have been found in a significant number of patients receiving anticonvulsants. Phenytoin is the drug of primary concern; however, therapy with phenobarbital, primidone, or carbamazepine is also associated with folate deficiency. Low serum folate levels accompanied by a fall in red blood cell folate and cerebrospinal folate levels have been reported in 27% to 91% of patients studied. Megaloblastic anemia is reported to occur in only a small number of patients. The mechanism by which these drugs cause a fall in folate concentrations is not understood. Suggested hypotheses include: malabsorption of folate, compromised transport of folate into the tissue, and depletion of folate from its use as a cofactor in some metabolic process.[15]

Administration of folate has been reported to precipitate seizures or to increase seizure frequency in some patients treated with anticonvulsants. In most patients no effect has been noted. At least eight different large controlled studies found no significant difference in seizure frequency between folate-deficient patients treated with folate and those treated with placebo.

Long-term anticonvulsant therapy may be associated with other vitamin deficiency states. Clinical evidence of cardiac beriberi and subclinical ascorbic acid deficiency has been noted in a 28-month-old black girl who allegedly was receiving a full diet in a nursing home and was receiving phenobarbital, phenytoin sodium (Dilantin), and primidone (Mysoline).[16]

MEGAVITAMIN THERAPY

For many years there have been claims that megadoses of vitamins and minerals will increase the intelligence of children who are developmentally delayed. Evidence supporting these claims is scant and unconvincing. Not much attention has been focused on this therapy. However, attention is refocused periodically on the hypothesis and parents have renewed hopes about the resolution of their children's problems and questions about the use of a variety of vitamin supplements for a number of disorders, including Down syndrome, mental retardation, autism, learning disabilities, and others.[15] A number of studies conducted on children and adults have not yielded any evidence of increases in intelligence, motor performance, or communicative abilities of the individuals involved. However, some who offer the supplements for sale continue to offer false hope at considerable expense to families of affected children.

PICA

Pica, an eating disorder noted in some institutionalized individuals but also found occasionally in the free-living population, has been shown to result in malabsorption of zinc and iron and can lead to lead poisoning depending on the nonfood items ingested. Individuals with pica have been shown to have low plasma zinc levels and low measures of iron status even though they had received an adequate dietary intake of the minerals.[17]

FEEDING CHILDREN WITH DEVELOPMENTAL DELAYS

Planning for feeding children who are developmentally delayed implies that recommendations for intakes of energy, nutrients, and textures of food, as well as expectations for the acquisition of self-feeding skills, must be individualized for each child. Some children may have oral, fine and gross motor, language, and personal-social development that is proceeding at a less than normal rate. Others may also have physical anomalies that imply the need for special equipment to sustain sitting posture to eat and to adapt utensils to self-feed.

Many of the problems of nutrient intake in children with developmental delays are preventable. Guidance and support for parents as they select nutritionally adequate foods for their children, and as they create an environment in which children learn to consume foods in a manner appropriate for their developmental level, are important. Parents may need instruction to understand the appropriate time at which to change the textures of food, to determine when to expect the child to self-feed, and to know the degree of messiness to expect when a child is self-feeding.

Factors That Influence Food Intake

Because of the many factors that interact to determine the food available to and accepted by children who are developmentally delayed, concerns about food and nutrient intake and feeding rarely result from a single cause; many factors must be considered. An understanding of those factors that contribute to problems of food intake is important in planning for feeding of such children.

Children with developmental delays experience the same responses to parental anxiety about their food intake as any child; they too can control their parents by their acceptance or rejection of food. Most normal preschoolers reduce their intakes of milk and vegetables, go on food jags, and have brittle, unpredictable appetites. It is not unreasonable to expect children with developmental delays to present the same food-related behavior. There may be, in addition, difficulties in feeding these children that are not encountered with typical children.

Developmental level. Delays in motor development may result directly or indirectly in an appropriate nutrient intake. The development and sequence of acquisition of feeding behaviors of children with delays proceed in the same orderly predictable sequence as that of typical children. The chronological age at which the developmental stages occur, however, is not predictable, and wide ranges are seen both in the timing at which stages occur and in the ultimate developmental level of function of children with delays. Abnormal motor and behavioral patterns may interfere with the sequence of development and acquisition of feeding skills.

Parents who fail to recognize developmental readiness often fail to provide children with appropriate stimuli. If this happens, parents do not encourage their children to progress in the oral motor skills of eating and the gross and fine motor skills of self-feeding. For example, parents may offer their children strained foods when they are capable of masticating coarser foods, or they may feed their children who have the ability to learn to feed themselves.

Readiness to accept solids is demonstrated blatantly in typical children and is difficult to ignore: they reach for food and bring it to their mouths. Children with disabilities may give more subtle clues, and as a result the stage is often ignored. Some parents do not realize the importance of the introduction of solids at the proper time. When these parents finally decide it is time for children to learn to eat table food, conflicts often occur between children and their parents that may appreciably reduce the children's nutrient and energy intakes. The children refuse to eat at all or skillfully spit out lumps while sucking and swallowing the soft, strained foods.

Some children are hypersensitive in the oral area. It may be important for an occupational, physical, or speech therapist to institute a program to normalize sensation before presenting more textured foods to the child.

Many children have such significant delays that they are totally dependent feeders. Feeding the infant is a culturally defined maternal role, but feeding a child with a disability over a period of many years may become a tedious process that interferes with other activities several times a day. Some parents become so overwhelmed with such a schedule that they continue feeding soft foods that do not support developmental progress; others cease their efforts at feeding their children before the children consume sufficient food.[18] Achieving self-feeding skills may appreciably increase the child's nutrient intake, self-confidence, and self-image.

Children whose delays in motor development impair their ability to learn to walk must be moved by their caregivers. The more weight the children gain, the more difficult they become to lift, move, and care for. Parents and caregivers of such children have expressed concern about the difficulties that may be created for them when children grow and gain weight; some have been known to limit inappropriately the amounts of food they feed. Obesity must be prevented, but children should have the advantage of nutrient and energy intakes that support the best possible growth and development for them. Parents may need information and counseling in methods of moving and caring for their children and in accepting their needs for increased amounts of nutrients and energy.

Abnormal oral-motor patterns and muscle tone. Children with developmental delays, particularly those who also have abnormalities in muscle tone and movement patterns, frequently also demonstrate abnormal oral-motor patterns. They may have pathological oral-motor patterns, that is, oral patterns that are never observed as part of the normal developmental sequence, or may show primitive oral patterns with the retention of primitive oral reflexes. These immature, primitive, or abnormal patterns can make the acquisition of mature feeding skills difficult. For example, a child who sucks reflexively when food is placed in the mouth cannot learn to chew until this reflexive behavior is integrated and more isolated movements of the lips, tongue, and jaw are developed.[19]

Abnormalities in overall muscle tone can exacerbate problems in oral control. Many pathological oral patterns are seen in association with specific types of abnormal muscle tone and are frequently heightened by these tonal abnormalities. A tongue thrust may be seen as part of increased **extensor** tone throughout the body. With **extension** of a child's head, the tongue thrust can be exaggerated. Hypotonia of the body and face may lead to inadequate stability of the oral musculature. The mouth will tend to be open and lip closure will be poor. Asymmetry in the distribution of muscle tone can be observed in jaw deviation toward the more involved side during chewing or during opening of the mouth for spoon insertion. In addition to abnormalities of tone and movement, children with developmental delays may have oral-facial structural anomalies. Clefts of the lip or palate or deviations in the shape or size of oral features, such as micrognathia, can significantly affect oral control. If these facial anomalies are also combined with abnormalities in muscle tone, feeding difficulties will be compounded.

Primitive oral reflexes. The full-term infant is typically born with a variety of well-established oral reflexes making the infant fully equipped to take in nourishment. The human fetus has a primitive swallow by 12.5 weeks' gestation and sucking behavior by 14 weeks' gestation, and the fetal swallow is sufficiently mature for functional use at roughly 36 weeks' gestation.[20] The child with motor and developmental delays, however, may retain the primitive oral reflexes and not develop the voluntary oral motor patterns that subsume the role of the primitive reflexes. Most of these primitive oral reflexes are involved in the sucking and swallowing of liquids or pureed foods. If they are retained, the child will be unable to develop the more mature oral movements involved in chewing higher textured foods.

In a child who has feeding difficulties, evaluation of individual primitive oral reflexes may provide some insight into the nature of the feeding difficulty. Ingram,[21] however, believes that merely testing oral reflexes provides little information about the individual's feeding abilities other than the presence of basic reflex arcs. Rather, Ingram states that one needs to consider how the primitive reflexes are integrated with breathing, adaptive feeding behavior, and vocalizations to adequately assess a child's feeding problems.

Protective oral reflexes. In addition to primitive oral reflexes, several important protective reflexes remain with the child through life and are not superseded by other functions. These are the cough and **gag reflexes.** The cough reflex protects against foods or liquids entering the airway or serves to remove them should they become aspirated. It is a violent expiratory effort preceded by a preliminary inspiration; the accessory muscles of expiration are brought into action as air is noisily expelled. When related to food, the stimulus is the presence of food or liquid in the laryngeal vestibule that must be expelled so that it does not enter the airway. The gag reflex serves to keep food items or foreign bodies that are too large and could potentially cause obstruction from entering the pharynx or the esophagus. Gagging occurs when the soft palate is stroked or pressure is applied to the posterior wall of the pharynx or the posterior half of the tongue; there is an arching of the tongue, mouth opening, head extension, and facial grimacing. Intense gagging may induce a vomit response.

In typical development, the gag reflex is frequently elicited when a baby puts a toy far into the mouth. Oral play helps the child to accommodate to a variety of sensations and aids in the normal reduction in the intensity of the gag reflex. Through oral exploration, the infant experiences a variety of textures, temperatures, shapes, and sizes that may lay the groundwork for future learning. The parent of a child with feeding problems, however, often reports that the child never participated in this usual mouthing stage of development. This fact should alert the professional to a potential problem with a hyperreactive gag response. In this case, gagging may be elicited to a wide variety of food tastes, textures,

A   B

FIG. 15-3 **A,** Child with cerebral palsy being tube-fed. Note the asymmetry of arms and legs and lack of head and trunk control. **B,** In a specialized chair she has better head and trunk control and can engage in more age-appropriate feeding behaviors.

or even smells that are new and unfamiliar to the child. This type of hypersensitive gagging may often be observed in children who have had a period of nonoral feeding such as gastrostomy tube feeding.

The gag reflex can also be inhibited or sensitized (increased) by physiological or psychological factors. A physiological sensitization may occur when a person is ill, dizzy, or emotionally upset. The normal reaction to these feelings is to avoid eating. If food were to be offered or forced, the reaction might well be a gag. Fear of choking resulting from a previous incident may cause a gag response at the sight of a particular food. This behavior usually receives attention from adults who frequently do not persist in offering the undesirable food. When there has been a lengthy period of nonoral feeding, the child may become unaccustomed to touch and taste within the mouth. When foods are introduced, gagging may result from lack of previous sensory experiences with foods. Children with these sorts of behavioral responses often severely restrict the variety of food textures in their diet, resulting in further sensory deprivation and

increased oral sensitivity. Treatment to decrease this hypersensitive response is needed to change feeding behavior and improve nutrition. This type of treatment is discussed in the next section.

Transition from tube to oral feeding. For many infants and children with developmental delays, feeding performance is so impaired that they require supplemental or total nonoral feedings. The need for nonoral feedings can stem from severe oral-motor dysfunction that impairs the ability to take appropriate quantity or quality of nutrition (fig. 15-3), from medical conditions that limit the child's endurance for feeding, from food refusals because of hypersensitive and aversive feeding behavior, or secondary to swallowing dysfunction. Nonoral feedings can occur through a gavage tube (through the nose or mouth), via a gastrostomy tube, or below the stomach via duodenal or jejunal tubes. Nonoral feeding may only be needed for a short period of time but frequently is required for lengthy periods to support overall good nutrition and appropriate growth.

Since oral/tactile hypersensitivity can result from the lack of oral experiences that occurs during tube feeding or may be the factor that resulted in the need for a tube, professionals should begin treating oral hypersensitivity at the time tube feedings are instituted and not wait until a transition off the tube is considered to deal with this problem area. Frequent, pleasurable oral experiences need to be continued even though feeding may occur via the tube. This can be done through oral play and mouthing of toys, through hygiene activities like toothbrushing, and through physical contact with the face and mouth.

The association between sensations in the mouth and sensations in the stomach can be maintained by using a pacifier during tube feedings. For the toddler or older child who is receiving gastrostomy feedings, the hunger-satiation cycle may be established by normalizing the volume at each gastrostomy feeding to approximate the usual mealtime schedule. Thus a gastrostomy-fed child who receives six equal-volume feedings per day might have the schedule changed to three larger gastrostomy "meals" and three smaller gastrostomy "snacks." This feeding schedule would approximate that of a typical child and would help the developmentally delayed child experience hunger and satiation while still maintaining the necessary energy intake per day. It will set the stage for the transition of not using the tube.

At some point the professionals managing the child's care may believe that a transition from the tube to oral feeding is indicated. The professionals need to establish that the child is indeed ready to make the transition off the tube. They need to determine that the original problem that necessitated the tube feeding has been resolved. If not, then some level of tube feeding may still be indicated. The child needs to have sufficient oral-motor control to allow food intake to occur safely and in a reasonable length of time. In addition, the professionals need to establish that the child's swallowing abilities allow for safe feeding. Not only does the child need to show readiness, but the parents and caregivers also need to be ready to participate in the process. Programs to make the transition from tube to oral feeding require a high level of parent and caregiver involvement and persistence to be successful. Their readiness

and commitment to the program are crucial to ensure success.

Once readiness has been established, a treatment program can be developed. It is at this point that problems with oral and tactile hypersensitivity may become apparent when the transition from nonoral to oral feeding begins. If oral treatment has always been a part of the child's feeding plan, this oral hypersensitivity may be manageable. If the oral hypersensitivity or aversive behavior is more significant, however, a treatment program under the direction of an occupational, speech, or physical therapist is indicated. Treatment for hypersensitivity to oral and tactile stimulation is a gradual, careful program of increasing the amount and variety of oral-sensory experiences.[22] The program is carefully graded according to the child's response because overstimulation could cause negative emotional and behavioral reactions or further increases in abnormal muscle tone that might interfere with feeding to a greater extent than the original problem. The therapeutic techniques used to normalize facial and oral sensitivity therefore are varied according to the individual child's reactions and needs.

Treatment programs designed to make the transition from the use of supplemental or tube feedings generally take a slow, more gradual approach. The child who has been fed via a tube for a long period may have missed the critical or sensitive period for the introduction of solid foods. Therefore the process can take months or several years to complete. Some programs, however, are designed to make this transition more quickly—in a matter of weeks. These types of programs generally require an inpatient stay. They are strongly behaviorally based and have an element of force-feeding to them. Patient selection criteria for these types of programs is stringent. The decision regarding what type of transition program is appropriate for each individual child should be made in consultation with a multidisciplinary team that may be involved with the child.

Components of feeding treatment programs
Oral-motor therapy. When oral-motor dysfunction is present and is interfering with feeding, a treatment program should be developed by an occupational, speech, or physical therapist

to improve oral control. These treatment programs often include facilitation or inhibition techniques to improve control of the lips, tongue, jaw, or cheeks. Hands-on support to the jaw during feeding is frequently used as a technique to improve the grading of jaw movement, improve tongue position, and increase lip control.[23,24] Specialized spoons, cups, or bottles may enhance oral control.

Alterations to the diet can be made to support the child's highest level of oral-motor control. This is particularly true for liquids. Thin liquids are frequently difficult or impossible for a child with oral-motor dysfunction to swallow. Thickening liquids may enable the child to drink by mouth. When liquids are thickened, they may hold together in a more cohesive bolus and move through the mouth and pharynx more slowly so that the child is better able to move the liquid from the front of the mouth to the back and prepare for swallowing. Liquids can be thickened with baby rice cereal, pureed foods, or commercially available thickeners such as Thick-it. If liquids are thickened, the amount of liquid consumed in the child's daily diet should be monitored carefully to ensure adequate hydration.

Positioning during feeding. The position of the child during feeding is of prime importance, since abnormal gross motor patterns can influence and impede oral control. Frequently a child's feeding difficulties can be greatly improved just by changes in the child's position during meals. Normalization of the child's muscle tone through positioning may minimize abnormal oral movement patterns and increase the child's voluntary oral control. Proper positioning considers the child as a whole—the relationship of the head position to the body as well as the overall body position.

Head position is especially important for children who have oral-motor dysfunction or swallowing difficulties and do not have a normally responsive gag or cough response. The child should never be fed with the head or body tipped backward in a position often referred to as a **"bird-feeding"** position. In this position normal swallowing and tongue control are impaired. The food bolus will slide into the pharynx without control, and the child is in danger of aspirating or choking. Acute or chronic aspiration could then lead to pneumonia or other respiratory difficulty. The head should therefore always be upright or slightly flexed forward 5 degrees to 10 degrees. The body should be upright or, if support is needed for head and trunk, within 30 degrees of vertical.

Children with feeding problems, especially those with abnormal muscle tone, are often difficult to position. It is essential that a pediatric, occupational, or physical therapist assess each child and recommend appropriate positioning. If the child has a customized, adapted seating device that is used at other times, it should also be used for feeding. Adapted positioning during mealtimes should be comfortable for both the child and the caregiver and should enable communication and interaction.

Figure 15-4 demonstrates some feeding positions that may be prescribed by occupational and physical therapists. Each position incorporates basic principles of appropriate, therapeutic positioning. The head is in good alignment with the body, and the mouth is in the midline. With the head aligned with the body or slightly **flexed** forward, abnormal head extension or pushing backward can be inhibited. In some children this pushing back with the head is not caused by increased extensor tone, but rather it is a compensatory behavior that reflects an inability to stabilize the head in an upright position. Whether the abnormal head position is caused by increased tone or by a lack of stability, proper head support during feeding can significantly affect oral-motor control.

The position of the arms is also related to and influences head and trunk control. When the arms and shoulders pull backward, the head tends to tilt backward and overall muscle tone increases. Therefore the shoulders and arms should be held forward and oriented toward the midline of the body. This forward position of the arms can be achieved by the manner in which the child is held near the feeder's body or by rolled towels or cushions placed behind the child's shoulders in the child's chair. Some children learn to stabilize their arms forward by grasping the far end of the wheelchair tray or supporting themselves with both elbows on the table.

FIG. 15-4 **A,** A young infant or child can be fed while being held in one's lap. The head is in line with body, and arms are forward. With left knee raised, hip flexion can be maintained. **B,** When firmly wedged, a young child can be fed while facing the feeder. Legs are abducted and flexed, which inhibits extension. The feeder's hands are freed to assist with jaw control. **C,** Rolls can be inserted into wheelchair to provide temporary trunk support and help keep arms forward and toward midline.

Trunk stability is essential because the trunk provides the base on which to achieve good head and arm control. If the child is unable to sit independently, support should be provided by the feeder or through the use of an adapted seating device. The position of the hips and legs affects trunk control and thus influences the position of the rest of the body. Extension at the hips can increase tone throughout the body and cause extension of the head, tongue, and jaw. Stiffness or spasticity in the legs can cause the legs to pull together, narrowing the child's sitting base and impairing the postural adjustments needed for sitting balance. Lateral support to the hips may be a component of the child's seating device, or a pommel can be placed between the child's legs to widen the base of support and to provide adequate leg separation.

The hips should be flexed to a 90-degree neutral position or slightly greater. This increased hip flexion can be provided by adding a wedge to the child's chair with the larger edge under the child's knees. Often just a seatbelt firmly fastened across the hips keeps the hips in a normal neutral position and provides a better base for trunk control. Finally, good stability at the feet can be achieved with a foot rest allowing the feet to be flat and flexed at the ankle.

Proper positioning during mealtime supports the child's highest level of oral-motor control. The relationship between the child's gross motor level at rest and during eating must be considered so that excessive demands are not placed on the child's gross motor skills. For example, a child may be able to sit independently with good head control when simply sitting and watching an activity. The level of the child's head and trunk control may deteriorate, however, when a child is eating or self-feeding. Mealtime should not be the time to make the child work on better head and trunk control. Rather, sufficient support should be provided through adapted positioning to reinforce the child's motor level while fostering better oral and feeding skills.

In addition to the type of static positioning used during meals, the environment and the placement of the food or spoon can influence the child's feeding skills. If the spoon and foods are presented above eye level, the child may tilt the head backward to orient toward the food and thus reinforce an extension pattern. Presenting the food in the middle, from a low angle, encourages slight head flexion and symmetry. Likewise, placing the container or plate of food at the side may encourage the child to turn sideways and increase asymmetry. By placing the food in front of the child, a symmetrical midline position can be encouraged. The manner in which the spoon is withdrawn from the mouth can also influence head position. If the spoon is lifted up and scraped against the upper front teeth, the head will tend to tilt backward and lip control will be impaired. In addition, if the feeder simply scrapes the food off on the upper teeth or lips, the child does not have the opportunity to use lip closure.

The foregoing information should prove useful in improving the quality of food intake when therapy services are not immediately available. It is important to use a problem-solving approach that includes ideas and feedback from the child and the caregiver. Consideration of the child's and the caregiver's comfort, feelings, and opinions when making changes in positioning or feeding techniques is likely to yield a workable plan with better follow-through. Changes in motor control may be slow to develop, but the quality of the daily feeding experience and the amount of positive interaction it allows the child will have great impact on the skills that develop.

Cerebral Palsy

Children with cerebral palsy have abnormal motor patterns that range from hypotonia to hypertonia and include spasticity and athetosis. They may or may not be developmentally delayed. Those who have average intelligence but no language may be treated as if they were delayed by those who do not recognize signs of typical intelligence. The frustration resulting from this behavior may affect an already fragile appetite.

Body composition of individuals with cerebral palsy may differ from those of typical individuals. Studies are limited but one indicated that such children have reduced cell mass resulting from atrophy of skeletal muscles as a result of disease and low levels of physical activity. If this is a valid judgment, reduced cell mass may reduce the requirement for essential nutrients and energy.

Children with cerebral palsy generally grow in height and weight at rates less than average. Weight may be greater than that of typical children in children with spastic cerebral palsy and less than average in children with athetoid cerebral palsy. Oral motor involvement may be associated with growth retardation. Most health care practitioners believe that mouth area involvement is closely associated with poor food intake, and that the extent of mouth involvement is limiting on nutrient and energy intakes, and as a result slow growth is associated. A relationship between oral motor involvement as defined by two or more of the following—weak suck, swallow, **tongue thrust,** tongue incoordination, **tonic bite reflex,** lip retraction, hypotonia of the tongue and lips, and growth retardation—has been noted.[20] Children with cerebral palsy who had oral-motor problems were significantly thinner for their age and height than their age-matched counterparts who had cerebral palsy but no oral-motor impairment. They were also shorter, but this was of borderline significance. Bone age delays of 2 to 47 months have been reported by several investigators indicating less than expected maturation for age.[13]

Studies of free-living populations of children with cerebral palsy have shown acceptable intakes of nutrients other than iron. Dietary intakes of less severely retarded children have been found to be markedly higher in all nutrients except vitamins A and C than intakes of the more severely delayed children. The energy value of the diets is influenced by the children's ability to self-feed. Children with motor involvements and mental retardation severe enough to interfere with their ability to feed themselves tend to consume fewer kcalories than do those who are able to self-feed.

Prader-Willi Syndrome

Children with Prader-Willi syndrome have nutritional problems both in infancy and in older childhood. An absence of the long arm of chromosome 15 is found in 60% of individuals with Prader-Willi syndrome. The remaining individuals with Prader-Willi syndrome have either maternal disomy, a submicroscopic deletion of chromosome 15, or an imprinting genetic mutation in the region of chromosome 15. Diagnosis is made on the basis of clinical symptoms.

Infants with the syndrome are hypotonic at birth; most have a weak suck. Failure to thrive is common in the first year. They often require tube feeding. Between 2 and 4 years of age these children become obese, unless aggressive intervention is instituted before the rapid rate of weight gain. An insatiable appetite will be noticed. Then food behaviors that include gorging, stealing, and hoarding food develop. They eat unusual food items such as raw hamburger and ornamental berries. One individual with Prader-Willi syndrome ate 12 pies at one sitting and 14 milkshakes at one time.

Most of these children gain excessive weight if permitted an energy intake recommended for typical children their age. Restriction of energy

intakes to approximately two-thirds of the RDA is necessary to maintain a weight gain within the growth channel. However, the ranges of appropriate intake are wide at any age. The following is one successful approach to management of weight control in children with this syndrome. Parents record (in household measures) all food offered and returned for 30 consecutive days. During this period individuals are weighed on a beam balance scale every 2 weeks. The energy value of the food consumed is calculated. The energy value of weight lost or gained is added to or subtracted from this energy value of that consumed (using the conversion figure of 7.7 kcal/gm of weight change). The individual's energy needs per centimeter of height are estimated by dividing the height into total energy expended, and a diet plan to effect weight maintenance or loss is prescribed.

Successful intervention requires control of the environment so that food is totally inaccessible to the child with Prader-Willi syndrome. Refrigerators and cupboards must be locked. Food must be removed from the table as soon as a meal is finished. The children must be supervised at school so that they do not steal others' lunches or rummage in the garbage.

Down Syndrome

Children with Down syndrome (trisomy 21) often have problems with nutrient intake. Some have conditions that require nutrition therapy or that can be prevented by anticipatory nutrition guidance. For example, there is a high incidence of cardiac anomalies among infants with Down syndrome. The child therefore may lack the endurance to ingest sufficient nutrients. Early or repeated cardiac surgery may lead to the use of supplemental tube feeding or the delayed introduction of solid foods. These children frequently have difficulty with tongue control and have tongue protrusion or a tongue thrust that impairs eating ability. Constipation secondary to hypotonia is not uncommon. Overweight has been suggested as a characteristic of children with Down syndrome from 2 to 3 years of age to adolescence. Some believe there is a constitutional but not inevitable tendency for individuals with this syndrome to be obese. A recent study has indicated that prepubescent children with Down syndrome have decreased metabolic rates compared with controls.[12] To prevent the onset of obesity, careful planning of energy intake is important.

Limited intakes of nutrients may create concern. One study of 47 children with Down syndrome from ages 6 months to 6 years noted 16% to have low intakes of calcium, 14% to have low intakes of iron, and 10% to have low intakes of vitamin D and ascorbic acid. Feeding problems were also identified. These children commonly refused to chew textured food when developmentally ready to do so. This resulted in the child accepting only a limited variety of foods. Social and emotional situations also resulted in feeding problems that compromised feeding and the children's nutrient intakes or developmental progress in feeding behavior or both.

Early individual or group intervention has proven effective in remediating these problems. Effective programs use an interdisciplinary approach including a nutritionist, an occupational or physical therapist, and a behaviorist. Counseling and therapy should focus on developmental readiness for the transition to appropriate textures of foods, the use of food to support developmental progress, parental feelings about and interaction with their children, physical growth, maintenance of appropriate weight for height, and foods that supply appropriate nutrients.

Rett Syndrome

Rett syndrome, a degenerative disorder affecting only females, results in a number of food, feeding, and nutrition issues as the children grow older. The girls grow and develop typically until 6 to 9 months of age when developmental stagnation begins and the rate of head growth declines. Previously acquired skills may be lost. Stereotypical hand movements that include hand wringing, clapping, tapping, and mouthing begin. The majority of the girls grow in channels below the 5th percentile on the NCHS growth charts. Many require long-term anticonvulsant therapy.

The etiology of the syndrome is unknown. There is speculation that an inborn error of carbohydrate metabolism may be the cause.

Oral-motor dysfunction is often a problem of girls with Rett syndrome. Over 50% have poor lip closure and drool. Most girls with Rett syndrome learn to feed themselves, although they may go through phases when self-feeding is lost and then regained. Most girls with Rett syndrome are undernourished even though they have good appetites and consume more energy than would be expected for their age. However, some adolescents and adults have been noted to be overweight during clinical observation. Constipation is a concern of all individuals with Rett syndrome.

The range of nutrition concerns presented in girls with this syndrome mandate that therapy be individualized. Therapy is most likely to focus on increasing weight of the undernourished and on resolving constipation through dietary approaches. Because an inborn error of carbohydrate metabolism is suspected, a high-fat diet may be suggested. In some instances a ketogenic diet to control seizures may be prescribed. Texture of the food offered to these individuals often has to be modified. Most girls are able to eat soft, well-cooked food. It is often mashed with a fork, but sometimes it must be pureed. Thickening liquids may make them more acceptable. Attention should also be given to the interaction of drugs and nutrients.

Phenylketonuria

Infants born with metabolic disorders are at high risk for developmental disorders. Early detection, intervention, and surveillance are urgent. Of the many disorders identified, programs for the hyperphenylalanemias are the most comprehensive because mental retardation can be prevented if treatment is begun immediately after birth.

Currently, all states have newborn screening programs for children with **phenylketonuria (PKU)** and other disorders. Blood samples obtained by heel prick and applied to Guthrie filter paper are taken from every infant before he or she leaves the nursery. Infants who leave the hospital before 24 hours of age are screened again at 1 week of age.[25] Newborns with a positive screening test are tested again by both qualitative and quantitative methods. Criteria for the diagnosis of PKU are blood levels of phenylalanine consistently above 16 to 20 mg/dl (900–1200 μmol/L) and normal tyrosine levels.

Nutrition therapy. Effective management of PKU requires special formulas, food products modified in their content of phenylalanine, and a cohesive team that includes the child, parent, nurse, social worker, psychologist, and pediatrician. Goals of nutrition therapy include both the provision of an adequate energy and nutrient intake and restriction of phenylalanine to maintain appropriate blood levels (2 to 6 mg/dl or 120–360 μmol/L) so that typical growth and development proceed. To achieve these goals blood levels are taken frequently, and the diet is adjusted until the exact prescription for the individual child is developed.

Several low-phenylalanine or phenylalanine-free formulas supplemented with tyrosine are available. These formulas are designed to meet age-specific nutrition needs, thus the manufacturers have developed formulas for infants and toddlers, and older children. In early infancy and childhood, these special formula or medical food mixtures should provide 90% of the protein and 80% of the energy needed by the individual. Foods with a low phenylalanine content are introduced when it is developmentally appropriate for the child and in amounts to maintain the desired blood phenylalanine levels.

Appropriate nourishment and maintenance of sufficiently low blood phenylalanine levels contribute to normal physical and cognitive development. Blood levels continue to be monitored frequently, and adjustments are made in children's phenylalanine intake to support their changing needs as they grow.

Current recommendations are to continue the diet throughout adulthood. Discontinuation of the diet has resulted in learning difficulties, progressively decreasing IQ, poor attention span, and behavioral difficulties. Structural changes in the white matter of the brain, which caused neurological difficulties, have been found in adolescents and young adults who have discontinued or relaxed dietary treatment and have allowed blood phenylalanine levels to rise.[25]

Environmental Deprivation

Children who are developmentally delayed from lack of appropriate stimuli are at risk for an inappropriate nutrient intake as well as environmental deprivation. These children frequently live in families that have limited economic resources and limited education. The parents may have poor interpersonal and parenting skills. They may abuse drugs or alcohol or both; they may have learning or developmental disabilities or both. Frequently the parents are young and single. Their children may also have experienced abuse or neglect; some may have experienced hunger, others inappropriate nutrient intake. Most families rely heavily on convenience and prepackaged foods. When food is offered, gorging or hoarding may be secondary to erratic feeding times. On the other hand, children may have familiarity with and accept only a few foods. Delayed feeding behaviors such as continued use of a bottle and eating of strained food when children are developmentally ready to consume food in a more mature manner may be noted.

When children who have experienced deprivation are identified, it is likely that a number of agencies will be involved in alleviating the cause of the environmental deprivation. Therapy will be intensive and prolonged. Surveillance will be provided, and efforts will be made to maintain children in their homes. However, in some situations foster placement is indicated. While the child is in a new environment and probably an early childhood stimulation program, efforts will be made to motivate and educate the parents to care for their children. Some parents will need help in planning food and mealtimes for their children, creating an environment for the children to learn nutritionally and socially appropriate food habits, and responding appropriately to their children's food behaviors. Efforts are usually made to return children to their natural parents. However, if they cannot be returned to a safe and nurturing environment, a permanent out-of-home placement or adoption may be planned.

Parents are often overwhelmed by the numbers of agencies and individuals involved in helping the child and family. In many instances, parents are given guidance from several individuals about what and how to feed their children. Often the advice is conflicting, and the parents then become confused and frustrated. To avoid this, a team approach is most appropriate. The nutritionist may be asked to provide education directly to the parent or other family members such as the grandparents. However, it may be more productive for the individual who is providing other services to include a nutrition and feeding plan as a part of their intervention efforts. In all instances, efforts should be made to see that the parents are instructed in only one approach on what and how to feed the children.

Bronchopulmonary Dysplasia

The number of children with bronchopulmonary dysplasia (BPD) in the community has increased in the last decade because of an increase in the survival of premature infants who have received oxygen and ventilation for the treatment of **hyaline membrane disease.** The problem may also be found in full-term infants. There may be medical problems such as heart disease secondary to BPD. Feeding difficulties and poor weight gain are also common.

Growth and development of new lung tissue can occur. The process is slow and may require continued oxygen, physiotherapy, medications, and nutritional support. It is likely that infants will remain hospitalized until they can tolerate feeds, even if they must be taken by tube.

Difficulties in achieving an adequate nutrient intake are common in these children. Most infants and children expend more than average energy in breathing. Respiratory infections also contribute to increased energy needs. Infants with BPD may expend as much as 25% to 50% more energy than typical, healthy babies. The elevated energy needs are likely to continue into childhood. There is, however, a subgroup of children with BPD who have lower than average energy needs. These include those who require mechanical ventilation, are steroid dependent, have a slow rate of linear growth, or have limited activity.

Eating difficulties, such as anorexia, secondary to illness or medication may create problems in achieving an appropriate intake. Infants may have difficulty coordinating sucking, breathing, and swallowing. They may tire easily during a feed. Gastroesophageal reflux and episodes of vomiting may make feeding aversive.

Heights and weights of children with BPD should be monitored frequently, and adjustments in nutrient and energy intakes should be made on the basis of medical status, growth

rate, and activity level. Fluid shifts need to be carefully evaluated. When children have difficulty meeting their energy needs, only food with high energy density should be offered. Small frequent feeds should be timed so that the effects of medication, chest physical therapy, and suctioning will not have an aversive effect on food intake. Diets should include at least 7% of the energy from protein to avoid excess fat and carbohydrate. Children with BPD may require multiple medications that necessitate monitoring fluid and electrolyte intakes.[26]

Acquired Immunodeficiency Syndrome

Pediatric acquired immunodeficiency syndrome (AIDS) was the 9th leading cause of death in children 1 to 4 years of age in 1987 and the 12th leading cause of death in children 5 to 24 years of age the same year. Of the children identified 80% had been infected in the gestational period. Evidence collected to date indicates that 25% to 35% of infants born to infected mothers will ultimately be infected. Postnatally, infants can become infected during breastfeeding. Most other cases have resulted from blood or plasma transfusions.[27]

The mean gestational age of infants born with **human immunodeficiency virus** (HIV) is less than those not infected. They are smaller for gestational age; their head circumference and length are less than those not infected. Also, they have a greater incidence of bacterial infection.[28]

Children with AIDS experience a number of medical problems that compromise their nutritional status and make the consumption of adequate nutrition difficult and in some cases impossible. Many live with parents who are also infected and often with low incomes. Abdominal pain, recurrent diarrhea, and failure to thrive are common in infected children. They may develop oral thrush, dysphagia, and a diminished appetite. A variety of bacterial infections determine the medical course of the children's therapy. Complications include infection, *Pneumocystis carinii* pneumonia, oral and esophageal candidiasis, herpetic gingivostomatitis, nonspecific diarrhea, and fever.[29] A pattern of developmental delays in infancy and progressive cognitive delays in older children, most pronounced in fine and gross motor and speech, occurs.

Acquired microcephaly and cerebral atrophy become evident as the disease progresses. School-age children become mildly to moderately retarded. There are problems with visual motor tasks. The majority have a pattern of plateaus and deceleration with a declining course.

Children with AIDS experience weight loss and decreased triceps skinfold thickness and arm circumference resulting from a greater decrease in lean body mass than fat. A decrease in serum protein levels indicates protein energy malnutrition.

A task force on nutrition support for AIDS has suggested nutrition goals for infected individuals (table 15-1). They include the preservation of lean body mass, provision of an adequate nutrient intake, and minimization of the symptoms of malabsorption. An energy-dense formula may be used for infants. Protein intakes of 1.5 times the RDA and a multiple vitamin and mineral supplement have been suggested. Frequent high-energy and nutrient-dense feeding should be readily available. During diarrhea adequate potassium must be provided. When children have oral lesions, soothing foods such as ice cream, nonacidic juices, and puddings should be offered. Nasogastric feedings may be used to supplement oral intakes.[30] If oral or tube feedings cannot support an adequate nutrient intake, total parenteral nutrition (TPN) may be used. However, oral or gavage feedings should continue to maintain sucking ability, mastication, and deglutition and to promote repair of the intestinal mucosa.

Fetal Alcohol Syndrome

Fetal alcohol syndrome (FAS), the birth defect that results when the fetus is exposed to the teratogenic effects of alcohol, is the most common known cause of mental retardation in the Western world. Since FAS is only the tip of the iceberg, many children exposed to alcohol in utero who do not have the syndrome may exhibit fetal alcohol effect (FAE). It is important to recognize that this syndrome is totally preventable by abstinence from alcohol during pregnancy.

Features of the fetal alcohol syndrome include craniofacial anomalies, growth deficiency, and central nervous system effects. The children have short palpebral fissures, a hypoplastic or long philtrum, a thin upper lip, a flat midface, a short upturned nose, a small chin, eye anomalies including strabismus and some minor anomalies of the external ear. Other anomalies that occur less frequently include heart defect and cleft lip and palate. Auditory and vision problems and malformed and misaligned secondary teeth are also frequently noted. FAS effects include learning disabilities, language delays, and attention deficit disorders. Children who have the fetal alcohol effect (FAE) do not have all of the abnormalities but have some of the symptoms of FAS.

Growth deficiency in height or weight is present at birth and continues during childhood. The growth deficiency results from the prenatal insult and is not usually associated with nutritional deficiency. In adolescence weight gain among females is so common that the short thin prepubescent phenotype may change into the obese adult. The short stature remains in both sexes into adulthood. During the preschool-age years hyperactivity, language, and motor problems become evident. During the school-age years attention and memory deficits are often noted.

Children with FAS have poor appetites secondary to their slow rate of growth. Most are finicky about the foods they will accept. Behavior problems often result from the parental concern about the child's slow growth and limited food intake compared with average children their age. Delays in the acquisition of feeding skills secondary to their delay in growth rate may be of concern to parents and may exacerbate feeding problems. If the children remain in homes with alcoholic parents, they may experience erratic meal patterns, the use of much convenience foods, and occasionally lack of an adequate nutrient and energy intake.

Nutritional intervention is not specific to FAS but approaches similar to these described for the environmentally deprived individual should be instituted. For children whose attention span is limited, small, frequent feedings may result in a more appropriate intake than three meals a day. During adolescence, weight gain should be monitored. Counseling should focus on teaching those individuals whose rate

TABLE 15-1   *Plan for Nutrition Intervention in the Pediatric Patient with AIDS*

Problem	Approach
Poor oral intake	Evaluate food preferences
	High-energy, nutrient-dense feedings
	Frequent snacks
	Nutritional supplements
	Multivitamin supplement
	Tube feedings—supplemental or total diet
	Parenteral nutrition
Oral lesions	Soft, nonirritating foods served cold or at room temperature
	Nonacidic juices
Infection/pneumonia	Increase energy and protein
	Multivitamin supplement
Receiving steroids	Sodium restriction
	Encourage foods high in potassium, calcium, and vitamin C
	Multivitamin supplement
	Folate supplement if indicated
	Avoid overconsumption
Diarrhea/malabsorption	Lactose restriction
	Elemental diet
	Slow, continuous drip tube feeding
	Parenteral nutrition
	Avoid long-term severe dietary restrictions, which cause poor intake
Abdominal distention	Elemental diet
	Parenteral nutrition
Fever	Keep patient hydrated (e.g., with popsicles, gelatin)
	Increase energy and protein
Developmental problems/ neurologic impairment	Utilize feeding therapist (knowledgeable speech, physical, or occupational therapist or dietitian)
	Bottle-feed or spoon-feed as necessary

From Bentler M: *J Am Diet Assoc* 87:488, 1987.

of weight gain is excessive an appropriate food intake and exercise pattern.

Children of Drug-Abusing Women

Children of mothers who abuse drugs during pregnancy are at high risk for a number of difficulties that affect physical growth, eating, and feeding. The infants are usually irritable and have a greater incidence of tremulous and hyperactive behavior and motor-impaired function than average children. Drug-exposed babies experience fetal growth retardation, lose more than average weight after birth, and take twice as long as average babies to regain birth weight. Interestingly, some infants exposed to cocaine in utero become obese before growing into typical weight. Delays in the acquisition of developmental milestones are often noted. Permanent disabilities may include attention deficits, difficulties in coordination, and atypical mood patterns. These infants are more likely to have medical problems, requiring four times as much medical care as unexposed babies. "Boarder babies," those who are medically ready but whose social problems contraindicate discharge, increase the census in many neonatal units.[30]

Withdrawal from the drugs, typically noted between birth and 4 days of age, usually continues until 2 to 4 weeks of age. Behavior problems that may result and affect feeding include irritability, vomiting, uncoordinated suck-swallow, sneezing and nasal stuffiness, and inability to sleep. Swaddling the infant may help. These infants are often orally hypersensitive.

Infants who are hypertonic, hyperactive, or excessive criers will have increased energy needs ranging from 150 to 250 kcal/kg/day in the neonatal period.[31] Frequent feeds of energy concentrated foods are usually offered. Nasogastric feeds or TPN may be required if oral feeding is unsuccessful. The infants will require monitoring and readjustments of their energy intakes until their energy needs become similar to those of unaffected infants. Breastfeeding may be contraindicated if the mother is still using drugs. Several drugs cross into breast milk and can be detected 12 to 60 hours after use.

Problems for these children are likely to extend beyond the neonatal period. Mothers may lack parenting skills to adequately feed and care for their infants or to provide psychosocial and emotional support for optimal growth and development. Many live on limited incomes and may continue to have problems associated with addictive behavior.

Management of Feeding

The diversity of concerns about the food and nutrient intake of children with disabilities and the many factors that affect such children's level of function and food acceptance imply that the skills of several disciplines may be necessary to find solutions to the concerns and to set priorities for therapy for individual children. The occupational, physical, or speech therapist will be called on to provide therapy for children with abnormal motor tone. The dentist will correct dental caries and malocclusions. A professional proficient in behavior modification techniques

may be required to change behavior. Table 15-2 defines many of the problems an interdisciplinary team serving children with special health care needs may encounter, team members needed to address specific concerns, and possible intervention strategies. Correcting these concerns may solve nutrient intake concerns. Parents may, however, still need help in planning appropriate foods for their children.

Behaviors. Children may have inappropriate nutrient intakes and food habits because of learned behavior. Children learn from the model set for them by their parents, peers, and relatives. If examples of poor food habits are set, the children will imitate them.

Disruptive and inappropriate feeding behaviors such as throwing food and utensils, stuffing the mouth before swallowing, and refusing to eat generally attract parental attention. These behaviors often compromise a child's nutrient intake. Resolution of the problems requires a structured, well-defined behavior modification program. Since, as a rule, behaviors get worse before they begin to get better, energy and nutrient intake should be monitored when the programs are implemented.

The behavior pattern and attention span of children affect their energy and nutrient needs and consumption. Hypoactivity reduces energy expenditure and needs. Lack of planned activity and stimulation for such children often results in boredom, which leads to children spending their days seeking and consuming excessive amounts of food.

Hyperactive children never appear to be quiet and expend much energy in their numerous activities. The attention span of hyperactive children may be as limited at the dinner table as in other activities resulting in very small intakes of food at one time. It may be important to offer hyperactive children frequent small feedings of high nutrient content.

Constipation. Constipation is a common problem in children with developmental delays, especially in those who are hypertonic or hypotonic. The infrequent passage of feces or the passage of unduly hard, dry fecal matter results from a variety of causes, such as lack of muscle

TABLE 15-2 *Nutrition Problems of Children with Special Health Care Needs*

Problem	Children "At Risk" Include Those with:	Team Members Needed	Intervention Strategies
Feeding problem (inability or refusal to eat certain foods or textures because of neuromotor dysfunction or behavioral or psychological factors)	Oral-motor disorders Inappropriate parent-child interaction with food	Nutritionist or dietitian Pediatrician Neurodevelopmental therapist Social worker or psychologist Nurse	Proper positioning Oral-motor feeding program Define reasonable expectations and developmentally appropriate feeding skills and food Behavior management programs
Overweight and obesity	Prader-Willi syndrome Spina bifida Down syndrome Spastic cerebral palsy Hypotonia Decreased mobility	Nutritionist or dietitian Pediatrician Social worker, psychologist, or family therapist	Define appropriate energy intake level for individual child to maintain or lose weight Increase activity Family counseling
Underweight	Athetoid cerebral palsy Oral-motor dysfunction Frequent infections Rett syndrome Attention deficit hyperactive disorder Dysfunctional parent-child interaction Parents who do not know what or how to feed	Nutritionist or dietitian Pediatrician Social worker, psychologist, or behavior therapist	Refer for appropriate therapy Promote appetite with behavior management approach Increase energy density of food offered If severe, may need to consider tube feeding
Constipation	Spina bifida Spastic cerebral palsy Hypotonia	Nutritionist or dietitian Pediatrician Nurse	Increase fiber Increase liquid Regular toileting schedule Stool softener Behavior management

Continued.

tone in the intestine or duodenal wall, excessive fatigue, anxiety, inappropriate dietary intake, or failure to establish a routine bowel pattern. When children are constipated, they usually complain of stomachache, distention, swelling of the abdomen, discomfort, or pain.

Increasing the amount of fluid and roughage in the diet may be useful for treating children who are constipated. Parents should also observe for individual food stimuli. Some children may need to limit milk intake to 1 pint/day. Prunes and prune juice are also frequently helpful.

TABLE 15-2 *Nutrition Problems of Children with Special Health Care Needs—cont'd*

Problem	Children "At Risk" Include Those with:	Team Members Needed	Intervention Strategies
Excessive fluid loss or poor fluid intake	Spastic cerebral palsy Hypotonia Drooling Refusing fluids	Nutritionist or dietitian Behavioral therapist Oral-motor therapist	Position child correctly Oral-motor intervention Thicken fluids, if appropriate Offer foods with high water content
Drug-nutrient interactions	Children who require: Anticonvulsants Tranquilizers Stimulant medications Diuretics AZT	Pediatrician Nutritionist or dietitian	Appropriate vitamin supplements Small, frequent meals and snacks (stimulants) Follow Na, K levels (diuretics) Cool, noncitrus juices for sore mouth (AZT)
Disorders in which early intervention is essential to prevent failure to thrive, mental retardation, and death	Inborn errors of metabolism (e.g., PKU, galactosemia, glycogen storage disease, urea cycle defects)	Nutritionist or dietitian Pediatrician Nurse Social worker Psychologist	Screen at birth to identify infants who need immediate intervention Adjust intake of specific nutrients to neutralize the impact of the metabolic defect while providing adequate nourishment for growth and development

Appetite. Central nervous system damage causes a lack of appetite in some children. These children never express hunger, and some mothers of such children have stated that setting alarm clocks helps them remember to feed their children. Children so affected are rarely pleased by any food and limit the volume of food they consume. The children's unresponsiveness gives the parents no positive reinforcement for their efforts to feed the children. This lack of positive interplay between parent and child may cause dissatisfaction in each; the parents may lose motivation to continue helping the child consume food, and the children may lose motivation to consume appropriate energy and nutrient intakes.

Damage to or developmental defects of the hypothalamus can cause insatiable appetites in children. Children so affected sometimes gorge, steal food, or eat animal food. Extreme measures, such as locking refrigerators and kitchen cupboards, have been necessary to control obesity in such children. Food-related behaviors of such children cannot be altered by behavior modification methods.

Parental Expectations

Parents need to have realistic expectations about the child's potential for physical growth. It is not possible to increase a child's height beyond his or her genetic potential; it is possible to increase a child's weight for height. Parental concern about a child's slow rate of growth may create anxiety about the volume of food the child is consuming. Counseling about expectations and growth response to food intake is important.

People who care for children with disabilities are often overindulgent, giving such children large amounts of preferred high-carbohydrate, sweet foods frequently. As with anyone, it is difficult to design a food intake pattern that provides necessary amounts of essential nutrients and maintains weight gain in growth channel if many of the foods consumed supply only carbohydrate and fat and few other nutrients. It may be important to help parents find ways to express their affection other than with food. Parents should also be aware of why they offer the foods they do.

Identifying readiness to progress. Assessing children's developmental levels of function and their readiness to progress in eating and self-feeding is necessary to define reasonable expectations for parents and caregivers. Parents often need help in accepting their children's disability and in recognizing their potential to progress.

Changes in food and feeding behavior should be effected when the children are developmentally 6 to 7 months of age, when they demonstrate readiness to self-feed and to use a cup. Table 15-3 defines important developmental landmarks and suggested foods appropriate for changes in feeding behavior.

Early intervention programs can aid in preventing later problems of food and nutrient intake.

Assessment of problems and suggested solutions. Efforts to prevent problems of nutrient intake are not always successful. Frequently expressed concerns about food and nutrient intake of children with developmental delays, factors that need to be assessed, and suggested solutions are provided in table 15-4.

Children with developmental delays frequently experience failure in their many efforts. It is therefore important that any plan to modify a child's food intake pattern be designed so that success is obtainable and the child and the parents are reinforced for each gain, however small. Adequate nutrition is important for every child to achieve his or her physical, mental, and emotional potential. Delayed and physically handicapped children should have the advantage of a nutrient intake that can support well-being, optimal growth, and development. Solutions to difficulties in attaining such goals may be complex and may require a multidisciplined approach.

Summary

Children who are developmentally delayed are vulnerable to the same problems of nutrient intake as other children. The incidence of feeding and nutrition problems appears to be greater than in the typical population, and they are often more severe. The causes of nutritional problems in children with developmental delays often involve motor abnormalities or delays, infantilism, and lack of attention to critical periods of development. Therefore an interdisciplinary approach to intervention is appropriate. Specific syndromes are associated with undernutrition; others, with obesity.

REVIEW QUESTIONS

1. List common problems of nutrient intake of children with disabilities.
2. What parameters not found in the average child must be considered when evaluating the adequacy of nutrient intake of a child with developmental disabilities?
3. What measure of physical growth can be used to assess the adequacy of energy and nutrient intake of children who have contractures?
4. What environmental controls are necessary to control the food intake of children with Prader-Willi syndrome?

TABLE 15-3   *Developmental Stages of Readiness to Progress in Feeding Behaviors*

Developmental Landmarks	Change Indicated	Examples of Appropriate Foods
Tongue laterally transfers food in the mouth	Introduction of soft, mashed table food	Tuna fish; mashed potatoes; well-cooked mashed vegetables; ground meats in gravy and sauces; soft diced fruit such as bananas, peaches, pears; liverwurst; flavored yogurt
Voluntary and independent movements of the tongue and lips		
Sitting posture can be sustained		
Beginning of chewing movements (up and down movements of the jaw)		
Reaches for and grasps objects with scissor grasp	Finger-feeding (large pieces of food)	Oven-dried toast, teething biscuits, cheese sticks (food should be soluble in the mouth to prevent choking)
Brings hand to mouth		
Voluntary release (refined digital grasp)	Finger-feeding (small pieces of food)	Bits of cottage cheese, dry cereal, peas
Rotary chewing pattern	Introduction of more textured food from family menu	Well-cooked chopped meats and casseroles, cooked vegetables and canned fruit (not mashed), toast, potatoes, macaroni, spaghetti, peeled ripe fruit
Approximates lips to rim of the cup	Introduction of cup	
Understands relationship of container and contained	Beginning self-feeding (messiness should be expected)	Food that when scooped will adhere to the spoon, such as applesauce, cooked cereal, mashed potatoes, cottage cheese
Increased rotary movement of the jaw	More skilled at cup and spoon feeding	Chopped fibrous meats such as roast and steak
Ulnar deviation of wrist develops		Raw vegetables and fruit (introduce gradually)
Walks alone	May seek food and get food independently	Food of high nutrient value should be available
Names food, expresses preferences; prefers unmixed foods		Balanced food intake should be offered (child should be permitted to develop food preferences without parents being concerned that they will last forever)
Goes on food jags		
Appetite appears to decrease		

TABLE 15-4 Assessment of Concerns About Foods and Nutrients

Symptom	Assessment	Action and Counseling Suggestions
Lack of appetite	What is child's total food and nutrient intake?	Counsel with parents about child's needs and help them obtain needed food
	Is some essential nutrient consumed in insufficient amounts?	Provide only between-meal snacks of high nutrient content at intervals that will not interfere with appetite at mealtime
	Is child receiving adequate amounts of food at other meals without having to eat large amounts?	Serve very small portions
	Is the food properly prepared?	Provide child with a quiet period before mealtime to prevent weariness
	Is child's rate of growth normal in spite of his or her apparent lack of appetite?	Reinforce child's acceptance of food with social reinforcement
	Is child reinforced?	Do not reinforce with food
	When he or she is eating? (appropriate) When he or she is not eating? (inappropriate)	Eat with child to provide a model
	Is child receiving too many snacks? (inappropriate)	Refer the emotionally deprived child to the nurse or social worker
	Is child too weary to eat at mealtime?	
	Is child attending to eating or is his or her attention diverted at mealtime?	
	Is child psychologically deprived?	
Refuses specific groups of foods	Is food properly prepared?	Continue offering very small portions of foods refused
	Has child had previous experiences with the foods?	Reinforce foods accepted with foods child likes
	Does child have a model (parents, teacher, peers) who eats these foods?	Provide a model for child by eating the foods
		Provide guidance in food preparation for children
Inappropriate feeding behavior	What started the behavior?	All inappropriate behaviors should be ignored even if it is necessary to remove child from feeding situation
Throwing	What follows the behavior?	
Gorging	Is child reinforced?	All attempts at appropriate eating should be encouraged through social reinforcement and food the child likes
Stuffing food in the mouth	Is child punished?	
Will not sit at the table	Is child ignored?	

Continued.

TABLE 15-4 *Assessment of Concerns About Foods and Nutrients—cont'd*

Symptom	Assessment	Action and Counseling Suggestions
Refuses to eat table food; insists on strained food	Has child had experience with table food? Has it been offered and refused? Has child eaten table food previously but refuses it currently? How is child positioned for feeding? Can he or she sit upright? Has a critical stage of development been ignored? Is child delayed so that strained foods are appropriate for his or her stage of motor development? Can child bite or chew? Is child hypersensitive in or around the mouth?	Consult with occupational, physical, or speech therapist regarding positioning, development, and hypersensitivity. Seat child in upright sitting position (using props if necessary) If child demonstrates readiness: Choose a food the child enjoys and place it between back molars (watch your fingers) Offer crunchy foods such as arrowroot biscuits, melba toast, crackers (be careful of foods that splinter, such as graham crackers)
Will not bite	Does child have a hypersensitive gag reflex? Does child have dental caries or malocclusion? Can child close the mouth? Has child been offered foods that require biting? Can child breathe through the nose?	Offer easy-to-bite foods such as arrowroot biscuits and melba toast Manually assist child in closing the jaw Provide social reinforcement when child takes a bite
Does not chew with a rotary motion	Is child delayed so that only munching or sucking is appropriate? Can child lateralize the tongue? Has child been offered foods that require chewing? Is child hypersensitive or hyposensitive? Are foods offered that are too tough to chew?	Consult an occupational, physical, or speech therapist regarding lateralization of the tongue and sensitivity Model for child by demonstrating chewing Manually move the jaw in chewing motions Encourage chewing with social reinforcement and with foods child likes
Refuses harder-to-chew foods	Is hypertonia or hypotonia preventing development of oral motor skills? Does child have dental caries? Is child sufficiently delayed that hard-to-chew foods are inappropriate?	Consult with occupational, physical, or speech therapist about oral motor skills; stimulate area around the lips and mouth before feeding as directed Consult about dental caries

❖ ❖ ❖

CASE STUDY

Tube Feeding: Is This Child Ready for Transition to Oral Foods?

The parents of P. C., a 21-month-old male who has quadriplegia secondary to spinal cord injury present at birth, request help because he is dependent on a gastrostomy tube, refuses to eat orally, and has chronic vomiting. He has limited lung capacity because of his quadriplegia and has been hospitalized frequently for pneumonia; a history of failure to thrive in infancy, resulting in the G-tube placement; continued refusal to eat orally; and limited motor ability to self-feed. He has received ongoing oral motor therapy. A videofluoroscopy at 1 month of age indicated normal suck and swallow with both very thin and thickened liquids. There was no evidence of reflux. His current height is 80.4 cm; his weight 20.23 kg.

P. C. currently is given 32 oz of a commercially prepared feeding for children providing 30 kcal/oz a day, and a continuous drip by pump at night, all by tube. In addition he receives a powdered infant and toddler vitamin in 2 oz of fruit juice daily. He gags and vomits often. He is included in the family's three meals and is offered a variety of table foods but does not consume any of the foods offered. He does explore them by touch and brief tastes. He is reported to take sips from a cup, taking turns with his godmother.

Recently P. C. has begun to have tantrums at mealtime. He pounds his G-tube site if more than 155 cc of formula is given. Even the sound of his pump starting will cause him to pound. Another concern is P. C.'s gagging and vomiting, which has been increasing since 15 months.

He gags himself by putting his finger in this throat and recently has been vomiting some at every feed.

Observations during the team evaluation included:

- He requires maximal trunk support for proper positioning during feeding, which is achieved by placement in an adaptive chair.
- He refuses to have any food in his mouth. He was observed bringing his lips together to make babbling sounds.
- Toward the end of the feeding session, after 150 cc has been tube-fed, he began fussing and banged on his tube site. Subsequently he arched and vomited.
- He brought a pretzel to his mouth but made no attempt to bite it. He played with both hands in a cup of water. He grasped a thin-handled toothbrush and moved it toward his face.
- No hunger cues were observed.
- During the tube feeding his mother was more subdued in her interactions with P. C. than at other times.

1. What effect is P. C.'s feeding problem having on his physical growth?
2. Is P. C. receiving an adequate nutrient intake?
3. What other information is needed to determine if P. C. is ready to make the transition from tube feeding to table foods?
4. What do you suspect is responsible for the pounding on the tube, gagging, and vomiting?

5. Why do children with heart and lung disease often have increased energy requirements?
6. Which nutrients must be carefully monitored if a child is taking anticonvulsant medications?
7. Why is an interdisciplinary team important in resolving problems of nutrient intake for children with special health care needs?

SUGGESTED LEARNING ACTIVITIES

1. Describe factors that must be addressed in evaluating the nutrient intake of a 3-year-old child with athetoid cerebral palsy.
2. Describe syndromes associated with both mental retardation and growth failure.
3. Define the nutritionist's role in early intervention programs for developmentally delayed children.

4. How would you respond to parents of a child with developmental delay who were considering megavitamin therapy?
5. Determine an appropriate energy intake for a 14-month-old girl with Down syndrome.
6. Observe a school lunch program in a school for special education. What motor problems of feeding do you observe? What adaptive equipment is being used to facilitate self-feeding?
7. To experience the effect of head position on eating, try to chew or swallow semisolid foods with your head tilted backward. Try to drink with your head tilted backward.
8. To experience the effects of the position of the body on the head and on feeding ability, try to eat with your hips slid forward in the chair without your feet touching the ground.

REFERENCES

1. Kozlowski BW, Powell JA: Position of the American Dietetic Association: nutrition services for children with special health needs, *J Am Diet Assoc* 95:809, 1995.
2. Thommessen M and others: Feeding problems, height and weight in different group of disabled children, *Acta Paediatr Scand* 80:527, 1991.
3. Thommessen M and others: Energy and nutrient intakes of disabled: do feeding problems make a difference? *J Am Diet Assoc* 91:1522, 1991.
4. Zorab PA, Prime FJ, Harrison A: Estimation of height from tibia length, *Lancet* 1:195, 1963.
5. Horton WA and others: Growth curves for height for diastrophic dysplasia, spondyloepiphyseal dysplasia congenita, and pseudoachondroplasia, *Am J Dis Child* 136:316, 1982.
6. Cronk CC and others: Growth charts for children with Down syndrome: 1 month to 18 years of age, *Pediatrics* 81:102, 1988.
7. Butler MG, Meaney FJ: Standards for selected anthropometric measurements in Prader-Willi syndrome, *Pediatrics* 88:853, 1991.
8. Hall JG, Froster-Iskenius UG, Allanson JE: *Handbook of normal physical measurements*, New York, 1989, Oxford University Press.
9. Meany FJ, Farrer LA: Clinical and medical genetics: a compilation of body measurements in genetic and congenital disorders, *Am J Med Genetics* 25:343, 1986.
10. Butler MG, Brunschwig A, Miller LK, Hagerman RJ: Standards for selected anthropometric measurements in males with fragile X syndrome, *Pediatrics* 89:1059, 1992.

11. Ekvall SW: *Pediatric nutrition in chronic disease and developmental disorders*, New York, 1993, Oxford University Press.
12. Luke A, Roizen NJ, Sutton M, Schoeller DA: Energy expenditures in children with Down syndrome: correcting metabolic rate for movement, *J Pediatr* 125 829, 1994.
13. Ekvall SW: *Myelomeningocele*. In Ekvall, SW, editor: *Pediatric nutrition in chronic disease and developmental disorders*, New York, 1993, Oxford University Press.
14. Bandini L, Patterson B, Ekvall SW: *Cerebral palsy*. In Ekvall SW, editor: *Pediatric nutrition in chronic disease and developmental disorders*, New York, 1993, Oxford University Press.
15. Springer NS, Shlafer M: *Drug-nutrient malnutrition*. In Ekvall SW, editor: *Pediatric nutrition in chronic disease and developmental disorders*, New York, 1993, Oxford University Press.
16. Klein G and others: Multiple vitamin deficiencies in association with chronic anticonvulsant therapy, *Pediatrics* 60:767, 1977.
17. Huber AH, Ekvall SW: *Pica and lead toxicity*. In Ekvall SW, editor: *Pediatric nutrition in chronic disease and developmental disorders*, New York, 1993, Oxford University Press.
18. Reilly S, Skuse D: Characteristics and management of feeding problems of young children with cerebral palsy, *Dev Med Child Neurol* 34:379, 1992.
19. Jones PM: Feeding disorders in children with multiple handicaps, *Dev Med Child Neurol* 31:404, 1989.
20. Hooker D: Fetal reflexes and instinctual processes, *Psychosom Med* 4:199, 1942.
21. Ingram TTS: Clinical significance of infantile feeding reflexes, *Dev Med Child Neurol* 4:159, 1962.
22. Arvedson JC, Brodsky L: *Pediatric swallowing and feeding assessment and management*, San Diego, Calif, 1993, Singular Publishing.
23. Tuchman DN, Walter RS: *Disorders of feeding and swallowing in infants and children: pathophysiology, diagnosis and treatment*, San Diego, Calif, 1994, Singular Publishing.
24. Ottenbacher K, Bundy A, Short MA: The development and treatment of oral-motor dysfunction: a review of clinical research, *Phys Occup Ther Pediatr* 3:1, 1983.
25. Report of Medical Research Council Working Party on Phenylketonuria: Recommendations on the dietary management of phenylketonuria, *Arch Dis Childhood* 68:426, 1993.

26. Adams E: Nutrition for the young child with bronchopulmonary dysplasia (BPD), *Nutrition Focus* 6 No. 3, Seattle May/June, 1991, Child Development and Mental Retardation Center, University of Washington.

27. Caldwell MB, Rogers MF: Epidemiology of pediatric HIV infection, *Pediatr Clin North Amer* 38:1, 1991.

28. Nair P and others: Maternal and neonatal characteristics associated with HIV infection in infants of seropositive women, *J Acquir Immune Defic Syndr* 6:298, 1983.

29. Bentler M, Standish M: Nutrition support of the HIV-infected pediatric patient, *J Am Diet Assoc* 87:488, 1987.

30. Barton SJ, Harrigan R, Tse AM: Prenatal cocaine exposure: implications for practice, policy development, and needs for future research, *J Perinatol* 15:10, 1995.

31. Rice-Asaro M and others: Nutritional concerns for children born to drug abusing women, *Nutrition Focus* July/August, 1990, Center on Human Development and Disability, Seattle, University of Washington.

APPENDIX

GIRLS: BIRTH TO 36 MONTHS
PHYSICAL GROWTH
NCHS PERCENTILES*

NAME_____   RECORD #_____

Ross
Growth &
Development
Program

MOTHER'S STATURE _____   GESTATIONAL
FATHER'S STATURE _____   AGE _____ WEEKS

DATE	AGE	LENGTH	WEIGHT	HEAD CIRC.	COMMENT
	BIRTH				

* Adapted from: Hamill PVV, Drizd TA, Johnson CL, Reed RB, Roche AF, Moore WM: Physical growth: National Center for Health Statistics percentiles. AM J CLIN NUTR 32:607-629, 1979. Data from the Fels Longitudinal Study, Wright State University School of Medicine, Yellow Springs, Ohio.

© 1982 Ross Laboratories

GIRLS: BIRTH TO 36 MONTHS
PHYSICAL GROWTH
NCHS PERCENTILES*

NAME _____ RECORD # _____

Adapted from: Hamill PVV, Drizd TA, Johnson CL, Reed RB, Roche AF, Moore WM: Physical growth: National Center for Health Statistics percentiles. AM J CLIN NUTR 32:607-629, 1979. Data from the Fels Longitudinal Study, Wright State University School of Medicine, Yellow Springs, Ohio.

© 1982 Ross Laboratories

DATE	AGE	LENGTH	WEIGHT	HEAD CIRC.	COMMENT

SIMILAC® Infant Formulas
in vivo performance
closest to mother's milk

ISOMIL® Soy Protein Formulas
When the baby can't take milk

ADVANCE® Nutritional Beverage With Iron
Instead of 2% lowfat milk

BOYS: BIRTH TO 36 MONTHS
PHYSICAL GROWTH
NCHS PERCENTILES*

NAME _____ RECORD # _____

*Adapted from: Hamill PVV, Drizd TA, Johnson CL, Reed RB, Roche AF, Moore WM: Physical growth: National Center for Health Statistics percentiles. AM J CLIN NUTR 32:607–629, 1979. Data from the Fels Longitudinal Study, Wright State University School of Medicine, Yellow Springs, Ohio.

© 1982 Ross Laboratories

Ross
Growth &
Development
Program

MOTHER'S STATURE _____ GESTATIONAL

FATHER'S STATURE _____ AGE _____ WEEKS

DATE	AGE	LENGTH	WEIGHT	HEAD CIRC.	COMMENT
	BIRTH				

BOYS: BIRTH TO 36 MONTHS
PHYSICAL GROWTH
NCHS PERCENTILES*

NAME _____ RECORD # _____

Adapted from: Hamill PVV, Drizd TA, Johnson CL, Reed RB, Roche AF, Moore WM.: Physical growth: National Center for Health Statistics percentiles. AM J CLIN NUTR 32:607-629, 1979. Data from the Fels Longitudinal Study, Wright State University School of Medicine, Yellow Springs, Ohio.

© 1982 Ross Laboratories

DATE	AGE	LENGTH	WEIGHT	HEAD CIRC.	COMMENT

SIMILAC® Infant Formulas
Because there's more to growth than just getting bigger™

ISOMIL® Soy Protein Formulas
When the baby can't take milk

ROSS LABORATORIES
COLUMBUS, OHIO 43216
DIVISION OF ABBOTT LABORATORIES USA

G105(0.05)/APRIL 1989   LITHO IN USA

GIRLS: 2 TO 18 YEARS
PHYSICAL GROWTH
NCHS PERCENTILES*

NAME _____   RECORD # _____

Ross
Growth &
Development
Program

*Adapted from: Hamill PVV, Drizd TA, Johnson CL, Reed RB, Roche AF, Moore WM: Physical growth: National Center for Health Statistics percentiles. AM J CLIN NUTR 32:607-629, 1979. Data from the National Center for Health Statistics (NCHS), Hyattsville, Maryland.

© 1982 Ross Laboratories

GIRLS: PREPUBESCENT
PHYSICAL GROWTH
NCHS PERCENTILES*

NAME _____   RECORD # _____

DATE	AGE	STATURE	WEIGHT	COMMENT

*Adapted from: Hamill PVV, Drizd TA, Johnson CL, Reed RB, Roche AF, Moore WM. Physical growth: National Center for Health Statistics percentiles. AM J CLIN NUTR 32:607-629, 1979. Data from the National Center for Health Statistics (NCHS) Hyattsville, Maryland.

© 1982 Ross Laboratories

SIMILAC Infant Formulas
Because there's more to growth
than just getting bigger™

ISOMIL Soy Protein Formulas
When the baby can't take milk

ROSS LABORATORIES
COLUMBUS, OHIO 43216
DIVISION OF ABBOTT LABORATORIES, USA

G108(0.05)/APRIL 1989   LITHO IN USA

BOYS: 2 TO 18 YEARS
PHYSICAL GROWTH
NCHS PERCENTILES*

NAME _____   RECORD # _____

Ross
Growth &
Development
Program

*Adapted from: Hamill PVV, Drizd TA, Johnson CL, Reed RB, Roche AF, Moore WM: Physical growth: National Center for Health Statistics percentiles. AM J CLIN NUTR 32:607-629, 1979. Data from the National Center for Health Statistics (NCHS), Hyattsville, Maryland.

© 1982 Ross Laboratories

BOYS: PREPUBESCENT
PHYSICAL GROWTH
NCHS PERCENTILES*

NAME_____ RECORD #_____

DATE	AGE	STATURE	WEIGHT	COMMENT

Adapted from: Hamill PVV, Drizd TA, Johnson CL, Reed RB, Roche AF, Moore WM: Physical growth: National Center for Health Statistics percentiles. AM J CLIN NUTR 32:607-629, 1979. Data from the National Center for Health Statistics (NCHS), Hyattsville, Maryland.

© 1982 Ross Laboratories

SIMILAC Infant Formulas
Because there's more to growth
than just getting bigger™

ISOMIL Soy Protein Formulas
When the baby can't take milk

ROSS LABORATORIES
COLUMBUS, OHIO 43216
DIVISION OF ABBOTT LABORATORIES, USA

ROSS

G107(0.05)/APRIL 1989   LITHO IN USA

Ross
Growth &
Development
Program

INCREMENTAL GROWTH CHARTS—GIRLS

Growth charts such as those that display the National Center for Health Statistics (NCHS) percentiles are used for routine assessment of physical growth.[1] Occasionally, growth rate (growth velocity or increment divided by time between measurements) should be assessed, eg, when an infant or preadolescent child is found to be at an extreme percentile or when a substantial shift of percentile has occurred on an NCHS growth chart. The accompanying incremental growth charts are useful for assessing growth rates. They do not replace written records of growth data or NCHS growth charts.

These incremental growth charts have been prepared from serial data for white US children whose growth is very close to that of children from whom the NCHS percentiles were derived.[1,2] Highly standardized anthropometric methods that conform to current recommendations were used to make all measurements.[3] Weight was measured as, or corrected to, nude weight. Recumbent length and stature were measured without shoes. Appropriate use of the incremental growth charts requires that similar methods be applied. Ideally, the same person should measure a child at the beginning and end of an interval.

References:

1. Hamill PVV, Drizd TA, Johnson CL, Reed RB, Roche AF, Moore WM: Physical growth: National Center for Health Statistics percentiles. *Am J Clin Nutr* 32: 607-629, 1979.

2. Roche AF, Himes JH: Incremental growth charts. *Am J Clin Nutr* 33: 2041-2052, 1980.

3. Fomon SJ: *Nutritional Disorders of Children. Prevention, Screening, and Follow-up.* Washington, DC: DHEW Publication No. (HSA) 76-5612, 1976.

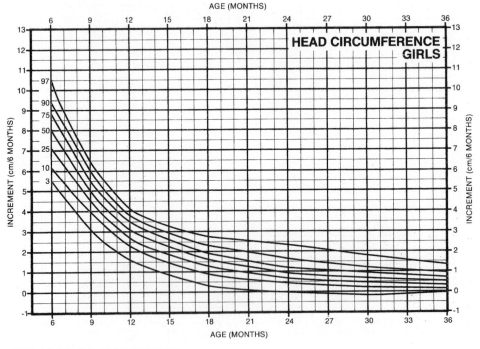

INSTRUCTIONS

1. Measure the child at the beginning and the end of a 6-month interval, if possible.

2. Subtract the initial measurement from the follow-up measurement to obtain the increment.

3. If the interval between measurements is not exactly 6 months (182 days), divide the increment by the interval in days and multiply by 182 to obtain the adjusted 6-month increment. The Table of Consecutively Numbered Days can be used to determine the interval between the measurements. If measurements are made in different years, add 365 to the day of the year for the follow-up measurement. Extrapolating increments from intervals of 3 months or less is not recommended.

4. Locate the intersection of the increment and the child's age at the **end** of the interval to determine the 6-month incremental percentile.

Interpretation: The accompanying charts permit definition of growth rate (growth velocity) relative to current reference data. Further investigation is indicated for children growing at rates markedly different from the 50th incremental percentile or for children whose incremental percentile changes rapidly.

Example 1 Girl at 5th NCHS* percentile at ages 6 and 12 months; aged 12 months at follow-up measurement.			
Measurement	**Length**	**Date**	**Day****
Follow-up	69.8 cm	July 16, 1981	197
Initial	61.8 cm	January 15, 1981	15
Increment =	8.0 cm	Interval =	182

Her increment is 8.0 cm/6 months.
Her increment is between the 25th and 50th percentile.
She is short but growing at a normal rate.

 * National Center for Health Statistics
** From Table of Consecutively Numbered Days

Example 2 Girl, aged 8 years at follow-up measurement.			
Measurement	**Stature**	**Date**	**Day***
Follow-up	118.0 cm	April 22, 1981	477**
Initial	116.9 cm	November 21, 1980	325
Increment =	1.1 cm	Interval =	152

Her adjusted 6-month increment is $\frac{1.1\ cm}{152}$ x 182 = 1.3 cm.

Her increment is below the 3rd percentile.
Further investigation is indicated.

 * From Table of Consecutively Numbered Days
** April 22 is day 112, to which 365 is added because follow-up measurement is in a different year (112 + 365 = 477).

Table of Consecutively Numbered Days

Day	JAN	FEB	MAR	APR	MAY	JUN	JUL	AUG	SEP	OCT	NOV	DEC	Day
1	1	32	60	91	121	152	182	213	244	274	305	335	1
2	2	33	61	92	122	153	183	214	245	275	306	336	2
3	3	34	62	93	123	154	184	215	246	276	307	337	3
4	4	35	63	94	124	155	185	216	247	277	308	338	4
5	5	36	64	95	125	156	186	217	248	278	309	339	5
6	6	37	65	96	126	157	187	218	249	279	310	340	6
7	7	38	66	97	127	158	188	219	250	280	311	341	7
8	8	39	67	98	128	159	189	220	251	281	312	342	8
9	9	40	68	99	129	160	190	221	252	282	313	343	9
10	10	41	69	100	130	161	191	222	253	283	314	344	10
11	11	42	70	101	131	162	192	223	254	284	315	345	11
12	12	43	71	102	132	163	193	224	255	285	316	346	12
13	13	44	72	103	133	164	194	225	256	286	317	347	13
14	14	45	73	104	134	165	195	226	257	287	318	348	14
15	15	46	74	105	135	166	196	227	258	288	319	349	15
16	16	47	75	106	136	167	197	228	259	289	320	350	16
17	17	48	76	107	137	168	198	229	260	290	321	351	17
18	18	49	77	108	138	169	199	230	261	291	322	352	18
19	19	50	78	109	139	170	200	231	262	292	323	353	19
20	20	51	79	110	140	171	201	232	263	293	324	354	20
21	21	52	80	111	141	172	202	233	264	294	325	355	21
22	22	53	81	112	142	173	203	234	265	295	326	356	22
23	23	54	82	113	143	174	204	235	266	296	327	357	23
24	24	55	83	114	144	175	205	236	267	297	328	358	24
25	25	56	84	115	145	176	206	237	268	298	329	359	25
26	26	57	85	116	146	177	207	238	269	299	330	360	26
27	27	58	86	117	147	178	208	239	270	300	331	361	27
28	28	59	87	118	148	179	209	240	271	301	332	362	28
29	29	—	88	119	149	180	210	241	272	302	333	363	29
30	30	—	89	120	150	181	211	242	273	303	334	364	30
31	31	—	90	—	151	—	212	243	—	304	—	365	31
Day	JAN	FEB	MAR	APR	MAY	JUN	JUL	AUG	SEP	OCT	NOV	DEC	Day

G517(0.50)/FEBRUARY 1987

Continued.

AGE (YEARS)

STATURE
GIRLS

INCREMENT (cm/6 MONTHS)

INCREMENT (cm/6 MONTHS)

97
90
75
50
25
10
3

AGE (YEARS)

AGE (YEARS)

WEIGHT
GIRLS

INCREMENT (kg/6 MONTHS)

INCREMENT (kg/6 MONTHS)

97
90
75
50
25
10
3

AGE (YEARS)

Ross
Growth &
Development
Program

INCREMENTAL GROWTH CHARTS—BOYS

Growth charts such as those that display the National Center for Health Statistics (NCHS) percentiles are used for routine assessment of physical growth.[1] Occasionally, growth rate (growth velocity or increment divided by time between measurements) should be assessed, eg, when an infant or preadolescent child is found to be at an extreme percentile or when a substantial shift of percentile has occurred on an NCHS growth chart. The accompanying incremental growth charts are useful for assessing growth rates. They do not replace written records of growth data or NCHS growth charts.

These incremental growth charts have been prepared from serial data for white US children whose growth is very close to that of children from whom the NCHS percentiles were derived.[1,2] Highly standardized anthropometric methods that conform to current recommendations were used to make all measurements.[3] Weight was measured as, or corrected to, nude weight. Recumbent length and stature were measured without shoes. Appropriate use of the incremental growth charts requires that similar methods be applied. Ideally, the same person should measure a child at the beginning and end of an interval.

References:

1. Hamill PVV, Drizd TA, Johnson CL, Reed RB, Roche AF, Moore WM: Physical growth: National Center for Health Statistics percentiles. *Am J Clin Nutr* 32: 607-629, 1979.

2. Roche AF, Himes JH: Incremental growth charts. *Am J Clin Nutr* 33: 2041-2052, 1980.

3. Fomon SJ: *Nutritional Disorders of Children. Prevention, Screening, and Follow-up.* Washington, DC: DHEW Publication No. (HSA) 76-5612, 1976.

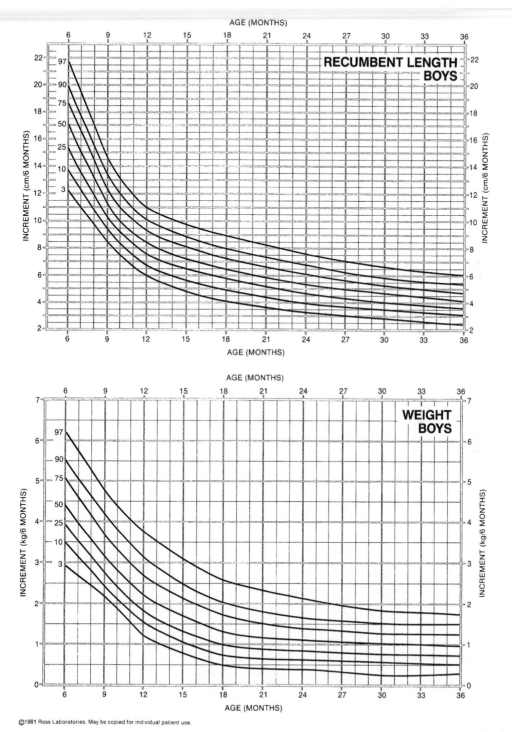

AGE (MONTHS)

RECUMBENT LENGTH BOYS

INCREMENT (cm/6 MONTHS)

97
90
75
50
25
10
3

AGE (MONTHS)

AGE (MONTHS)

WEIGHT BOYS

INCREMENT (kg/6 MONTHS)

97
90
75
50
25
10
3

AGE (MONTHS)

Continued.

AGE (YEARS)

STATURE
BOYS

INCREMENT (cm/6 MONTHS)

INCREMENT (cm/6 MONTHS)

97
90
75
50
25
10
3

AGE (YEARS)

AGE (YEARS)

WEIGHT
BOYS

INCREMENT (kg/6 MONTHS)

INCREMENT (kg/6 MONTHS)

97

90

75

50

25

10

3

AGE (YEARS)

©1981 Ross Laboratories. May be copied for individual patient use.

Ross
Growth &
Development
Program

Midarm Circumference and Skinfold Thickness Measurement Instructions and Percentiles

Midarm circumference and skinfold thickness measurements may be made on infants and children with an Inser-Tape™ Ross Insertion Tape and an Adipometer™ Skinfold Caliper. The measurements may be compared with age- and sex-specific percentiles prepared by the National Center for Health Statistics (NCHS) to facilitate their interpretation.[1] The NCHS data were collected on some 20,000 children between 1963 and 1974 in National Health Examination Surveys and in the first National Health and Nutrition Examination Survey (NHANES I).

The NCHS percentiles describe the distribution of these measurements for American children. The percentiles may be used as reference data but should not be considered "standards," "norms," or "ideals."[2] It is inappropriate to conclude that a measurement above or below an arbitrary percentile or value is unacceptable, because data are insufficient to validate associated risks. However, midarm circumference and skinfold measurements are useful for screening and for monitoring the progress of individual children who have been identified as having a potential or real problem of undernutrition or overnutrition.

Instructions

Measurements may be made on the right or the left side; measurements for the NCHS percentiles were made on the right side. Midarm circumference and triceps skinfold thickness are measured at the level of the midpoint between the acromion and olecranon. To locate the midpoint, use the side of the Inser-Tape labeled MIDPOINT MEASURE. With the child's arm bent at the elbow and palm up, position the tape vertically along the posterior arm so the same figure appears at the acromial process of the scapula and at the olecranon process of the ulna. The midpoint is at zero. Mark the midpoint to identify the level to measure midarm circumference and triceps skinfold thickness.

To measure midarm circumference, slip the loop of the Inser-Tape up the arm to the midpoint. With the arm hanging freely at the child's side, tighten the loop without compressing the arm. Measure to the nearest 0.1 cm.

To measure triceps skinfold thickness, grasp a fold of skin and subcutaneous tissue between the thumb and index finger about 1 cm above the midpoint, with the long axis of the skinfold parallel to the long axis of the arm. Place the jaws of the Adipometer over the skinfold at the previously marked midpoint. Holding the Adipometer in a horizontal position, apply force with the thumb and index finger until the lines on the caliper are opposite each other. After 2 or 3 seconds, read the measurement on the scale opposite the pointer to the nearest millimeter.

Subscapular skinfold thickness is measured by grasping a fold of skin and subcutaneous tissue just below the angle of the scapula and applying the jaws of the Adipometer. The child's shoulder and arm should be relaxed. The skinfold should parallel the natural cleavage lines of the skin, approximately 45° from the horizontal extending medially and upward. Apply force with the thumb and index finger until the lines on the caliper are opposite each other. After 2 or 3 seconds, read the measurement on the scale opposite the pointer to the nearest millimeter.

References

1. Johnson CL, Fulwood R, Abraham S, et al: Basic data on anthropometric measurements and angular measurements of the hip and knee joints for selected age groups, 1-74 years of age, United States, 1971-1975. *Vital and Health Statistics* Series 11, No. 219. DHHS Publication No. (PHS) 81-1669, 1981.
2. Owen GM: Measurement, recording, and assessment of skinfold thickness in childhood and adolescence: Report of a small meeting. *Am J Clin Nutr* 35:629-638, 1982.

Continued.

AGE (YEARS)

SUBSCAPULAR SKINFOLD
THICKNESS—BOYS

SUBSCAPULAR SKINFOLD (mm)

95th
90th
75th
50th
25th
10th
5th

SUBSCAPULAR SKINFOLD
THICKNESS—GIRLS

SUBSCAPULAR SKINFOLD (mm)

95th
90th
75th
50th
25th
10th
5th

AGE (YEARS)

Recommend the formulation you prefer
with the name you trust
SIMILAC®
SIMILAC® WITH IRON
SIMILAC® WITH WHEY + IRON
Infant Formulas

The **ISOMIL®** System of
Soy Protein Formulas

ADVANCE®
Nutritional Beverage

Figures adapted from Johnson CL, Fulwood R, Abraham S, et al: Basic data on anthropometric measurements and angular
measurements of the hip and knee joints for selected age groups, 1-74 years of age, United States, 1971-1975. *Vital and
Health Statistics* Series 11, No. 219. DHHS Publication No. (PHS) 81-1669, 1981.

© 1983 Ross Laboratories, Columbus, Ohio 43216. May be copied for individual patient use.

ROSS LABORATORIES
COLUMBUS, OHIO 43216
Division of Abbott Laboratories, USA
P552/DECEMBER 1983
LITHO IN USA

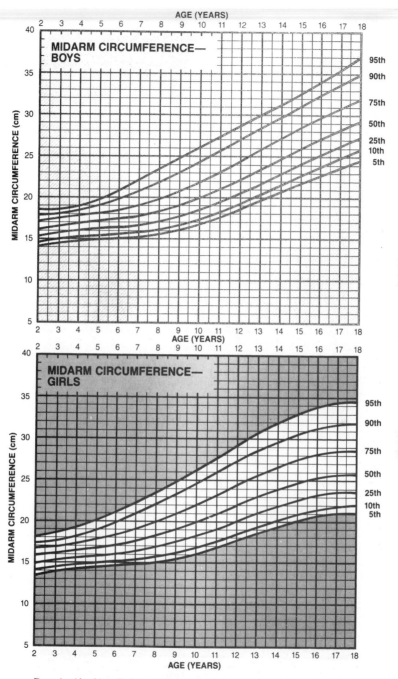

AGE (YEARS)

MIDARM CIRCUMFERENCE—
BOYS

MIDARM CIRCUMFERENCE (cm)

95th
90th
75th
50th
25th
10th
5th

AGE (YEARS)

MIDARM CIRCUMFERENCE—
GIRLS

MIDARM CIRCUMFERENCE (cm)

95th
90th
75th
50th
25th
10th
5th

AGE (YEARS)

Figures adapted from Johnson CL, Fulwood R, Abraham S, et al: Basic data on anthropometric measurements and angular measurements of the hip and knee joints for selected age groups, 1-74 years of age, United States, 1971-1975. *Vital and Health Statistics* Series 11, No. 219. DHHS Publication No. (PHS) 81-1669, 1981.

Continued.

AGE (YEARS)

TRICEPS SKINFOLD THICKNESS—BOYS

TRICEPS SKINFOLD (mm)

AGE (YEARS)

95th
90th
75th
50th
25th
10th
5th

TRICEPS SKINFOLD THICKNESS—GIRLS

95th
90th
75th
50th
25th
10th
5th

AGE (YEARS)

Figures adapted from Johnson CL, Fulwood R, Abraham S, et al: Basic data on anthropometric measurements and angular measurements of the hip and knee joints for selected age groups, 1-74 years of age, United States, 1971-1975. *Vital and Health Statistics* Series 11, No. 219. DHHS Publication No. (PHS) 81-1669, 1981.

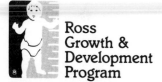

Ross
Growth &
Development
Program

PARENT-SPECIFIC ADJUSTMENTS FOR
EVALUATION OF LENGTH AND STATURE–GIRLS AND BOYS

Recumbent length and stature (standing height) are affected by both genetic and nongenetic factors. The genetic component should be considered when concern arises that diet or disease may have retarded or accelerated growth. Adjustment of length or stature to take parental stature into account may help identify or explain the nature of a growth problem. Such adjustment may prompt diagnostic studies or suggest a genetic basis for the growth problem.

Parent-specific adjustment procedures have been developed for US children by Himes, Roche, and Thissen.* The accompanying tables of adjustments are adapted from their research. Parent-specific adjustments need not be done routinely but should be considered when a child has unusual length or stature. As a guideline for applying parent-specific adjustments, "unusual" may be defined as below the 5th percentile or above the 95th percentile in length or stature for age.

Occasionally, a child's length or stature may appear normal, but the parents (one or both) are very tall or very short. Under such circumstances, parent-specific adjustment also is appropriate. Rapid decrease or increase in a child's percentile for length or stature generally is not an indication for applying parent-specific adjustments because the cause is more likely to be nongenetic than genetic.

*Himes JH, Roche AF, Thissen D: *Parent-Specific Adjustments for Assessment of Recumbent Length and Stature.* Monographs in Paediatrics. Basel, Switzerland: S Karger, 1981, vol 13.

Table 1.   Metric Equivalents (cm) for Length and Stature

INCHES	0	¼	½	¾	INCHES	0	¼	½	¾	INCHES	0	¼	½	¾
12	30.5	31.1	31.7	32.4	36	91.4	92.1	92.7	93.3	60	152.4	153.0	153.7	154.3
13	33.0	33.7	34.3	34.9	37	94.0	94.6	95.2	95.9	61	154.9	155.6	156.2	156.8
14	35.6	36.2	36.8	37.5	38	96.5	97.2	97.8	98.4	62	157.5	158.1	158.7	159.4
15	38.1	38.7	39.4	40.0	39	99.1	99.7	100.3	101.0	63	160.0	160.7	161.3	161.9
16	40.6	41.3	41.9	42.5	40	101.6	102.2	102.9	103.5	64	162.6	163.2	163.8	164.5
17	43.2	43.8	44.4	45.1	41	104.1	104.8	105.4	106.0	65	165.1	165.7	166.4	167.0
18	45.7	46.4	47.0	47.6	42	106.7	107.3	107.9	108.6	66	167.6	168.3	168.9	169.5
19	48.3	48.9	49.5	50.2	43	109.2	109.9	110.5	111.1	67	170.2	170.8	171.4	172.1
20	50.8	51.4	52.1	52.7	44	111.8	112.4	113.0	113.7	68	172.7	173.4	174.0	174.6
21	53.3	54.0	54.6	55.2	45	114.3	114.9	115.6	116.2	69	175.3	175.9	176.5	177.2
22	55.9	56.5	57.1	57.8	46	116.8	117.5	118.1	118.7	70	177.8	178.4	179.1	179.7
23	58.4	59.1	59.7	60.3	47	119.4	120.0	120.6	121.3	71	180.3	181.0	181.6	182.2
24	61.0	61.6	62.2	62.9	48	121.9	122.6	123.2	123.8	72	182.9	183.5	184.1	184.8
25	63.5	64.1	64.8	65.4	49	124.5	125.1	125.7	126.4	73	185.4	186.1	186.7	187.3
26	66.0	66.7	67.3	67.9	50	127.0	127.6	128.3	128.9	74	188.0	188.6	189.2	189.9
27	68.6	69.2	69.8	70.5	51	129.5	130.2	130.8	131.4	75	190.5	191.1	191.8	192.4
28	71.1	71.8	72.4	73.0	52	132.1	132.7	133.3	134.0	76	193.0	193.7	194.3	194.9
29	73.7	74.3	74.9	75.6	53	134.6	135.3	135.9	136.5	77	195.6	196.2	196.8	197.5
30	76.2	76.8	77.5	78.1	54	137.2	137.8	138.4	139.1	78	198.1	198.8	199.4	200.0
31	78.7	79.4	80.0	80.6	55	139.7	140.3	141.0	141.6	79	200.7	201.3	201.9	202.6
32	81.3	81.9	82.5	83.2	56	142.2	142.9	143.5	144.1	80	203.2	203.8	204.5	205.1
33	83.8	84.5	85.1	85.7	57	144.8	145.4	146.0	146.7	81	205.7	206.4	207.0	207.6
34	86.4	87.0	87.6	88.3	58	147.3	148.0	148.6	149.2	82	208.3	208.9	209.5	210.2
35	88.9	89.5	90.2	90.8	59	149.9	150.5	151.1	151.8	83	210.8	211.5	212.1	212.7

*The term "girl" is used throughout, however the process is the same for boys.

Continued.

Table 2.   Parent-Specific Adjustments (cm) for Stature of Girls From 3 to 18 Years

Age (Years)	Stature (cm)	150	152	154	156	158	160	162	164	166	168	170	172	174	176	178	180	182	184
3	82.0– 83.9	6	5	4	4	3	2	1	1	0	−1	−1	−2	−3	−3	−4	−5	−6	−6
	84.0– 93.9	6	6	5	4	3	3	2	1	1	0	−1	−1	−2	−3	−4	−4	−5	−6
	94.0–102.9	7	7	6	5	4	4	3	2	2	1	0	−1	−1	−2	−3	−3	−4	−5
4	92.0– 93.9	6	6	5	4	3	3	2	1	0	0	−1	−2	−3	−3	−4	−5	−6	−7
	94.0–103.9	7	6	6	5	4	3	2	2	1	0	−1	−1	−2	−3	−4	−4	−5	−6
	104.0–112.9	8	7	7	6	5	4	3	3	2	1	0	0	−1	−2	−3	−3	−4	−5
5	100.0–101.9	8	7	6	5	4	3	2	1	1	0	−1	−2	−3	−4	−5	−5	−6	−7
	102.0–111.9	8	7	6	6	5	4	3	2	1	0	−1	−1	−2	−3	−4	−5	−6	−7
	112.0–120.9	9	8	7	7	6	5	4	3	2	1	1	0	−1	−2	−3	−4	−5	−6
6	106.0–109.9	9	8	7	6	5	4	3	2	1	0	−1	−2	−3	−4	−5	−6	−7	−8
	110.0–119.9	9	9	8	7	6	5	4	3	2	1	0	−1	−2	−3	−4	−5	−6	−7
	120.0–128.9	11	10	9	8	7	6	5	4	3	2	1	0	−1	−2	−3	−4	−5	−6
7	112.0–117.9	9	8	7	6	5	4	3	2	1	0	−1	−2	−3	−4	−5	−6	−7	−8
	118.0–127.9	10	9	8	7	6	5	4	3	2	1	0	−1	−2	−3	−4	−5	−6	−7
	128.0–136.9	11	10	9	8	7	6	5	4	3	2	1	0	−1	−2	−3	−4	−5	−6
8	116.0–123.9	9	8	7	6	5	4	3	2	1	0	−1	−2	−3	−4	−5	−6	−8	−9
	124.0–133.9	10	9	8	7	6	5	4	3	2	1	0	−1	−2	−3	−4	−5	−7	−8
	134.0–142.9	11	10	9	8	7	6	5	4	3	2	1	0	−1	−2	−3	−4	−6	−7
9	122.0–131.9	10	9	8	7	6	5	3	2	1	0	−1	−2	−3	−4	−5	−6	−7	−9
	132.0–141.9	11	10	9	8	7	6	4	3	2	1	0	−1	−2	−3	−4	−5	−7	−8
	142.0–150.9	12	11	10	9	8	6	5	4	3	2	1	0	−1	−2	−3	−5	−6	−7
10	126.0–127.9	10	9	7	6	5	4	3	2	1	0	−1	−2	−3	−5	−6	−7	−8	−9
	128.0–137.9	10	9	8	7	6	5	4	2	1	0	−1	−2	−3	−4	−5	−6	−7	−8
	138.0–147.9	11	10	9	8	6	5	4	3	2	1	0	−1	−2	−3	−4	−5	−7	−8
	148.0–156.9	12	10	9	8	7	6	5	4	3	2	1	0	−1	−3	−4	−5	−6	−7
11	130.0–133.9	10	9	8	6	5	4	3	2	1	0	−1	−2	−3	−4	−6	−7	−8	−9
	134.0–143.9	10	9	8	7	6	5	4	3	1	0	−1	−2	−3	−4	−5	−6	−7	−8
	144.0–153.9	11	10	9	7	6	5	4	3	2	1	0	−1	−2	−3	−5	−6	−7	−8
	154.0–162.9	11	10	9	8	7	6	5	4	3	1	0	−1	−2	−3	−4	−5	−6	−7
12	134.0–139.9	10	9	8	7	6	5	3	2	1	0	−1	−3	−4	−5	−6	−7	−8	−10
	140.0–149.9	11	10	9	7	6	5	4	3	2	0	−1	−2	−3	−4	−6	−7	−8	−9
	150.0–159.9	12	10	9	8	7	6	5	3	2	1	0	−1	−3	−4	−5	−6	−7	−8
	160.0–168.9	12	11	10	9	8	6	5	4	3	2	0	−1	−2	−3	−4	−5	−7	−8
13	140.0–145.9	10	9	8	7	6	4	3	2	1	0	−1	−3	−4	−5	−6	−7	−8	−10
	146.0–155.9	11	10	9	7	6	5	4	3	2	0	−1	−2	−3	−4	−6	−7	−8	−9
	156.0–165.9	12	10	9	8	7	6	5	3	2	1	0	−1	−3	−4	−5	−6	−7	−8
	166.0–174.9	12	11	10	9	8	6	5	4	3	2	1	−1	−2	−3	−4	−5	−7	−8
14	146.0–149.9	10	9	8	6	5	4	3	2	1	0	−1	−3	−4	−5	−6	−7	−8	−9
	150.0–159.9	11	9	8	7	6	5	4	3	1	0	−1	−2	−3	−4	−5	−7	−8	−9
	160.0–169.9	11	10	9	8	7	6	5	3	2	1	0	−1	−2	−3	−5	−6	−7	−8
	170.0–178.9	12	11	10	9	8	6	5	4	3	2	1	0	−2	−3	−4	−5	−6	−7
15	146.0–151.9	10	9	8	7	5	4	3	2	1	−1	−2	−3	−4	−5	−6	−8	−9	−10
	152.0–161.9	11	10	9	7	6	5	4	3	1	0	−1	−2	−3	−4	−6	−7	−8	−9
	162.0–171.9	12	11	10	8	7	6	5	4	2	1	0	−1	−2	−4	−5	−6	−7	−8
	172.0–180.9	13	12	11	9	8	7	6	5	3	2	1	0	−1	−3	−4	−5	−6	−7
16	146.0–151.9	11	10	8	7	6	5	3	2	1	−1	−2	−3	−4	−6	−7	−8	−10	−11
	152.0–161.9	12	10	9	8	7	5	4	3	2	0	−1	−2	−4	−5	−6	−7	−9	−10
	162.0–171.9	13	12	10	9	8	6	5	4	3	1	0	−1	−3	−4	−5	−6	−8	−9
	172.0–180.9	14	13	11	10	9	7	6	5	4	2	1	0	−2	−3	−4	−5	−7	−8
17	148.0–153.9	11	10	9	7	6	5	3	2	1	0	−2	−3	−4	−6	−7	−8	−10	−11
	154.0–163.9	12	11	10	8	7	6	4	3	2	0	−1	−2	−4	−5	−6	−8	−9	−10
	164.0–173.9	13	12	11	9	8	7	5	4	3	1	0	−1	−3	−4	−5	−6	−8	−9
	174.0–182.9	14	13	12	10	9	8	6	5	4	2	1	0	−1	−3	−4	−5	−7	−8
18	148.0–149.9	10	9	8	7	5	4	3	2	1	−1	−2	−3	−4	−6	−7	−8	−9	−10
	150.0–159.9	11	10	8	7	6	5	4	2	1	0	−1	−3	−4	−5	−6	−7	−9	−10
	160.0–169.9	12	11	9	8	7	6	4	3	2	1	0	−2	−3	−4	−5	−6	−8	−9
	170.0–178.9	13	11	10	9	8	7	5	4	3	2	1	−1	−2	−3	−4	−5	−7	−8

Table 3. Parent-Specific Adjustments (cm) for Stature of Boys From 3 to 18 Years

Age (Years)	Stature (cm)	150	152	154	156	158	160	162	164	166	168	170	172	174	176	178	180	182	184
3	86.0– 87.9	7	6	5	5	4	3	2	1	1	0	−1	−2	−3	−3	−4	−5	−6	−7
	88.0– 97.9	8	7	6	5	4	4	3	2	1	0	−1	−1	−2	−3	−4	−5	−5	−6
	98.0–106.9	8	8	7	6	5	4	4	3	2	1	0	0	−1	−2	−3	−4	−4	−5
4	90.0– 93.9	7	6	5	4	4	3	2	1	0	−1	−1	−2	−3	−4	−5	−5	−6	−7
	94.0–103.9	8	7	6	5	4	3	3	2	1	0	−1	−1	−2	−3	−4	−5	−6	−6
	104.0–112.9	8	8	7	6	5	4	3	3	2	1	0	−1	−1	−2	−3	−4	−5	−6
5	96.0–103.9	8	7	6	5	4	3	2	1	0	0	−1	−2	−3	−4	−5	−6	−7	−8
	104.0–113.9	9	8	7	6	5	4	3	2	1	0	0	−1	−2	−3	−4	−5	−6	−7
	114.0–122.9	9	9	8	7	6	5	4	3	2	1	0	0	−1	−2	−3	−4	−5	−6
6	102.0–111.9	8	7	7	6	5	4	3	2	1	0	−1	−2	−3	−4	−5	−6	−7	−8
	112.0–121.9	9	8	7	7	6	5	4	3	2	1	0	−1	−2	−3	−4	−5	−6	−7
	122.0–130.9	10	9	8	7	6	6	5	4	3	2	1	0	−1	−2	−3	−4	−5	−6
7	108.0–117.9	9	8	7	6	5	4	3	2	1	0	−1	−2	−4	−5	−6	−7	−8	−9
	118.0–127.9	10	9	8	7	6	5	4	3	2	1	0	−1	−2	−4	−5	−6	−7	−8
	128.0–136.9	12	10	9	8	7	6	5	4	3	2	1	0	−1	−2	−4	−5	−6	−7
8	114.0–115.9	10	9	8	6	5	4	3	2	1	−1	−2	−3	−4	−5	−6	−8	−9	−10
	116.0–125.9	11	9	8	7	6	5	4	2	1	0	−1	−2	−3	−5	−6	−7	−8	−9
	126.0–135.9	12	10	9	8	7	6	5	3	2	1	0	−1	−2	−4	−5	−6	−7	−8
	136.0–144.9	13	12	10	9	8	7	6	5	3	2	1	0	−1	−2	−4	−5	−6	−7
9	120.0–121.9	11	9	8	7	6	4	3	2	1	0	−2	−3	−4	−5	−7	−8	−9	−10
	122.0–131.9	11	10	9	8	6	5	4	3	1	0	−1	−2	−3	−5	−6	−7	−8	−10
	132.0–141.9	12	11	10	9	7	6	5	4	2	1	0	−1	−2	−4	−5	−6	−7	−9
	142.0–150.9	13	12	11	10	8	7	6	5	4	2	1	0	−1	−3	−4	−5	−6	−7
10	124.0–127.9	11	10	9	7	6	5	3	2	1	−1	−2	−3	−5	−6	−7	−9	−10	−11
	128.0–137.9	12	11	10	8	7	6	4	3	2	0	−1	−2	−4	−5	−6	−8	−9	−10
	138.0–147.9	13	12	11	9	8	7	5	4	3	1	0	−1	−3	−4	−5	−7	−8	−9
	148.0–158.9	14	13	12	11	9	8	7	5	4	3	1	0	−1	−3	−4	−5	−7	−8
11	128.0–133.9	12	10	9	8	6	5	4	2	1	0	−2	−3	−5	−6	−7	−9	−10	−11
	134.0–143.9	12	11	10	8	7	6	4	3	2	0	−1	−2	−4	−5	−6	−8	−9	−10
	144.0–153.9	14	12	11	10	8	7	5	4	3	1	0	−1	−3	−4	−5	−7	−8	−9
	154.0–162.9	15	13	12	11	9	8	7	5	4	3	1	0	−2	−3	−4	−6	−7	−8
12	132.0–141.9	12	10	9	8	6	5	4	2	1	0	−2	−3	−4	−6	−7	−8	−10	−11
	142.0–151.9	13	11	10	9	7	6	5	3	2	1	−1	−2	−3	−5	−6	−7	−9	−10
	152.0–161.9	13	12	11	9	8	7	5	4	3	1	0	−1	−2	−4	−5	−6	−8	−9
	162.0–170.9	14	13	12	10	9	8	6	5	4	2	1	0	−2	−3	−4	−6	−7	−8
13	136.0–139.9	12	10	9	8	6	5	4	2	1	−1	−2	−3	−5	−6	−7	−9	−10	−12
	140.0–149.9	12	11	10	8	7	6	4	3	1	0	−1	−3	−4	−6	−7	−8	−10	−11
	150.0–159.9	13	12	10	9	8	6	5	4	2	1	−1	−2	−3	−5	−6	−7	−9	−10
	160.0–169.9	14	13	11	10	8	7	6	4	3	2	0	−1	−3	−4	−5	−7	−8	−9
	170.0–178.9	15	13	12	11	9	8	6	5	4	2	1	0	−2	−3	−5	−6	−7	−9
14	142.0–145.9	13	11	10	8	7	5	4	2	1	−1	−2	−4	−5	−7	−8	−10	−11	−13
	146.0–155.9	14	12	11	9	8	6	5	3	1	0	−2	−3	−5	−6	−8	−9	−11	−12
	156.0–165.9	15	13	11	10	8	7	5	4	2	1	−1	−2	−4	−5	−7	−8	−10	−11
	166.0–175.9	15	14	12	11	9	8	6	5	3	2	0	−1	−3	−4	−6	−7	−9	−11
	176.0–184.9	16	15	13	12	10	9	7	6	4	3	1	−1	−2	−4	−5	−7	−8	−10
15	148.0–151.9	14	13	11	9	7	6	4	2	0	−1	−3	−5	−7	−8	−10	−12	−14	−15
	152.0–161.9	15	14	12	10	8	7	5	3	1	0	−2	−4	−6	−7	−9	−11	−13	−14
	162.0–171.9	17	15	13	11	10	8	6	4	3	1	−1	−3	−4	−6	−8	−10	−11	−13
	172.0–181.9	18	16	14	13	11	9	7	6	4	2	0	−1	−3	−5	−7	−8	−10	−12
	182.0–190.9	19	17	16	14	12	10	9	7	5	3	2	0	−2	−4	−5	−7	−9	−11
16	156.0–163.9	17	15	13	11	9	7	5	3	1	−1	−3	−5	−7	−9	−11	−13	−16	−18
	164.0–173.9	19	17	15	13	10	8	6	4	2	0	−2	−4	−6	−8	−10	−12	−14	−16
	174.0–183.9	21	19	17	15	12	10	8	6	4	2	0	−2	−4	−6	−8	−10	−12	−14
	184.0–192.9	23	21	19	17	14	12	10	8	6	4	2	0	−2	−4	−6	−8	−10	−12
17	162.0–165.9	17	15	13	11	9	7	4	2	0	−2	−4	−7	−9	−11	−13	−15	−17	−20
	166.0–175.9	20	17	15	13	11	9	6	4	2	0	−2	−4	−7	−9	−11	−13	−15	−18
	176.0–185.9	22	20	18	16	13	11	9	7	5	3	0	−2	−4	−6	−8	−11	−13	−15
	186.0–194.9	25	23	20	18	16	14	12	9	7	5	3	1	−1	−4	−6	−8	−10	−12
18	160.0–165.9	18	16	13	11	9	6	4	2	0	−3	−5	−7	−10	−12	−14	−17	−19	−21
	166.0–175.9	20	18	16	13	11	9	7	4	2	0	−3	−5	−7	−10	−12	−14	−17	−19
	176.0–185.9	23	21	19	16	14	12	9	7	5	3	0	−2	−4	−7	−9	−11	−14	−16
	186.0–194.9	26	24	22	19	17	15	12	10	8	6	3	1	−1	−4	−6	−8	−11	−13

Continued.

INSTRUCTIONS

1. Measure and record mother's stature.

2. Measure and record father's stature.

3. When one parent's stature cannot be measured, the measured parent's estimate of the other parent's stature (in cm) can be substituted for measured stature, and midparent stature can be calculated as in instruction 4. Alternatively, the measured parent's perception of the other parent's stature (short, medium, or tall) can be used to determine midparent stature directly from Table 4.

Table 4. **Midparent Stature (cm) When Measured Parent Reports Other Parent's Stature as Short, Medium, or Tall**

Measured Parent's Stature (cm)	When Mother Reports Father's Stature as*			When Father Reports Mother's Stature as*		
	Short†	Medium†	Tall†	Short‡	Medium‡	Tall‡
146	156	162	166	150	154	158
148	158	162	166	152	154	160
150	158	164	168	152	156	160
152	160	164	168	154	158	162
154	160	166	170	154	158	162
156	162	166	170	156	160	164
158	162	168	172	156	160	164
160	164	168	172	158	162	166
162	164	170	174	158	162	166
164	166	170	174	160	164	168
166	166	172	176	160	164	168
168	168	172	176	162	166	170
170	168	174	178	162	166	170
172	170	174	178	164	168	172
174	170	176	180	164	168	172
176	172	176	180	166	170	174
178	172	178	182	166	170	174
180	174	178	182	168	172	176
182	174	180	184	168	172	176
184	176	180	184	170	174	178
186	176	182	—	170	174	178
188	178	182	—	172	176	180
190	178	184	—	172	176	180
192	180	184	—	174	178	182
194	180	—	—	174	178	182
196	182	—	—	176	180	184
198	182	—	—	176	180	184

* All midparent statures are rounded to the nearest 2 cm to facilitate use of Tables 2 and 3.

† Values for father's stature used in calculations of midparent stature: short, 167.6 cm (5 ft 6 in.); medium, 176.3 cm (5 ft 9½ in.); tall, 185.4 cm (6 ft 1 in.).

‡ Values for mother's stature used in calculations of midparent stature: short, 154.9 cm (5 ft 1 in.); medium, 162.8 cm (5 ft 4 in.); tall, 170.7 cm (5 ft 7¼ in.).

4. Calculate midparent stature by adding the mother's stature and the father's stature in cm and dividing by two. Metric equivalents for stature are shown in Table 1.

5. Measure, record, and plot the girl's length (birth to 36 months) or stature (3 to 18 years) in cm on the appropriate growth chart that displays the National Center for Health Statistics (NCHS) percentiles. Metric equivalents for length and stature are shown in Table 1.

6. Calculate the girl's adjusted length or stature by using the parent-specific adjustments from Table 2 for length or from Table 3 for stature:

    a. Locate the age closest to that achieved by the girl.

    b. For that age, locate the horizontal row that includes the girl's length or stature.

    c. Locate the vertical column closest to the midparent stature for the girl's mother and father.

    d. The parent-specific adjustment (in cm) appears at the row-column intersection.

    e. Add the parent-specific adjustment to the girl's length or stature if the factor has no sign; subtract the adjustment if it has a minus sign.

7. Determine the girl's parent-specific adjusted percentile by plotting adjusted length or stature on the appropriate NCHS growth chart. Clearly label plotted measurements as being actual or adjusted values.

Interpretation: A girl at a low percentile for actual length or stature whose parents are short probably is genetically short. However, her shortness, particularly if it is extreme, may have additional contributing factors that should be considered.

If the girl's adjusted percentile is low, her growth probably has been slowed by nongenetic factors, and diagnostic studies should be considered. If the parents are tall, the girl's adjusted percentile will be lower than her actual percentile, and her shortness is more likely due to malnutrition or disease.

A girl at a high adjusted percentile for length or stature most often will be found to have accelerated maturation. Rarely, a specific disorder such as Marfan's syndrome or pituitary gigantism may be responsible for the girl's unusual length or stature.

Follow-Up: Counseling may be advisable when a girl is judged to be genetically short or tall. Additional contributing factors should be considered and growth monitored to confirm the relative stability of the girl's length or stature percentile.

Further investigation and modification of diet or specific therapy are indicated for a girl with unusual length or stature due to malnutrition or disease. Growth should be monitored to evaluate the effectiveness of dietary management or drug therapy.

Example	Girl aged 8 years, stature 46¾ in., mother's stature 68½ in., and father's stature reported as "tall."

Daughter's actual stature in cm is 118.7 (from Table 1).
Daughter's actual percentile is 10th (from NCHS growth chart).
Mother's stature in cm is 174.0 (from Table 1).
Midparent stature is 180.0 cm (from Table 4).
Adjustment is −6 cm (from Table 3).
Daughter's adjusted stature is 118.7 cm − 6 cm = 112.7 cm.
Daughter's adjusted percentile is below the 5th (from NCHS growth chart).
Interpretation: Probably nongenetically short. Further investigation is indicated.

Example	Boy aged 8 years, stature 47¼ in., mother's stature 68½ in., and father's stature reported as "tall."

Son's actual stature in cm is 120.0 (from Table 1).
Son's actual percentile is 10th (from NCHS growth chart).
Mother's stature in cm is 174.0 (from Table 1).
Midparent stature is 180.0 cm (from Table 4).
Adjustment is −7 cm (from Table 3).
Son's adjusted stature is 120.0 cm − 7 cm − 113.0 cm.
Son's adjusted percentile is below the 5th (from NCHS growth chart).
Interpretation: Probably nongenetically short. Further investigation is indicated.

In vivo performance confirms . . .

SIMILAC®
SIMILAC® WITH IRON
Infant Formulas
closest to mother's milk

ROSS LABORATORIES
COLUMBUS. OHIO 43216
Division of Abbott Laboratories. USA

P145 (0.25)/MARCH 1985

LITHO IN USA

IHDP Growth Percentiles: LBW Premature Girls[1,2]

Head Circumference (cm) vs. Gestation-Adjusted Age (mo)

Head Circumference — percentiles: 95th, 75th, 50th, 25th, 5th

Growth of very-low-birth-weight (VLBW, ≤ 1500 g) and low-birth-weight (LBW, 1501 to 2500 g) premature (≤ 37 weeks, GA) infants differs from that of normal-birth-weight term infants during infancy and early childhood. Because these infants may not catch up to term infants in growth during the early years, their growth should be compared to that of premature infants of similar birth weight.

The growth percentiles presented here are based on a large sample of infants enrolled in the Infant Health and Development Program (IHDP).[1,2] Some infants most likely to experience growth problems from biologic or environmental causes, premature infants with birth weight greater than 2500 g, and small-for-gestational-age term infants were excluded.[1] Study infants, however, are probably typical of premature infants who receive modern neonatal intensive care.

References

1. The Infant Health and Development Program: Enhancing the outcomes of low-birth-weight, premature infants. *JAMA* 1990;263(22):3035–3042.
2. Casey PH, Kraemer HC, Bernbaum J, et al: Growth status and growth rates of a varied sample of low birth weight, preterm infants: A longitudinal cohort from birth to three years of age. *J Pediatr* 1991;119:599–605.

IHDP studies were supported by grants from the Robert Wood Johnson Foundation, Pew Charitable Trusts, and the Bureau of Maternal and Child Health, US Department of Health and Human Services. These graphs were prepared by SS Guo and AF Roche, Wright State University, Yellow Springs, Ohio. IHDP, its sponsors, and the investigators do not endorse specific products.

Instructions for Use

1. Measure and record weight, length, and head circumference.
2. Calculate gestation-adjusted age by subtracting Adjustment for Prematurity in weeks from postnatal age in weeks. Adjustment for Prematurity equals 40 weeks minus GA. For example, at 12 wk postnatal age, an infant born at 30 wk GA would be 2 wk (0.5 mo) gestation-adjusted age.
3. Plot data at the gestation-adjusted age on the appropriate graph.
4. When possible, plot serial data on the same graph to permit detection of change in growth percentiles with age.

Interpretation

These graphs permit comparison of a LBW premature girl's growth relative to current reference data. Further investigation may be indicated when the plotted measurements are markedly different from the 50th percentile, or growth percentile changes rapidly.

Provided as a service of

SIMILAC® NeoCare™
Premature Infant Formula With Iron

ROSS PRODUCTS DIVISION
ABBOTT LABORATORIES
COLUMBUS, OHIO 43215-1724

LITHO IN USA

IHDP Growth Percentiles:
LBW Premature Girls[1,2]
(1501 to 2500 g BW, ≤37 wk GA)

Name_____

Record #_____

ROSS
PEDIATRICS

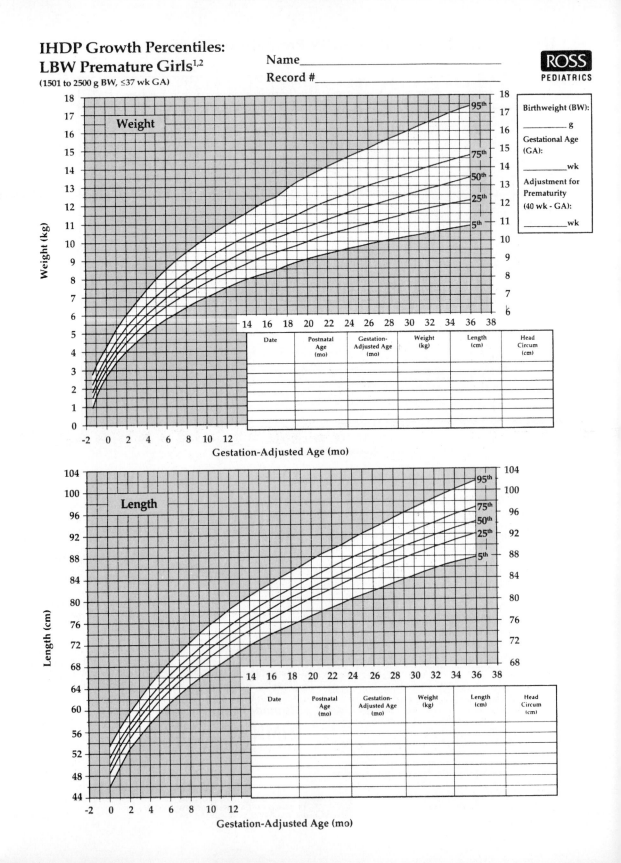

Birthweight (BW):
_____ g

Gestational Age (GA):
_____ wk

Adjustment for Prematurity (40 wk - GA):
_____ wk

Weight

Weight (kg)

Gestation-Adjusted Age (mo)

95th
75th
50th
25th
5th

Date	Postnatal Age (mo)	Gestation-Adjusted Age (mo)	Weight (kg)	Length (cm)	Head Circum (cm)

Length

Length (cm)

Gestation-Adjusted Age (mo)

95th
75th
50th
25th
5th

Date	Postnatal Age (mo)	Gestation-Adjusted Age (mo)	Weight (kg)	Length (cm)	Head Circum (cm)

IHDP Growth Percentiles: LBW Premature Boys[1,2]

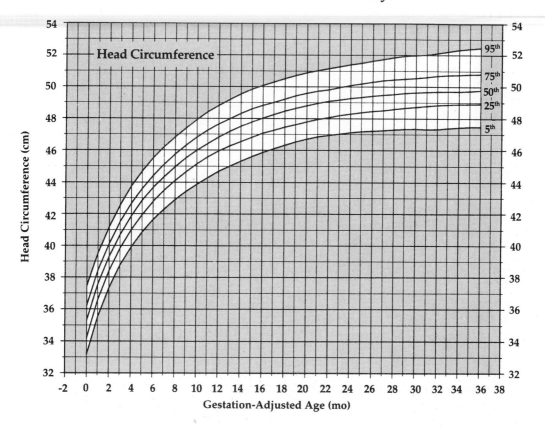

Head Circumference

Head Circumference (cm) — vertical axis: 32, 34, 36, 38, 40, 42, 44, 46, 48, 50, 52, 54

Percentile curves (right side, top to bottom): 95th, 75th, 50th, 25th, 5th

Gestation-Adjusted Age (mo) — horizontal axis: -2, 0, 2, 4, 6, 8, 10, 12, 14, 16, 18, 20, 22, 24, 26, 28, 30, 32, 34, 36, 38

Growth of very-low-birth-weight (VLBW, ≤ 1500 g) and low-birth-weight (LBW, 1501 to 2500 g) premature (≤ 37 weeks, GA) infants differs from that of normal-birth-weight term infants during infancy and early childhood. Because these infants may not catch up to term infants in growth during the early years, their growth should be compared to that of premature infants of similar birth weight.

The growth percentiles presented here are based on a large sample of infants enrolled in the Infant Health and Development Program (IHDP).[1,2] Some infants most likely to experience growth problems from biologic or environmental causes, premature infants with birth weight greater than 2500 g, and small-for-gestational-age term infants were excluded.[1] Study infants, however, are probably typical of premature infants who receive modern neonatal intensive care.

References

1. The Infant Health and Development Program: Enhancing the outcomes of low-birth-weight, premature infants. *JAMA* 1990;263(22):3035–3042.
2. Casey PH, Kraemer HC, Bernbaum J, et al: Growth status and growth rates of a varied sample of low birth weight, preterm infants: A longitudinal cohort from birth to three years of age. *J Pediatr* 1991;119:599–605.

IHDP studies were supported by grants from the Robert Wood Johnson Foundation, Pew Charitable Trusts, and the Bureau of Maternal and Child Health, US Department of Health and Human Services. These graphs were prepared by SS Guo and AF Roche, Wright State University, Yellow Springs, Ohio. IHDP, its sponsors, and the investigators do not endorse specific products.

Instructions for Use

1. Measure and record weight, length, and head circumference.
2. Calculate gestation-adjusted age by subtracting Adjustment for Prematurity in weeks from postnatal age in weeks. Adjustment for Prematurity equals 40 weeks minus GA. For example, at 12 wk postnatal age, an infant born at 30 wk GA would be 2 wk (0.5 mo) gestation-adjusted age.
3. Plot data at the gestation-adjusted age on the appropriate graph.
4. When possible, plot serial data on the same graph to permit detection of change in growth percentiles with age.

Interpretation

These graphs permit comparison of a LBW premature boy's growth relative to current reference data. Further investigation may be indicated when the plotted measurements are markedly different from the 50th percentile, or growth percentile changes rapidly.

Provided as a service of

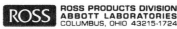

SIMILAC® NeoCare™
Premature Infant Formula With Iron

ROSS **ROSS PRODUCTS DIVISION**
ABBOTT LABORATORIES
COLUMBUS, OHIO 43215-1724

LITHO IN USA

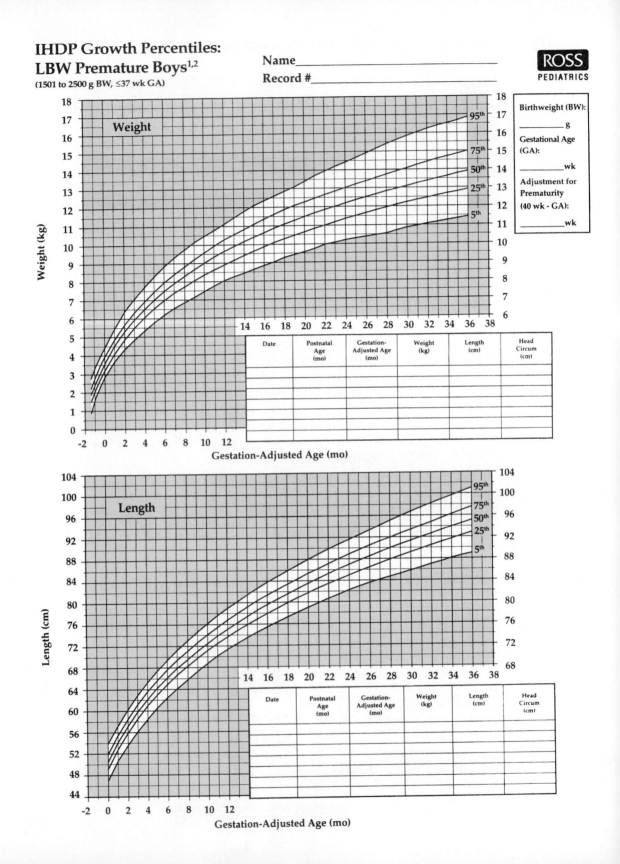

IHDP Growth Percentiles:
LBW Premature Boys[1,2]
(1501 to 2500 g BW, ≤37 wk GA)

Name_____

Record #_____

ROSS
PEDIATRICS

Birthweight (BW):

_____ g

Gestational Age
(GA):

_____wk

Adjustment for
Prematurity
(40 wk - GA):

_____wk

Weight

Weight (kg)

Gestation-Adjusted Age (mo)

Date	Postnatal Age (mo)	Gestation-Adjusted Age (mo)	Weight (kg)	Length (cm)	Head Circum (cm)

Length

Length (cm)

Gestation-Adjusted Age (mo)

Date	Postnatal Age (mo)	Gestation-Adjusted Age (mo)	Weight (kg)	Length (cm)	Head Circum (cm)

IHDP Growth Percentiles: VLBW Premature Girls[1,2]

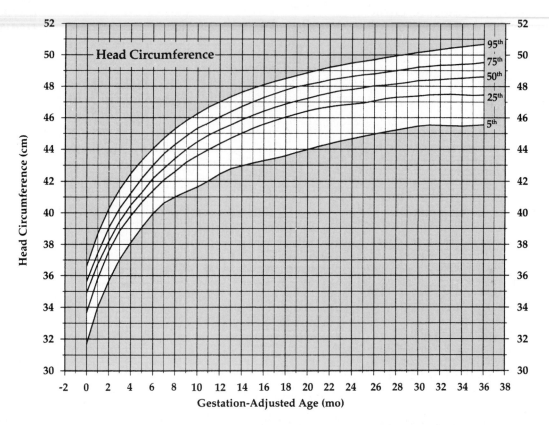

Growth of very-low-birth-weight (VLBW, ≤ 1500 g) and low-birth-weight (LBW, 1501 to 2500 g) premature (≤ 37 weeks, GA) infants differs from that of normal-birth-weight term infants during infancy and early childhood. Because these infants may not catch up to term infants in growth during the early years, their growth should be compared to that of premature infants of similar birth weight.

The growth percentiles presented here are based on a large sample of infants enrolled in the Infant Health and Development Program (IHDP).[1,2] Some infants most likely to experience growth problems from biologic or environmental causes, premature infants with birth weight greater than 2500 g, and small-for-gestational-age term infants were excluded.[1] Study infants, however, are probably typical of premature infants who receive modern neonatal intensive care.

References

1. The Infant Health and Development Program: Enhancing the outcomes of low-birth-weight, premature infants. *JAMA* 1990;263(22):3035–3042.
2. Casey PH, Kraemer HC, Bernbaum J, et al: Growth status and growth rates of a varied sample of low birth weight, preterm infants: A longitudinal cohort from birth to three years of age. *J Pediatr* 1991;119:599–605.

IHDP studies were supported by grants from the Robert Wood Johnson Foundation, Pew Charitable Trusts, and the Bureau of Maternal and Child Health, US Department of Health and Human Services. These graphs were prepared by SS Guo and AF Roche, Wright State University, Yellow Springs, Ohio. IHDP, its sponsors, and the investigators do not endorse specific products.

Instructions for Use

1. Measure and record weight, length, and head circumference.
2. Calculate gestation-adjusted age by subtracting Adjustment for Prematurity in weeks from postnatal age in weeks. Adjustment for Prematurity equals 40 weeks minus GA. For example, at 12 wk postnatal age, an infant born at 30 wk GA would be 2 wk (0.5 mo) gestation-adjusted age.
3. Plot data at the gestation-adjusted age on the appropriate graph.
4. When possible, plot serial data on the same graph to permit detection of change in growth percentiles with age.

Interpretation

These graphs permit comparison of a VLBW premature girl's growth relative to current reference data. Further investigation may be indicated when the plotted measurements are markedly different from the 50th percentile, or growth percentile changes rapidly.

Provided as a service of

SIMILAC® NeoCare™
Premature Infant Formula With Iron

IHDP Growth Percentiles:
VLBW Premature Girls[1,2]

(≤1500 g BW, ≤37 wk GA)

Name_____

Record #_____

ROSS
PEDIATRICS

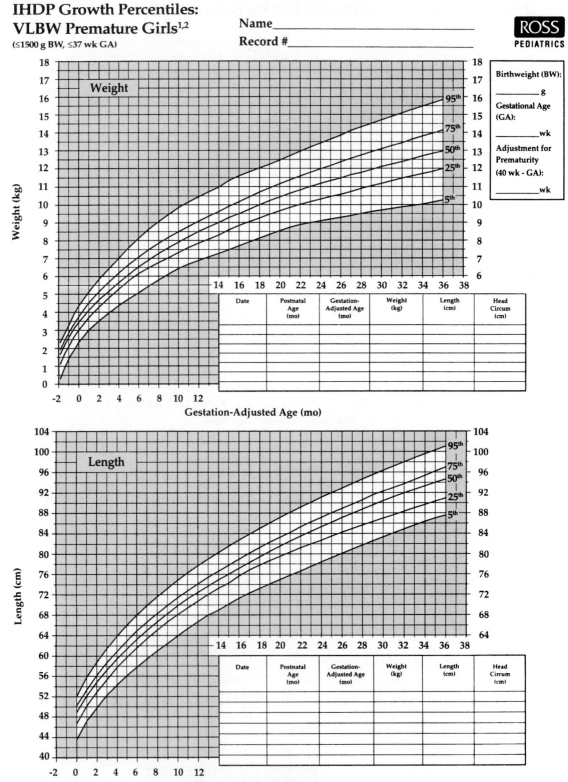

Birthweight (BW):

_____ g

Gestational Age
(GA):

_____ wk

Adjustment for
Prematurity
(40 wk - GA):

_____ wk

IHDP Growth Percentiles: VLBW Premature Boys[1,2]

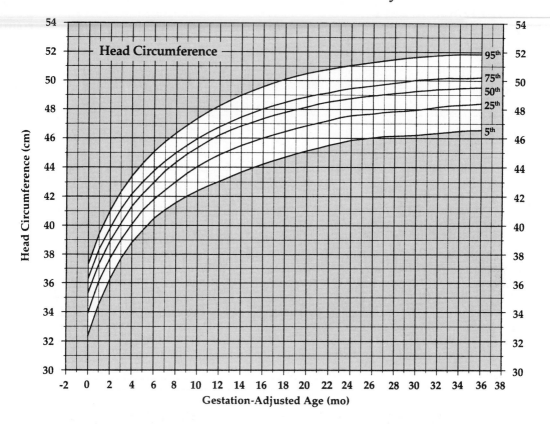

Head Circumference

Head Circumference (cm)

95th
75th
50th
25th
5th

Gestation-Adjusted Age (mo)

Growth of very-low-birth-weight (VLBW, ≤ 1500 g) and low-birth-weight (LBW, 1501 to 2500 g) premature (≤ 37 weeks, GA) infants differs from that of normal-birth-weight term infants during infancy and early childhood. Because these infants may not catch up to term infants in growth during the early years, their growth should be compared to that of premature infants of similar birth weight.

The growth percentiles presented here are based on a large sample of infants enrolled in the Infant Health and Development Program (IHDP).[1,2] Some infants most likely to experience growth problems from biologic or environmental causes, premature infants with birth weight greater than 2500 g, and small-for-gestational-age term infants were excluded.[1] Study infants, however, are probably typical of premature infants who receive modern neonatal intensive care.

References

1. The Infant Health and Development Program: Enhancing the outcomes of low-birth-weight, premature infants. *JAMA* 1990;263(22):3035–3042.
2. Casey PH, Kraemer HC, Bernbaum J, et al: Growth status and growth rates of a varied sample of low birth weight, preterm infants: A longitudinal cohort from birth to three years of age. *J Pediatr* 1991;119:599–605.

IHDP studies were supported by grants from the Robert Wood Johnson Foundation, Pew Charitable Trusts, and the Bureau of Maternal and Child Health, US Department of Health and Human Services. These graphs were prepared by SS Guo and AF Roche, Wright State University, Yellow Springs, Ohio. IHDP, its sponsors, and the investigators do not endorse specific products.

Instructions for Use

1. Measure and record weight, length, and head circumference.
2. Calculate gestation-adjusted age by subtracting Adjustment for Prematurity in weeks from postnatal age in weeks. Adjustment for Prematurity equals 40 weeks minus GA. For example, at 12 wk postnatal age, an infant born at 30 wk GA would be 2 wk (0.5 mo) gestation-adjusted age.
3. Plot data at the gestation-adjusted age on the appropriate graph.
4. When possible, plot serial data on the same graph to permit detection of change in growth percentiles with age.

Interpretation

These graphs permit comparison of a VLBW premature boy's growth relative to current reference data. Further investigation may be indicated when the plotted measurements are markedly different from the 50th percentile, or growth percentile changes rapidly.

Provided as a service of

SIMILAC® NeoCare™
Premature Infant Formula With Iron

ROSS PRODUCTS DIVISION
ABBOTT LABORATORIES
COLUMBUS, OHIO 43215-1724

LITHO IN USA

IHDP Growth Percentiles:
VLBW Premature Boys[1,2]

(≤1500 g BW, ≤37 wk GA)

Name_____

Record #_____

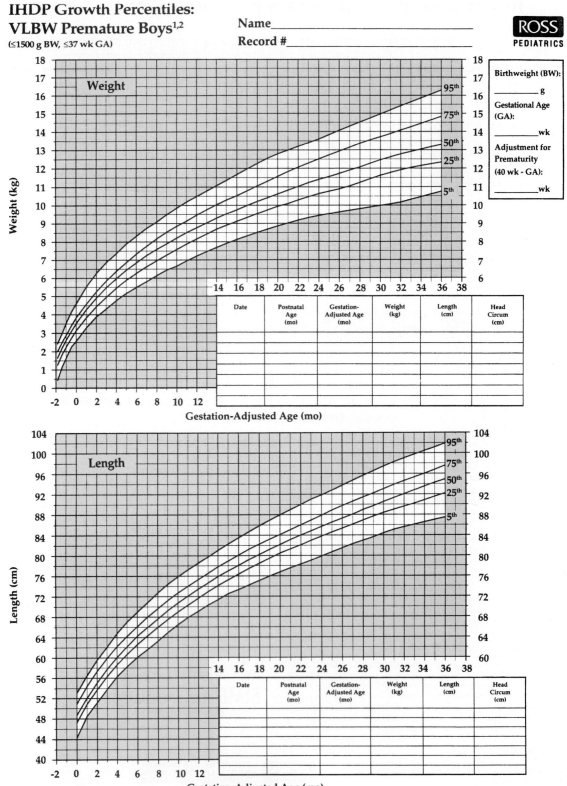

Birthweight (BW):

_____ g

Gestational Age (GA):

_____ wk

Adjustment for Prematurity (40 wk - GA):

_____ wk

Weight

Date	Postnatal Age (mo)	Gestation-Adjusted Age (mo)	Weight (kg)	Length (cm)	Head Circum (cm)

Gestation-Adjusted Age (mo)

Length

Date	Postnatal Age (mo)	Gestation-Adjusted Age (mo)	Weight (kg)	Length (cm)	Head Circum (cm)

Gestation-Adjusted Age (mo)

Glossary

ABC analysis a method of analyzing interactional behavior between two individuals utilizing antecedents, the behavior being analyzed, and the consequences of that behavior

acidosis a pathological condition resulting from accumulation of acid or depletion of alkaline reserves

acquired immunodeficiency syndrome (AIDS) a syndrome caused by the human immunodeficiency virus, which causes cell dysfunction or death after the virus replicates

acrocyanosis a condition characterized by cyanotic discoloration, coldness, and sweating of the extremities

adolescence the period of maturation of a child's mind and body terminating with attainment of adulthood

affectional ties emotional attachment and degree of psychological involvement between parent and child

allergens substances that cause an altered response of cells and, as a result, allergies

alopecia partial or complete loss of hair

alopecia totalis complete loss of hair

amenorrhea absence of menstruation

amylase an enzyme that catalyzes the hydrolysis of starch to glucose

anabolic steroids compounds derived from testosterone to promote body growth and masculinizing effects

anorexia lack of appetite for food

anorexia nervosa a disorder characterized by prolonged refusal to eat, resulting in amenorrhea, emaciation, and distorted body image

anthropometry scientific measurements of various parts of the body

appetite the natural desire or craving for food

arteriosclerosis hardening, thickening, and loss of elasticity of the arteries

aspiration inhaling

assessment a critical analysis of the status or quality of a condition

asymmetry dissimilarity in corresponding parts or organs on opposite sides of the body that are normally alike

atherosclerosis a term denoting a number of different processes resulting in patchy deposition of various materials in the intima of the arteries

athetosis a condition characterized by constant but slow and recurrent movements of the hands, feet, and other parts of the body

attention deficit hyperactivity disorder (ADHD) a clinical diagnosis in children characterized by fidgeting and squirming, easy distractibility, excessive talking, and other disruptive behaviors

basal energy needs energy expended in maintenance of basal metabolic processes or involuntary activities in the body (respiration, circulation, gastrointestinal function, muscle tone, and body temperature) and functional activities of organs

behavior modification a therapeutic tool often employed to extinguish socially unacceptable behavior

bioavailability the degree of availability of a substance to the organism

"bird-feeding" feeding an individual with his or her head thrown back

body image a mental picture a person has of his or her physical self

body image distortion an abnormal or untrue view of one's body size

bonding development of a close emotional tie to another individual or to a newborn infant

botulism food poisoning caused by the toxin produced by *Clostridium botulinum*

bronchopulmonary dysplasia (BPD) a disorder characterized by hypoxia, hypercardia, and oxygen dependency: a complication of hyaline membrane disease

bulimia nervosa an insatiable craving for food, often resulting in periods of continuous eating followed by depression and self-deprivation and purging

cachexia general ill health marked by weakness and emaciation

carotenemia the presence of high levels of carotene in the blood resulting in yellow appearance of the skin

Carpenter syndrome a syndrome of abnormalities which include obesity, mental deficiency, and abnormalities of the hands, feet, and craniofacial area

casein the principal protein of milk

catch-up growth increased growth velocity after remediation of medical or nutritional insult which precipitated growth failure

cell differentiation diversification of cells

central vs. peripheral vascular routes techniques for administering parenteral solutions to the preterm infant; the route chosen depends on the energy needs of the infant and the expected duration of parenteral support

cephalocaudal from head to toe, the sequence in which a normal developmental pattern occurs

cheilosis fissures of lips and mouth due to dietary riboflavin deficiency

chylomicron the largest and lightest of blood lipids

cineradiographic the making of motion picture record of successive images appearing on a fluoroscopic screen

clinical malnutrition (clinical signs of malnutrition) changes in skin, hair, membranes, or growth that can be attributed to an excessive or deficient intake of a nutrient or nutrients

Cohen syndrome a syndrome of abnormalities including obesity, moderate mental retardation, narrow hands and feet, lumbar lordosis, and facial abnormalities

colostrum the first milk secreted by the mammary gland after parturition

congenital existing at, and usually before, birth

convenience foods foods requiring little or no preparation

creatinine a substance formed from the metabolism of creatine, commonly found in blood, urine, and muscle tissue

cultural paradox when two conflicting situations prevail in a society, such as when abundant food is available and used lavishly while at the same time slimness is highly valued

de Lange syndrome (Cornelia de Lange) a syndrome associated with short stature, thin downturned upper lip, and micrognathia

desquamation the cornified layer of the skin is shed in fine scales

developmental obesity obesity that results primarily from psychological factors in the family

Down syndrome a congenital condition caused by trisomy 21, a chromosomal abnormality; characterized by a small, anteroposteriorly flattened skull, short flat-bridged nose, epicanthus, short phalanges, widened space between the first and second digits of hands and feet, and moderate to severe mental retardation

Duchenne's muscular dystrophy a sex-linked recessive genetic disorder involving progressive degeneration of skeletal muscle and resulting weakness

dysplasia congenita a congenital condition resulting in abnormal reduction in cell size and small stature

eating disorder to have an abnormal use of food, that is, to eat too little, too much or to purge and accompanying psychological problems

enteral by way of the intestine

enteroglucagon a gastrointestinal hormone

epiphyseal closure the final calcification of the ends of the long bones causing cessation of growth

erythropoiesis the production of red blood cells

extension movement that brings the members of a limb into or toward a straight condition

extensor any muscle that extends a joint

extinction removing a positive reinforcer to decrease negative behaviors

fading a technique used to teach new behaviors in which the entire behavior must be completed before reinforcement

family-style service meal service where individuals select their portions from serving containers that are passed

fast food food items that are cooked and ready to be eaten immediately

feedback chains of response between parent and child

ferritin an iron complex found in liver, spleen, bone marrow, and reticuloendothelial cells; it is the chief storage form of iron in the body

fetal alcohol syndrome (FAS) a syndrome resulting from fetal exposure to the teratogenic effects of alcohol

flexed bent or put into a state of being bent

food asphyxiation loss of consciousness from too little oxygen and too much carbon dioxide in the blood; brought about by a piece of food lodged in the throat

food idiosyncrasies individual or peculiar food habits or choices

gag reflex elevation of the soft palate and retching elicited by touching the back of the tongue or the wall of the pharynx

gastrin a hormone elaborated by the pyloric mucosa that stimulates hydrochloric acid secretion by the parietal cells

gavage feeding by insertion of a stomach tube through the mouth and into the stomach

gestational age the age of the infant calculated from the beginning of conception, often used with low birth weight infants

gluconeogenesis the formation of glucose or glycogen from non-carbohydrate sources such as glycerol and glycogenic amino acids

glucosuria the presence of sugar in the urine

goitrogenic effect an effect of substances in some foods capable of producing goiter

Healthy People 2000: Nutrition Objectives based on Dietary Guidelines for Americans, proposes achievable goals for improved nutritional status

hematocrit the volume percentage of red blood cells in the blood

hemoglobin the oxygen-carrying pigment of the erythrocytes

high-density lipoproteins protein combined with lipids that carries cholesterol in the blood to the liver where it is released and excreted

hirsutism excessive body hair in a masculine distribution

human immunodeficiency virus (HIV) a retrovirus that presents with unusual opportunistic infections or rare skin cancer and severe depression of cellular immunity (AIDS)

hunger craving for food more pronounced than appetite

Hurler syndrome a condition described by Hurler in 1919 characterized by deceleration of growth between 6 and 18 months, gross retardation, and a number of physical malformations

hyaline membrane disease respiratory distress syndrome occurring most frequently in premature infants

hydroxyproline an amino acid that is elevated in the urine in diseases of the bone and certain genetic disorders

hyperactivity abnormally increased activity

hyperammonemia an abnormally high level of ammonia in the blood

hyperbilirubinemia excess bilirubin in the blood that may lead to jaundice

hypercholesterolemia a condition in which blood cholesterol is above normal limits

hyperglycemia increased glucose concentration in the blood above normal limits

hyperglycinemia increased glycine concentration in the blood

hypernatremia high level of sodium in the blood

hyperplasia an abnormal increase in the number of cells composing a tissue or organ

hypertension elevation of blood pressure above normal

hypertonia a condition of excessive tone, tension, or activity

hypertrophy increase in cell size

hypocalcemia below normal levels of calcium in the blood

hypocholesterolemia a condition in which blood cholesterol is below normal limits

infectious complications difficulties in providing adequate parenteral nutrients due to infection

insensible water loss loss of water nonperceptible to the senses

ketones compounds derived from the oxidation of a secondary alcohol

lacto-ovovegetarian a vegetarian who consumes dairy foods and eggs in addition to plant foods

lacto-vegetarian a vegetarian who consumes dairy foods in addition to plant foods

Laurence-Moon-Biedl syndrome a syndrome characterized by obesity, mental retardation, polydactyly, genital hypoplasia or hypogonadism (or both), and retinitis pigmentosa

linoleic acid essential fatty acid; a polyunsaturated fatty acid with 2 double bonds and 18 carbon atoms

low-density lipoproteins a plasma protein containing high levels of cholesterol that appears to damage the arteries

macrobiotic vegetarian persons who consume vegan or vegetarian diets that also involve nonanimal food avoidances and extensive use of unprocessed, unrefined foods

megadose an amount of a substance, i.e., nutrients or vitamins, that vastly exceeds the typical amount

menarche the beginning of the menstrual function

metabolic acidosis a disturbance in which the acid-base status of the body shifts toward the acid side because of changes in the fixed acids and bases

metabolic complications problems arising in provision of nutrients via parenteral nutrition because of changes in metabolic response to the solution being administered

methemoglobinemia the presence of methemoglobin, a compound formed after poisoning by some substances, in the blood

microcytic abnormally small red blood cell

modified fast a provision of a small percentage of the energy and nutrients needed to maintain nourishment

morbidly obese to be so overweight that the condition interferes with health and physical function

motilin a gastrointestinal hormone

motility effects effects on motility of gastrointestinal tract

myelomeningocele a developmental defect in which a hernial sac containing a portion of the spinal cord, its meninges, and cerebrospinal fluid protrudes from the back.

narcissism an abnormal interest in oneself, especially one's body and sexual characteristics

National Cholesterol Education Program a federal program that provides guidance and education to reduce coronary heart disease in the general population, including health screening and dietary changes

National School Lunch Program a uniform federal school feeding program administered by the USDA

necrotizing enterocolitis a disease seen in infants that involves degeneration of a part of the intestinal tract

neonatal growth pattern the three phases of growth of neonates are (1) weight loss, (2) regaining of birth weight, and (3) sustained growth

neurotensin a gastrointestinal hormone

neutrophil a cell that stains easily with neutral dye

Nutrition Education Training Program a federally funded program administered by the USDA to improve nutrition education and knowledge for school children, teachers, and school feeding staff

nutritional adequacy the provision of all essential nutrients in amounts necessary for the individual

obese about 20% or more above normal weight-height ranges with a high degree of fatness

obesity a state of malnutrition in which the accumulation of depot fat is so excessive that function is disturbed

occiput the back part of the head

omphalocele hernia of the navel

oral motor skills the motor coordination of tongue, lips, mandible, cheeks, and other parameters that affect sucking, chewing, and the coordination of other skills with swallowing

osmotic diuresis increased secretion of urine due to difference in concentration gradient across a membrane wall

osteomalacia inadequate mineralization of the organic matrix of the bones resulting in skeletal deformities and fractures

osteopenia insufficiency of bone resulting from reduced production or increased breakdown of the bone

osteoporosis decreased density of bone

overweight the term applied to a person who is about 10% to 20% above desirable weight

palmar grasp grasp of objects with the palm of the hand

paraprofessional a trained aide who assists a professional person

parenteral injection of substances into the body through any route other than the alimentary tract

passive response pattern behavioral patterns that subordinate the individual's own interest to the demands of others

pharynx the muscular and membranous tube extending from the oral cavity to the esophagus

phenylketonuria (PKU) inactivity or absence of phenylalanine hydroxylase in the liver; early and continuous restriction of dietary phenylalanine can prevent mental retardation

photodegradation the breakdown of nutrients in a solution due to exposure to light

Piaget's theory of learning a theory of cognitive development in children based on progressive developmental stages

pica an abnormal craving to consume unusual substances such as clay, chalk, laundry starch, and dirt

pincer grasp grasp of small object with the thumb and index finger

plasma amino acid levels/patterns the amino acid concentration in plasma; often measured as an index of protein quality

plate waste food items refused or discarded from the standard menu

poverty line guidelines for family income for eligibility for federal supplemental income or food programs; these guidelines are periodically revised to reflect the economic status of the nation

Prader-Willi syndrome a syndrome characterized by small genitals, mental retardation, and obesity; affected individuals have an abnormal craving for food

prehension the act of seizing or grasping

propensity to interact the ability and desire of parent or child to give and receive communication

protein energy malnutrition the generic term to cover any protein energy deficiency state; infants and children are particularly vulnerable; early symptoms include loss of appetite, easy fatigability, loss of weight, and retarded growth

prothrombin the protein in blood plasma needed for blood clotting

pseudoachondroplasia a group of disorders producing short-limb short stature, moderately severe retardation of trunk height, and normal face

puberty the period of sexual development terminating with capability to reproduce

punishers consequences applied after a behavior that decrease the behavior

punishment something aversive added or applied in response to an undesired behavior

raking grasp grasp of objects by raking with palm of the hand

reciprocity the activity of one that occurs as a direct result of stimuli from another

reflex total sum total of any particular involuntary activity

reflux backward or return flow

reinforcers an individually designed consequence that increases the behavior that precedes it

renourishment to provide appropriate nourishment to an individual who is malnourished

resting metabolic rate the energy expended by a person at rest under conditions of thermal neutrality

Rett syndrome a degenerative disorder affecting only females; characterized by autistic behavior, dementia, seizures, ataxia, and loss of purposeful use of the hands

roentgenographic studies diagnostic studies using X rays

rooting a food-seeking movement that occurs in response to stimulation of the lips or cheeks; the head turns toward the stimulus and the mouth opens

Russell-Silver syndrome a syndrome of malformation with short stature of prenatal onset, skeletal asymmetry, and small incurved fifth finger

School Breakfast Program a federal breakfast feeding program for school children in the U.S.

secondary sexual characteristics outward features of male or female sexuality

secular trend (of menarche) tendency for women to menstruate at younger ages throughout the world

sedentary inactive

self-esteem satisfaction in oneself

separation anxiety to be fearful of being independent, especially of one's parents

sepsis infection in the blood stream

set-point theory the theory that a certain body weight is physiologically normal for each person

sexual maturity the stage of development in reproductive capability toward the maximal development

shaping the reinforcement of successive approximations to a desired behavior

spasticity a state of hypertonicity or increase over normal tone in the muscles

specific dynamic action increase in metabolism as a result of extra heat production when food is digested, absorbed, and metabolized

spermarche initial semen production

"sports anemia" iron deficiency anemia associated with a high level of physical activity

staple food a primary food in the diet

stomach capacity the volume of fluid or masticated food that the stomach is able to contain at one time

superobesity the definition of children with triceps skinfold measurements greater than or equal to the 95th percentile in the NHANES cycle 3 or 3 sample of children

supraorbital situation above the bone cavity that contains the eyeball

tactile pertaining to the sense of touch

tactile sensitivity a state or quality of being unusually responsive to touch

tasks of adolescence goals of psychological and social development

technical complications difficulties in providing parenteral nutrition precipitated by the technique in use

tetany a syndrome characterized by muscle twitchings, cramps, and convulsions

three levels of neonatal care nurseries are classified as level I, II, or III based on care they can provide, e.g., Level I nurseries provide uncomplicated care, Level II nurseries care for normal newborns and screen and refer high-risk infants, and Level III nurseries cope with the most serious neonatal illnesses

tongue thrust moving the tongue through the lips when swallowing, normally associated with suckling in infants less than 4 months of age; an abnormal reflex in some individuals with motor coordination difficulties

tonic characterized by continuous tension

tonic bite reflex an automatic clamping of the teeth on any food, implement, or other article placed in the mouth

tonic neck pattern when the head is turned forcibly to one side the arm and leg on that side will extend while the opposite arm and leg will be flexed; described as the fencing position

total parenteral nutrition provision of all nutrients into a large central vein, usually the superior vena cava

toxicity the quality of being poisonous

toxicology the study of poisons

transferrin serum β-globulin that binds and transports iron

trisomy three of a particular chromosome

trisomy 13 a congenital condition caused by triple chromosome 13; characterized by severe brain malformations, midline abnormalities that affect face, brain, and heart, and death within the first year of life

trisomy 18 a congenital condition caused by triple chromosome 18; characterized by severe mental retardation, prominent occipital shelf, overlapping fingers, and frequently death within the first year of life

trophic effects the stimulation of cell reproduction and enlargement

Turner syndrome a syndrome resulting from chromosomal abnormalities characterized by short stature, sexual infantilism, and a webbed neck in females

vegan (pure vegetarian) a person who consumes only foods of plant origin and excludes all animal protein from the diet

vegetarian a person who consumes primarily plant foods (grains, legumes, vegetables, and fruits) and eliminates meats, poultry, and fish from the food pattern; dairy foods and eggs may be consumed

very low-density lipoproteins protein that in combination with fat transports endogenous triglycerides in the blood

weaning changing nourishment to another form other than breastfeeding

weight management to provide nourishment to maintain a person's weight at a stable and appropriate level

whey the residue of milk remaining after the curd and cream have been removed

Williams syndrome a syndrome characterized by mental retardation, unusual facies, and cardiovascular abnormalities

Index